CW01603544

| | |
|---|---|
| **Order Date** | **: 2014-11-22** |
| **OrderId** | **: 026-3253141-2206700** |
| **Email** | **: cjkjj7cgch413ng@marketplace.amazon.co.uk** |
| **Venue** | **: ECAUK** |
| **Shipping** | **: Standard** |

**Items : 1**

| **Qty** | **Item** | **Locator** |
|---|---|---|
| 1 | Gentle Cures For Tough Cancers: Non-Toxic, God-Giv<br>ISBN : 1603831150 | MUL-2-DA-03-000-7<br>LE |

RCode:

# Electric Chicken

Unit 2, Holm Oak, Goring By Sea, West Sussex, BN12 4QY
Email: fba@electricchicken.co.uk

# Gentle Cures For Tough Cancers

## Non-Toxic, God Given, Natural Cures That Work

Deanna K. Loftis, RN, BBA

All Scripture quotations, without exception,are taken from the AV 1611 King James Bible



ISBN: 978-1-60383-115-4

Published by:
Holy Fire Publishing
717 Old Trolley Road
Attn: Suite 6, Publishing Unit #116
Summerville, SC 29485

www.ChristianPublish.com

Printed in the United States of America and the United Kingdom

# DEDICATION

Dedicated to "the high and lofty One that inhabiteth eternity, whose name is Holy;" and to His Son, The Lord Jesus Christ, "In whom are hid all the treasures of wisdom and knowledge."
*(ISA 57:15 & COL 2:3 KJV)*

May He impart to you and your loved ones, His hidden treasures of wisdom and knowledge, His wonderful healing, and His excellent promises as you read this book and offer up to Him the eternal praise & worship that He alone deserves!

# MY APPRECIATION TO:

I wish to express my heartfelt gratitude to the many people who helped make this book possible; first and foremost: my Redeemer, the Lord Jesus Christ, who has never forsaken me, and who has blessed me with an inexplicable desire to write, even amidst some of the most difficult circumstances. Also, my deepest gratitude to my loving devoted sisters, Chris and Shelby, who have never given up on me and continue to encourage me, and without whom this new book would have never been possible; my sister, Patsy, for her encouragement; and my terrific friends who shared with me some of the experiences that would one day prompt me to be a writer: Dee, Mary, Ann, Carol, Antoinette, Gwen, and Tina.

## DISCLAIMER

This book is neither a medical guide, nor a manual for self-treatment. It is for informational purposes only and is not intended to be a substitute for medical diagnosis, treatment or health care, nor should it be construed as practicing medicine. None of the websites mentioned in this book consider themselves self-treatment medical guides, but are for informational purposes only. Nutrients given herein are dosage suggestions and are for your information only. You should always check with your physician for your own individual needs regarding any supplements. Anyone with a chronic disease or illness should consult a physician before initiating a change in treatment or before beginning any new treatment, or if you have health questions regarding the use of any information in this book. Many of the items in this book would be considered cancer prevention measures, rather than cures. Many are actual treatments that have cured very aggressive cancers, even in children. The author and publisher do not prescribe and assume no liability for any adverse effects or consequences resulting from the use of any of the suggestions, preparations, recipes, therapies, or procedures discussed in this book, nor for the reliance thereon, nor for interpretation errors or transcription errors. Many of the statements and treatments regarding various therapies and substances herein have not been thoroughly evaluated by the FDA, and most websites referenced have the FDA disclaimer on them. It is also noted that some people are allergic to, or may have allergic responses to herbs, vitamins, minerals, and their preparations, so caution is advised. If you ever develop breathing problems after taking any substance, regardless of what it is, you should seek immediate medical help as this can be an indication of a potentially life-threatening reaction. Be aware that some herbs and supplements can interfere with the action of prescription medications, or may be incompatible with certain drugs. Just as an example, taking large quantities of soy products can interfere with the body's ability to absorb thyroid medication. This is why you should always consult with your physician before taking any herb, supplement, vitamin, hormone or treatment, regardless of your health condition. The publisher and author of this book are not affiliated with the websites mentioned herein (except the author's own website), nor their products, nor do the author and publisher of this book attest to the reliability of any of those products, except those items the author herself has used (e.g., Maureen Kennedy Salaman's products, Dee Simmon's Products, Swanson® Vitamins, Kyoto® Chlorella, Green Magma® Kamut®, Ola Loa™ Energy Drinks, and Flor Essence® Essiac. What you choose to do with this information is up to you. The publisher and author of this book assume no liability for those decisions. Should you use products or therapies from those websites, or those described in this book, you do so at your own discretion and risk.

# TABLE OF CONTENTS

INTRODUCTION ........ 8
CHAPTER 1
HEALING—HOW & WHERE TO START ........ 9
CHAPTER 2
NATURAL VERSUS SYNTHETIC ........ 26
CHAPTER 3
AMAZING CURES FROM A COMMON TABLE FRUIT ........ 43
CHAPTER 4
GENTLE CURES FOR TOUGH BREAST CANCERS ........ 51
CHAPTER 5
GENTLE CURES FOR TOUGH PROSTATE CANCERS ........ 102
CHAPTER 6
GENTLE CURES FOR TOUGH COLON, COLORECTAL & ABDOMINAL CANCERS ........ 130
CHAPTER 7
GENTLE CURES FOR TOUGH CERVICAL, UTERINE, OVARIAN & VULVA CANCERS ........ 169
CHAPTER 8
GENTLE CURES FOR TOUGH LEUKEMIAS & MULTIPLE MYELOMAS... 198
CHAPTER 9
GENTLE CURES FOR TOUGH LIVER CANCERS ........ 237
CHAPTER 10
GENTLE CURES FOR TOUGH LUNG CANCERS & MESOTHELIOMA ........ 269
CHAPTER 11
GENTLE CURES FOR TOUGH MOUTH, NOSE, THROAT & THYROID CANCERS ........ 299
CHAPTER 12
GENTLE CURES FOR TOUGH PANCREATIC CANCERS ........ 315
CHAPTER 13
GENTLE CURES FOR TOUGH BLADDER & KIDNEY CANCERS ........ 331
CHAPTER 14
GENTLE CURES FOR TOUGH BRAIN CANCERS, ASTROCYTOMAS & NEUROBLASTOMAS ........ 349
CHAPTER 15
GENTLE CURES FOR TOUGH SKIN CANCERS (MELANOMA) ........ 383
CHAPTER 16
GENTLE CURES FOR TOUGH LYMPHOMAS & SARCOMAS ........ 401
CHAPTER 17
GOD'S GREAT GRASSES ........ 426
CHAPTER 18
FLAX & OTHER MIRACLE OILS ........ 437
CHAPTER 19
ANTI-CANCER HERBS & FOODS ........ 448
CHAPTER 20
MORE CANCER-FIGHTING SUPER ANTI-OXIDANTS ........ 462

CHAPTER 21
CURING WITH CAROTENOIDS & OTHER HEALING FOODS & NUTRIENTS......477
CHAPTER 22
PRESCRIPTION HRT – CANCER CULPRIT VERSUS BHRT......489
CHAPTER 23
WATER, WATER EVERYWHERE, BUT ARE YOU GETTING ENOUGH?..510
CHAPTER 24
PREVENT CANCER WITH OXYGEN, EXERCISE, SUNSHINE & REST......518
CHAPTER 25
CURING WITH SOME AMAZING MUSHROOMS......524
CHAPTER 26
WHAT HAPPENED WITH DAIRY?......530
CHAPTER 27
ORTHOMOLECULAR MEDICINE, MACROBIOTICS, PROBIOTICS, MOLASSES & SEED FOODS......540
CHAPTER 28
FLUSH THE BUGS......545
CHAPTER 29
HEALING FROM BEES......552
CHAPTER 30
ALKALIZE FOR HEALTH......557
CHAPTER 31
SPICES TO PREVENT & CURE......562
CHAPTER 32
THOSE AWESOME TEAS!......567
CHAPTER 33
THE TRUTH ABOUT CLINICAL TRIALS & NATURAL PRODUCTS......573
CHAPTER 34
MISCELLANEOUS ALTERNATIVE CANCER THERAPIES......582
CHAPTER 35
FASTING & DETOX......631
CHAPTER 36
WHAT'S NEXT?......637
APPENDIX I......655
APPENDIX II......656
REFERENCES......659
INDEX......718

If any of the italicized words in this book are direct quotes, they are always followed by a reference.

# INTRODUCTION

I lost three family members that I loved dearly to cancer, all of them to conventional medicine. I also lost many cancer patients during the years I worked in a clinical background and in a case management setting, all to conventional medicine. Many of my case management patients were going through bone marrow transplants for cancer. I began researching alternative medicine which prompted an endless study of the subject. I discovered that there are many people, thousands of them, using non-toxic, alternative therapies to cure themselves of deadly cancers and chronic illnesses, yet none of my loved one's physicians had ever mentioned any of these natural, gentler cures to me or my family members when they were fighting cancer. They were all told that their only hope for recovery was chemo, radiation or surgery, yet they all died within months of receiving these treatments.

I decided to put my research results into an easy-to-read format so that others fighting this disease (or having loved ones battling cancer), could reference this material without having to spend years in research as I had done. My first book, *Painless Cancer Cures & Preventions Your Doctor May Not Be Aware of*, was a result of that decision. The book was out only three months before it won a first prize, trophy, and cash award (non-fiction category) in the *International Jada Book of the Year awards*, (Jan. 2006), then in 2007, it was a finalist in the *Indie Excellence Book Awards* (in the health category.)

Many people have written to me or contacted me personally to tell me how much this book has helped them. I have even had conventional physicians tell me that they are giving the book to their patients to inform them about alternative therapies. This new book is an updated look at what is most current and most successful at treating all major forms of cancer from an alternative standpoint (with a few of the newer, gentler standard treatments mentioned), and also contains specifics about other diseases that are being successfully treated using natural, non-toxic methods. It mentions a few of the newer, safer drugs that are being developed for treating cancer, as well as new diagnostic tests for earlier detection. Many of the items in this book would be considered cancer prevention measures, rather than cures, while many others have been used by cancer patients to cure aggressive cancers, even those in children.

# CHAPTER 1

## HEALING—HOW & WHERE TO START

*"Who forgiveth all thine iniquities; who healeth all thy diseases." (Ps 103:3)*

For the sake of your immune system, it is safer to heal through non-toxic means than resorting to substances that increase your risk for secondary cancers like leukemia. If you have been diagnosed with cancer, you must start immediately to restore your body's harmony and balance, and you can do so with many of the natural, non-toxic, gentle, God-given items described in this book. Realize that healing involves your entire body, soul, and spirit—something I refer to as ***HARMONY*** Healing. Seven letters, but each one is so important!

- **H**—is for HARMONY and a HEALING HEART. You must put your whole heart into your healing;
- **A**—is for ATTITUDE. You must believe that you are healing, and you must keep a positive attitude to bring your body into a healing balance. This involves body, soul and spirit.
- **R**—is for REST. You can learn to rest upon the promises of God. Give your anxieties over to him and rest in the assurance that he can and WILL heal you. It is also important that you reduce stress in your life and learn to rest at the end of your daily activities.
- **M**—is for the MIND. We are told in the Bible that "…as he thinketh in his heart, so is he." (Prov. 23:7.) Also: "And all things, whatsoever ye shall ask in prayer, believing, ye shall receive." (Matt: 21:22.) "Without faith it is impossible to please him." (Heb. 11:6.) Faith comes first, then comes healing. You must picture your healing, while believing that God can and will heal you.
- **O**—is for OVERCOMER. You CAN overcome all obstacles. It is so important that you remove from your life any obstacles that will prevent you from healing completely (you may be on the wrong diet, you may not be getting enough rest, you may be handling stress inappropriately, etc.)
- **N**—is for NATURAL. You will be using gentle, non-toxic God-given natural substances to heal your body, and one of the most important of these is what you EAT. The food choices that you make truly can determine whether you live or die!

- **Y**—is for YOU—the most important person in your life to help you get well! It is you who must make the choices and decisions to follow in getting yourself well, and it is up to YOU to be informed! No one can force you to eat the wrong foods or choose the right foods. This book will give you a head start with information that you can use to help you get completely well and regain your body's natural harmony and balance, just as your Creator intended. Throughout this book you will find websites and resources for more information and nutritional supplies. Also, see Appendix II for important links to help you find Naturopaths and Alternative physicians in your area, and resources for health information and supplies.

## I. SEVEN STARTING STEPS—Harmony Healing

### 1. Harmony Healing from the Heart

Putting your whole heart into your healing involves the body, soul, mind and spirit. When you are ill, your body is out of balance. Doing the right things will bring back the harmony and healing into your life. You will find in this book many natural ways to boost the body's immunity. You will discover amazing case studies of people who used the methods in this book to completely cure themselves of cancer and other illnesses without using toxins. You will read about the best foods, nutrients, vitamins, and supplements to eat that will restore a healthy alkalinity to your cells. Most cancer patients are very acidic. There is an entire chapter in this book on restoring the body's healthy alkaline/acid balance. The best way to start is with raw foods. Raw foods contain healing enzymes that are destroyed with cooking. Juicing is one of the very best ways to restore your body's healthy alkalinity and remove damaging excess acid, which pours harmful free radicals into your system.

### 2. Attitude—As You Think In Your Heart —So You Are

Do you get up every morning certain that it is going to be a horrible day filled with disappointment, failure and stress? If this is how you start your day, you are probably right—your day WILL end up that way! Take your favorite Bible verse promises and tape them on your bathroom mirror. Read them aloud every morning and declare them over your day, and do this every day. God's word is powerful, quick, sharp and strong. As a matter-of-fact, it is so powerful that he said in the Book of Psalms "*...for thou hast magnified thy word above all thy name*" (Ps 138:2). God has actually put his word ABOVE the importance of his name—that is POWERFUL—especially when you realize that demons tremble at the name of Jesus! If you are ill, declare Psalm 118:17 every morning and throughout the day as you go about your routine: *"I shall not die, but live, and declare the works of the Lord."* When you are praying for healing, BELIEVE God and declare aloud every day where he states in his word: *"For with God nothing shall be impossible"* (Luke 1:37). Declare Isaiah 53:5 everyday: *"...with his stripes we are healed."* Realize that I am not advocating that someone who is ill not seek medical attention. I believe God still heals today, but I have also read horror stories of parents with sick children (e.g., diabetes), who refused medical attention for their child, which resulted in the death of their child! This is not God's intention.

## 3. Rest, Prayer & the Healing Touch

It is critical that you find time every day to REST. God considered rest so important that he set aside six days for work and the seventh day for a Sabbath of REST. Modern society thinks that they can circumvent this planned rest and the results have been disastrous. We are constantly bombarded with warnings of how harmful stress is to the body. Inadequate rest = stress. Burning the candle at both ends will burn you out rapidly and cause your health to deteriorate.

Scientific studies prove that stress is a killer. Limiting stress in your life will decrease your risk for all cancers and help your immune system to fight disease. There are times when we cannot avoid stress. For example, the stress caused by a radio tower looming over your community, and molds growing in buildings where you work, or the stress of losing a loved one. Researchers know that a diagnosis of cancer, for example, greatly increases stress in a person's life (159). If they cannot deal with the stress, they will deteriorate much faster than people who have learned how to deal effectively with stress in their lives.

Scientists from Rutgers School of Environmental & Biological Sciences describe a peptide that is released from the brain (the *BEP or beta-endorphin-peptide*) when you are doing something enjoyable, and their belief is that this peptide helps control the body's immunity and reactions to stress (159). They have found that insufficient levels of this substance in the brain occur in those who are physically ill, and even in those who are emotionally depressed. When this peptide was given to animals exposed to prostate cancer, their immune systems produced more killer cells to fight the cancer, giving them a *90 percent* protection against the cancer. The BEP also lowered inflammation in the animals (159). Widespread studies have not yet been done on humans; however, it is a well-known fact that those who effectively handle stress live longer, healthier, happier lives—proof that relaxation techniques and stress-relief WORKS (159). This is why so many cancer centers are now using light, music, laughter, relaxation, colors, imagery, touch, vibration, and other techniques to help their patients cope with stress.

Jesus used words and touch more than anyone when it came to healing people instantly. Just be aware that there are many touch therapies that involve various ***New Age*** healing techniques. Recall that there were 12 disciples and one of them was Judas. Jesus called Judas a *devil,* yet all of the disciples were able to heal the sick and work miracles! One of the most deceptive characteristics of the devil is to masquerade as an *angel of light* to deceive people. **Laying on of hands and prayer** for healing is scriptural! Just watch to whom it is that you are directing your prayers. Guard your soul, do not be deceived. Be wary of who it is that is laying hands on you for prayer. Are they a born-again Christian or a New Age devotee?

Don't open doorways for the occult for you or for your children. Some alternative therapies (e.g., yoga) are blended with Eastern philosophies. At their very heart, they may be worshipping Buddha, Hare Krishna, a Hindu God, or any number of non-Biblical deities. Be sure to research anything you get involved in very thoroughly before embracing it. Be like the Bereans, who searched the scriptures daily to test all things.

I caution Christians to avoid all forms of New Age teaching, regardless of the appeal it may have. Eastern religions have many levels that they use for indoctrinating the gullible, and they keep changing their tactics. Some of their modalities include the use of channeling and *CHI* (or *Ki)* and reaching levels of *enlightenment,* centering, the Kundalini force (serpent power), and reincarnation. Be aware of anyone or anything that has to do with people who refer to or call themselves *Ascended Masters, Grand Masters, Spirit Guides, Illuminated Ones*, or *Enlightened Ones.* You may see other names for this channeling, including *radiance technique, Reiki (or anything with the name of Reiki), Usui, Karuna, Quantum Touch, or Seichem.* Remember the Rajneesh cults? Well, they are still pushing their Eastern religion doctrines. Sad but true, many people keep falling for the same old lies, same old deception.

Studies continue to show that there is something very powerful that occurs when we pray. Jesus himself was continuously lifting up prayers to his heavenly Father, and he often used touch and laying on of his hands to bring total healing and recovery to the ailing. He even instructed his disciples to do the same, yet how often is this avenue of healing used by his modern day followers? Scientists know that human touch is so important that if you withhold touch from newborn infants, they will get so ill that they will eventually die. Fortunately for us, this type of experimentation is no longer being allowed, but it was done in the past, and there are negligent mothers in the world, even today, who do not hold and cuddle their babies in a natural, bonding manner, which can cause failure to thrive in newborns (though there are other causes). Seeing that these things are true, how much more should we be seeking God's face in prayer and laying our hands on those who are sick, and claiming God's wonderful healing promises over them? Be sure that you belong to a church where the elders teach and BELIEVE in healing, anointing the sick with oil, laying on of hands, and intercessory prayer.

## 4. Mind—A Powerful Tool—Words, Thoughts, Actions for Healing

Many people are not aware of the fact that we live in a world that is more than three-dimensional. We are surrounded by a fourth dimension, a spirit world that the Bible clearly describes as present all around us, affecting us for good or evil, positive or negative. We must acknowledge what God says about this unseen world in order to stay under his protective power. Tampering with the occult, for example, can bring you out from under God's protection, as can drunkenness, drug abuse, pornography, murder, blaspheming God, abusing others, abusing yourself, and worshipping other gods. God knows what things bring us wellness. He has our best interests at heart.

Studies have shown that boosting the immune system is possible, for example, with laughter. We are told in the Bible that *"a merry hearth doeth good, like a medicine"* (Prov 17:22). Did God know something that we don't about our physical makeup? Of course! He knows everything! Even our thoughts can affect our lives for good or bad. It is a known fact that harboring anger, resentment, and unforgiveness in your heart against others depresses the body's immune system and can make you ill! God is the expert, yet many people run their day-to-day lives with little or no interest in what their Creator has to say about their physical well-being, or about them, for that matter. Is it true that the words you speak can affect your health or the well-being of those around you? Consider these words from Proverbs 16:24: *"Pleasant words are as an honeycomb, sweet to the soul, and* ***health to the bones.****"* (God's word can affect your very bones!) The words of Jesus himself are so important that he said of them *"…the words that I speak unto you, they are spirit, and they are life"* (John 6:63). We are also told in Proverbs 18:21 *that: "Death and life are in the power of the tongue…"* The words of God are quick, sharp and powerful, and they have the ability to heal. Doubt this? Then consider Psalm 107:20*: "He sent his* ***word****, and healed them, and delivered them from their destructions."* God's word has the power to heal! Want to get well? Memorize scripture so that it is within you. Claim the promises of God aloud over your life every single day. You can claim these promises over your children and loved ones as well. Also, start doing things to help those who are less fortunate than you are. You can then claim the wonderful promises found in Psalm 41: *"Blessed is he that considereth the poor: the Lord will* ***deliver him*** *in time of trouble. The Lord will* ***preserve him, and keep him alive;*** *and he shall be* ***blessed*** *upon the earth: and thou wilt not deliver him unto the will of his enemies."*

Did you know that God's words are so powerful that they have a cleansing and a healing effect? Jesus himself told us this when he said: "*Now ye are* ***clean*** *through the* ***word*** *which I have spoken unto you"* (John 15:3). God's word actually has a purification effect. Are you seeking healing from God? Start declaring his word every day in your life. Get a tape player and a copy of the gospels and go to sleep listening to them at night. Also, use praise and prayer as described later in this chapter.

## 5. Overcomer - You CAN Overcome Obstacles—Getting Help from High Places

As a covenant child of God, you can expect God to keep his word to you. If you are already ill, healing is promised in his word in many places. For example, we are told in Isaiah 53:5 that Jesus *"was wounded for our transgressions, he was bruised for our iniquities: the chastisement of our peace was upon him; and with his stripes we are healed."* There are many other verses in the Bible, too numerous to list here, where God promises healing to his people. Not only that, but there are certain avenues that you can take to increase the effectiveness of your petitions before God. Combining fasting with your prayers is one very important way, and is discussed in greater detail later in this book. When you combine prayer with fasting, something supernatural happens. Don't believe it? Then read the story of

Esther in the Old Testament and the story of Daniel as well. Esther prayed and fasted three days and saved a nation! Daniel prayed and fasted 21 days and was given a panoramic view of the entire future of this world! Jesus fasted 40 days before he began his powerful ministry of miracles. There are many stories in the Bible of miracles of healing, deliverance and salvation attributed to times of prayer and fasting. As Christians, we are commanded to pray and fast at certain times. Read Isaiah 58, verses 6—14 for all the terrific promises from God that you can claim when you fast, including the **restoration of your health!** There are many ways that you can expect blessings from God. If you are tithing to your local church, God promises to *"...open you the windows of heaven, and pour you out a blessing, that there shall not be room enough to receive it"* (Mal. 3:10). Are you a tither?

We are also promised a blessing if we help feed and clothe the poor, for *"...he that hath mercy on the poor, happy is he* (Prov. 14:21), and *"He that hath pity upon the poor lendeth unto the Lord; and that which he hath given will he pay him again"* (Prov. 19:17).

Have you been told by your physician that your condition is hopeless? Terminal? Read the first part of Psalm 41! If you have been helping the poor, you can claim those verses! If you haven't been helping the poor, then start doing so, and you can claim those verses:

> ***"Blessed is he that considereth the poor: The Lord will deliver him in time of trouble. The Lord will preserve him, and keep him alive; and he shall be blessed upon the earth: and thou wilt not deliver him unto the will of his enemies."*** **(Ps. 41:1-2)**

Do you support your local church's missions? Have you done anything lately to help someone less fortunate than yourself? Are you a cheerful giver, or a miserable miser?

## 6. Natural Means *God-Given, Nature-Made*

You will mainly be concerned about using natural, God-given substances from nature for your healing. There are some conventional treatments discussed in this book for informational purposes, and because there are some newer drugs coming on the market for treating cancer which are less toxic than some of the older chemo drugs—so while it is true that every single item in this book is not completely *gentle*, *God-Given*, *non-toxic*, or *nature made*—most of them are. Before you even think of starting a conventional protocol, boost your immunity with natural products. Start

TODAY! There are many you can choose from in this book. If you already have cancer, be sure to read the rest of this chapter, chapter three, and the chapter that pertains to the type cancer you have FIRST, and then read the rest of this book. Don't skip any chapters. There are wonderful treatments described in my chapters on mushrooms, bee products, healing teas, carotenoids, and flax, for example, that you don't want to miss. Many of the newest, non-toxic cancer treatments are given in chapter 34 of this book. Most are natural, God-given items—a few are man-made.

## 7. It Starts With YOU—Only You Can Determine Your Destiny

You may already be struggling against an illness, or perhaps you just want to stay well. Our physical bodies were created by a mighty King—the Creator and King of the Universe. If you are seriously ill, you should be consulting your Creator in prayer for your recovery. If you are going to consult your Creator for your healing, where do you start? Do you know who your Creator is? Do you know God? Do you know what he has said about you and about himself? Not only did he give you life, but he gave you the right kind of food that you need for your body to sustain itself in the very best mode of operation possible! If you want your car to perform at maximum capacity, you feed it quality fuel. Start putting garbage into the gas tank and the car will sputter and die, yet this is what we sometimes do to our bodies without even realizing it. Our bodies are composed not just of flesh and blood, but soul and spirit as well! Many people are struggling to maintain their health, but they have never consulted the Bible to see what God has said about health and healing.

You may be fighting a deadly disease and find an alternative approach in this book that could prolong or save your life, but even if you do, you are not going to live forever in the body you are now in. You will merely prolong the life God himself has been gracious enough to give you! Eventually, somewhere down the road, if Jesus delays his return, you will die just like your ancestors did, just like the rest of humanity. Jesus himself asked, *"For what is a man profited, if he shall gain the whole world, and lose his own soul?" (Matt: 16:26.)* It is your soul that makes you **YOU**. All your dreams, aspirations, desires, loves, dislikes, fears, emotions and memories make up your soul. It is what makes you unique! There is only ONE of you and there will never be another person to cross this earth again exactly like YOU. You truly are special and unique. However, even if you pray for healing and you are healed, unless you have accepted God's provision for your soul, you would be better off had you never been born! God told us in the Bible that one day our own words will save us or condemn us. God tells us in his Word that he is a **great King**! *(Mal. 1:14.)* He rules a vast domain far beyond anything you or I could possibly imagine. His throne is encompassed with splendor, honor, majesty, beauty, justice, wisdom and glory unimaginable by mortal man.

We are told in the Book of Revelation that a rainbow encircles his throne, and that out of his throne proceeds thunder, lightning and voices. John, the apostle, was caught up into heaven in Revelation chapter four and saw God's great throne. This mighty Sovereign King created everything, including you, and everything that you have. Angelic beings with a splendor brighter than the sun worship and bow before him. He made you, your loved ones, your children, the world you live in and the food that you eat every day, in spite of what you may have been told, or what you believe about coming from a tadpole or a monkey.

Darwin himself knows by now that God exists, but it is too late for him; **don't let it be too late for you!** As long as you still have breath in you, it is not too late for you. God is totally just and totally holy. When sin entered the world through Adam and Eve's transgression, there was no way that a holy God could justify man and be just himself, unless—and there's the catch. There was a way—only **one way for God to do it**. Man could only be redeemed by someone who had never transgressed the laws of God—someone completely perfect, totally pure, blameless, and willing to take our place. God himself was the only one qualified. He had to pay the price for our transgression, because of the total justice that he demands. He incarnated his only Son into the body of a young virgin, producing Immanuel, God in the flesh, Christ Jesus, our Messiah.

Jesus was born with **God's blood in him** because he was and is God. Not Mary's blood, not Joseph's blood, but God's blood. Pure, immortal blood! You see, Jesus could never die as long as his blood coursed through his veins and arteries! He had sinless, immortal **LIFE** in his blood! He was and is **God in the flesh**. When he was crucified by the Romans, they had no idea that the only way Jesus could die was for all of his blood to be drained from his body. As long as his eternal, sinless blood kept coursing through that beating heart, he could not die. Only after his precious blood had been drained from his body through the crucifixion, did he expire. You can see the awful representation of that in the movie, *The Passion,* by Mel Gibson. That same blood is physical, spiritual, immortal and pure! When you turn from your sins (repent) and accept Jesus' sacrifice on your behalf, a spiritual *circumcision* takes place between your body and your soul. Your sins are forever cut loose from your soul. The blood of the Lamb of God is applied to your body, soul and spirit. When you die, you are free to join God in heaven, your soul forever free from the sins that Jesus himself paid for. You are justified by the blood of the Lamb. If you never repent and turn from sin, and do not accept God's free gift of pardon, when you die, your sins are still attached to your soul. God is holy, perfect and just. He cannot allow sin into his presence. Your soul is forever consigned to hell—a place of the **lost**—a place where your sins are a permanent part of your eternal soul.

Your soul never dies, neither do you! You may look different at sixty than you did at fifteen, but inside you don't feel any different. (Apart from a few aches and pains, maybe!) Ever wonder why? It is because your soul never ages. Go ahead—pay for it yourself, if you like. Don't you know—that's what all those other "religions" are doing out there? They are trying to pay their own way without JESUS. The Buddhists think Buddha will save them, but Buddha did not have immortal blood and he wasn't resurrected! Neither were any of the other prophets of the world's major religions. Their bones are still in the grave awaiting the great resurrection. The bones that have never been **found** were those belonging to Jesus. That's because all those other "gods" out there are still in the GRAVE! Jesus is alive today because he is the only one that was resurrected. He had immortal blood. Your blood is stained with Adam's sin. You need a "blood transfusion!" You need a Savior with **pure, immortal** blood!

You can follow every guideline in this book and help your body stay well and recover from serious illness, but it won't do a bit of good if your soul is still black as death. If you have terminal cancer, and you are not healed, you will be meeting God face-to-face in the very near future. Think about that. Are you ready? None of us are promised tomorrow, even if we are strong and healthy. This chapter will prepare you to meet God tomorrow or twenty years from now. Simply bow your head where you are—tell God that you are sorry for your sins and that you repent (forsake your sins and determine to leave them behind you)—change of heart, change of attitude—you are turning your life over to him and turning against sin. We are instructed in his word: *"That if thou shalt confess with thy mouth the Lord Jesus, and shalt believe in thine heart that God hath raised him from the dead, thou shalt be saved."* (Romans 10:9-10.) For a sample of a prayer that you can pray, see ***Appendix I*** at the end of this book.

You should be willing to tell others that you are a new Christian, confessing it with your mouth as God requires. Find a spirit-filled local Bible-believing church to join; be willing to follow the Lord's example in baptism, and begin growing in faith by reading your Bible every single day. It is your lifeline to the future! As a Christian, you can claim the Blood of Jesus over your mind, spirit, soul and body for divine protection, instruction and wisdom, and you need to be under the guidance of a shepherd (or pastor) of a local Bible-believing Church.

## II. Learn the Language of Heaven

There is another avenue of gaining power in your prayer life that is sadly overlooked by many people in today's world. I believe it is possibly the most powerful avenue of all when it comes to getting God's attention, and that is through **PRAISE and WORSHIP**! Ask yourself this: how much time did you spend **today** worshipping God? Yesterday? This week? This month? Your entire life? Did you know that our God is a God who desires our worship? Think about it! Why do you think you were created? What do you think your purpose is in this life and the next? I can tell you in one word—WORSHIP! You were made to worship God! God desires that you lift your hands up toward heaven to exalt and worship him! Men are compared to TREES in the Bible. You have built-in PALMS (branches) in your hands to wave before God in worship! You have a voice to sing with  a built in trumpet  lungs to breathe with. You were made to worship and sing to God! Do you drive back and forth to work every day? Then you have time to worship God! Get a worship CD and sing along with it, or sing without one! It will change your life! (I guarantee you, if everyone in your town or city would do this, there would be no such thing as crime or *road rage, ever!)* Your whole body is a temple made to worship God!

What can you possibly give God that he hasn't first given you? Can you give him wealth, riches, joy, purpose, strength, love, beauty, talent, power, wisdom, creativity, generosity, compassion, benevolence? There is absolutely nothing that you can give God that doesn't already belong to him. When you contemplate just for a moment all that he has done for you (he gave you LIFE!), the enormity of it is overwhelming. There is nothing left for you to do, but to worship him! He is worthy! He has angelic beings that stand before him singing endless praises to him, songs of adoration and worship, yet he still desires ***your worship!*** Never be led to believe that God does not care for you as an individual. Believe me, God is BIG ENOUGH to go around! He has time for you! He knows every thought you will think tomorrow before you even get up in the morning! He has numbered the hairs of your head. You are precious to him! So precious, in fact, that he willingly gave his life for you.

Worship is the language of heaven. We are given a glimpse of God's throne room in the Book of Revelation when John the apostle is caught up into heaven in chapter four. It is a noisy place! There are thunderings, voices, lightnings, shouts and songs of praise filling God's throne room! I am happy to say that the church I belong to has a powerful worship service. I can barely sing a tune, but I still like to sing. You don't have to sing like a bird to sing in God's presence. He says in ***Psalm 66:1: "Make a joyful noise unto God, all ye lands. Sing forth the honor of his name: make his praise glorious."*** Can you make a joyful **noise?**

Have you ever been in a church service where the people around you acted like they were fearful of lifting their arms during the worship and praising God audibly? They need to be educated about worship, or you might want to find a church that isn't afraid to physically worship God! I am amazed that so many people (even those who call themselves *Christians),* can attend ball games, car races, and golf outings, and they will jump up and down, stomp their feet, scream at the top of their lungs, wave their hands frantically, and shout for joy when their team scores, but get them in the worship service Sunday morning and they are blank, empty, silent, staring, spectacles of gloomy inhibition when it comes to glorifying their Creator! Suggest to them that they raise or clap their hands and shout to God and they will look at you like you just crawled out from under a dark rock for even suggesting such a thing!

There are many ways that the Bible gives us to worship God. You can worship him through singing (the most common form of worship), through playing stringed instruments, with shouts of praise, by clapping your hands while you are singing, leaping before the Lord, and through the dance, such as David did when the Ark of God was returned to Jerusalem.

Worship is noisy! Make a joyful NOISE when you come in God's presence! If you recall, David's wife, Michal, was filled with contempt when she saw him singing loudly and dancing about, and she accused him of making a fool of himself. David scolded her, telling her he was dancing to please God, not the crowd *(II Sam. 6:20).* Throughout the entire Bible, it was very common for people to worship God by singing psalms to him. Most of the psalms in the Old Testament were written by King David himself, and you can be certain, that he sang them out before God! David was a man after God's own heart, primarily because he was a **worshipper!** What about you? Are you a worshipper? Do you get to church late to miss half the worship service because you don't think it's important? It is critical for you to realize as a Christian, that God desires you to worship him not only in the congregation of saints, but privately in your own home as well. When popular pastor, evangelist, Darlene Bishop, was a guest speaker at our church, she said that God explained to her that he lives, moves, and operates within the atmosphere of WORSHIP. He BREATHES in praise and worship, like you and I inhale oxygen! Dr. Norvel Hayes, a successful businessman, author, teacher, preacher and worshipper of God, believes that the most important time we spend in worship is the time that we spend alone with God when no one else but God sees us. Dr. Hayes explains in his book *Worship—Your Foundation For the Victorious Life,* that God revealed to him that he desires all humans to make a covenant of worship with him. He said that God revealed to him that those who worship God and make him their God, they will receive whatsoever they desire, for God himself has made a worship covenant with the human race (427).

Are you seeking healing from God? Are you a woman who is trying to have a child and you are still childless? Try worshipping God. Then, bring your petition before God for a child, after you have spent daily time in worship. God always tests us to see how sincere we are. He isn't your personal vending machine. You don't just murmur a few words to him, praise a few minutes, then—*presto!* You get your *wish!* You may spend eight months or a year or more worshipping him and praying before him for a certain request before you see results. Are you being obedient to his word? Are you tithing as he commanded in both the Old and New Testament? Are you doing what you can to help those who are less fortunate than yourself? Are you fasting, praying and seeking God? Are you a worshipper? Are you a Christian who isn't afraid to tell someone else about Jesus?

It amazes me how many people who claim to be *Christians* never darken the door of their local church; never give a dime to help the needy; balk at the thought of tithing their income; would rather die than fast for one meal; watch T.V. for two or more hours a day (then claim they haven't time for prayer or for church); cringe at the thought of any sort of open expression of praise and worship to God; then come and ask **you** to pray for them because they need healing, all the while expecting God to give them a miracle and heal them when they haven't obeyed a single thing that Jesus commanded of them! Remember, God knows that we are far from perfect. He knows the framework of our bodies—that we are just clay, but he also knows what we are capable of. As his creation, we are to worship God with all of our hearts and with our lives. His Word tells us that "*Whoso offereth praise glorifieth me" (Ps. 50:23).*

We are also to worship God with our thoughts. What's on your mind during your free time? Do you want peace of mind? Try worshipping God with your thoughts. Exalt him, think about him, memorize his words and think on them, for he promises: *"Thou wilt keep him in perfect peace, whose mind is stayed on Thee: because he trusteth in thee" (Isa 26:3).* Try renting nature movies, just so you can admire God's great creation. Keep your mind on God and you won't lose it! Did you know that if you are depressed, Isaiah 61:3, says that you can actually lift DEPRESSION by putting on the "garment of praise!" Been depressed lately? Start PRAISING GOD! Are your children depressed? Teach them to PRAISE and worship God! You may argue that you have no idea HOW to worship God. Well, here is a good way to get started—take each of the verses below and memorize one of them every day until you know them all by heart. Memorize them by SINGING them!

*Sing unto him, sing psalms unto him, talk ye of all his wondrous works. (I Chron. 16:9.)*

*Let us lift up our heart with our hands unto God in the heavens (Lamentations 3:41.)*

*O give thanks unto the Lord; for he is good; because his mercy endureth forever. (Ps 118:1.)*

*O clap your hands all ye people; shout unto God with the voice of triumph. (Ps 47:1.)*

*In God we boast all the day long, and praise thy name forever...(Ps. 44:8.)*

*Thus will I bless thee while I live: I will lift up my hands in thy name. (Ps. 63:4.)*

*Thou art my God, and I will praise thee: thou art my God, I will exalt thee. (Ps. 118:28.)*

*Great is the Lord, and greatly to be praised; and his greatness is unsearchable. (Ps. 145:3.)*

*Every day will I bless thee; and I will praise thy name forever and ever. (Ps. 145:2.)*

*Heal me, O Lord, and I shall be healed; save me, and I shall be saved; for thou art my praise. (Jer. 17:14.)*

*...Blessed be the name of God forever and ever: for wisdom and might are his. (Daniel 2:20.)*

*I will praise thee: for thou hast heard me, and art become my salvation. (Ps. 118:21.)*

Or, if you would rather, just pick a psalm, such as *Psalm 149,* and memorize it. It is only nine verses—or *Psalm 150*—which is only six verses. There is even a promise from God you can claim when you are worshipping him. It is Psalm 37:4: "*Delight thyself also in the Lord; and he shall give thee the desires of thine heart.*" God even revealed to Dr. Norvel Hayes, author of *Worship—Your Foundation For the Victorious Life,* if you learn to be a worshipper of God, you will never go hungry. Are you hungry or do you know someone who is? Who are they worshipping? Who is their God? Are they worshipping the true God, or idols? God actually desires and seeks your worship. When Jesus was speaking to the woman at the well, he made the remarkable comment that his father actually SEEKS people to worship him.

Worship is so powerful that God actually used praise and worship to win a battle for him in the Old Testament: *II Chronicles 20:17-22.* It reveals the story of Jehoshaphat who was concerned about being surrounded by powerful enemies that he felt were going to overwhelm him and his small army. God revealed through one of his prophets that he himself would fight the battle. Jehoshaphat ***"appointed singers unto the LORD, that they should praise the beauty of holiness, as they went before the army, and to say, Praise the LORD; for his mercy endureth forever."*** When these praisers began singing and praising, their enemies were soundly defeated, yet Jehoshaphat and his army never lifted one finger against them—just their voices and musical instruments were all that was needed, and God did the fighting. Notice that they used SCRIPTURE to praise God.

## III. Health & Healing From God

God sometimes heals instantly—other times—he heals gradually, but either way, he expects you to cooperate with him in your healing. If you are praying to him to heal you of some disease, such as cancer, you need to be doing your part. If God has healed you and you go back to eating fast-food burgers and fries every day, and living a very unhealthy lifestyle, don't expect to maintain your good health. You have to do your part in staying healthy. Praise God that he has more compassion on us than we sometimes have on each other. He is very forgiving, but he requires accountability and responsibility on our part. If you want healthy kids, feed them a healthy diet. Reach them with good nutrition while they are small, so it will stick when they are adults. I made the mistake of researching alternative health and nutrition when my child was already a teenager. Try to convince a teen to eat a nutritious diet! They already know everything, so you are wasting your time! Our society has become a fast-food, package-crazed society, not caring, nor thinking about what we ingest. We let our tastes enslave us. God did not design all the dead foods that clutter our modern supermarket shelves, nor did he ever intend that we give these items to our children on a regular basis. Occasional treats are one thing, but living on them day-after-day will depress the immunity and cause illness, diabetes, and other disorders. Our God has already provided for us exactly what we need in the most natural, nutritious form possible.

There is an old expression which states that we spend the first half of our lives acquiring wealth and the second half using our wealth to regain our health! How many of us have spent twenty or more years living on "dead foods," only to wind up complaining that we are beset with arthritis, gout, diabetes, high blood pressure, fatigue, coronary artery disease, poor circulation and migraine headaches, yet we continue to live this way and wonder why we can't get well, feel better, or get more energy! (Note that there are some GOOD foods that get packaged, such as potatoes, onions, some fruits (bags of oranges and apples), fiber breads, and frozen fruits, so all "packaged" foods are not bad. Even fresh sprouts that you purchase in a health food store may be packaged, as well as frozen cubes of wheat grass juice, etc.).

Only **live** food has the **enzymes** already within it that enables you to digest it. If you take a raw vegetable, like an onion, with the roots still attached and put it in the ground, it will sprout and live. Cook it, then put it in the ground and it will rot. Why? Because, once cooked, you have destroyed all the life in the vegetable and it is dead. It no longer has within it the living enzymes needed for the body to digest it. Thus, your body will have to produce the enzymes to digest it—a taxing process on your entire digestive system. Not only that, cooked food moves through the bowels sluggishly, fermenting on the way. Raw food moves through the bowels much quicker, its roughage acting as a broom to sweep out the colon along the way.

Researchers are finally realizing that a diet high in fat and low in fiber (e.g., cooked vs. raw food) contributes to cancer. This is because bodily wastes from these foods move slowly through the intestines allowing time to release toxins back into the body, causing illness, eventually leading to the breakdown of the immune system, auto-immune disorders, and other problems. We drown our meals with carbonated pop or water, wondering why we can't digest our food, when what we have done is to neutralize all the hydrochloric acid in the stomach that was intended to digest the food in the first place. It is best not to take fluids with meals. There will be exceptions to this. For example, if you are taking certain vitamin/mineral supplements with your meals, or medicines taken with food, you will need enough fluids in order to swallow them.

# CHAPTER 2

# NATURAL VERSUS SYNTHETIC

*"For by me thy days shall be multiplied and the years of thy life shall be increased." (Proverbs 9:11)*

## Cancer Statistics

- **Are They Changing?**

Statistics show that most cancers are on the rise, though it is possible that some cancers may regress on their own. Little has changed in the pharmaceutical industry over the years, except that a handful of companies have, after much public pressure, begun to develop a few new drugs for cancer treatment that are not as toxic as the old, standard conventional chemo drugs. Aware of the public outcry over toxic substances used to fight disease, some pharmaceutical companies are responding by working on safer, non-toxic drugs for fighting cancer. However, some of the older drug companies haven't changed a bit. Many of them are coining new diseases to convince the public it has the disease so that they must use their pharmaceutical remedy. Some of the adverse side effects are almost laughable, if not so tragic. I saw a television ad a few weeks ago for a new drug—and I kid you not—one of the possible side effects was increased *gambling urges!*

Man is basically an electronically-functioning individual, yet we are daily being told by the medical society and big pharma that we are mostly composed of chemicals, so chemicals can cure us. Drug companies spend millions on pharmaceutical ads trying to convince the populace that it is fine to risk your life taking a drug to treat osteoporosis, restless legs, stress incontinence or clogged sinus' and in the same ad, they very hurriedly recite an entire list of potentially lethal side effects that these same drugs may have. Just one example is a popular drug pushed for arthritis, which has potential side effects of septic arthritis, osteomyelitis, lymphomas, breast cancer, lung cancer, prostate cancer, and colon cancer. Now I ask you—what would you rather battle? Arthritis or cancer? Yet, we are being led to believe by this particular drug company that it is okay to fight your arthritis with a drug that may leave you with CANCER. This sort of insanity (among others), is doing much to erode the public's confidence in the FDA and the drug industry.

- **Newer, Safer Drugs, Treatments & Radiation?**

I am not putting down all medications, because many drugs have been developed by pharmaceutical companies that save lives every day—diabetic medications, heart drugs, kidney drugs, anti-rejection drugs for transplant patients—to name a few. If given credit for nothing else, the drug industry can be credited (lately) for more research and development into less toxic drugs. There are also less toxic forms of treatment being developed (e.g., see chapter 34 on CyberKnife®) which pinpoints tumors more precisely), and chapter 34 for information on the new Nano-Knife™.

Another example is Rexin-G™, which is being tested on pancreatic cancer patients, and it is claimed that it does not have the side effects that are commonly found in chemo drugs (256). It was developed by *Epeius Biotechnologies* (257), and is discussed later in this book in more detail.

Another example is CMA-676 (Mylotarg®), also known as Gemtuzumab for AML, and Sprycel® or Dasatinib. Sprycel® is still undergoing testing for chronic myeloid leukemia, usually given to those who have not been helped by Gleevec®. It is claimed, thus far, that side effects are mild (bone and muscular aches and pains). More will be known when further tests are complete.

Mylotarg® is a type of targeted-antibody therapy, a chemo agent. There are also less toxic and damaging forms of radiation discussed in this book, such as *IMRT (Intensity Modulated Radio Therapy),* which uses more precise beams of radiation to target cancer cells than conventional older treatments. IMRT is discussed in later chapters in this book, and is also used extensively for children's cancers. Others that are still in the clinical trials are drugs for ovarian cancer, such as Karenitecin, which developers hope will be less toxic than older chemo drugs have been.

Monoclonal antibodies, such as 3F8 used for neuroblastoma, can be received at Memorial Sloan-Kettering Cancer Center (205). For more information on this treatment, see website *http://www.mskcc.org/mskcc/html/3215.cfm.* At the same website, this cancer hospital does admit that "Chemotherapy itself causes leukemia…in 5 to 10 percent of patients, and leukemia is very hard to cure" (205). Other monoclonal antibodies currently in various trials are drugs like Epratuzumab, which is being tested on children with acute lymphocytic leukemia (241). If interested, you can find details at *Bio-Medicine.org's* website. Just realize that many of these less toxic drugs are sometimes combined with chemo drugs which ARE very toxic to the immune system. Also, be sure if you have chosen chemo drugs, to follow your physician's advice (e.g., you may be warned against sun exposure while on chemotherapy and radiation).

## Cancer & Radiation

There are many types of radiation being used now for conventional cancer therapy, some very intense and toxic, others milder and less risky (e.g., the CyberKnife® for hard-to-reach brain tumors and other cancers).You may hear your physician refer to radiosurgery systems, such as cobalt systems (Gamma Knife®); tomotherapy; 3D radiotherapy; Modified Linear Accelerator Systems (e.g., X-Knife); and Shaped Beam Systems (e.g., IMRT or Intensity Modulated Radiation Therapy) (286a). You may also hear your physician refer to external beam radiotherapy (EBRT or XBRT); gamma ray radiation or x-rays; photon beam (a type of particle beam radiation); proton beam; internal radiation, such as using radioactive seeds implanted in the body (also referred to as brachytherapy and interstitial radiation); radioactive isotopes, and other various names.

There are going to be rare times when it may make sense to use radiation. If your doctor tells you that you have a rapidly-growing brain glioma and you have three days to live—and using radiation to shrink it may extend your life—this may be the most sensible immediate choice for you. Many people with "inoperable" brain tumors have been helped with Gamma Knife® and CyberKnife® which actually do not use a knife, nor is it considered "surgery," as there is no incision, but it is a form of radiation. CyberKnife® and Gamma Knife® have also been successfully used to treat trigeminal neuralgia and AV malformities. It is often used on hard-to-reach tumors, such as pituitary tumors and acoustic neuromas (schwannomas). CyberKnife®, when used on brain tumors, is painless and without the intense side effects normally found in chemo and traditional radiation, though it can cause damage to nearby healthy tissues. Gamma Knife® does use a painful stereotactic frame that is attached to the skull with screws, and is only used for brain tumors, while CyberKnife® can also be used for tumors elsewhere in the body, especially hard-to-reach tumors. (See chapter 34 for more details and for information on when it might be considered painful.) Also, look under NanoKnife™. Just remember that your best defense is to be informed. This book will arm you with the knowledge you need about many of the most effective natural therapies used to treat tough, aggressive cancers and other illnesses. Remember too, if you are diagnosed with cancer, whether or not you choose to go the conventional medicine route, or alternative route (or a combination of both) will ultimately have to be YOUR decision. It is a decision that I cannot make for you.

Chemo drugs (and conventional radiation) can be a double-edged sword. The cancers may return twice as deadly as they were before, and they can inflict an enormous blow to an immune system that is already ill. The purpose of this book is to give you enough information so that you will know what is available in alternative therapies; which conventional treatments may be less harmful than others; as well as how to use preventative measures to assist your immune system in keeping you well and getting you well if you are already sick. You will also read many case histories about gentle, nature-made cancer CURES and preventatives that multitudes of people have experienced without ever using toxins.

## Cancer & Surgery

There are times when you must have surgery for cancer. For example, with a cancer that is obstructing the bowel, unless the mass is removed, you will not regain life-sustaining bowel function. Some studies even show that removing a secondary lung tumor may help extend your life if you are struggling with osteosarcoma. There are times, as described earlier, when it may make sense to have radiation. There are also other types of radiation you will read about in this book that you may want to choose to discuss with your physician, such as IMRT or *Intensity Modulated Radiation Therapy*, which has reportedly much less severe side effects than standard radiation. IMRT is discussed in several chapters of this book. It is also being used for many children's cancers.

Though some surgeries are unwarranted, I do believe that in certain instances, surgery may be the best choice for cancer. A surgical removal can often bring about total remission in some cancers, and sometimes surgery (for example in the case of a bowel being obstructed by a large tumor) is needed immediately. However, if a lifetime of bad habits and poor choices is the reason you have cancer, unless you change those habits, the cancer may return. If you have a cancerous tumor growing (for example, in your lung), you have a systemic disease, not an isolated problem in one organ. Your entire immune system is ill. There are, of course, some cancers that are considered genetic and some people are more prone to develop them; however, even these cases can benefit by treating the immune system to make it a more efficient disease-fighting machine, including the use of good nutrition.

There are some types of cancer that can be caused by allergies, for example, *gluten-sensitive-enteropathy,* a type of t-cell lymphoma in an abdominal cancer that is actually a result of being allergic to wheat gluten. See chapter four in this book (on breast cancer) for information on a genetically-induced type of breast cancer that can be fought with a common natural mineral, selenium.

You will hear very little about natural or alternative remedies in mainstream medicine. During the time that I worked as an R.N. Transplant Coordinator for a major insurance company, I followed cancer patients telephonically as they underwent bone marrow (or stem cell) transplants, as well as various solid organ transplants. Many of them had very appalling side effects from the massive doses of chemotherapy and/or radiation used to obliterate their immune systems. This book is meant to arm you with knowledge about today's current cancer prevention measures and natural cures. You will find from reading this book that there are many non-toxic cancer therapies that people are using every day to cure themselves without harming their bodies.

## Current Cancer Testing - What's New?

Note that there are many diagnostic tests that your physician may do to check for cancer. Be aware that there is a new blood test that is greater than 95% accurate in finding any type of cancer, even small amounts. It is known as the **AMAS** or "Anti-Malignin Antibody in Serum" test. It will detect cancer anywhere in the body—even tiny amounts—and many physicians do not know it exists. It can be found under the name of *Target Reagent,* and if you need to get this test done (and see if your insurance covers it), tell your physician (and insurance company) that the CPT code for the test is **86-317**. See chapter seven in this book (on ovarian cancer) for some new diagnostic tests that are coming out for earlier detection. LabCorp has developed a test that they say is 99% effective in detecting early onset of ovarian cancer, something that, hopefully, will save thousands of lives! Strange as this sounds, there are even dogs that trainers say can detect the presence of breast and ovarian cancer in humans, as well as impending seizures and blood sugar drops.

## FDA Atrocities

You will read in this book, about many of the heart-breaking fights that people have undergone with the FDA when they bucked the system and tried to treat people with non-toxic cancer therapies. A good example is Dr. Stanislaw Burzynski in Houston, Texas. His treatment is discussed in greater detail in chapter 16 on lymphomas, and chapter 14 on brain cancers. You will read the amazing story of Maryjo Siegel, who was completely cured of a fatal non-Hodgkins lymphoma using non-toxic antineoplastons developed by Dr. Burzynski (see chapter 14, 15 and 16).

Ms. Siegel was diagnosed in 1991. She is very much alive and well today (as of June 2009), completely cancer-free and living a healthy, normal lifestyle. She was so appalled at the treatment that Dr. Burzynski has received from the U.S. government, that she testified before the U.S. House of Representatives Government Reform and Oversight Committee on February 4, 1998 in defense of him. See chapter 16 on lymphomas and sarcomas for Maryjo's testimony. Anyone who thinks that the FDA has the public welfare at heart has to be totally unconscious! Read the full story of Maryjo's experience in chapter 16 of this book, and at website: *http://burzynskipatientgroup.org/maryjo.htm.*

You can also read about a massive coverup involving the drug maker, MERCK, in a scheme to take their own company authors and *disguise* them in such a way that the FDA and public thought that they were *independent* and *unbiased* (327). How was the coverup unraveled? Only because of litigation from private citizens who said that pharmaceuticals from MERCK harmed them. We now know that MERCK lied about their research on Vioxx®, and did so intentionally. Could it be because in one year alone (per a Senate investigation), Vioxx® brought them 2.3 billion dollars in sales? This drug may have been responsible for the deaths of more than 50,000 U.S. citizens, and many thousands more that have also experienced heart attacks (327). Can you think of anyone else in this country, private or commercial, who would still be allowed to stay in business after they produced a product that was responsible for 50,000 deaths (apart from the abortion industry)? Yet the FDA will try to convince you that they want to control the sale and distribution of all vitamins and natural supplements to keep you safe (327)! See chapter 15.

## Gene Therapies

Many scientists are currently testing various gene therapies for their use in fighting cancer. They are working at ways to turn off some of the genes they believe are responsible for causing cancer.

## Modern Medicine

Medical school graduates are taught how to alleviate and treat symptoms, and which drugs to prescribe for which illnesses. If you go to your doctor and tell him or her that you are having abdominal pain, you will often be scheduled for diagnostic testing. By the time you leave the office, you may very well have in hand several FREE drug *samples* (left by pharmaceutical sales reps), or a written prescription to treat your *symptoms* until your follow-up visit. Some doctors will even give a patient sample drugs and tell them to "try them out" to see if they help their symptoms before they even perform any diagnostic tests. How safe is this?

Forget about alternative therapies. Your insurance company, working with beaurocrats in Washington, D.C., as well as leaders in the medical establishment, can guarantee that your cancer regimen won't include alternative medication and cancer treatments by classifying them as *experimental* and *unconventional.* This is because many alternative treatments involve natural products, and natural products cannot be patented. Pharmaceutical companies cannot make a profit from a *naturally-occurring* herb or nutrient because the FDA will not allow them to patent natural substances, so it is not considered an accepted treatment and not a *covered benefit,* and you are denied coverage! Do you see how the *system* works? Believe me, the AMA wants as little competition from alternative medicine as possible. Many of these potentially lifesaving alternative therapies, such as Burzynski's antineoplastons, that have proven successful in treating cancer are not easily accessible or affordable to the public, and make no mistake, this is an intentional effort by the FDA to blacklist alternative, non-toxic treatments—it is no accident!

Conventional Medicine often accuses those who advocate alternative cancer therapies as providing *false hopes* and *untested cures.* They often list all natural treatments as *quackery*, with little evidence to prove their accusations. Nothing could be further from the truth. Many times, people who participate in clinical trials are given false hopes about a cure, and many of the chemo drugs on the market could be classified as "untested" because very little testing is done with some of them and—as pointed out earlier—those participating in their trials often have no idea how the trial is going to come out. Drugs that are given "fast track" approval status have very little testing done before they are unleashed on the public. Dr. Burzynski has tested his non-toxic cancer therapy extensively and he has brought about many cures, even in many children with terminal cancers who were sent home to die. Realize that some individuals can have side effects from antineoplastons, but they are quickly reversible, unlike toxic chemo drugs that often cause fatal adverse reactions.

## Must Have—Good Immunity

Your major hope of getting well is boosting your depressed immune system and the intervention of God's help in your behalf. Though cancer can result from a lifestyle of poor diet and wrong choices, do not be too hasty in blaming your cancer on yourself. The last thing any cancer patient needs is a guilt trip. Realize that environmental surroundings can cause cancer. Because of the FDA allowing many carcinogens into our food and water supply, we are constantly being bombarded with chemicals that can make us sick.

Food handlers spray vegetables with wax to make them look shiny and attractive. Dyes are even used in oranges to make them a brighter orange and more appealing to consumers. Foods are genetically changed to make them fungus and bug-resistant. Hormones are injected into cattle and poultry to make them gain weight before they are slaughtered. These same hormones end up in the meat, poultry, and dairy products that consumers ingest every day. Did YOU get to vote on whether or not any of these products could be added to your food supply?

The FDA allows what they consider acceptable traces of poisons in the food supply, but small amounts of poison in everything you consume multiplies into a deadly array of toxins ingested every day by millions of people, including children, who have been led to believe that their food supply is safe. We are importing plastics from other countries that are used in toy manufacture that have lead and other carcinogens in them. They are being used for making children's toys and baby bottles. When people are subjected to overwhelming environmental toxins and pollutants beyond their control, illness follows. Such is the case of those with mesothelioma and leukemia and other cancers that are caused by toxins, pollutants, chemicals, certain work environments, or those who have genetic cancers. The job of the immune system is to destroy defective cells, and cancer cells are *defective* cells. We are so inundated with chemicals in our environment and food supply that cancer has become an epidemic. Perhaps it will not be long before everyone in the nation succumbs to some sort of cancer. Millions of times a day, our cells are attacked with free radicals generated by the chemicals in our food and environment. The only way to fight this onslaught is to continuously nurture and fortify the body's immunity, trust in our Creator God, and stay in the battle!

## Ongoing Saga of Current Chemo Drugs

It is not unusual for patients who faithfully adhere to a prescribed chemo or radiation regimen for one type of cancer, to discover a year or two later (when they think that they are in remission) that a second, even more sinister cancer than the one that they started with, has invaded their system—just one of the *little* side effects of their toxic treatment. I would strongly recommend that you read the rest of this book and the book by Dr. Ray D. Strand, M.D., *Death By Prescription,* before you begin a chemo regimen.

It is also becoming more and more common for people to find out AFTER an expensive drug has been on the market for months and even years, it may not be living up to its expectations. A good example is the drug Avastin® (produced by Genentech), which is said to starve tumors by cutting off their blood supply, however, the drug can cost upwards of *$100,000 per year* (450). The drug companies sell the drugs to physicians and hospitals, then the physicians and hospitals mark up the price and make a hefty profit as well. With a gold mine like this for the drug company, physicians, and hospitals, is it any wonder that they might be somewhat reluctant to admit that it isn't all it's cracked up to be? The drug company sold *$3.5 BILLION* worth of this drug in 2007 (450). What incentive would the medical establishment have NOT to use this drug (which can be very toxic) when they are making so much money from it?

In an article from the New York Times (July 8, 2008), writers Gina Kolata and Andrew Pollack stated that even though Avastin® has "become one of the most popular cancer drugs in the world…there is another side to Avastin®. Studies show the drug prolongs life by only a few months, **if that**…And some newer studies suggest the drug might be **less effective** against cancer than the Food and Drug Administration had understood when the agency approved its uses" (450). (Emphasis mine.) The writers of this article state that "some patient advocates are…troubled by very expensive treatments like Avastin® coming into routine use on what they see as little more than a hope and an expensive prayer." They also question the meaning of success with such a drug. Is it truly successful if the drug cannot extend lives or improve them (450)?

How many people receiving this drug were given false hopes? This is another drug that has potentially lethal side effects, like dangerous blood clots, but a drug company had 3 billion in sales on this drug in one year! Do you think that THEY are going to be the ones to admit that—"gee, maybe it isn't working as well as we thought?" Well, neither did Vioxx®. As a matter-of-fact, Vioxx® KILLED a lot of people and so did Propulsid and Baycol before they were finally removed from the market, but not before the drug companies made a fortune on them.

Consider recent reports and warnings from the FDA that a pain patch known as *Fentanyl* may be responsible for the deaths of *3500* people (421). The slow-release patch may empty its contents much more rapidly during exercise and hot weather, causing respiratory arrest (421).

How many toxic drugs that "might be less effective against cancer," than the FDA THINKS, will be given to unsuspecting victims before enough is enough? What will it take for the American consumer to put two-and-two together to figure out that the FDA is in bed with the drug industry and that they have no concern for the welfare of the public? Folks, they are in the business of making money and make no mistake about it—they are NOT concerned with the safety of the general public. (How many people are told by their physicians that shark cartilage also cuts off the blood supply to growing tumors, but without toxic side effects? Shark cartilage is discussed in several chapters in this book, as well as information about when it should not be taken. Also see the herb *bindweed* discussed later in this book.)

## Other Treatments

Note that some of the alternative treatments in this book (and my first book) are not *natural, painless* or particularly *gentle* (since they may be given by injection or require anesthesia), but they are mentioned for informational purposes, and because some of them have achieved commendable results without the use of toxic substances. This book is by no means an exhaustive work on natural cancer therapies (but it's close)!

There are many alternative and conventional therapies—some tested and some not—some toxic and some not—which I have not included in this book in detail, such as Carnivore, IGF-I receptor antagonists, B-cell biology, intercalating agents, Target GI™ (diagnostic involving colon cancer testing), Antibody-Drug Conjugates (ADCs), all the chemo combo drugs, Contortrostatin, Greenbriar, A-Type Lamins, Bemer 3000, EFT (Emotional Freedom Technique), Anodyne Therapy (for pain reduction and to help with circulatory problems), new cancer markers for early disease diagnosis (e.g., surface plasma resonance, spectrum technology, gene chip sensors and many more), German New Medicine®, GEMM Therapy, the rodent tuber plant, 2ME2, Acemannan (from aloe vera, though I do discuss glyconutrition and RM-10), Flex-Het drugs (flexible heteroarotinoids), Holt Microwave Therapy, S3I-201 or S3I-2001 (for breast cancer), Dicer and Drosha genes (in regards to ovarian cancer), nanobombs, Zalypsis® (for multiple myeloma), TSACH (for liver cancer), oncogenic protein studies, Nieper Therapy, Wasabi, Sun Farms Soup, DR70 blood test for cancer, GRP receptors (in fighting neuroblastoma), ground ivy, REOLYSIN® (a drug made from the respiratory enteric orphan virus or reovirus) for gliomas, Bowman-Birk inhibitor (for oral leukoplakia), Merlin (for gliomas), Iressa, Gc-MAF, Annexin A3 (a diagnostic test for prostate cancer), PTPRD gene, pangamic acid (B15), Urea, Cansema black topical salve (Tumorx), MENS (musculoskeletal nerve stimulation), Reams Biological Theory of Ionization, IVDMIA (in vitro diagnostic multivariate index assay testing), Seneca Valley Virus trials, the Ayurvedic treatments, tribulus herb, Fosteronia refracta, BNCT (Boron Neutron Capture Therapy), bitter melon, Reossification Therapy, Krebiozen, Tong Ren Therapy (for leukemia), Alsihum, Aveloz, Dries Cancer Diet, IAT, Wiedbrande Treatment, some plant-based cancer vaccines, the Scenar (aka *Skenar*) healing machine, Degarelix, MDX-1106, Qigong cancer therapy, the ACSL3 gene, Somocystinamide A (ScA), the PAPION Magnetic Inductor (PAPIMI©), lactoferrin, Osiecki Treatment, therapy that targets excess TG-2 in the body, Xeloda, Yuccalive, TVZ-7, the ADH-1 trials for advanced melanoma, cDPCP (for colorectal cancer), investigational drugs (e.g., phenoxodiol, under testing for chemo-resistant ovarian cancers, given *fast track* status by the U.S. FDA), some of the new colon cancer vaccines getting ready to come on the market, or already there (e.g. Trovax and Avicine), steroid sulfatase inhibitors, benzodiazepinone inhibitors, C-MET/HGFR inhibitors (such as ARQ-197), HDAC (Histone Deacetylase inhibitors), gossypol, Tibetan herbal remedy (PADMA-28 for lymphocytic leukemia), chemokines, molecular breast imaging, drugs that target interleukin-8, comfrey plant (which is very toxic when taken internally), peptide vaccines for myloid leukemia, tetraplex binding molecules, and many others too numerous to list here.

I have also not discussed in detail galectin inhibitors; radiolabeled monoclonal antibodies, which you may see or hear referred to as *antibody-directed-enzyme therapy* or *pro-drug antibody therapy*; though I do discuss 3F8 (for children with neuroblastoma), a monoclonal antibody treatment at Memorial Sloan-Kettering Cancer Center. See website *http://www.mskcc.org/mskcc/html/3215.cfm* for more information on this therapy. I did talk about Epratuzumab and 131-I-Labetuzumab very briefly. I did not discuss in detail some of the protein inhibitors, such as PX-12, or many of the biologically-targeted therapies, like Erbitux. I did talk about targeted therapy and targeted chemotherapy, but not drugs like Prolarix™, nor did I discuss Antigenics vaccine, the NOVO-TTF device, Kangra herbs (e.g., Immunokan), blood electrification, Alzheimer's drugs for cancer, anti-depressants for cancer, or radiation balloon implants.

Many health institutions are completely against using natural products for cancer and insist on using chemo and radiation as their only *recognized* treatments, meaning that they have been tested on humans, and making you think that no natural products have had human testing, which is not true. Please read chapter 33 in this book (on clinical trials) before you decide on the mode of treatment that you will use. If you do an internet search, you will find many articles written against alternative medicine, and most of them are written by people who represent the FDA, which is not surprising, because the FDA is in bed with the pharmaceutical companies. Thus, it does not take a mental heavyweight to figure out where the loyalties of the FDA lie. They always manage to incorporate the word "fraud" into their articles to give them an air of detective-like credibility and sophistication, so the public will THINK that they are telling the truth and have their best interests at heart. Don't count on it! The FDA does NOT have the public's best interests at heart. If they did, drugs like Vioxx® and Propulsid would never have killed so many people before they were removed from the market! Read chapter 33 in this book for more information about what goes on in many clinical trials that big pharma would prefer be unknown.

There are many cancers that are not described in great detail in this book, such as Wilm's tumors, LCH, pleuro-pulmonary blastoma, spindle cell carcinomas, myelofibrosis, desmoid tumors, acral and lentigo maligna melanomas, rhabdomyosarcomas, MPNSTs, MALT tumors, pNETs, mantle-cell lymphomas, non-rhabdomyosarcoma soft tissue sarcomas (NRSTS), leydig cell and sertoli-cell tumors, thecomas, DiGuglielmo's Syndrome, megakaryoblastic leukemia, Burkitt's lymphoma, Merkel cell cancer (a type of carcinoma, that you may also hear referred to as a form of nerve cell or neuroendocrine skin cancer), sarcoma botryoides, mycosis fungoides, Sezary Syndrome, pleomorphic rhabdomyosarcomas, thecomas —and others—nor do I discuss cancer staging; however, the alternative therapies (with some conventional treatments) described herein, have been used for all types of cancers, even some considered rare.

## Pharmaceuticals

In chapter 22 of this book (on Prescription HRT), you will discover that for decades physicians have been prescribing a synthetic form of progesterone and estrogen to their female patients. This synthetic hormone replacement was developed by a pharmaceutical company because they could not patent the NATURAL form of the hormones. They changed molecules in the natural hormone, patented the end result and created a new drug. There was, however, one very BIG problem with their new creation! It was foreign to the human body. Progesterone and estrogen in their natural forms (taken in correct doses) do NOT have the **toxic side effects of the synthetic formulas.** The synthetic hormones that the pharmaceutical companies had created caused major side effects that physicians were supposed to warn their patients about. Why did they create these hybrid mutants? Because they could not make a profit from natural estrogen and progesterone—natural products cannot be patented. If they cannot corner the market with a product, they are not interested in promoting it.

Have you ever been on hormone replacement therapy (HRT)? Did your physician tell you about all the potential deadly side effects of taking them? Did your physician ever tell you that there are NATURAL forms of estrogen and progesterone that you can walk into your local health food store and purchase without a prescription? They are applied topically to your skin in a cream form and absorbed through the skin, and when used in normal dosages, there are **no toxic side effects**. See chapter 22 of this book for more information on natural progesterone and the deadly problems associated with using synthetic progesterone and estrogen.

If you have any doubts about the flippancy with which the FDA treats our safety, all you have to do is research what happens with their drug approval system. The internet abounds with horror stories related to drugs like Propulsid, Baycol, Rezulin, and Vioxx®, and recently, a vaccination called *Gardasil®*, supposedly to help prevent cervical cancer caused by the HPV virus. The pharmaceutical company that produced Gardasil® is trying to get it state-mandated for all young girls, yet there have already been several deaths linked to this vaccine, and thousands of cases of people who have been made ill, some irreversibly so. Where is the outcry when these vaccines and drugs kill and maim people?

Did you know that the media is still reporting about the fact that the producers of Vioxx® KNEW this drug could be fatal YEARS before it was ever removed from the market!? Do you know what would have happened if this had been a natural, alternative herbal supplement not owned by a billion dollar drug conglomerate? Those who manufactured the natural supplement would be in jail facing prison terms, their records would be in the hands of the FDA, and the story would be making headline news every single day for weeks before it would finally die down! The FDA would be screaming about the need to place all vitamins, herbs, and supplements under their direct control. (To protect you and I, of course! The same way that they protected us from Propulsid, Vioxx®, and Baycol!?) Some of these drugs have been on the market for years. Why has it taken so long for this critical news to be made public? Because every day it wasn't made public meant more sales for the companies producing the drugs. The longer the delay before a drug is removed from the market, the longer the drug company can pull in sales.

## Targeted Therapy & Targeted Gene Therapy

Suffice it to say that some drugs are considered *targeted* chemotherapy drugs (aka chemoembolization), indicating that they are supposed to hit the cancer cells more precisely without as much damage to surrounding healthy cells as other chemo drugs. You may hear them referred to *as molecular-targeted-drugs* or *molecular-targeted-therapies*. Some of these drugs block the enzymes cancer cells produce, or the epidermal growth factor receptors (EGFR) that promote cancer growth (also referred to as HER1). Some of these drugs have the same basic potential for toxicity to the liver, kidneys or immune system that any chemo drug has. Some of the newer drugs being developed are said to be less harmful to the body's immunity—for example Rexin-G™ discussed later in this book—is even considered a non-chemo drug since it does not have the side effects usually seen in chemo drugs (256).

Tarceva®, also known as Erlotinib, is a targeted therapy drug that works on EGFR, and is given by conventional medicine for *non-small cell lung cancer* (108). It may not cause the total hair loss and immune system harm that many other chemo drugs cause, but there is always the potential for minor side effects (rashes and diarrhea) and very serious side effects, including kidney or fatal liver damage, anaphylactic reactions, and death (108).

Be certain that you never take any herbs, vitamins or other substances while taking targeted therapy or other drugs without consulting your physician. Even drinking grapefruit juice can cause serious reactions with some of these drugs. Before you undergo treatment, simply look the drug up and check the side effects or ask your physician about side effects and toxicity as well as **success rates**.

If you or someone you know has already been diagnosed with cancer (for example a brain tumor), and told that it is inoperable and your situation hopeless, PLEASE read chapter 14 of this book immediately! Some of the treatments in this book would come under the heading of immunotherapy (giving the body substances to boost the immune system to enable it to fight disease). You may also hear it referred to as *biological response modifier therapy, biological therapy, immunological therapy, and/or biotherapy*. Sometimes chemical items are used to facilitate the immune system in healing the body—things like interleukin, cytokines, interferon, and other substances—some of which have undesirable side effects. Many herbs are also discussed in this book (botanical medicine). This book does not discuss in detail homeopathic remedies, which would take a book in itself. Naturopathic physicians often use homeopathic treatments which are actually extracts taken from minerals, enzymes and plants to boost the body's natural immune system. You can find homeopathic remedies in most natural health food stores and books about how to use them.

## Trusting With Your Life

The next time you go to your physician's office, you may be loaded down with *free* samples of the latest new drug on the market, or pressured into taking that promising new vaccine someone just developed. Don't be surprised if your doctor sends you merrily on your way with no advice about side effects to these new drugs, except maybe a printed pamphlet with microscopic-sized warnings on line 135 of the drug label. Do you know how the FDA and the pharmaceutical companies will determine the extent of serious side effects involved with the new drug? If **you** don't have serious side effects from taking it, and it doesn't kill **you**, then it stays on the market, and even if it does kill you, or a loved one, or make you deathly ill, it could still stay on the market for years before it is forced off! The drug companies depend on your physician to contact them if **you** have a serious side effect to a medication you are taking, and this means a lot of paperwork for physicians that they do not have the time to do.

While there are many life-saving medications on the market (insulin, heart medications, drugs that extend the lives of dialysis and transplant patients and others very ill), be sure that you, your spouse, or your child are not the next guinea pig for the latest new drug. Do not automatically feel that you can trust that chemotherapy drug your physician wants to try out on you. Do not feel secure taking it simply because it was approved by the FDA. What about those *freebies* your doctor dispenses at your next visit? Are you going to eagerly accept them without question, simply because they are free? What might they ultimately cost you? A kidney? Your liver? Your life?

## Vaccines - Are They Really SAFE?

Are you aware that there are many health issues related to vaccinations? Childhood vaccinations have been suspected in Crohn's Disease, autism, juvenile diabetes, other auto-immune disorders, brain tumors in children, and many other illnesses, yet your school officials will tell you that you MUST have your child vaccinated, when in reality you can always request a *waiver* from your school to opt out of the vaccination. If vaccinations are effective, *why are booster shots needed for some vaccines?* You may wish to read the book by Neil Z. Miller, *Vaccines: Are They Really Safe & Effective,* before you take that next flu shot or take your child for their next vaccination.

There are many news articles circulating regarding a preservative in vaccines (thimersol or mercury) causing autism in children, and many websites have information about the dangers associated with flu shots. A Hollywood celebrity recently came out and admitted that she believed her young child's autism was caused by a recent vaccination. Though this is all being ignored by the CDC, T.V. news abounds with the gestapo-like tactics the U.S. government has resorted to in order to force vaccinations on children.

If you have a child who has recently been diagnosed with autism, Crohn's disease, type I diabetes, meningitis, Gullain-Barre syndrome, or you've lost a child to SIDS (sudden infant death syndrome), ask yourself this question: when was the last time that they were vaccinated, and what was it for? For those parents who have been lulled into believing that they MUST have their pre-teen and teen daughters vaccinated against cervical cancer with the new drug Gardasil®, which is already responsible for the deaths of several young girls, be sure you read up on the stories of young girls who have suffered irreversible, declining health after they received this new "promising" vaccine, including many cases of Gullain-Barre syndrome. Some pediatricians are demanding that childhood vaccines be spread out over a longer period of time, with children receiving fewer vaccines at any given time to reduce the risk of overwhelming their young immune systems. See this article about a young teen who developed total paralysis after vaccination with Gardasil®: *http://articles.mercola.com/sites/articles/archive/2008/08/02/hpv-vaccine-blamed-for-teen-paralysis.aspx?source=nl.*

Also, see the article about twelve babies that died in Argentina after receiving an experimental pneumonia vaccine. Website is: *http://www.theoneclickgroup.co.uk/news.php?start=2300&end=2320&view=yes&id=2819#newspost*, as well as the story of three young girls who say that they were paralyzed by the Gardasil® vaccine and are seeking damages from the drug manufacturer: *http://www.theoneclickgroup.co.uk/news.php?start=2300&end=2320&view=yes&id=2816#newspost.*

Be aware that I am **not** telling you that you should not take vaccines, pneumonia shots or flu shots. There are even new vaccines in the making for colon cancer and other cancers. How effective they will be is anybody's guess. There are some new individualized vaccines being produced to boost the body's immunity against cancer and some of those are working miraculously. (I am not speaking of Gardasil!) I have discussed those later in this book. As for taking vaccines for childhood diseases and for the flu, that is a decision **you will have to make and live with.** I am telling you to do the research on vaccinations. Be informed about the health decisions that you make, and be sure that your doctor is informed as well. Read and research everything you can before allowing yourself, or your child, to be the next guinea pig.

# CHAPTER 3

# AMAZING CURES FROM A COMMON TABLE FRUIT

*"And call upon me in the day of trouble: I will deliver thee, and thou shalt glorify me." (Psalm 50:15)*

## Old News - Good News

In her book, *The Grape Cure*, Johanna Brandt says that she came to America in 1927 to describe her amazing cure for cancer using common table grapes and a raw foods diet. She cured her own abdominal cancer when physicians had advised her that she would die without surgery. The story of her cleansing, fasting, raw diet is given in detail in a powerful little book known as *The Grape Cure*. Johanna experienced a complete cure from her abdominal cancer by consuming fresh grapes and drinking fresh grape juice, as well as a total raw foods diet. It did not seem to matter what type of grape she consumed—the more the variety—the better. She healed herself completely without surgery, radiation or chemotherapy (355). Her diet is discussed in great detail in her book, which can be purchased on internet book stores and at Ehret Literature Publishing Co., Inc. (for $4.95), PO Box 24, Dobbs Ferry, N.Y. 10522. Their website is *www.arnoldehret.org*.

Johanna was a great believer in raw foods, and felt that a total raw food juicing diet was healthiest, especially for those already fighting cancer. We are living, electronically-functioning organisms. When you feed your body raw foods, you are giving your cells electrically-balanced food that can be recognized, processed, and used optimally. Once foods are cooked, the live enzymes within them are destroyed. Johanna's book, though written more than 70 years ago, is still very relevant today!

## Bacteria & The Raw Foods Diet - Which Foods Are Safer?

There are a lot of safety concerns regarding consumption of raw foods (fruits & vegetables), especially in light of the fact that the FDA has no risk-free guarantees on raw food in the U.S. marketplace. There have been many outbreaks in the past few years from bacteria in raw food (spinach, tomatoes, peppers, salsa, lettuce, peanut butter), and in undercooked meats from fast-food restaurants that have sickened and even killed people. Even though organic is better because of lack of insecticide and herbicide use, this is no guarantee that organic raw foods will be safe from threats, such as salmonella, e-coli and other dangers. During the bubonic plague in Europe, many people saved their lives by soaking their food in wine before consumption. If you cannot get organic foods in your area, some of the non-organic foods that have the least amount of pesticides, herbicides, and other chemical sprays (the lowest amounts) were found by *foodnews.org* to be the following: (in order of lowest amount of pesticides to highest) "Onions (lowest pesticide load), Avocado, Frozen Sweet Corn, Pineapples, Mango, Frozen Sweet Peas, Asparagus, Kiwi, Bananas, Cabbage, [and] Broccoli…" (117a)

Some raw food proponents recommend filling a previously-scrubbed sink with cold water and putting in two ounces of regular 3% solution hydrogen peroxide, then letting (e.g., leafy greens, carrots) soak in the solution for twenty minutes, and vegetables with thicker skins for 30-35 minutes, then rinsing them thoroughly before consuming or refrigerating. You can also make a spray with a few ounces of 3% hydrogen peroxide diluted in six to eight ounces of water for your countertops. Remember, this is NOT food grade peroxide you are using. It should not be ingested. You are only using it to kill parasites! Always rinse thoroughly. Even this is not a total guarantee. I always recommend that people (especially if eating out) take with them cinnamon, cloves, garlic capsules, and even oil of wild oregano capsules, or grapefruit-seed extract, and consume the capsules with their meals for added protection. Milk thistle and alpha lipoic acid can protect the liver from toxins. These substances won't give 100% protection when eating out, but it is possible that they could save your life or the life of a loved one. Some people advocate sipping wine with meals as an added safety measure to help kill bacteria in food, however, even unfermented grape juice will kill bacteria. Alcohol will eventually harm the liver. Never consume raw seafood or raw, undercooked meat, fish, fowl, or eggs! You are taking a risk!

I believe the day will come when people will be forced to have their own backyard gardens to grow their family's food in order to be safer about raw food consumption. With all the new trade laws in effect, foods are being sent across international lines faster and more adamantly than ever before in the history of the world. There are times when you purchase vegetables in a local grocery store, and you have no idea if they are from the U.S., Mexico, Thailand, Pakistan, Columbia, Canada, Peru,

Egypt, Australia or Kenya. Does anyone know the farming practices of these countries? Even foods grown in the U.S. cannot be guaranteed safe for consumption. How can foods imported from foreign countries—where we have little intervention in growing standards—be guaranteed safe?

Realize that it won't do you one bit of good to practice scrupulous scrubbing and soaking of your fruits and vegetables to kill bacteria if your personal hygiene habits are poor. Human beings GROW e-coli in their intestines. The best way to prevent the spread of bacteria has always been proper hand-washing!

## Grapes & Abdominal Cancer

In my first book, *Painless Cancer Cures*, I also discuss a gentleman suffering from a malignant tumor of the abdomen who opted out of conventional medicine and used a diet much like the one advocated by Johanna Brandt. He went on a juice fast, staying with the raw fruit and vegetable juices until his cancer had completely disappeared (386). Grapes also contain another super anti-oxidant known as *caffeic acid*, and they are rich in ellagic acid, as are raspberries, pomegranates, strawberries, pecans, walnuts, cherries, cranberries, and other fruits. Ellagic acid helps boost the body's own immune system, giving it the ability to fight cells that are running amuck in the body and causing disease (493). Cranberries also cut the risk for ulcers and bladder infections, and help fight leukemia (22).

## Grapes & Alkalinity

The healthiest state for the human body is one of moderate alkalinity. The ideal blood pH of the body is 7.35—7.45. The lower the number, the more acid your body is; the higher the number, the more alkaline. If you keep your body in a state of alkalinity, rather than acidity, you will drastically slash your risks for getting cancer and other diseases, because diseases thrive when the body is kept in a state of acidity. A diet high in meat, dairy products, and cooked foods keeps the body in a state of constant acidity, increasing the risk for cancer and all chronic diseases. When the blood is acidic, it will try to alkalize on its own by pulling calcium and magnesium into the bloodstream. Where does it get these minerals? Well—usually from your BONES! This is why a cooked diet rich with meats, dairy, processed foods, and refined sugars causes joint pain, osteoporosis, and other ailments. Raw fruits and vegetables contribute to the body's alkalinity. Any cooking of foods immediately reduces their alkalinity and makes them more acidic. Grapes alkalize the blood. See chapter 30 for more information on the acid/alkaline balance and what those numbers represent.

Diets that promote acidity also cause large amounts of free radicals to circulate in the human body. Free radicals are a type of aberrant electron, and though some are good for us, most are not. Those that are harmful have the capacity to cause chaos within the DNA, leading to mutations that can result in cancer and chronic diseases.

Those who criticized Johanna Brandt during her lifetime did so out of ignorance. They knew nothing of free radicals, proanthocyanidins, carotenoids, or super anti-oxidants. As time goes by, more and more amazing properties of Johanna's miracle grapes are being discovered.

## Grape Power

During her day, many people adopted Johanna's grape cure, but others were critical, disbelieving that something this simple could affect disease so profoundly. Modern researchers, however, have isolated an amazing ingredient in grapes, known as ***resveratrol.*** It is a very powerful anti-oxidant that not only inhibits the growth of cancer cells, but contains healing and blood-thinning properties (337). Johanna Brandt's remarkable cure from abdominal cancer certainly proved that she was ahead of her time, and that there is something miraculous in the healing power of fasting, detoxification, and the lowly grape.

The reason white wine is white is because the resveratrol-rich grape skins are not used in white wine—only in red wines (386). For an excellent 58-page study on resveratrol's role in fighting cancer, which was conducted by M.D. Anderson Cancer Center and the UCLA Center for Human Nutrition, see website: *http://www.agrawal.org/PDF/ACR-Resveratrol1.pdf*, (346). Resveratrol is also being touted as a way to fight obesity, since it keeps the body from storing fat. Studies at the University of Virginia Health System recently unraveled how resveratrol works at fighting cancer. Apparently, the resveratrol in red wine and grape skin blocks the effect of a very important protein that cancer cells can't live without; however, it only takes a small amount of wine (about 8 ounces a few times a week); too much, and the risk for cancer increases. Non-alcoholic wine works just as well (252) (255), can be used by kids, and is much safer for the liver. Better yet, use the grape skins in their original packaging as prepared by our Creator.

Another very powerful anti-oxidant comes from the seeds and skins of grapes (as well as acai berries, raspberries, cranberries, strawberries, and other fruits) and the bark of the pine tree. It is pycnogenols. While the green and white grapes are higher in pycnogenols, the purple and red grapes are higher in resveratrol and we need both (337).

Most of us are familiar with recent health studies showing the lack of heart disease and lack of harmful cholesterol levels found in the French (known as the *French paradox*), yet they enjoy rich foods and consume wine with most of their meals. As mentioned in Reese Dubin's *Miracle Food Cures From the Bible*, this is because wine can raise good cholesterol levels, and also helps to scour harmful fats from the arteries (386). Grape extracts appear to strengthen the walls of blood vessels, thus preventing vein variscosities and degenerative diseases of the eye, such as diabetic retinopathy and many others. When cholera broke out in the 18th century, many lives were saved when it was shown that wine killed bacteria. People used it to soak their foods, especially meat, fish, and fruits. During the 1970's when viruses were tested against grape extract, a day later, none of them were alive (386), and this is the juice we are talking about, BEFORE it is fermented into wine!

Although wine kills harmful germs and bacteria, you don't need alcohol-containing wine to do this. Fasting, juicing, fresh grape juice, and a detox regimen can do the same thing. Try to use organic whenever possible. Many commercial grapes are heavily sprayed. Be aware that any drink containing alcohol is harmful to the liver, not to mention what it does to the brain. Grape extract also kills viruses and bacteria without harming the liver or the brain, and it inhibits cancer rather than increasing its risks. No adverse side effects have been reported from taking grape seed extract. Just don't mix it with vitamin C supplements. Research suggests that taking them at the same time may raise blood pressure in some individuals. This extract has been useful in the treatment of many disorders, including those affecting the circulatory system.

## Grapes Help Fight Lung Cancer, Colon, Breast, Prostate, Pancreatic, Liver Cancer & Leukemia

This isn't the end of the miraculous grape and resveratrol. According to an article at website *CancerProject.org,* resveratrol can slow down the spread of many types of cancer, including those in the *breast, liver, colon, lungs,* and even *leukemia* (117). Grape seed extract can help kill colorectal cancer cells. Is it any wonder that Johanna Brandt's grape cure diet was such a potent enemy against so many forms of cancer? She was considered a *genius* by some in her day while others scoffed at her. It appears that where the scientific community is concerned, Johanna Brandt has had the last laugh. It is very unfortunate that her *Grape Cure* blessing never reached the majority of Americans for which it was intended. How many people have ever heard of it before now? **(Have you?)**

## Grapes & Resveratrol, the Super Flavenol

Research on this compound has shown that resveratrol can inhibit the cancer process in any of its three stages of development from beginning to end (375). It also has anti-inflammatory properties similar to some chemo drugs, but without the damaging effects that they cause. Even concord grapes have been shown to repress tumors as effectively as the common chemo drug *methotrexate* (375).

According to website *http://www.mnwelldir.org/nw_current.htm,* "some call resveratrol the Fountain of Youth" (255a). More and more studies continue to be done on this amazing anti-oxidant found in the "skin of grapes, berries and red wines" (255a):

> Dr. Stuart Richer OD, PhD, Chief, Optometry Section at the Veterans Medical Center in North Chicago, speaking at the 111th annual American Academy of Optometry meeting in Seattle, says this may be the first time an intervention has been shown to reverse aging changes in the retina. The patient, an 80-year-old male, came to the eye clinic complaining of loss of night vision. Commonly prescribed nutriceuticals, such as lutein, vitamin E and fish oil were employed with no positive result. After 5 months on the dietary supplement regimen [resveratrol], five measurable parameters of vision improved to varying but significant degrees including night (contrast) vision, visual acuity, color and side vision....it was also found the patient's mental capacity had improved (255a).

Harvard studies have recently shown that resveratrol "Cleans your arteries of plaque making them smooth and youthful; gives you a boost of energy, helping to burn more calories; boosts the immune system, and might even reverse the damage from a lousy diet and lifestyle" (255a).

Researchers even found, to their amazement, that they could feed half a group of aging mice a *high...trans fat, junk food diet*, and all of them "developed the same symptoms of humans who ate the same diet:" liver problems, "diabetes and cardiovascular issues…" (255a). The rest of the mice ate the exact same diet, but were given resveratrol. They gained weight, were much healthier…functioned normally, looked healthier. All the rodents in the first "group died prematurely." Those in the "second group lived 15% longer than normal" and "…another related study showed that mice on resveratrol were able to run twice as fast as normal, healthy mice not taking resveratrol" (255a). More research keeps coming forth on the amazing rejuvenation powers of resveratrol. Dr. Robert Rowan's findings show that "rats who were given wine compounds for eight weeks maintained healthy blood pressure; One study shows resveratrol" outperformed "Pepto-Bismol in combating three strains of bacteria that cause diarrhea" (255a). It is also an antifungal, offering some protection from pathogens, not just in the *grape plant*, but *in humans* as well and was shown to help prevent "cataracts (taken in the form of red wine)" (255a).

## Other Health Benefits of Eating Grapes

Organically grown grapes should be purchased whenever possible. Grapes are often one of the most highly sprayed fruits in production. Organically grown grapes are certified to be free of pesticides and herbicides. Grapes are a rich source of quercetin, a potent anti-oxidant. They also contain the important anti-inflammatory, anti-oxidant—pycnogenol®. Pycnogenol® helps fight debilitating disorders, such as cardiac and circulatory problems, arthritis, stress, and even inhibits allergies and cancerous growths.

A research group recently reported that resveratrol protects against both liver and breast cancer, but don't look for resveratrol in white wine, because it is found only in the pulp and seeds which are excluded when white wine is processed from the juice. However, as stated earlier, alcohol consumption in itself can increase the risk of certain cancers. The cancer-fighting chemicals are found in grapes before they are ever fermented into wine. Why not consume them the way our Creator God gave them to us—in their healthiest and most natural state? Resveratrol supplements are available in health food stores and many local supermarkets. If taking resveratrol, consult with your physician first, especially if you are on prescription meds, are expecting, breast feeding, or fighting a chronic illness, and find a good Naturopath!

## Pterostilbene - Another Healing Ingredient Discovered in Grapes

In our annuals of modern medicine, every single day seems to bring more amazing discoveries about the healing properties of natural foods, such as grapes and their cancer-fighting nutrients. Yet another compound has recently been discovered in grapes that may not only fight cancer, but diabetes as well (86). The compound is known as *pterostilbene.* It is supposed to work much like resveratrol, but also lowers blood sugar (86). Blueberries are even higher in pterostilbene content than grapes (86). Pterostilbene also enhances memory and fights heart disease and harmful cholesterol (37).

One researcher noted that this compound could prevent cancer-causing changes in DNA, especially against malignant breast cells. For some reason, this particular nutrient—though found in blue, red, and black grape skins—is destroyed when the juice is made into wine; another reason to consume the grape in its natural, God-given, raw form.

## Sources of Resveratrol

A very rich source of resveratrol is the root of the Japanese knotweed plant known as *hu zhang*. Some resveratrol supplements are taken from hu zhang, others use ground-up purple grape skin. Blueberries, peanuts, mulberry, cranberries, and many other food sources contain resveratrol. I am seeing more and more resveratrol supplements available in health food stores, pharmacies, and local supermarket shelves.

## Which Grapes Are Best?

I believe the best advice, as given by Johanna Brandt, is to eat a **variety**, because you will get more **resveratrol** in the red and purple grape skins, and, as noted by James F. Balch, M.D., author of *The Super Anti-Oxidants,* there are more **OPCs** (super anti-oxidants, also known as *oligomeric proanthocyanidins),* in the "green and white grapes," and **you need both** (337). Remember that for OPCs, you need to eat the entire grape along with the SEEDS. It is the seeds that are so rich in OPCs (337).

# CHAPTER 4

# GENTLE CURES FOR TOUGH BREAST CANCERS

*"For I will restore health unto thee, and I will heal thee of thy wounds, saith the Lord;" (Jeremiah 30:17)*

## Types of Breast Cancer

The most commonly diagnosed breast cancer is infiltrating ductal carcinoma. There are other types of breast cancer, including invasive lobular carcinoma and ductal carcinoma in-situ, and rare types, such as papillary carcinoma, mucinous carcinoma (aka colloid breast cancer), tubular carcinoma, and medullary breast cancer. This chapter has some amazing cases of complete breast cancer cures, some of them without surgery, chemo or radiation. Many are finding that switching to a raw foods, vegan diet can help begin the healing process for the body's immune system. Even the American Cancer Society has finally agreed, after decades of controversy and earlier statements to the contrary (that there was no connection between dietary intake and cancer), that eating a diet high in fiber, fresh fruits and vegetables will reduce your cancer risk. (WHERE have they been for the past 30 years?)

## Breast Cancer Testing — NEW Tests for Greater Accuracy

* **BSGI (Breast Specific Gamma Imaging) –** This diagnostic imaging is cheaper than an MRI, yet it shows up details that can be missed in mammograms, finding breast cancers earlier. Breast density is not an issue.

* **CURE – Computed Ultrasound Risk Evaluation Device** – for details on this new test for detecting early breast cancer, see website: *http://www.nbc10.com/health/17556752/detail.html* (215b).

* **DiaGenic -** is a company in Norway, which has produced a *blood test* for detecting breast cancer. It is said to be far superior to tests that seek out genetic defects, and relies on very *specific...proteins* produced only by the cancer cells (215a). We have no idea how long it will take the FDA to approve this one; however, if you happen to be traveling in The *United Kingdom*, you can get the test done there at *Opaldia*, their *largest cancer center* (215a). It is a sad, but true fact (for Americans), that many nations are far ahead of the U.S. when it comes to cancer diagnostics and treatment.

* **MBI -** This Molecular Breast Imaging is yet another choice over mammogram for breast diagnostics; however, those who undergo this type imaging need to beware—because this test will give you up to ten times more radiation than your routine mammogram—while a thermogram (see below) delivers NO radiation and is totally painless.

* **MR - Magnetic Resonance Elastography** - developed by the Mayo Clinic in Rochester, Minnesota, this combo of using *sound waves and MRI* may be a good screener to use in conjunction with mammograms, especially for situations where mammograms are not as effective (188).

* **3TP System - Cadscience MRI** - this *new MRI machine* is a way that physicians can diagnose cancers of the breast *earlier,* especially for those who are *high risk* and concerned about a genetic tendency for breast cancer (94). See details at: *http://www.sciencedaily.com/videos/2006/0102-detecting_breast_cancer_early.htm* (94).

* **Oncotype DX™ -** this is a "genomic test" that peeks at 21 of your cancer genes to figure out what your "recurrence score" is (9a). Score is *0-100.* The higher the score, the higher your risk for the return of your cancer (9a). If you have "node-positive breast cancer," this test will also, not only help your doctor determine if you are at greater risk for recurrence, but whether or not you will (or won't) *benefit* from *chemotherapy* (9a). Be sure first, however, to read the rest of this book!

* **PEM (Positive Emission Mammography) –** this is a new diagnostic test which could prove to be more accurate at diagnosing breast cancers than MRI machines.

* **Saliva Testing -** It could be another *five years* before this test gets *FDA* approval, but as noted by Dr. Charles Streckfus at the University of Texas, since having *breast cancer* causes significant changes in *proteins* that come *from the salivary gland...*, and since we now know that there are at least *49 different proteins in saliva* that can determine the presence of *malignan*t versus *benign breast tumors*, there is no reason why the FDA should drag its feet on this one (215a).

## Thermogram Versus Mammogram

Thermograms, popular in California (also known as thermography), can detect suspicious breast changes much earlier than the routine mammogram can, yet they are not easily available in many states, and some states that DO have this tool, only have ONE location in the entire state where a thermogram can be obtained. Mammography uses radiation, thermography does not. Thermography uses infrared sensory detectors to find abnormalities. Mammograms compress the breast, which is often painful, but during thermography, there is no breast contact, thus making thermograms not only safe, but painless and *gentle*. It is the earliest means of screening for breast changes, yet women in the U.S. are consistently pressured into having only mammograms because thermography has not yet been made widely available to them, nor do some insurance companies cover them. This is an outrage and should NOT be the case! Thermography is the ONLY painless procedure that can tell a woman if she has excess estrogen within her breasts, something a mammogram cannot do. I am not saying that thermograms should replace mammograms, but every time a woman gets a mammogram, she is getting a huge dose of radiation, which accumulates in the body over the years. How many women are aware that when the breasts are pressed in a mammogram, if a tumor IS present, crushing it can SPREAD the cancer!? Very often, this is what a mammogram actually does!

Women should be able to have a choice of having either or BOTH of these procedures, yet in most cases they do not. (The next time you choose a mammogram, ask the radiologist to provide you with a topical lidocaine gel, which will make the procedure much less painful.)

When more and more women are being diagnosed with breast cancer, there is no reason that thermography should not be available as an adjuvant second choice with mammograms, especially since so many lives are at stake. Neither a mammogram nor a thermogram can diagnose cancer, but their findings can let women know if they are at risk.

Mammograms miss a higher percentage of cancers than thermograms. If a woman has fibrocystic breast disease, this may interfere with the results of her mammogram, but will NOT interfere with the results of a thermogram. All women should be demanding that their insurance companies and their physicians make thermograms as easily available to them as mammograms are! Thermograms can also detect disease processes in the rest of the body, not just the breasts.

## I. Dietary Changes & Breast Cancer Cures

Eydie Mae Hunsberger was given up by the medical establishment when she developed breast cancer. However, within one year of changing her diet and lifestyle, her cancer was in remission and has not returned since. She has been cancer-free for many years. In her book, *HOW I CONQUERED CANCER NATURALLY,* she describes how she reversed her cancer by switching to a raw fresh fruit and vegetable diet, which included juicing fresh juices and wheat grass. Though her surgeon wanted her to have a mastectomy, she agreed to a simple lumpectomy only, with no other treatment (436). She followed the vegan raw foods, juicing diet as popularized by Ann Wigmore in her books: The *Hippocrates Diet And Health Program,* and *The Wheat Grass Book* (420, 422). Also, see the book by Ann Wigmore, *THE SPROUTING BOOK: How to Grow and Use Sprouts to Maximize Your Health and Vitality* (599).

It is interesting to note that Ann Wigmore and Eydie Mae both followed a raw foods vegan diet, as did others discussed in this chapter. Wheat grass is very detoxifying to the body. It can only be tolerated in small amounts when first beginning the raw foods program. During her stay at Ann Wigmore's mansion, Eydie was consuming two ounces of wheat grass juice up to four times a day, besides using wheat grass implants rectally (599), directions for which can be found in her book (above).

## Rita Myers Cures Her Stage IV Breast Cancer

When Rita Myers was told that she had Stage IV invasive "ductal cell carcinoma," which had gone into her bone, physicians gave her six months to two years to live. She began to prepare to die. Her doctors recommended surgery, radiation and chemotherapy. She started on chemotherapy until her husband, Leon, discovered the *Hallelujah Acres* diet. Rita realized that she did not want a lymphectomy—that she needed the nodes for "her immune system to function properly" (475). She stopped chemo abruptly, told them that she would not allow any radiation, and started on the *Hallelujah Acres* program of biblical nutrition. Rita believes that it was prayer and the *Hallelujah Acres* program that saved her life and healed her completely. She remains cancer-free and following a raw foods program, juicing about "50 pounds of carrots…" a week (475). In Rita's words:

> People who hear my story have rarely heard of anyone with stage IV cancer surviving. They are in wonder and amazement. They realize the traditional way is not working and want the same kind of miracle in their life that I experienced (475).

The *Hallelujah Acres* diet can be found at their website, *www.hacres.com,* and is discussed in more detail in this book in chapter six. It is mainly a raw food vegan diet as advocated by Eydie Mae, Ann Wigmore, and Johanna Brandt.

## Green Drinks Fight Cancer

My first book, *Painless Cancer Cures & Preventions Your Doctor May Not Be Aware Of*, contains several descriptions of people who used anti-oxidant-rich green drinks, such as fresh wheat grass, for fighting breast cancer and other cancers. Also, see articles later in this new book on chlorella, chlorophyll and chlorophyllin.

## Fungus Cure Also Cures Cancer, Says Oncology Physician

See chapter 34 of this book for the amazing cancer cure that Italian Oncologist, Dr. Simoncini, is using to cure his cancer patients within just days! Cancerous growths are usually WHITE. He says that they are a fungus, which can be killed with a non-toxic soda bicarb solution that quickly alkalizes the tumor for destruction (582). (& see pp 591-594.)

## The Raw Foods Diet & Oxalates

A note on the raw foods diet—be aware that there are many raw foods, such as rhubarb, kiwi, berries and spinach that are considered high-oxalate foods. They contain a form of acid that can aggregate to form kidney stones or gallstones (173). These foods should not be used in large amounts by those who may be prone to develop gallstones or kidney stones. These acid crystals can irritate joints, as in the case of gout or rheumatoid arthritis (173). Also, avoid taking calcium with high oxalate foods, since oxalates can inhibit calcium's assimilation by the body. Wait a few hours in between (173). Many times, stone formation could be avoided by simply increasing fluid intake, and making sure that sufficient amounts of B vitamins and magnesium are taken daily; however, there will always be some folks who are prone to develop stones, regardless of what they do.

The majority of people have no problem with oxalate foods. There are many websites that give complete lists of all the foods that contain oxalates.

If you are prone to develop stones, and are able to obtain one of them, have it analyzed to find out the stone's composition. Depending on what the stone consists of, will tell you how to prevent a reoccurrence. For example, if you have stones that consist mostly of calcium phosphate or magnesium ammonium phosphate (sometimes called *struvite stones*), keeping your urine acidic with things like cranberry juice and/or ascorbic acid (vitamin C) will help prevent, and in some cases, even dissolve these type stones. If you have cystine stones or calcium oxalate stones, keeping your urine acidic will not help dissolve them, nor if you have uric acid stones. Even though vitamin C may increase oxalate formation, it won't cause you to form these type stones. If you have a problem with gout caused by uric acid and purines, try eating sour cherries, increasing your intake of vitamin C, and decreasing meat, sugar, and coffee intake. It is also important to maintain good water hydration and restrict sugar consumption and carbonated sodas to prevent stones. Be sure to get adequate B vitamins. Alkalize your body.

## Burzynski's Antineoplastons

See chapter 14 of this book for amazing cases of cancer patients completely cured of *terminal* cancers; people who were basically sent home to die, then chose non-toxic antineoplastons from the Burzynski Clinic in Texas. Also, see many of the patient's own stories about their success in fighting cancer with antineoplastons at website: *http://burzynskipatientgroup.org/stories.html*. Many of these cases were breast cancer patients.

Many were hopeless, very aggressive brain tumors. The main Burzynski Clinic website is at: *http://www.burzynskiclinic.com.*

## Chlorella & Protein in the Vegan Diet

Chlorella alga is vitamin and mineral-rich, and for those concerned about protein (in a vegetarian diet, or vitamin B12), it is high in protein and vitamin B12 as well. It is discussed in more detail later in this book. Also, realize that you don't need meat to get complete proteins in your diet. Combining grains and legumes (beans) gives complete proteins. In animal research with chlorella, tumor masses completely vanished in half the subjects receiving chlorella. All of the animals not on the extract worsened as their cancers continued to grow. All those not given chlorella died.

Be sure, when using chlorella, to get the *broken cell-wall* chlorella, otherwise your body will have a difficult time with absorption. Chlorella has the highest concentration of chlorophyll of any green food, and since it is an alga—and not a seaweed—it does not contain iodine.

## Curing Breast Cancer by Eliminating Dairy

A physician scientist, after being diagnosed with breast cancer, going through chemo, then having it return, discovered that her cancer completely disappeared when she eliminated all dairy products from her diet. Studies have shown that high amounts of dairy in the diet can contribute to many forms of cancer, including those of the breast and prostate. There has been some recent hype in the news about milk preventing colon cancer, which is totally absurd, because it is CALCIUM that prevents colon cancer, not MILK. Proponents of this idiotic reasoning argue that since milk has SOME calcium, it can prevent colon cancer, never mind all the other problems associated with dairy products (see chapter 26)!

## Essiac Tea for All Cancers

You can obtain Flor-Essence® Essiac tea at many natural health food stores in an already prepared drinkable form, or a powdered form that you brew yourself, and Essiac® Resperin Canada tea is also available in some health food stores and internet sites. See chapter sixteen in this book for the amazing story of a young man healed of lymphoma using 714X injections and Essiac® Resperin's tea (as well as dietary changes and nutrients described in that chapter).

See chapter six for more details on Rene Caisse, a Canadian nurse, who healed hundreds, possibly thousands of people, of every imaginable cancer using her amazing herbal tea blend. Many of them came to her after conventional medicine considered them incurable and hopeless.

One of the most amazing books describing the effectiveness of this tea and how it was suppressed by the health industry in Canada, is called *The Essiac Report Canada's Remarkable Unknown Cancer Remedy,* by Richard Thomas, who claims that Flor-Essence® is the original (drinkable) formula that Rene Caisse used. In his book, he documents a letter from Anna T. whose mom was suffering from advanced breast cancer that had gone into several areas throughout her body (580). She was given six months to live. After a couple of months, her mom worsened, and Anna was told that her mother might live another two weeks. She began giving her the Flor-Essence® formula tea. Four weeks later, her mom was still alive, and improving. After being an invalid in bed for many months, she was now walking and began gaining weight. This was in 1994. Anna's letter a year later to the maker's of Flor-Essence®, informed them that her mom was now living by herself, pain-free, and getting ready for the arrival of a new grandchild (580)!

In his book, Thomas says that Rene shared the original recipe with Dr. Brusch, the physician that she worked closely with. The drinkable formula was perfected to the point that injections no longer needed to be given. He claims that the original formula was developed into Flor-Essence® tea, which you will find at most health food stores (580).

May H., who is discussed in Mr. Thomas' book, was treated with the Essiac formula for bilateral breast cancer and uterine cancer. She had been sent to Rene by her physician as a *hopeless* case. Within 90 days, she had returned to work. **40 years later**, she was still alive and doing very well, without ever having cancer again (580). Another patient (Annie B.) was treated with the Essiac formula for uterine and bowel cancer. She had received radiation, which caused extensive swelling and discoloration in her arm. She was supposed to have her arm *amputated,* but went to Rene for treatment instead. Four months later, after receiving the Essiac formula, Annie regained the 60 pounds she had lost, and her arm was completely normal (580).

Note that there is some competition between the tea produced by Resperin of Canada, known as Essiac®, and Flor-Essence® Essiac tea. Both companies claim that they have the original Essiac formula (the drinkable formula, not the injectable) that Rene Caisse used in treating her cancer patients. See chapter six of this book for more detailed information on Essiac tea.

In spite of the fact that the U.S. FDA would not allow claims (for many years) that folic acid prevented birth defects, physicians are now recommending that all women who are pregnant should be on folic acid supplements (413). When claims are made for any vitamin or herbal formula (such as Essiac), the FDA announces that it is now a DRUG, removes it from the public availability, and insists that it goes through a series of drug trials that can take years! (This is what Canada and the U.S. tried to do with Essiac.) In the meantime, the public does not have access to the product. This is exactly what the FDA has been trying to do for years with all supplements. They want to make it impossible for you to go into a health food store and buy a vitamin or herb. They want to control every supplement on the market so that you have to go to a pharmacy or a physician to get a PRESCRIPTION for a vitamin or herb. Once that happens, the price goes through the roof and availability and brand selection dwindles drastically.

When is the last time that you had a ten minute diagnostic procedure done (without general anesthesia) that you or your insurance company was charged three-thousand dollars for? Do the math. If you are being billed three-thousand dollars for a ten-minute procedure, that comes out to $18,000 an hour. How many OTHER professions besides the medical profession do you know that can get away with charging fees of $18,000 an hour?

## Flax Fights Breast Cancer

Lignans found in ground flax seed are protective against breast cancer. Many nutritional experts are recommending that women have *one to three tablespoons* a day *of Omega-3-rich ground flax seed* (389). Apparently, the flax oil is not as rich in lignans as the ground seeds for fighting not only breast cancer, but other chronic diseases as well. Studies show that flax not only prevents new cancers, but inhibits those already formed, and fights their spread. Flax has *800 times* the *lignans* of *any other plant* (389)!

The body has estrogen-receptors on cells. Natural plant estrogens lock onto the receptors and BLOCK out the harmful estrogens. This is how flax fights hormone-positive cancers.

I use an inexpensive coffee-grinder, get the whole, organic flax, and grind it myself in small amounts daily as needed. You won't get the essential Omega-3 without grinding up the flax seed. You can use the ground flax in cereals, whipped drinks, casseroles, and recipes (389).

## New Non-Toxic Drugs for Breast Cancer

### • BSI-201

This is a new drug, still in testing phases, developed by BiPar Sciences, Inc., that is said to have no toxic side effects (561a). Tests thus far involve those cancers (e.g., breast and ovarian) that are fast-growing (561a).

### • Nanotechnology—*Lodamin*—Curing Breast Cancer without Side Effects

Also a new drug, Lodamin works by halting the blood vessel growth that tumors need to survive, and was shown (in animal testing) to be effective against many tumor types, including those of the breast, brain, ovaries, uterus, prostate, neuroblastoma and glioblastoma (401). It also worked very well in preventing cancer from going into the liver (401). The discovery of the drug, using *nanotechnology* and a derivative from a fungus, was quite accidental. Reports say that it can be taken orally without *side effects* (401). The drug also inhibited melanoma and lung cancer in mice (401). (Shark cartilage and bindweed, discussed later in this book, starve tumors by cutting off their blood supply without adverse side effects.) Lodamin is still in the testing phases, and is also being considered for treating macular degeneration and arthritis.

### • Onconase—New Non-Toxic Drug for Breast Cancer

This drug (aka *Ranpirnase*), is a new pharmaceutical drug developed for treating mesothelioma, and is claimed to be *free* of the adverse effects that are normally seen in common chemo drugs (222). It is said to work on other cancers, such as those of the breast. It was developed by a company known as *Alfacell* (222). The drug is also supposed to make it possible to give lower dosages of standard chemo drugs with the same cancer-killing effects. It is said to fight *solid tumor cancers,* such as *carcinomas*, as well as those of the *kidney, breast, lung, and prostate* (222). Just be aware that even though this new drug is said to be relatively free of toxic side effects, drugs such as this one, are sometimes combined with conventional chemo drugs that **do have** toxic side effects. Human trials are currently underway on Ranpirnase. Check with your Oncologist.

## Raw Food Vegan Diet & Vitamin B12 Concerns

Vegetarians are often told that they will suffer a vitamin B12 deficiency without consuming meats. B12 can be destroyed by gastric acid in the stomach, though some amounts of B12 are created by *friendly* bacteria in the intestines. For concern about gastric acid destruction of vitamin B12, this vitamin is available in **sublingual** tablets at most health food stores. You simply put the small tablet under your tongue, and it is dissolved and absorbed directly into the rich supply of blood vessels there, completely bypassing the stomach acid. It is also now possible to get B12 patches where the vitamin is absorbed directly into the top layer of the skin.

## II. Hormones Can Cure—Or Kill

One of the most important ingredients for breast cancer prevention in women is the right balance of hormones in the body. See chapter 22 in this book. It explains how millions of women were prescribed hormone replacement therapy in the last forty-fifty years that have had deadly side effects because they were given SYNTHETIC hormones created by pharmaceutical companies. Their physicians never told them that there are NATURAL hormones (estrogen as well as progesterone) that are available to them without **TOXIC side effects** when given in normal dosing. What was the reason for this very blatant cover-up? The natural hormones can be bought at any health food store and they cannot be PATENTED, so the huge drug companies could not make a profit from selling them. Instead, they pushed their synthetic versions of the hormones onto the unwitting public, and thousands have paid the price with their health and their lives due to the deadly side effects of these drugs—effects like blood clots, strokes, uterine cancer and breast cancer. Chapter 22 will also tell you how a simple and safe natural hormone, found at your local health food store, may reduce your risk for uterine cancers, breast cancers, fibroids, endometriosis and may even help cure problems with cystic breasts, migraines, irregular periods and infertility!

## III. Nutrients That Help Prevent & Treat Breast Cancer

### AHCC—Mushroom Combo Enhances Immunity

AHCC (*Active hexose correlated compound)* is actually a complex compound composed of the mycelia of many mushrooms. In human testing, it was found (when given to patients in doses of *3g/day orally for 2-6 months)* to significantly increase the body's natural immunity, killing abnormal cells (206). This compound is found at many natural health food stores and online supplement providers (e.g., *www.discount-vitamins-herbs.net).*

### CoQ10 for Breast Cancer

CoQ10, though not a vitamin, has often been referred to as a vitamin because it is so essential to every cell in our body. All cells have some amounts of CoQ10, but unfortunately, as we grow older, our bodies manufacture less and less of this nutrient. How healthy you are can often be determined by how much CoQ10 is in your body. CoQ10 is such an important nutrient, it has even been used to cure breast cancers that have metastasized.

Stephen T. Sinatra, M.D., tells in his informative book, *The Coenzyme Q10 Phenomenon,* how anti-oxidant CoQ10 affects breast cancer so dramatically, that *390 mg per day* produced total *remission* in several women having late stage disease (564). For prevention purposes, a starting dose is usually recommended at 30 mg per day, then gradually working up to higher doses over a period of time, depending on what your health care practitioner has determined. I do recommend that you see a naturopathic or alternative health physician about going on CoQ10, because many conventional doctors have no idea what this nutrient is, nor how important it is in fighting cancer.

One major factor present in nearly all cancer patients (discovered by the late Dr. Karl Folkers) has been a profound deficiency in CoQ10 (as well as B6). He discovered that the lowest levels of CoQ10 were found in those having cancer of the breast (564).

Dr. Folkers tested CoQ10 in Denmark on two women with breast cancer. He gave one of them "300 mg daily and the other 360 mg daily." They *both recovered.* He suggested *500 mg of CoQ10 daily* for any cancer patient fighting a malignancy (435). Dr. Folkers treated two other breast cancer patients with CoQ10, both of whom were also suffering from congestive heart failure brought on by their cancer, as well as four others who had lung cancer. All six of them went into remission (435)!

When my mother-in-law was in the hospital fighting heart failure, I asked her cardiologist to place her on daily CoQ10. He had no idea what it was. He said it was not on the hospital formulary and he had no intention of giving it to his patients!

## CoQ10 with Selenium for Breast Cancer

For optimum health, CoQ10 should be taken in conjunction with selenium, because animal testing has shown that being deficient in selenium reduces liver levels of this nutrient, as well as cardiac levels (507). Selenium can be found in many food sources, such as fresh leafy greens, *garlic…egg yolks* and *Brazil nuts* (507); however, if the soil that produced them is selenium-poor, there is no guarantee you will profit from eating them. Most adults find it difficult, if not impossible, to get an adequate amount of CoQ10 daily without supplementing.

Current research conducted by the Leonard M. Miller School of Medicine in Miami, under Nevain, et al, revealed that CoQ10 has the ability to kill cancer cells without damage to healthy cells. Take CoQ10 with selenium and alpha lipoid acid. The NCI (National Cancer Institute) acknowledged in 2005 that CoQ10 can extend the lives of those with breast cancer and other cancers. CoQ10 is used at the Issels Treatment Centers. You can reach Issels at: #888-447-7357 (290).

## • Selenium & Iodine Deficiencies Linked To Breast Cancer

Besides the work of super anti-oxidants in preventing and curing cancers, such as breast cancer, the fact that our soils have been leached of minerals is the focus of much concern in cancer prevention. Maureen Kennedy Salaman warns in her excellent book, *Nutrition: The Cancer Answer II,* of the disastrous consequences we face as a nation due to the lack of essential minerals in our soils. Many of our soils are leached of vital cancer-preventing nutrients, such as iodine and selenium, both important breast cancer preventatives. Ms. Salaman has an excellent line of health products, including a super, easily-absorbable mineral drink, *Mineral Rich*®, that I recommend to others and use myself. You can find it, along with many other nutritional products, at her website, *www.mksalaman.com.* Her health products are also available at many health food stores. Also, see Dr. Mark Sircus' book on *Iodine Bringing Back the Universal Medicine* at website *http://www.winningcancer.com,* and information on a gentle, superior form of oral iodine called *Magnascent* or *Nascent* iodine (566a), and see chapter 34 of this book for more details.

Human studies have shown that insufficient levels of selenium in the diet can lead to type II diabetes, as well as gestational diabetes. A recent study involving men who took selenium for cancer prevention, stated that those men who took selenium only (as opposed to those who took it with vitamin E) had a higher incidence of diabetes. It is apparent from looking at both studies, that we need all the nutrients and vitamins as given by our Creator, not just isolated supplements working alone.

## • Selenium Fights the BRCA-1 Gene (Genetic Mutation that Increases Breast Cancer Risk)

In a human study, described by *Cancer Epidemiology, Biomarkers & Prevention,* researchers studied subjects who were identified as having the BRCA-1 gene, which dramatically increases the risk for ovarian and breast cancer in women (as well as breast cancer and prostate cancer in men). They discovered that the chromosome damage in those who carry this gene could be normalized by giving them selenium supplements by mouth (451). Though the study was conducted over a small span of time (just 90 days), this is indeed encouraging news for those who carry this gene, as well as confirmation that nutrition can play an important role in cancer prevention, even where there is a genetic tendency! For specific details on this human study, see website: *http://cebp.aacrjournals.org/cgi/cont ent/full/14/5/1302.*

## • Selenium, Keshan's Disease, & HIV

Dr. Ralph Moss, author of *Anti-oxidants Against Cancer,* says that selenium is so important that Chinese scientists are using it to heal a virus known as *Keshan's disease. Vitamin E* helps as well (507). Too much selenium, however, can be toxic. Though the FDA recommends 40-55 micrograms per day for adults and adolescents, much higher levels than those have been used in some cancer patients. It is difficult to overdose on selenium through dietary measures (eating certain foods). Overdosing usually occurs from taking too much in supplement form. This mineral has also been helpful with HIV patients.

## D.I.M., Broccoli & Breast Cancer

As described at website *www.cancertutor.com*, cruciferous foods (e.g., cabbage, brussel sprouts and broccoli), contain substances known as *indoles* that the digestive acids convert into *DIM, I3C*, or *diindolymethane* (96). They also contain sulforaphane (SFN) substances. Indoles have been considered one of the most advanced anti-cancer agents discovered. Found in all the cruciferous vegetables, it has the capacity to act like a chelating agent in eliminating harmful estrogens from the body. This is critical, because most women have excessive amounts of estrogen in the body, resulting in a deficiency of **natural** progesterone, increasing their risk for breast cancer and other cancers.

Other cancer-fighting ingredients in these vegetables are known as *isothiocyanates,* found in greater concentrations in broccoli sprouts and broccoli itself, important in fighting breast cancer (299b). SFN in these isothiocyanates, is now known to work at the cellular level much like *Taxol and Vincristine* (299b).

## Folate Deficiency - More Risky for Cancer Than Having BRCA-1 & BRCA-2 Mutation

New research published by Oxford University Press indicates that those who have abnormally low blood levels of folic acid may be at higher risk for genetic damage than people who have the BRCA-1 and BRCA-2 mutation (343), which increases the risk for ovarian and breast cancer in women and prostate and breast cancers in men. The BRCA-2 mutation can cause an especially lethal form of prostate cancer. What does all this mean? Not having enough folic acid in your body can put you at a greater risk for cancer than inheriting faulty genes! This is how important nutrition is in the diet (343).

## Grape Seed Extract

See chapter three for more information on the ingredient in grapes *(resveratrol)* that has a history of curative properties for many types of cancer. Grape seeds should be consumed with the grapes, rather than discarded. If you are fighting cancer, your nutritional arsenal for healing your immune system should include grape seed extract, CoQ10, resveratrol, Flor-Essence®, *liposome-encapsulated vitamin C* (see page 544), and green tea, as well as other supplements described in this book. (Do not take grape seed extract at the same time that you take Vitamin C; research suggests that taking them at the same time may raise blood pressure in some individuals.) Resveratrol is also being touted as a way to fight obesity, since it keeps the body from storing fat.

For an excellent 58-page study that was done on resveratrol's role in fighting cancer, including breast cancer, see website: *http://www.agrawal.org/PDF/ACR-Resveratrol1.pdf.* The study was conducted by M.D. Anderson Cancer Center and the UCLA Center for Human Nutrition (346).

## IP6 (Inositol Hexaphosphate) for Breast Cancer

Cancer cells use a lot of iron and must have iron to survive; however, drugs that remove iron from the body, thus fighting cancer cells, have adverse side effects. A natural substance, known as IP6, effectively robs cancer cells of iron without depleting the body's natural stores of iron. It is a safe ingredient, without the high toxicity of chemo drugs, and it is relatively inexpensive. Human trials have yet to be done on IP6 (554). This nutrient, derived from rice bran, is discussed later in this book.

## Jamun Berry for Breast Cancer

This powerful little purple berry (aka the *Jambolana* berry), was able to fight a type of breast cancer that has a high *recurrence* rate, triple negative breast cancer (573a). It is referred to as *triple negative,* according to researchers Caroline Killian and *URI professor* Navindra Seeram, because identifying and treating some types of breast cancer "require the presence or absence of three key indicators or receptors," however, in *triple negative* breast cancer, these *indicators* can't be found. Killian says that "though these berries have been used in the past as a pre-insulin treatment for diabetes," no one had previously tested them for cancer (573a). The berries have been found, thus far in laboratory testing, to fight "most types of breast cancer, including" the "triple negative" (573a). Will the jamun berry soon become as popular as the acai berry? Time will tell.

## LifeMel Honey for Cancer Patients

This amazing honey is also discussed in chapter 29 of this book. It is a special honey that is used from the nectar taken from 40 herbs, including *Echinacea, Siberian ginseng,* and *Uncaria tomentosa* (with some other natural ingredients), and was developed in Israel. Two teaspoons per day (one in the morning and one in the evening) are recommended (614). This special honey has been shown (in **human testing**) to help in the prevention of neutropenia (severe drop in white blood cells) caused by chemotherapy and to lower the risk of severe platelet drop (thrombocytopenia), often found in chemo patients (614). You can find out more about this amazing honey at website *http://www.lifemelisrael.com* (614).

## Magnesium Important (Can Help Prevent Cerebral Palsy in Premies)—But Too Much Calcium Increases Cancer Risk

Studies involving more than 47,000 men showed that a high daily calcium intake (*1500 and 1,999 mg of calcium per day*) could double the chance for advanced cancer of the prostate. Using 2000 mg or more quadrupled the risk (as compared to men ingesting *less than 500 mg* daily), and another study involving over 20,000 men, revealed that those who ingested greater amounts of *dairy products* in their diet increased their risk for this type cancer by *32%* (566).

Many people, women especially, are aggressively encouraged to take calcium for their bones as they age, but some health care professionals do not emphasize the importance of magnesium, without which the cells cannot use calcium efficiently. Many of the most important nutrients in our cells must have magnesium to perform their anti-oxidant properties (566). Studies with animals prove that keeping them magnesium-deficient raises free radical activity and will result in malignant cancers (566). Not only that, but recent studies have shown that moms who are at a greater risk for having premies, can help prevent cerebral palsy in their child by having sufficient amounts of magnesium sulfate. See the full article at *http://www.washingtonpost.com/wp-dyn/content/article/2008/08/27/AR20080882702634.html* (385a). Besides magnesium, your calcium supplements should also contain boron, and some include zinc.

Women are warned against drinking alcohol due to the increased risk for breast cancer; however, alcohol consumption uses up magnesium in the body, so is it possible that the magnesium deficiency thus created is the real culprit in causing the cancer (566)? Stressors in the body (e.g., giving a person chemo and/or radiation) also decrease magnesium levels (566). Why is it that, according to Mark Sircus Ac., OMD, a whopping *78%* of children diagnosed with leukemia have a past record of *anorexia*, and these same children are also very deficient in magnesium (566)?

Human studies have even shown that high magnesium amounts in the body can help prevent stomach cancer (566). Many chronic illnesses are attributable to magnesium deficiencies, including migraine headaches.

To find out more, including information on a way of delivering magnesium chloride directly into the skin, see website: *http://www. ancient-minerals.com* (566b). Epsom salts, that some people use in their bath water, contain magnesium, but it is inferior to magnesium chloride.

## Modified Citrus Pectin

Research described in the *Journal of the National Cancer Institute* revealed that giving citrus fiber (pectin) to animals slashed the size and metastasis of breast tumors, as well as cancers of the colon (383).

## MonaVie™

MonaVie™ is a high anti-oxidant health drink made with the acai Amazon berry plus 18 other fruits including pomegranate, passion fruit, bilberry, wolfberry, blueberry, kiwi, banana, cranberry, apricot, prune, acerola, dark and white pigment grapes and others, in a proprietary blend. It was developed by Dr. Ralph Carson, and many people are lauding its healthy contents and claiming its benefits. (Note that bilberry thins the blood. Use bilberry supplements with caution, especially if you are already on blood thinners.)

Realize that some nutritional drinks are pasteurized, which can decrease heat-sensitive nutrients, such as vitamin C, while others are considered *flash-pasteurized*, which is not as harmful to the enzymes and nutrients within, but they also have a short shelf-life.

## Nutrients & Breast Health

This chapter does not have an all-inclusive list of nutrients needed for breast cancer prevention or treatment. There are many minerals and vitamins needed for optimum health and recovery. If you are juicing every day, eating a nutritious diet, and taking vitamin-mineral supplements, you will obtain the many important vitamins, minerals and enzymes needed for optimal health. I do recommend if you are taking supplements, whenever possible, choose organic whole food supplements. A good example would be Dee Simmons' ***Green Miracle*** powdered drink (available at her website: *http://www.ultimateliving.com/Dee Simmons.asp)* and other drinks, such as *Kamut®*, *Green Magma®* and *Just Barley®* powdered green drinks.

There are many other nutrient-dense drink mixes on the market. See later information on an amazing nutrient called *Poly-MVA* that many cancer survivors are crediting with curing their *terminal* cancers. For testimonials of cancer patients using Poly-MVA to cure their cancers, see *http://www.polymvasurvivors.com/testimonials.html.* Many of these testimonials are given ten or more years ago and all survivors are still here as of March 2007. There is even a testimonial for anaplastic carcinoma. (Also see: *cancercompass.com/messageboard/message/all,15401,0.htm.)*

## Orange Juice & Quercetin Fight Breast Cancer

According to a study reported at the National Library of Medicine's PubMed website, from the University of Western Ontario, laboratory testing reveals that orange juice, especially when it is combined with the nutrient, *quercetin*, can halt the growth of breast cancer cells (568b). Quercetin can be found in many foods, such as black and green tea, onions, apples (378), cayenne, beans (551), and leafy green vegetables. Other sources of quercetin are olive oil, grapes and berries (568b).

## Vitamin D Prevents All Forms of Cancer

Recent studies have shown that insufficient amounts of natural sunshine (resulting in vitamin D deficiency) increases the risk for nearly all types of cancer, including cancer of the breast, and may even promote other chronic illnesses, such as MS, *Type I diabetes* (311), and lupus. Nutritional experts are now concluding that most people need *1,000 to 2,000 IU* per *day* of vitamin D for maintaining health and preventing disease. This is a much higher amount than the RDA of *200 to 600 IU* (311). Adequate amounts of this vitamin are crucial for preventing colon, breast and gastric cancers. The best natural source is sunshine. A nutritious diet and *supplements* can also help keep vitamin D levels normal (311). A research study that spanned eight years and involved more than 3000 people, showed that those people having the lowest vitamin D levels were twice as likely to die from all causes. They concluded that insufficient levels of vitamin D greatly increases the risk for early death (575). Most people need ten to twenty minutes a day of natural sunshine (without sunscreen) for vitamin D synthesis. Recent studies also show that increased levels of vitamin D can help prevent heart attacks.

Darker-skinned individuals usually need more sun exposure to get sufficient vitamin D (484). Always check with your doctor, especially if you have a history (or family history) of skin cancer. Human studies have shown that the majority of Type I diabetics have deficient levels of vitamin D.

## Vitamins Important for Breast Cancer Prevention & Treatment

Vitamins A, C, D and E are important in the prevention and treatment of breast cancer. Studies have shown that deficiencies in these vitamins can contribute toward not only breast cancer, but many other types of cancer, including colon cancers. Mega-dosing with vitamin C has been used to treat some cancers, including breast cancer and pancreatic cancer. This is also known as *Orthomolecular Medicine* and requires intravenous dosing in high amounts, from 80-120 grams or more per day. When given intravenously, sodium ascorbate is commonly used. When taken by mouth, it is usually taken in the form of ascorbic acid.

Huge vitamin C doses usually cannot be tolerated by mouth because they cause diarrhea (ascorbic acid) (430). When given intravenously in the form of sodium ascorbate (see below article), there is normally excellent tolerance. The human body can tolerate vitamin C (ascorbic acid) by mouth in large enough doses until diarrhea occurs. Once diarrhea occurs, this tells you your *tolerance level* (430). For example, if you take 3500 mg of vitamin C and have no problems with it, then take 4000 mg of vitamin C four hours later and it gives you diarrhea, your tolerance would be below 4000 mg. Your body is tolerating less than 4000 mg doses and will not tolerate doses higher than that. If you have stomach irritation from vitamin C, take it with food and in divided doses, or use the non-acidic *Ester-C®* (calcium ascorbate), or the sodium ascorbate non-acidic form, rather than the ascorbic acid form of vitamin C.

## Vitamin C - Megadosing Intravenously to Destroy Breast Tumor & Lung Cancer

When 59 year-old Arlindo O. was told that his advanced lung cancer had gone into his brain, physicians sent him home to die (149a), yet today he is *cancer-free* (149a), and he credits his survival to vitamin C. Recent studies *from the National Institutes of Health* showed that vitamin C given *intravenously* could halt the growth of "aggressive brain, ovarian and pancreatic tumors…" in mice (149a). The treatment is non-toxic to healthy cells, with none of the adverse, damaging side effects associated with standard *chemotherapy and radiation.* According to Dr. Scott Greenberg, who treated Arlindo with high intravenous doses of vitamin C, "it is a valuable option for those who don't respond to other treatments," and "can be used along with traditional chemo and radiation" (149a). He said that the vitamin C creates "hydrogen peroxide," which kills the cancer cells much "like chemotherapy does" (149a), except that vitamin C is non-toxic to healthy cells. He even talked about a woman he treated with massive intravenous vitamin C, who had "a large breast mass protruding out of her chest" (149a). Within just "a few months of treatment," the mass disappeared. It has been five years and she has had no further "sign of cancer whatsoever," says Dr. Greenberg (149a). (See page 544 of this book for exciting news about a new oral form of vitamin C that is said to be clinically more effective than intravenous C. It is called *liposome-encapsulated vitamin C.)*

## IV. Other Breast Cancer Helps

### Abajeru (*Chrysobalanus icaco*) for Breast Cancer & Other Cancers

Isolated from a tropical plant of the Brazilian Rain Forest (aka as *coco-plum*), abajeru was once used by the locals for fighting arthritic pain and diabetes (145a). When researchers first conducted lab testing, they found that the extract killed not only pancreatic, brain, and breast cancers, but those of the *lung-bowel- [and] larynx* as well, including some difficult-to-treat leukemia cells. In testing humans, they were surprised to see that the substance was effective in *90% of the cases* (145a).

### Algae & Breast Cancer

There are many different algae important in breast cancer prevention and treatment. These include kelp, chlorella, dunaliella and spirulina, all available in supplement form. A blue-green alga known as ***Aphanizomenon flos-aquae*** (**AFA**), harvested from Klamath Lake in Klamath Falls, Oregon, is also very rich in chlorophyll, beta-carotene and many other vitamins and minerals. (It is best to take algae supplements on an empty stomach.)

## Avemar *(MSC)* for Fighting Breast Cancer

Avemar is an extract taken from fermented wheat germ, which has undergone many **human** studies and shown to be most effective at fighting breast cancer when combined with the drug, *Aromasin*. Lab studies revealed that even Tamoxifen, a widely used cancer drug, worked better when combined with Avemar. Avemar, which is given by mouth, has been approved for use in Hungary. All studies thus far have shown Avemar to be safe and non-toxic. You may also hear it referred to as *fermented wheat germ extract* or *MSC* (318).

## Black Cohosh May Spell Death for Breast Cancer Cells

Also referred to as *Cimicifuga* species, this herb may be very important in breast cancer prevention and treatment. Researchers concluded that compounds from black cohosh could help in preventing and treating cancer (379). The in vitro study was publicized in *Phytomedicine* (379); however, be aware that new reports are surfacing that this herb could cause liver problems in some people. Always check with your physician.

## CyberKnife® & NanoKnife™ Therapy for Tumors

See chapter 34 in this book for details on CyberKnife® therapy, which is being used successfully for many cancers. It is a gentle, painless procedure that does not require an incision, surgery, sedation or inpatient stay. It takes very little time, and as soon as the procedure is over, the patient is able to walk out and return home. It does involve some radiation (89a) and can cause damage to nearby healthy tissue. Also, see information on the non-toxic NanoKnife™ in chapter 34.

## Ginseng & Breast Cancer Testing

Ginseng has been used to fight breast cancer and prostate cancer cells in animal testing. Ginseng should always be used with the advice of a health care practitioner. Some people using ginseng have blood pressure elevations, especially with the *Panax* ginseng type (494).

## Graviola Supplement & Breast Cancer Cures

See chapter six in this book for information on the herb, *graviola,* and its preventative and curative properties.

## Non-Toxic Immunotherapy - Global First of a Kind Miracle Cure for Acute Myeloid Leukemia

See chapter 34 under this title for a new immunotherapy treatment, where a woman was put into total remission from *acute myeloid leukemia* by *natural killer cells* taken from her own daughter. Her cells were treated, then injected into her mom (568a). It is hoped that this treatment (a first in the world - in London) is on its way to America and other countries), and that it will be just as successful against other cancers, such as breast and ovarian cancer (568a).

## Lapatinib – New, Safer Drug for Those With HER-2 Protein

A new drug that is being tested for women with breast cancer having the *Her-2 protein* (who adherents say have not responded to conventional treatment), may benefit from Lapatinib, which is claimed to be *safe* with *minimal side effects* (e.g., *rash…fatigue…diarrhea*), (168) and rarely some severe side effects could occur that are heart-related. (It is also know as *Tykerb*® and is discussed below in this chapter.)

## New Breast Cancer Treatment Destroys Cancer Cells Without Toxins

A new breast cancer treatment that is said to be *non-toxic* has been developed and used successfully (in animal testing) by researchers at the University of Missouri (209). Human testing is planned. The treatment uses a *molecular drug*, known as *PRIMA-1,* that fights cancerous cells with an *antibody* (known as *2aG4*), which also starves the cancer by cutting off its blood supply. Alone, they are ineffective; however, once combined, they work—and reportedly—with few *side effects* (209).

## Olive Oil Reduces Breast Cancer Risk 46%

Laboratory studies have revealed that ingesting a lot of olive oil (such as found in the *Mediterranean Diet)* could possibly slash a woman's chances of breast cancer by as much as 46%. Apparently, the oleic acid in the oil has a protective genetic benefit similar to that experienced by women who are given the drug *Herceptin*, which fights effects of the *Her-2/neu* cancer gene. The same protective benefit is also found in *evening primrose oil* (595). In choosing olive oil, always use organic. Note that it was extra virgin olive oil that proved beneficial in recent studies for fighting breast cancer, with its ability at suppressing the HER2 gene.

## PARP Inhibitors – New, Safer Drug for Women with BRCA1 - BRCA2 Mutations

A new drug undergoing clinical trials in "Europe, the United States and Australia by…pharmaceutical giant, AstroZeneca, involved women who were at death's door with end-stage cancer" (348a). Most had failed standard treatments of "surgery, chemotherapy and radiotherapy," as noted by William Birnbauer in an article at *theage.com.au* website 08/17/2008 (348a). The drug, known as a *PARP inhibitor,* was able to "reduce tumour sizes in 46% of the cases, and 59% of the" women experienced "tumour shrinkage or stabilization" (348a). Though the "international trials involved just 63 people with advanced breast cancer" and 63 "with advanced ovarian cancer," results are encouraging and trials are continuing. This drug "mainly targets cancer cells," so the usual side effects seen by standard chemo (e.g., "hair loss and nausea") don't occur because chemo attacks both cancer cells and healthy cells (348a).

## Tykerb® for Women with HER-2 Gene with Advanced Breast Cancer

Though Tykerb® is a drug and not what I consider a *gentle, natural, or non-toxic* treatment, it is being mentioned here because developers, GlaxoSmithKline, claim that the drug has few side effects ("mild skin rashes and diarrhea"), and half the women in the clinical trials, done by Israeli researchers, experienced tumor shrinkage (168). In spite of the positive report for this drug, note that according to the article, Tykerb® is given together with a chemo drug known as Xeloda (168), which has many of the same adverse side effects (some potentially severe) as with other chemo drugs. Most physicians leave it up to their patients to weigh the risks, but they usually do not give them much information on natural, non-toxic cancer therapies, along with their conventional suggestions. Tykerb® is also know as *Lapatinib* (discussed earlier in this chapter).

## V. Fruits That Can Save Your Life

### Berries - Little Fruits, BIG Lifesavers

Researchers have discovered that compounds taken from fruits inhibited not only cancer of the cervix, but two types of breast cancer. The fruits tested were blueberries and strawberries. Animal testing has also shown cranberries important in breast cancer prevention. (Cranberries also help prevent ulcers and bladder infections, and they fight leukemia (22.)

### Cherries Fight Cancer

An ingredient in cherries has been found, in animal testing, to inhibit several types of cancer. The compound is considered even more potent than limonene against cancer. Always try to get organic cherries if possible. Conventionally-grown cherries are often heavily-sprayed with pesticides and herbicides. (Cherries, especially sour cherries, have long been used to relieve the symptoms of gout.)

Cherries and other fruits also contain cleansing agents that act like chelators or tiny little brooms or strainers to remove harmful toxins, including heavy metals from the blood and organs of the human body (552). Other foods that do this are vegetable juices and sulfur-containing foods, such as cabbage, eggs, garlic, peppers, broccoli, brussel sprouts and onions (552). The Budwig diet (mentioned in several chapters of this book) also contains sulfur. Cilantro works much the same way in removing toxins from the blood. It can also help kill salmonella.

### Concord Grapes Inhibit Breast Cancer

Animal testing has shown a dramatic decrease in breast tumors in animals fed purple grape juice and concord grapes (129). Yet another study that supports Johanna Brandt's use of grape juice in curing cancer (see chapter three).

## Ellagic Acid & Other Compounds that Fight Breast Cancer

Grapes, berries, and other fruits (and some nuts) contain amazing substances that cleanse the body of toxins and prevent cancer. These include pomegranates as well as raspberries, cranberries, pecans, walnuts, cherries, and tangerines. All vegetables and fruits should be washed thoroughly before consumption, because many are sprayed with pesticides and insecticides and may also contain parasites. Even organic produce should be washed thoroughly.

## Limonene Destroys Breast Cancer Cells

There is an ingredient known as *limonene*, which is found in citrus fruits (as well as the skin of oranges, limes, and grapefruits), that can block the formation of breast and lung cancers (604). Limonene is also available as a supplement at natural health food stores. You should know that before you start grating raw citrus peelings for this nutrient, take caution. Raw fruit peelings, such as lemons, limes and grapefruits are fine in small amounts, but they do have chemicals that can be toxic if ingested in excessively large quantities. (I can't imagine anyone wanting to eat a lot of lemon or lime peel!) One of the best ways to take advantage of citrus peelings is to steep them in hot tea. Juicing enthusiasts often juice entire lemons and limes along with the peel.

Note that some juicer manufacturers brag about the ability of their machines to juice an entire apple or pear without slicing, however, there is one very BIG problem with this. An apple, for example, can look beautiful on the outside and have an ugly decayed spot in the middle that you would never see unless you, at least, cut it in half. If you juice the entire fruit, you are juicing the decayed area along with the rest of the fruit, and you could end up with worms in your juice!

## Mangosteen Fruit for Breast Cancer

The fruit of this plant (when tested in lab experiments on breast cancer), had the ability to cause the abnormal cells to self-destruct, making it a candidate for breast cancer prevention (185). Mangosteen is not the same thing as mango.

## Papaya for Breast Cancer

Papaya, according to Harald Tietze, author of *Papaya The Healing Fruit*, can help in the prevention of breast cancers. It works like a chelating agent in ridding tissues and cells of poisonous substances, and is widely valued and used in the tropics for disease prevention and healing (581). See chapter 20 of this book for more detailed information on papaya and cancer. Also, note that papaya enzymes can thin the blood.

## Resveratrol - How Grapes May Save Your Life

Refer to chapter three for information on this amazing ingredient in grapes that has shown the ability to not only suppress the growth of cancer cells, but in many cases, even destroy them once they have already developed. Resveratrol is also being touted as a way to fight obesity, since it keeps the body from storing fat.

Studies have recently unraveled how resveratrol works at fighting cancer (252) (255). Apparently, the resveratrol in red wine and grape skin blocks the effects of a very important protein that cancer cells can't live without known as *nuclear factor - kappa B (NF-kB)*; however, it only takes a small amount of wine (about 8 ounces a few times a week). Use too much and the risk for cancer increases (252) (255). Better yet, use the grape skins in their original package as prepared by our Creator.

As described by *http://www.mnwelldir.org/nw_current.htm*, this powerful anti-oxidant (in lab studies) fights the type of aberrant cell that morphs into breast cancer (255a). Is it possible that this amazing substance from our Creator is, as *some call it the Fountain of Youth* (255a)?

**More Miracles from Grapes**: Researchers at Madrid University took an extract of red grapes made, not from the juice, but its *by products*—the *skins and seeds*—(which many people discard) and made a *cocktail* from it that they referred to as *GADF* (*Grape Antioxidant Dietary Fibre*) (91a). "Tests on human volunteers found the extract was extremely rich in both fibre and antioxidants which reduce the risks of cardiovascular disease - the world's biggest killer" (91a). Red grapes help fight high cholesterol and high blood pressure.

## Vitamin D Prevents Breast Cancer

Multiple **human studies** have proven that a lack of vitamin D will raise the risk for nearly all types of cancer, including breast cancer. The best source of vitamin D is natural sunlight, about 20-30 minutes a day with no sunscreen on, or—at the very least—two or three times per week. Those who have a tendency toward skin cancer (hereditary or otherwise) will need to check with their physician about sun exposure. Natural sunlight boosts the body's immunity, reduces blood pressure, and has a relaxing effect on the body. Those living in colder, northern climates are most likely to be deficient in this essential vitamin, and darker-skinned people need more time in the sun to generate vitamin D in their skin (484). The only vegetables that contain natural vitamin D are mushrooms. Recent **human** studies show that women getting adequate daily amounts of vitamin D can cut their risk for breast cancer in half.

## VI. Soy Products & Breast Cancer

There is a lot of information circulating regarding impurities in soy, and studies showing that soy can harm the thyroid. I would recommend fermented soy only. Avoid GMO (genetically-modified) soy products. Weak phyto-estrogens, such as those found in fermented soy products, like Haelan, may help remove harmful estrogens from the body in estrogen-positive cancers.

For information on Haelan, see the company's website at *www.haelan 951.com*. The information on Haelan's Research Foundation website was accumulated from clinical studies performed on fermented soy beverages manufactured by Haelan Products, Inc. of Woodinville, Washington. The Haelan fermented soy beverages are sold in the United States, without medical claims, and are available directly from the company or one of their distributors (143).

## VII. Other Life Saving Nutrients & Vegetables

### Anti-Cancer Nutrients in the Cabbage Family

Cruciferous vegetables, mentioned earlier (e.g., broccoli, cauliflower, cabbage and brussel sprouts), are receiving a great deal of publicity in the world of nutrition for their cancer-fighting properties. These vegetables contain *sulforaphane,* which apparently helps by assisting the body to flush free radicals from the system before they can cause damage (604). See the information earlier in this chapter on D.I.M. IC3, also discussed earlier, can cause the excretion of toxic estrogens from the body, thus protecting against hormone-sensitive cancers of the breast and prostate.

Pound-for-pound, cauliflower contains more vitamin C than tangerines or white grapefruits, but it is best to eat it raw, as cooking destroys much of the vitamin C and indole content. The high sulfur content in many of these foods inhibits cancer cells (604). A *synthetic* substance recently isolated from broccoli, known as *oxomate*, fights breast cancer much like another popular natural ingredient from broccoli (and other *cruciferous* foods) known as *sulforaphane* (208). These two substances work to neutralize carcinogens. Animals receiving the oxomate experienced half as many cancerous breast tumors as their counterparts (208).

## Beta-Glucan - The Yeast & Shiitake Mushroom Extract that Fights Breast Cancer

Beta-glucan is a substance found in yeast and mushrooms. When a human study was done (from 1975) on several people with cancer, injection of the substance into the growths caused the tumors to shrink in less than a week (354). This happened in every patient without exception; however, it did not catch the attention of mainstream medicine (354). According to C. Borek, Ph.D, a beta-glucan (known as *lentinan*) from *shiitake*, is widely used in Japan for human cancer treatment (354). *Lentinan* injections given intravenously have been able to increase the lifespan of patients receiving them (354).

## Bromelain (From Pineapple) Helps Fight Breast Cancer

See chapter 34 of this book for information on the importance of bromelain, a substance found in pineapple, for fighting breast cancer.

## Curcumin (Turmeric) Fights Breast Cancer

This common table spice was shown, in animal testing, to have the ability to restrict many types of cancer, including breast cancer. You will find more curcumin in turmeric than you will in curry powder. Use organic turmeric rather than curry. If you want a turmeric capsule that is free of magnesium stearate additive, see *Nature's Way*® brand. Also, see chapter 20 for instances when you should never use curcumin (turmeric). Yellow mustard is very high in turmeric. If you want your body to absorb turmeric more easily, eat it with pineapple and/or an oil source.

## Lutein & Lycopene for Breast Health

Lutein helps in cancer prevention. Good sources of lutein are dark green leafy vegetables such as spinach, collards and turnip greens, as well as egg yolks, but if using eggs, be sure they are organic. Avocados are also very high in lutein. Look for lycopene in red vegetables and berries. Lycopene and lutein can be found in supplement form in most health food stores, however, getting them from natural, organic food sources is always best, when possible. (Lutein is also a critical nutrient for maintaining eye health.)

## Mushroom Cures Breast Cancer

*The Maitake Mushroom AND D-Fraction,* a book by Shari Lieberman, Ph.D., and Ken Babal, C.N., documents the story of a woman who was cured of breast cancer taking maitake D-fraction. The patient opted for breast removal in 1992, then she received chemo over a period of two years (469); however, in spite of the surgery and the chemo, her **cancer returned** two months after finishing up the chemo. She opted out of another surgery and took approximately 100 drops of the maitake D-fraction per day. She also ingested daily doses of maitake tablets *(5 grams)* for a period of six months, after which she reduced her intake to *50 mg* daily. In 1995 she was told by her doctor that her cancer was in remission (469). You can find maitake supplements (including the maitake D-Fraction) at natural health food stores. This supplement is not recommended for people suffering with MS (184). Maitake mushroom (*grifola frondosa*) is also known as the *Hen-of-the-Woods*, and goes by several other names.

## Pomegranate for Breast Health

Pomegranate is the newest superstar among the anti-oxidants. A fruit that you rarely saw in stores ten years ago is appearing everywhere and for good reason. This biblical fruit is packed with nutrients and anti-oxidants that fight free radicals in the body (376). It is now being touted as a deterrent for all types of cancer, including prostate and breast cancer (376). Just 8 ounces a day is all that you may need to keep your immune system healthy (376). The seeds and juice from the seeds also promote heart health by fighting arterial plaque, lowering cholesterol, and preventing the type of inflammation in the colon that can lead to cancer (376). You can also find pomegranate juice and supplements in health food stores. Laboratory testing revealed that extracts from pomegranate (in combination with genistein) could kill breast cancer cells (18). Genistein is one of the main substances found in soy. It is available as a supplement. I would take the genistein as a supplement, rather than ingesting soy. I no longer recommend soy, unless fermented.

## Shiitake Mushroom & Karawatake

The shiitake mushroom, also called the *black forest mushroom,* has demonstrated anti-cancer properties in human research.

A powerful extract taken from this mushroom, often given by injection and mentioned earlier, is *lentinan* (354). The karawatake mushroom (also called *Coriolus versicolor* and the *turkey tail* mushroom) has shown anti-cancerous, anti-bacterial, and anti-viral properties.

In a human study involving hundreds of Korean postmenopausal women, researchers found that eating mushrooms could cut their incidence for having breast cancer (434). It is noteworthy that mushrooms help fight breast cancer by lowering the body's estrogen levels (301). Use fresh or dried mushrooms (reconstituted). Mushrooms are the only vegetables that contain natural vitamin D.

## Soy (Fermented) for Breast Cancer

According to an article by Donna Sage, M.S.S.A., at website *http://www.buyhaelan.com*, Haelan is a soy drink that has been fermented (541). Other types of fermented soy are soy sauces, natto, miso, tempeh and fermented tofu. Some cancer patients are using Haelen to help boost their body's immunity in fighting the disease.

The Chinese originally produced the drink for nutrition purposes over two decades ago. It has high amounts of isoflavones known as *diadzein* and *genistein* (541). You can purchase Haelan at this same website (above). Fermented soy contains many important vitamins and minerals. (Note that genistein can also lower blood pressure.) Many case studies are available of people who say that they have used Haelan to cure their cancers.

Nina P. of Russia was diagnosed with cancer of the breast that had spread to several bones and muscles in 1996. She refused surgery and was considered terminal. Nina implemented several dietary changes, began drinking Haelan (one bottle daily) and began a moderate exercise program involving daily walks (541). She had already outlived her six month life expectancy, so of course her Oncologist was quite shocked when she walked into their office in March of 1997 and no trace of cancer could be found, all her diagnostic tests returning completely normal! She used a maintenance dose of four tablespoons of Haelen per day. Her son, Alexander, used Haelan (two tablespoons daily) and reported excellent results reducing his Parkinson's tremors (541). A report from 2000 noted that Nina was still cancer-free at age 82 (541). (In April 2005, Donna Sage informed me that Nina passed away, but not from cancer, from old age.)

Another case history described by Ms. Sage is that of Patti Soccoman who was diagnosed with breast cancer. This case is described at *http://www.buyhaelan.com* website. After a biopsy, which confirmed the malignancy, her physician recommended lumpectomy and lymphectomy or a mastectomy. Ms. Soccoman underwent the lumpectomy, however, she argued against the lymph node removal. When she told her doctor, he then insisted on breast removal. She was referred to an Oncologist of whom she said absolutely insisted that she undergo the surgery (541). She never returned to that Oncologist. In early November 1997, Ms. Soccoman started to ingest the Haelan drink, one bottle daily. During this same time, she also took vitamin C, CoQ10, flax oil, and began a mostly organic raw food (fruits and veggies) juicing program, as well as chelation therapy. Six weeks went by and diagnostics showed that the breast tumor had decreased remarkably. Subsequent mammograms revealed that the tumor was progressively shrinking in size (541). A mammogram in the summer of 1999 showed no spreading of the cancer and a drastic shrinkage of the original tumor. Her radiologist was shocked by the results. He also admitted his concerns about chemo, stating that when the FDA approves a chemo regimen, this is no indicator of the safety of the treatment. When asked if he recommends Haelan, he said that his wife, a liver and colon cancer survivor, was taking Haelan (541).

According to an update from Ms. Soccoman in 2000, at age 65, she was still cancer-free. She also stated that since starting Haelan, her cataracts had disappeared. During her illness, she drank Haelan for a period of seven months, then used a daily preventative dose of two ounces. She credits her dietary changes, renting comedy movies to boost her immune system, and her religious convictions to helping her overcome cancer (541). I last spoke to Ms. Soccoman in June of 2005 and she was doing wonderfully and still drinking the Haelan as a preventative. She never had the radical surgery her physician recommended (just a lumpectomy), no radiation and no chemo. (Note that Haelan is usually taken on an empty stomach for maximum absorption.)

For information on Haelan, also see the company's website at *www.haelan951.com*. Information on Haelan's Research Foundation website was accumulated from clinical studies performed on fermented soy beverages manufactured by Haelan Products, Inc. of Woodinville, Washington. The Haelan fermented soy beverages are sold in the United States, without medical claims, and are available directly from the company or one of their distributors (143).

## VIII. Miracle Oils for Cancer Prevention

See chapter 18 for the amazing curative properties of flax oil for cancer.

## CLA - Conjugated Linoleic Acid Prevents Cancer Spread

CLA is a fatty acid that helps prevent the formation of tumors, as well as their spread throughout other areas of the body. It also promotes the self-destruction of tumor cells (43). Particularly impressive was a report published in *Anti-cancer Research* that in vitro and animal testing showed CLA blocked not only the growth, but the spread of human breast cancer (43). From the studies done, this fatty acid worked even better when combined with beta-carotene (43). (CLA supplements can be found at most natural health food stores, and though it is promoted in weight loss supplements, I do not recommend CLA in supplement form.) It is available naturally in GRASS FED beef and dairy products. If you are going to consume beef and dairy, use only organic products whenever possible. Many people are resorting to finding farmers with healthy herds who will provide them with raw, organic milk, since they are having problems with homogenized, pasteurized milk. See chapter 26.

Note that the human body can manufacture monounsaturated and saturated fats; however, we cannot make what are known as EFAs or *essential fatty acids*, such as alpha-linolenic and linoleic acid, so they must be obtained from the diet. Most people get too much omega-6 or linoleic acid (found in processed foods and oils) and insufficient amounts of alpha-linolenic acids, which are often referred to as the *good fats*, the omega-3 fats (found in fish, flax seed oil, green leafy vegetables, walnuts and other foods). A good rule of thumb is to eat natural foods, rather than processed foods to get the good fats.

## Flax Seed Fights Breast Cancer

Flax seed is discussed in many chapters of this book for its health benefits. In a **human** study, conducted by the University of Minnesota in 2001 on postmenopausal women, this potent form of lignan reduced estrogen levels (116). See chapter 22, later in this book, about hormone replacement therapy for an explanation of why most women (especially those who are post-menopausal) have too much estrogen and how to correct this imbalance. Just realize that there are rare cases of women who cannot metabolize extra estrogen or progesterone of any kind. The best way to tell if you are estrogen or progesterone-deficient is to have your physician check your levels of both.

## Gamma-Linolenic Acid Inhibits Gene That Causes Breast Cancer

This is another type of fatty acid, and it is commonly found in black currant seed, borage oil and evening primrose oil. GLA works best when taken in combination with fish oil. This fatty acid was shown, in laboratory studies, to suppress a genetic type of cancer-causing gene (known as the *Her-2/neu)* when combined with Herceptin, a common drug given for breast cancer (121). The study showed that the Herceptin worked best when given with the GLA (121). GLA can be found at natural health food stores and online supplement stores, such as *www.discount-vitamins-herbs.net.* I am not advocating the use of Herceptin, just informing you of the GLA study and its effects. Note that some of the richest sources of omega-3 are krill oil, avocado, chia seeds, flax, Lyprinol, and salba. You can find all these products in health food stores and on the internet.

# IX. Herbs & Other Nutrients for Breast Health

## Andrographis

According to website *www.herbs2000.com,* this is not a widely known herb, but it has been used extensively for medicinal purposes, including cancer and infections (20). Recent studies show favorable outcomes with this herb against breast cancer cells. *Androtech* (produced by *BioTherapies*) combines this herb with enchinacea (20). Andrographis can contribute toward infertility. Do not use herbs without consulting your physician, especially if you are pregnant, lactating, or have a chronic illness (20). Toxicity is rare, but may include cardiac irregularities in some people.

## Aspilia

Aspilia, also known as *Wild Sunflower*, not only kills parasites, but acts much like an antibiotic. This herb has demonstrated the ability to destroy malignant cells in breast and lung tissue (27).

## Bindweed & Breast Cancer

See chapter 34 of this book for more information on an herb known as *bindweed* (and chapter 12 for its use against pancreatic cancer) that is said to have *100 times* the ability at blocking blood vessel formation in tumors as that found in shark cartilage (301a). For an amazing case study of a woman with stage IV "terminal" breast cancer that had gone into her *liver and bone,* see website: *http://organicpharmacy.org/products/VascuStatin* (301a). Always check with your physician before using, as with any herb.

## Cat's Claw

Cat's claw, also known as *Uno de Gato,* can be found growing in the forests of the Amazon. It is known for its ability to enhance the body's immunity (393). This herb is popular in Europe for treating a variety of ailments, and it is being investigated there in cancer treatment (393). As noted by Rita Elkins, author of *Cat's Claw (Uno de Gato),* one physician in particular had great success using this herb (and others) for more than a dozen types of cancer in hundreds of patients during a four-year period in the eighties.

The herb is also a source for pycnogenol®, a potent anti-oxidant (393). See chapter 20 for instances when you should not take this herb.

## Coffee May Help Reduce Breast Cancer Risk

Researchers in Sweden have discovered, in human testing involving 460 women with breast cancer, that women with a certain type of genetic marker may cut their breast cancer risk by coffee consumption; however, scientists involved in the study said that more testing is needed to verify findings before they can make any definite *recommendations* for drinking the beverage (82). Though coffee may also ward off Type II diabetes (80), excess consumption may increase the risk for rheumatoid arthritis (81) and gout. (Vitamin K also helps fight Type II diabetes by helping to increase insulin resistance.)

## D-Ribose for Energy Level

Cancer patients suffering from fatigue may benefit from d-ribose supplements. D-ribose, though a sugar substance, does not raise the body's blood sugar; however, it has been studied in humans for its effectiveness in improving the stamina and energy levels of those suffering from fibromyalgia and chronic fatigue syndrome, as well as congestive heart failure patients and those about to undergo bypass surgery. You can find d-ribose in health food stores. It is usually sold as *D-ribose* or under other supplement names, such *as CORvalen®, COR-valenM®*, or *Bioenergy RIBOSE™* (4) (35) (253).

## Dandelion for Breast Cancer

The people of China have used this herb medicinally to treat breast cancer for many centuries (93). The herb is a very concentrated source of vitamin A and beta-carotene. The greens were found, during studies in Japan, to boost the body's cancer-fighting strength (93). This is important for patients fighting cancer, because many cancer patients suffer from abnormally low levels of vitamin A. Dandelion greens are also rich in vitamins and minerals, such as iron (93).

Since dandelion can have diuretic properties, be sure that if you drink dandelion tea or eat dandelion greens, you are getting extra potassium in your diet, even though dandelions do contain some potassium. You can sometimes find organically-grown dandelion greens at local health food stores reasonably priced. If you yank the greens from your front yard or some country roadside, first be sure that they haven't been sprayed with chemicals! You should not use dandelion if you have any type of billiary disease (or ulcers) since the herb can stimulate bile flow and increase gastric acid. Do not consume any herb high in iron if you suffer from a rare genetic disorder known as *hemachomatosis*. (As always, before beginning any herbal regimen, consult with your physician or Naturopath.)

## Fenugreek for Breast Cancer

Triterpenes, or plant saponins extracted from the herb, fenugreek, were found (in laboratory tests), to have amazing anti-cancer properties against breast cancer cells. You can find fenugreek supplements at most health food stores and even some pharmacy and supermarket shelves.

## Garlic for Cancer Prevention

Though some people consider it more of a *spice* than an herb, garlic has proven effective in the prevention of many types of cancer—and apparently it does not take much—less than one clove per day can boost the immune system (591). According to Optimal Diet Healthy Eating website (at *http://homodiet.netfirms.com)*, just one clove has the bacteria-fighting equivalent of thousands of units of penicillin (591). Garlic can lower blood pressure and increase clotting time, so consult with your physician if you are on blood-thinners or blood pressure medications before taking large amounts of fresh garlic or garlic supplements, or if you are contemplating surgery, or just recovering from a surgical procedure. Garlic is able to inhibit substances that cause cancer development, and has demonstrated the ability to greatly reduce tumor growth. It is believed that mashing the bulb releases the compounds that fight cancerous cells. The same is true of using cloves to fight parasites. It is best to chop them up immediately before consuming them.

In animal tests using garlic, scientists also discovered that uncooked garlic could destroy cancerous breast cells (363). Use fresh, organic garlic bulbs whenever possible.

## Ginkgo Fights Breast Cancer Growth

Animal studies at Georgetown University Medical Center in Washington D.C., showed that this herb (which was taken from ginkgo leaves) restricted cancerous cells by 80%. Not only was the extract used on breast cancer cells, but it worked at slowing cancers of the brain (125).

## Green Tea for All Cancers

Green tea is such a potent anti-oxidant, it is discussed in detail in several other chapters of this book. It is said to boost the body's metabolism, and it may also be important in helping to prevent cancer of the breast and gastric cancer. This tea also fights prostate cancer, lung cancers (135), and leukemia. When drinking tea, decaffeinated is best for its non-dehydrating effects, but the downside is that it may not fight arterial plaque as well. Drinking several cups per day of decaffeinated, organic green tea for anyone with cancer, auto-immune disorders, or simply for health maintenance, can be beneficial.

Green tea has also been found, in animal testing by Israeli researchers, to actually regenerate brain cells, something hitherto thought impossible (169). Be sure if consuming large amounts of tea, you are also getting adequate vitamins and minerals in your diet, especially if you opt for tea with caffeine. Caffeine can strip the body of minerals and nutrients due to its diuretic effect. As noted earlier, the downside is that the caffeine-free tea may not fight arterial plaque as well.

## Milk Thistle Inhibits Breast Cancer

This herb blocks harmful estrogen from entering the cells; however, if excess milk thistle causes diarrhea, reduce the amount you are taking (46). The diarrhea will generally disappear within a few days and only occurs in some individuals, since the herb promotes bile flow (197). Extracts from this herb have been used in fighting cancers of the breast (351). Milk thistle is also discussed in chapter nine of this book on liver cancer because of its amazing ability to rejuvenate and heal the liver. See the case history in that chapter of a terminal liver cancer patient totally cured using milk thistle. It is also being used to help fight colon and skin cancers.

Beware that if you have a chronic disorder, such as hemochromatosis, the body absorbs too much iron. This is a genetic disorder that you would have been born with, and you need to be sure that your physician approves your using milk thistle and other herbs. You want to be sure that if you are approved to take it, the herb you use is a standardized extract that is not high in iron. Anyone with hemochromatosis should not take large amounts of vitamin C either, since doing so can increase iron in the body. Also, if you are awaiting a transplant, or have already had one, you should never take any herbal preparations, hormones, minerals or vitamins without consulting your physician, since they may interfere with your anti-rejection medications.

## Myrrh - Biblical Plant for Fighting Cancer

In laboratory testing, compounds from this biblical herb not only killed breast, brain, and prostate cancer cells, it killed the cancer cells that were drug-resistant, without harming nearby healthy cells. Large-scale human testing has not yet been done on myrrh.

## Pau d'Arco to Enhance Immunity & Fight Cancer

Pau d' Arco (also known as *taheebo*) has proven useful in immunity boosting for several types of cancer, including breast cancer, and especially, leukemia (151). It is often considered equivalent to Asian ginseng and echinacea. When used, the **entire herb** (lapacho) should be used, not just the extract *(lapachol)*. It was also found to inhibit *Yoshido's sarcoma,* without causing toxicity (151). Most health food stores have pau d'arco tea. This tea is also known as *lapacho.* Be aware that lapachol is just one of the compounds extracted from pau d'arco tea, and that this herb can thin the blood. Use it in the whole tea format.

## Red Clover & Rosemary

Rosemary, because of an ingredient that it contains, known as *carnosol,* may help cut the risk for malignancies of the breast and skin (57). Red clover contains a compound which restricts blood vessel formation, thus blocking nutrition to tumors (387). Note that this effect of blocking blood vessel formation is exactly how shark cartilage works (see later in this chapter). Do not use red clover in excessive amounts without consulting your doctor. It can thin your blood. The compound that does this, genistein, can also help lower blood pressure.

## Rhodiola Rosea for Cancer

Rhodiola is a great anti-oxidant and is found growing freely in the high mountain ranges of Eastern Siberia (258). Folklore credits the herb to extraordinarily long lifespans for those drinking the tea (258). In Russia, scientists found that the herb (given by mouth) not only stopped cancers in animals tested, but prevented the cancers from spreading (258). Lifespans were also increased in test subjects having lung and breast tumors (258). The herb can be found at Planetary Formulas Online Store. See website *www.planetherbs.com* for the full article (258). Be aware that this herb can stimulate the body, having an effect much like that of caffeine. Recently, I have seen rhodiola as a supplement in health food stores.

## Schisandra

Schisandra herb may help fight fatigue (56). Many patients undergoing chemo have problems with exhaustion. Schisandra seeds have numerous anti-oxidant ingredients that help prevent liver damage. It is used by the Chinese to treat liver disease and inflammation (387).

## St. John's Wort

St. John's Wort helps keep cancer from metastasizing in the upper thorax (46). It should not be used by those taking any type of MAO inhibitors, nor during pregnancy or lactation. This herb also causes sun-sensitivity, so be sure to avoid prolonged sun exposure when using it (46). (MAO inhibitors are anti-depressant medications, though not all anti-depressants are considered MAO inhibitors. If you are taking any type of antidepressant medication, your physician or pharmacist can tell you whether or not it is a MAO inhibitor and which foods and/or medications are dangerously incompatible with them.)

Researchers in Germany have discovered, in animal testing, that a compound called *hyperforin* (from the herb St. John's Wort) was able to halt breast cancer and performed very much like the chemo drug *paclitaxel*. The main difference was that there were no **adverse** effects from the St. John's Wort (277).

## Turmeric & Breast Cancer

Turmeric, rich in curcumin, can stimulate the production in the body of a cancer-fighting gene known as the *p53 gene* (31). This gene is important because it has the ability to suppress the genes that are responsible for causing cancer (31). Turmeric and curry are safe when used as a spice; however, as with any herb or spice, organic is best. Check with your health care practitioner first. Do not use turmeric if you have gallbladder problems (571) or ulcers. You will find more curcumin in turmeric than you will in curry powder. Use organic turmeric rather than curry. Yellow mustard is very high in turmeric. Take turmeric with pineapple (bromelain) and an oil source for best absorption.

## Wormwood Used in Fighting Breast Cancer

According to website *www.cancertutor.com,* an herb known as *sweet wormwood* (containing the active ingredient *artemisinin*), has been laboratory tested for its effectiveness against breast cancer cells and found to be lethal against cancer, but safe to normal cells (282). Wormwood has long been a popular remedy for killing parasites and worms, and it is a cure for some forms of malaria; however, it was not allowed for treating malaria without first being compounded into a prescription (282). The website also points out the fact that malaria is caused by a parasite, and since wormwood kills cancer cells, perhaps there truly is a link between parasites and cancer (282). It is already believed that being infected with *H-pyloric* bacteria can increase your risk of stomach cancer. Researchers from the University of Washington recently discovered that they could outfit wormwood (artemisinin) with a *homing device* that sends the substance to cancer cells only, keeping normal cells unharmed (75a). The substance gets inside the cells and acts like a *bomb inside the cell*, as described by Professor Tomikazu Sasaki. It works against the high iron content found in cancer cells (75a).

This herb should not be taken on an empty stomach. Be sure to consult with your physician or Naturopath before taking artemisinin if you recently received or are currently on radiation therapy. Note that in a clinical trial with hundreds of children having the *H-pylori infection,* cranberry juice was also able to kill H-pylori. This bacteria can cause gastritis and increase your risk for lymphoma and stomach cancer (102). Use organic, unsweetened cranberry juice and add stevia or eXcella™ sweetener. (You can find eXcella™ at: *www.liveonlabs.com.*

# X. Miscellaneous Items for Breast Cancer

## Calcium D–Glucarate™ Fights Breast Cancer

D-Glucarate is a normal component of many foods, especially greens like broccoli and sprouts. It is also found in some fruits, including apples (394). This substance can help rid the body of unneeded estrogen, very important for those with estrogen-sensitive breast cancers (394). In some animal studies, this ingredient was actually shown to reverse the cancer (394). There have been no human reports of toxicity in using D-Glucarate, even in those who receive massive doses; however, since the nutrient works as a detoxifier in the body, beware, because it may neutralize the effects of medications that you are taking (394).

## Cartilage for Breast Cancer Remission

Shark cartilage contains proteins that prevent tumors from forming new blood vessels and works exceptionally well at shrinking tumors, starving them of the nutrition that they need for survival. Shark cartilage is more concentrated in these compounds than bovine cartilage—by as much as one thousand times (158). Cancers that form tumors, especially those of the breast, are more successfully treated with shark cartilage (158). See your natural health physician for specific dosing for your own particular condition.

Do not use shark cartilage or bovine cartilage without consulting with your physician, especially if you are on prescription medications, have high blood pressure, a recent history of heart attack, surgery, transplant, or pending surgery or are pregnant, nor if you are taking chemo or radiation. It is not recommended for children. It is not for those with pheochromocytoma (adrenal tumor which can cause excessively high blood pressure), seafood allergies, ulcers or circulatory diseases. It is not for those with liver disease, except that it has been used successfully against some liver cancers. For more information on dosing, see chapter seven in this book. (For treating hard-to-reach adrenal tumors, see CyberKnife® therapy in chapter 34.) Also, look under NanoKnife™.

## Clodronate Fights Spreading Breast Cancer

According to *www.cancertutor.com*, this compound is said to prevent the metastasis of cancer of the breast into bone cells, however due to FDA inhibition, it cannot be obtained in the U.S. in spite of a 1998 article in the *New England Journal of Medicine* which said of clodronate that it could halt the spread of this disease (79). Clodronate is a *biophosphonate* (79). You can get clodronate in Mexico and Canada. Note that there are biophosphonate drugs on the market to prevent osteoporosis (e.g., *Fosamax*) that have been discovered to have the potential side effect of deteriorating the bones of the jaw! (See chapter 22 of this book for natural, non-toxic ways of preventing osteoporosis.)

## Colcy's Toxins for Breast Cancer

William B. Coley, M.D., was responsible for the development of *Coley's Toxins* in the late 19th century (504). They were actually developed from bacteria and were effective not only with breast cancer, but Hodgkin's, ovarian cancer, and melanoma as well (504). In human studies involving breast cancer patients, more than half of the terminal patients using the compounds lived another five years. Coley's toxins are still being used today, predominantly in European countries and China (504). This procedure worked on Coley's patients because injecting them with the bacteria caused them to run high fevers and the immune stimulant boost resulted in the death of their cancers. (See chapter 34 on Malaria cancer treatment, which works much the same way.)

Even today, some physicians disagree about childhood (and adult) fevers. Some believe that you should not try to bring a fever down with medications, but let it run its course (as long as it does not get so high that the patient develops seizures), because a high fever in the body will often KILL the disease that is causing the fever! Fever is part of the body's immune system response to fight disease.

I believe it is best to use natural treatments for cancer prevention and treatment whenever possible. Coley's toxins are not natural, but are being included here for informational purposes, and because of their reported success at prolonging the lives of some cancer patients.

You can get this type cancer therapy at Issels Treatment Centers and others. Their website is *http://www.issels.com,* and their ph# 888-447-7357. They may also use it for other types of cancer (290).

## Cytotron Therapy - Non-Toxic & Non-Invasive

A new cancer (and arthritis) treatment developed and available in India that you will not yet be able to get in the U.S., is being successfully used on humans and is known as *Cytotron Therapy*. It is completely painless and non-toxic. See chapter 34 in this book for more details on what is also called *QMR* or *Quantum Magnetic Resonance* (90).

## ECT - ElectroChemical Therapy for Breast Cancer

Also described as *direct-current* ECT, this therapy originated in China (474). Widespread human testing has not yet been carried out in the U.S. In animals, *platinum electrodes* are placed on the tumor and treated with direct current (474). Animals with *colorectal carcinomas* that have spread to the liver were tested, and it was found that the treatment caused tumor shrinkage (474). More studies are planned in the U.S. on this therapy.

Currently, an ECT machine developed by *Solco Biomedical* (known as the "Solco SET-C21") by Swedish Professor, Nordenstrom, is claimed to have minimal side effects, boosts the immunity, and changes the pH of cells via electrochemical reaction. It is available from Korea. The therapy is being used for most cancers, including those of the G.I. tract, breast, lung, skin, and liver (275). It is widely used in Chinese hospitals, Korea, Germany and some cancer treatment centers in the U.S.

## Hydrazine Sulfate & Breast Cancer

For an excellent article about this substance and Dr. Joseph Gold, who developed it, go to website *http://www.hydrazinesulfate.org* and read the article: *THE TRUTH ABOUT HYDRAZINE SULFATE - DR. GOLD SPEAKS*, from July 14, 2004 (last amended Oct. 13, 2007). Also, see the link there: *MedTruth A commentary on truth in medicine.* Many people have successfully been treated for cancer, including breast cancer, with hydrazine sulfate. You will see the obvious tendency that the NCI has for covering up positive test results using this compound when you read the article above.

Kathy K. successfully fended off stage IV breast cancer using hydrazine sulfate and cured her cancer. She later died, but not from cancer, from surgery complications. A relative of hers considered a lawsuit against a prominent cancer organization for covering up information about the efficacy of hydrazine sulfate (490).

Be aware that hydrazine sulfate is a MAO inhibitor. As noted earlier in this chapter, there are certain foods and drugs that you can never combine with MAO inhibitors or the results can be deadly. Your physician can give you a complete list of foods and drugs that should not be taken in conjunction with MAO inhibitors. Dr. Joseph Gold and hydrazine sulfate are discussed in more detail later in this book.

## Hypofractionated Radiation Therapy for Breast Cancer

Though this is certainly not a non-toxic, God-given, gentle, or natural treatment for breast cancer, it is being touted in some clinics as an improved form of breast cancer treatment. What it really means, in a nutshell, is that you get fewer treatments, but the dose you get is stronger, thus, it has the same potential for toxic side effects as any radiation treatment, so the choice is yours. It is generally promoted as a way to get radiation over with more quickly and more conveniently - that's about it. I have seen no studies showing it to be any safer, with any better results or outcomes than standard treatments. If your oncology doctor tells you it's "safer" or has less "side effects," ask for documented studies from the radiologists who are "selling" it to him or her.

## Intensity Modulated Radiotherapy (IMRT) for Breast Cancer

This radiation treatment is currently under testing in Europe and is being used in the U.S as well. It uses targeted radiotherapy to help minimize damage to nearby normal cells. It is used for lung tumors, thyroid and breast cancers, as well as prostate, esophageal, nasal, head cancers, liver, brain, ovarian, cervical cancers and uterine growths. You may also see this treatment referred to as ***TOMO Therapy*** or *TOMO Treatment*—they are the same thing.

IMRT was first used at Memorial Sloan-Kettering Hospital for treating cancer of the prostate (163a). This type radiation uses many beams to target cancer tumors more precisely, thus (hopefully) preventing excess damage to nearby normal cells; however, it is still considered radiation, and will have some of the same side effects as any radiation would cause. IMRT has been popular at treating tumors located around or near hard-to-reach vital organs (163a).

## IOERT - Intraoperative Electron Radiation Therapy - The Mobetron

Though this is still considered a form of radiation treatment, and will have possible side effects, just as any radiation treatment does, Mobetron is being included here because it can be used right during surgery, while the tumor is open and exposed, thus minimizing damage to healthier nearby cells (165a). It is cost-efficient, portable and *less risky* for the patient. It is already being extensively used on humans and said to have few adverse effects. This treatment, also known as IOERT or "Intraoperative Electron Radiotherapy," has been used for cancers of the GI tract, throat, kidney, and many other sites. The IOERT machine is known as the ***Mobetron*** (165a).

## Marijuana Substance Halts Spread of Breast Cancer

Researchers from California Pacific Medical Research Institute have just recently discovered that a compound in marijuana known as *CBD* can restrict the spread of breast cancer, and without toxic side effects; however, the scientists cautioned that this is not a green light for smoking marijuana, because doing so won't achieve the same results (186). The study can be found in the journal *Molecular Cancer Therapeutics.* More research is planned (186). Marijuana smokers are not only at risk for brain degeneration, but the drug can also cause genetic defects in their children.

## Melatonin Anti-Oxidant

Melatonin is discussed in several other chapters in this book. It is a hormone produced by the pineal gland (some is formed in the gastrointestinal lining) during the darkest hours of the night during sleep time. It helps regulate the wake-sleep cycle and is a powerful anti-oxidant and anti-depressant. Recent studies have shown that having insufficient levels of this hormone can cause a greater risk for breast cancer in women. People who work swing-shifts are often deficient in melatonin. Most health food stores have supplements in the range of 2—3 mg capsules or pills. Some people use this supplement for a sleep aid.

It is not recommended that patients with *leukemia, lymphoma and myeloma* take melatonin; there is a possibility that melatonin may accelerate these type cancers (507). In addition to this precaution for melatonin, the supplement could cause depression and worsening of allergies in some individuals, and it should not be taken by those on cortisone, nor those who are pregnant (192). It is also possible that the hormone can have a narrowing (temporary) effect on *blood vessels* and interfere with libido and fertility. It may also lower the temperature of the body and could harm the retina in some individuals (192). Significant amounts of natural melatonin can be found simply in eating tart cherries (61).

## Poly-MVA

See later chapters in this book for more detailed information on Poly-MVA. For testimonials of people who used this substance to cure their cancers, see website: *http://www.polymvasurvivors.com/testimonials.html.* Many of these testimonials are given ten or more years ago, and all survivors are still here as of March 2007. This substance can cross over into the brain, making it helpful at fighting brain cancers. Many cancer-fighting drugs and other substances do not cross into the brain, the *blood-brain* barrier.

## Rexin-G™ for Metastatic Cancers

Rexin-G™ has been undergoing clinical trials at Mayo Clinic, M.D. Anderson, and a few other facilities. It is a drug for cancers that have spread and those types of cancer that conventional medicine says do not respond to chemo (256). **Human** clinical studies, thus far, have had good results. In the very first **human** trial, 83% of the patients experienced tumor shrinkage. The patients all had spreading pancreatic cancer (256). Good responses were also achieved in human studies involving several other types of metastatic cancer. Due to the reports, this drug is now used for treating all forms of *solid tumors* in the Philippines that are resistant to conventional therapy (256). The U.S. FDA has given the drug its *orphan drug status* for use with pancreatic cancers in the US, as well as other types of cancer metastases, which means that trials will continue (256). It is given intravenously, so isn't exactly natural or painless, but could be considered gentler than older chemo drugs. This is because it is said to be a non-chemo drug, showing itself in **human** clinical trials, not to have the adverse side effects normally associated with chemo drugs (256). You can get more information on this drug at *epeiusbiotech.com/rexin_g-factsheet.asp*. Epeius Biotechnologies produce Rexin-G™ (257).

## Ukrain: Effective Non-Toxic Cure for Breast Cancer

Ukrain is a combination of two compounds which are both toxic when used alone, but when combined, they are only toxic to cancer cells (287). The main Ukrain website, *www.ukrin.com*, described a **human trial** involving hundreds of people with dozens of different types of cancer that all received Ukrain treatment over a period of 5.5 years (287). Every patient, without exception, had already received everything that conventional medicine had to offer, and nothing had stopped their cancers. All were terminal. *31%* of the *breast cancer* patients went into total *remission* as well as hundreds of the other cancer sufferers (287). Ukrain is only available through alternative health clinics in the U.S., Canada, and Europe.

2009 update: note that because Ukrain is not authorized in Austria, the website has been changed (since my first book came out) and is now called *Nowicky Pharma; however,* you can read detailed information about Ukrain now in the book*: Anti-Cancer Agent Ukrain—The Crime Story of an Obstruction* by Eleonore Thun-Hohenstein. For pictures of how Ukrain works, see website: *http://www.ukrain-drug.net/webspeed/index.htm.*

Human testing on breast cancer patients showed that Ukrain is important in the increase of certain amino acids in the body. One of the amino acids that Ukrain helps to increase is glutamine (515). Many cancer patients are glutamine-starved, which causes the typical wasting away that is associated with this disease (507) (515). (L-glutamine taken by chemo patients can also help lessen the severity of mucositis.)

## Ukrain Brings About Complete Remission in Recurrent Spreading Breast Cancer

A human case study on a patient having stage IV breast cancer (that had spread to the lung) can be found at National Library of Medicine's website, *www.pubmed.com* (PMID 8899340). The cancer was treated with Ukrain, which is non-toxic. The patient went into complete remission from all traces of cancer (442). Another human study involved a patient who received Ukrain treatment only, and has had 12 years without further pathology (556). This case study can be found at NCBI PubMed website (PMID 8899341). Another woman, age 50, with stage IV breast cancer, who was not able to undergo chemo or radiation, was able to successfully have the main breast tumor removed, along with nearby *lymph nodes* after only one Ukrain treatment. After two more rounds of Ukrain, the patient was cancer-free (610). This case study can also be found at the National Library of Medicine PubMed NCBI website (PMID 11345033). Ukrain has proven to be completely safe, non-toxic, and without adverse side effects. Ukrain's cancer-killing effect does not harm the body's hormone balance (584). Using the advantage of an electron microscope and light microscopy, research also revealed that Ukrain boosts the body's natural immune system, causing severe cellular changes in tumor cells, killing them. See PubMed study PMID: 8899319 for details (585). Another large human study involving 75 breast cancer participants, revealed that Ukrain was very beneficial in pre-surgery use when they were given either 50 mg or 100 mg of the substance (586).

## XI. Low Fat Diet Inhibits Breast Cancer

The American Cancer Society has finally admitted, after years of denying that diet could influence cancer rates, that increasing fresh fruits and vegetables in your diet, and eating less fat can decrease cancer risk (550).

## XII. Other Treatments

### Mammosite Treatment - Brachytherapy

This is not a natural, non-toxic treatment, nor is it considered *gentle* or *painless*; however, it is being included here because it is being used more frequently for breast cancer treatment in lieu of other more toxic forms of treatment. Mammosite treatment involves putting radiation in the form of *seeds* into the area of the breast affected by the cancer. The treatment is usually for five days. Just realize that radiation of any kind depresses the body's natural immunity. This is also called *brachytherapy* or *internal radiation therapy*. It is also used for prostate cancer and other types of cancer.

### TAP—Tumor-Activated Prodrug or TAP Technology for Breast Cancer

Dr. Anne Kellogg, a pathologist and researcher from East Carolina University, is the developer of a new type of monoclonal antibody that may pave the way for treating breast, ovarian, and *other cancers* more effectively, perhaps with fewer side effects as mainstream chemo (207). She calls the new antibody *DS-6* and describes it as a *delivery vehicle* for a cancer-killing agent that was produced by a company known as *ImmunoGen*. The antibody works by hitching onto tumor cells and allowing itself (as well as the cancer-killing agent) to get inside the cell where it then destroys the cell (207). It is only *activated* once it gets into the abnormal cell (207).

## Visica2™ Treatment System for Breast Cancer

This therapy is for invasive ductal breast cancer and is from Sanarus Medical. It uses a type of cryoablation to destroy the cancer. For more information, see website: *www.marketwatch.com/news/story/Cryoablation-Early-Invasive-Ductal-Breast/story.aspx?grid=%B945AE573-00F8-408B-8B18-BAECFA8F3767%7D*.

## Zeolites for a Stage IV Breast Cancer

See website *http://liquidzeolite.zoxic.com* for the report of a woman who used zeolites to cure her stage IV breast cancer.

# XIII. Important Lifestyle Changes

Eydie Mae Hunsberger, Rita Myers, Johanna Brandt and others, discussed in this book, did not cure their cancers merely with a raw foods diet. Their diet plan incorporated a total way of living that involved many other aspects of health, besides dietary changes. Several of these are discussed later in this book. For example: proper rest, exercise, oxygen, fresh air, adequate water, prayer, a positive attitude, unselfishness, stress reduction, and faith in God are all critically important in helping the body get well. Though diet itself is the main focus of this chapter, it is not intended that the rest of these ingredients, so important for optimal health, be minimized.

## The Importance of Water

According to the late Dr. F. Batmanghelidj, M.D., in his book, *Your Body's Many Cries For Water*, cancer patients are dehydrated (341). It is important that you get adequate amounts of water on a daily basis. This quantity of water requires extra salt. He recommended that, "For every 10 glasses of water (about two quarts)" you drink, you need an extra "half teaspoon of salt per day" (341). Always check with your physician.

## XIV. Help for Lymphedema & Neuropathy

Lymphedema often occurs when cancerous lymph nodes are removed or damaged, or it can be a hereditary disease. The disease, or lack of lymph nodes, causes limbs to swell from inadequate drainage of the lymphatic system. Many treatments are given, from elevating the limb to avoiding tight clothing, lymphedema pumps, sleeves, lymphedema therapists, acupuncture, pycnogenols, garlic, ginkgo biloba, niacin, ginger, CoQ10, ALA, and many other items that help with circulation.

Some people have had good results using prescription *low dose* Naltrexone for lymphedema (596). For this purpose, it is usually given at *bedtime* in small doses. (You may need a *compounding* pharmacist.) This prescription has been used for auto-immune disorders, Crohn's disease, MS, and larger doses are generally given for helping those with addictions (596). It is also being tested for use in fighting cancer (see chapter 34).

Research noted in the *Journal of Clinical Investigation* (Dec. 20, 2007) that a hormone the body normally secretes (*adrenomedullin*) could help alleviate this painful condition, as well as work toward cancer prevention (527). Also, a human study showed that patients using the supplement, Wobenzyme, had good results with alleviating lymphedema. Wobenzyme, an enzyme, has an anti-inflammatory effect on the body (321). It also helps prevent blood clots, lowers LDL, and is used in treating auto-immune disorders and arthritis pain. It contains natural ingredients, and there are no known adverse effects. It is usually taken between meals (321) and is available on the internet.

For those who develop neuropathy from chemotherapy (or other illnesses), you may wish to try a new *Nerve Support Formula* from website: *http://www.mcvitamins.com/neuropathy.htm#A*, which contains a fat-soluble form of the B-1 vitamin (known, not as thiamine, but as *benfotiamine*), and *methyl-12* B vitamin. High blood pressure before having surgery for cancer (especially breast cancer), can increase your risk for lymphedema afterwards. Also, try MAGNESIUM! The wonderful Magnesium Chloride oil that you simply spray onto your skin for transdermal absorption or their bath flakes that you can use for foot soaks or in your tub. Most cancer patients (and most Americans) are seriously magnesium deficient. You can find this product at: *http://www.magneticclay.com*, as well as website: *http://www.swansonvitamins.com*. (See Appendix II)

# CHAPTER 5

# GENTLE CURES FOR TOUGH PROSTATE CANCERS

*"Behold, I will bring it health and cure, and I will cure them, and will reveal unto them the abundance of peace and truth." (Jeremiah 33:6)*

## Case #1—The Prostate Cancer That Vanished

An herb from the rain forest, known as *Graviola,* has shown promise in the fight against several forms of cancer. Many documented cases of complete cures are being reported as a result of using this herb, including one from the *Health Sciences Institute* newsletter that tells of a Texan businessman by the name of Daryl S., who discovered *Raintree* products while he was researching natural remedies for *prostate cancer* (34). Diagnostic testing had confirmed that he had over 20 growths. Though his physician recommended surgery, Daryl refused, knowing that surgery might mean a lifetime of urinary tract problems and other health issues (34). As explained by Health Sciences Institute, he opted for something besides surgery for his cancer. He was treated with a hormone regimen and the **graviola** herb contained in the supplement known as *N-Tense* (34). Within 8 weeks, Daryl's PSA was normal and multiple diagnostic tests were negative for any prostate tumors. The 20 growths were gone (34).

Be sure to check with your physician or Naturopath before taking Graviola, especially if you already have any type of health disorder. Graviola supplements are now available in health food stores.

## Case #2—Another Prostate Cancer Disappears

Dr. Abram Hoffer was able to bring about a complete prostate cancer cure in a patient with prostate *sarcoma*, who was told by his conventional medicine doctors that it was too late for therapy (432). His cancer had already spread to the *pelvic bone*. When the patient came to seek treatment from Dr. Hoffer, he was only able to tolerate 10 grams of vitamin C daily by mouth, so Dr. Hoffer suggested injections of vitamin C in the same amount as he was taking orally, except that the injections were to be given twice a week. He was to keep taking the daily oral doses (432). His cancer totally disappeared within *six months* and he survived his ordeal, living cancer-free for many years. When he expired, it was not from cancer (432). See the complete story at Dr. Abram Hoffer's webpage: *http://www.islandnet.com/~hoffer/*.

## Abiraterone for Advanced Prostate Cancer

This is a new drug for treating advanced prostate cancer that is not *natural,* but gentler (thus far) than chemo and radiation, since side effects include "loss of libido, breathlessness, fatigue, fluid retention and weight gain," reportedly not as severe as some of those caused by older, conventional chemo drugs and radiation (482).

Preliminary trials, headed up by Dr Johann de Bono in *South-West* London's *Royal Marsden Hospital,* remarked that "patients there had been able to control the disease with just four pills a day and very few side effects" (482). They have shown that the drug "can reverse even the most aggressive, resistant and deadly cancers," and could save thousands of lives per year (242), and offer palliative relief as well. In human studies, many of the cancers had already gone into "the liver, lungs or bones" (242).

Early tests show that the treatment (given in pill form) "can shrink tumors in up to 80 per cent of cases," and may even "end the need for damaging chemotherapy and radiotherapy." They are hoping it could also work with other cancers, such as "breast and bowel cancers" (482). The downside is that it may not be available for widespread use for another two or *three years*, except in *clinical trials* (482).

## Ablatherm® HIFU—Non-Invasive Ultrasound Treatment for Prostate Cancer (Sonablate®)

This ultrasound therapy is being sought out in Canada and Mexico, as it has not yet been approved in the U.S. The treatment, first used in Europe, uses a form of concentrated ultrasound which produces heat that destroys tumors (63). The procedure has been successfully used to treat prostate cancer in hundreds of people, and has also been used on liver tumors in Europe (63). You may hear this called *Sonablate® therapy*, though the Sonablate® machine itself is not yet approved in Canada or the U.S. Most patients need only one of these treatments, and it is considered less risky than conventional radiation and *cryotherapy* (63). In several years usage, it has not caused injury to the rectal area (63). (Note that the procedure is only used on those with T-1 and T-2 prostate cancer, not for those with T-3 and T-4.) Though it does not require surgery, it does require spinal anesthesia and the probe that delivers the therapy is done rectally (63). Side effects that may occur include incontinence, which is usually temporary, narrowing of the urethral opening (which may or may not require later widening), and/or impotence that usually responds to pharmacological treatment (63).

## AHCC - Mushroom Combo Enhances Immunity

AHCC (*Active hexose correlated compound)* is actually a complex compound composed of the mycelia of many mushrooms (206). In human testing, it was found (when given to patients by mouth) that doses of "3g/day…for 2-6 months" could significantly increase the body's natural immunity, thus enabling the death of prostate cancer cells and several other types of cancerous cells (206). This compound is found at many natural health food stores and online supplement providers, such as *www.discount-vitamins -herbs.net.*

## Avoid Dairy - Cut Your Risk of Prostate Cancer

Another way to be sure to cut your risk of getting prostate cancer is to avoid milk and dairy products entirely. An eleven-year study involving more than 20,000 men, revealed an apparent risk in the ingestion of dairy products. Drinking milk can dramatically raise the risk for prostate cancer (91).

Studies also show that the alpha lipoic acid (ALA) found in some processed foods can lead to an increased risk for prostate cancers (73). Be sure your source for ALA is natural foods or supplements, rather than processed foods.

Studies have also proven that high amounts of hormones being injected into cattle in the U.S. are increasing cancer statistics. Some countries have banned hormones in cattle and poultry, but not the U.S., because the FDA still considers them harmless! If you do use cow's milk, buy organic raw milk if you can find it. In some states of the U.S., organic raw milk has been banned. Unless you are a farmer with your own dairy cows (or live next to one), you may find it impossible to obtain!

Health site *http://www.yourhealthbase.com/prostate_cancer.html* warns men that having vasectomies also increases their risk for prostate cancer (73).

## Baicalein Against Prostate Cancer (Skullcap Extract)

An extract from the Chinese herb skullcap (baicalein), a type of mint, was able (in laboratory and animal testing) to inhibit bladder cancer (488). The herbal extract was also used in human studies to help stabilize and extend the lives of advanced prostate cancer patients who were not helped with conventional treatment. The extract was given by mouth (488).

## Beans & Peas for Prostate Health

Studies have shown that men who have two or more servings of garden peas and beans a week have a 37% less risk of this type cancer (73).

## Bee Pollen Extract for the Prostate

A common extract of bee pollen, *Cernitin,* helps prevent hyperplasia of the prostate and helps neutralize toxins (394). Animal research revealed that cernitin prevented poisonous cadmium from being absorbed into the body, and it also reduced harmful cholesterol (394).

## Beta-Carotene Protects the Prostate Against Cancer

Beta-carotene (as well as lycopene) has been shown to reduce the risk of prostate cancer. As described by Jack Challem in his book, *All About Carotenoids Beta-carotene, Lutein & Lycopene,* in one research group (*The Harvard study*) involving thousands of physicians over a period of many years, an analysis was made on the dietary levels of beta-carotene that they consumed (366). Results showed that low dietary consumption of beta-carotene increased the men's cancer risk dramatically (366). Mr. Challem has a new book out, *Stop Prediabetes Now,* (with co-author Ron Hunninghake, M.D.) Also see his new book*: The Food-Mood Solution.* For information on both books, see website*: http://www.thenutritionreporter.com.*

## Beta-Sitosterol Decreases Prostate Tumor Growth

In her book, *D-Glucarate, Powerful Protector Against Breast and Prostate Cancers,* Rita Elkins, M.H., reports that this nutrient could dramatically reduce prostate malignancies within just one week of treatment (394). You will find that many health food stores have combination herbal blends for prostate health. One example is Zyflamend from *New Chapter, Inc.*, in

Brattleboro, Vermont. This is a compound containing several herbs, including green tea and turmeric (404). Laboratory testing with Zyflamend against prostate cancer cells revealed a dramatic reduction of the cancers within just three days (404). This compound has blood-thinning effects. Always consult with your physician or Naturopath before beginning any new herbal regimen such as Zyflamend. (Note that hu zhang, another herb in Zyflamend, is a very popular source of resveratrol, as are red, black, and purple grape skins.)

## Boron Can Help Prevent Prostate Cancer

Studies reveal that adequate boron in your diet (from fruits and nuts) can help prevent prostate cancer (153). When dozens of men having prostate cancer were compared to thousands of those without cancer, it was discovered that those with the highest boron consumption had the lowest cancer risk (153). Boron-rich foods include not only nuts, but grapes and their juices, as well as several other food sources (153).

## Broccoli & Cabbage for Prostate Cancer Prevention

A human study involving 600 participants, showed that eating not just broccoli and cabbage, but any of the cruciferous vegetables three times per week can cut your risk of prostate cancer by 50%. It may be due to the I3C or *indole-3-carbinol* that these veggies contain. Leafy greens and seed foods were also protective (499). Other cruciferous vegetables include: arugula, collards, kale, turnips, brussel sprouts, mustard, rutabaga, garden cress, bok choy (tatsoi), wasabai, daikon radish, watercress and cauliflower.

## Burzynski's Antineoplastons for Advanced Prostate Cancer

Kenneth B. was diagnosed with *advanced untreatable prostate cancer* in 1999, which had spread throughout his body, causing unrelenting *pain*. A few months later, he turned 70. Within just two weeks of starting on Dr. Burzynski's antineoplastons, his PSA was normal at 1.3. His cancer was cured and, at last report in May of 2005—6 years after he was told he was terminal—he was still cancer-free. He received no other treatment for his cancer. For details on his case, see website: *http://burzynskipatientgroup.org/kenb.html.*

See chapter 14 of this book for more amazing cases of cancer patients completely cured of *terminal* cancers, people who were basically sent home to die, then chose non-toxic antineoplastons from the Burzynski Clinic in Houston, Texas. Also, see many of the patient's own stories about their success in fighting cancer with antineoplastons and PBs (sodium phenylbutrates) at website: *http://burzynskipatientgroup.org/stories.html.* Many of these cases were prostate cancer patients; many were hopeless, very aggressive brain tumors. The main Burzynski Clinic website is at *www.burzynskiclinic.com.* The FDA has finally approved the oral form of antineoplastons (sodium phenylbutrates or PBs) for off-label use, but you will need to ask your physician about prescribing them. Some individuals can have side effects from antineoplastons, but they are quickly reversible, unlike toxic chemo drugs that often cause fatal adverse reactions. (Antineoplastons can now be used for gliomas.)

## Calcium D-Glucarate™ for Prostate Cancer

Calcium D-Glucarate™ can be found as a natural ingredient in many foods, including leafy greens, sprouts and some fruits, like apples (394). It has the ability to decrease harmful estrogen (estradiol) and testosterone in the body, and in 1990, it was revealed that the compound could stunt tumors, thereby preventing their spread (394). In fact, D-Glucarate is so efficient at removing harmful compounds from the body, that Japanese researchers discovered when they dosed rats with *Kanamycin* along with the D-Glucarate, that the nutrient prevented the kidney toxicity that *Kanamycin* usually causes! Calcium D-Glucarate has shown no adverse effects in **human** testing, not even with excessive amounts (394). You can find it at natural health food stores.

## Cherries Stop the Growth of Prostate Cancer Cells

Studies conducted at Iowa University by Dr. Raymond Hohl revealed that *perillyl alcohol* in cherries can help prevent cancer in many forms (61). Perillyl alcohol apparently works by cutting off the protein supply that cancer cells need. The scientists studying the compound said that it worked, without exception, against all the cancers exposed, including those of the ovaries, breast and prostate, even in advanced stages (61). Raspberries are very high in this nutrient, as are pomegranates. Also, see more information on ellagic acid later in this chapter and book.

## CoQ10 & Prostate Cancer

Current research conducted by the Leonard M. Miller School of Medicine in Miami, under Niven R. Nerain, revealed that CoQ10 has the ability to kill cancer cells without damage to adjacent healthy cells. Not only that, but the NCI (National Cancer Institute) acknowledged in 2005 that CoQ10 can extend the lives of those with prostate cancer and other cancers, as described at the Issels Treatment website *http://www.issels.com.* Their phone #888-447-7357 (290). Karl Folkers Ph.D., studied CoQ10 extensively for many years and used it for his patients. He funded the work of Dr. William Judy (Brandenton, Florida) to use CoQ10 on his hormone-independent prostate cancer patients (435). Note that prostate cancers can start as hormone-dependent, then after hormone treatment, they can become hormone-resistant or hormone-independent) (435). Dr. Judy tested 30 such cancer patients (half of them had cancer that had spread to their lungs and bone and half did not), giving them Dr. Folker's recommended dose of CoQ10 at 500 mg a day. 14 of the 15 without spreading cancer enjoyed a PSA *return to normal,* while eight of the 15 patients with metastases had a PSA that also went back to *normal* (435). Dr. Judy also treated six other prostate cancer patients with the same dosage as above for four months, and all six had normal PSAs at the end of the treatment (435).

## Cruciferous Vegetables Protect Against Prostate Cancer

As described earlier in this chapter, the cruciferous veggies (broccoli, cabbage, brussel sprouts, kale, arugula, daikon, watercress, mustard, bok choy, wasabai, and others) all contain ingredients that prevent and attack prostate cancer cells. New studies show that they can also help prevent diabetes. Raw fresh juices are terrific. Cooking and pasteurization destroys many of the live enzymes and beneficial nutrients found in juices.

## Cryotherapy

Usually guided by doppler imagery, cryotherapy involves freezing cancer with a controlled method that seeks to leave healthy tissue undamaged. It has been used effectively in many types of cancer. It usually causes less damage to the body than radiation or chemo and is less invasive. Normally it cannot be considered natural, painless or gentle, but it is being mentioned here simply because it may be a more favorable choice than chemo or radiation, depending on the type cancer. It has been successfully used for abnormal cells of the cervix, retinoblastoma, skin growths (before they become malignant), prostate cancer, liver growths and others, and is sometimes used in combination with other therapies.

## CyberKnife® Therapy for Prostate Tumors

See chapter 34 in this book for details on CyberKnife® therapy, which is being used successfully for prostate cancers and other cancers, including hard to reach brain tumors. It is a gentle, painless procedure that does not require an incision, surgery, sedation or inpatient stay. It is quick, and as soon as the procedure is over, the patient is able to return home. There are very few risks and side effects, though it does involve varying amounts of radiation (89a) and it can cause damage to nearby healthy tissue. Also, look under NanoKnife™, chapter 34.

## Cytotron Therapy

See chapter 34 in this book for more details on this gentle, painless, non-invasive cancer therapy that many people are also using to restore cartilage in their joints, making joint-replacement surgeries completely unnecessary (90). You may hear this referred to as *QMR* or *Quantum Magnetic Resonance*—they are the same thing.

## DHEA & Prostate Cancer

This hormone, in animal testing, was shown to prevent cancer and cause regression of cancers of the prostate; however, be sure to consult with your physician before taking DHEA, because he or she will want to draw blood first to be sure that your levels of DHEA are subnormal before recommending supplementation (95).

## Diet & Lifestyle Change Used to Cure Prostate Cancer

When Eric Gardiner was diagnosed with prostate cancer, he began a search for a natural alternative. He had no desire to go the cut, poison and burn route. He credited the cancer to a lifetime filled with stress, improper diet, and inadequate exercise, which damaged his immune system (405). When his physician recommended conventional treatment (surgery, chemo, or radiation), he was less than enthusiastic and wrote about the experience in his book: *How I Conquered Cancer – A Naturopathic Alternative* (405).

When he opted out of conventional treatment, Mr. Gardiner met with the same resistance that Eydie Mae Hunsberger experienced when she butted heads with the current health system. He found himself questioning the wisdom of orthodox treatment when statistics show that current methods of cancer treatment produce a dismal survival rate (405).

Eric also knew full well that if he did not change his diet and lifestyle, his cancer would likely return (405). When Rita Myers, Eric Gardiner, Eydie Mae, and Ann Wigmore were diagnosed with cancer, and other diseases (e.g., gangrene and bowel disease in the case of Ann Wigmore), they did not return to the same lifestyle. They did not take up where they left off and resume their old habits. They completely changed their diet and lifestyle.

Eric Gardiner changed his diet and his lifestyle and conquered his cancer. He began a regular exercise program, cut down his fat intake, increased his intake of fresh fruits, vegetables and water, and cut the junk food out of his diet (405). He used a bowel-cleansing program and began using nutritional supplements. He also used Dr. Hulda Clark's herbal program to successfully kill parasites. Eric also recommends buying organic produce (405). Dr. Clark's program of killing parasites in the body is discussed later in my book (see chapter 28).

A national news report in 2007 stated that organic foods are, indeed, better for the body. The pesticides, hormones, and herbicides found in non-organic crops take a toll on the liver and other vital organs. Why has it taken so long for this to be admitted? This is common sense.

## Ellagic Acid Prevents Cancer Cells From Dividing

Ellagic acid (discussed earlier in this chapter) occurs naturally in many types of berries and in some nuts (105). According to *mnwelldir.org*, the richest source of this nutrient is raspberries, in whatever form they are found, cooked or raw (105). According to their sources, halting prostate cancer cells for seven days can be helped by weekly consumption of eight ounces of raspberries (105). A recent laboratory study from the Hollings Cancer Institute reported that this compound kills cancer cells in many types of cancer, including those of the prostate, and also kills the human papilloma virus. All they recommended was a cup of raspberries daily (105). Apparently, ellagic acid is also powerful enough to kill a pathogen that has long been associated with causing ulcers, the infamous *H. pylori* (105). Another natural source of ellagic acid is pomegranates.

See the article in this chapter on using pomegranate juice for recurring prostate cancer. If raspberries are not in season, you can usually find them in the frozen section of your store. Many health food stores carry organic frozen berries. Cherries are also high in ellagic acid, as are cranberries, pecans, walnuts, and strawberries. (Cranberries also cut the risk for ulcers and bladder infections, and they help fight leukemia (22.)

## Essiac Tea & Prostate Cancer

See chapter six of this book for detailed information about a natural herbal tea formula, developed by a Canadian nurse, who cured hundreds (perhaps even thousands) of her cancer patients with an herbal tea she developed, despite the years of harassment she endured from the Canadian Health Department.

In the book by Richard Thomas, *The Essiac Report Canada's Remarkable Unknown Cancer Remedy,* he included a letter from patient Fred W., who had been diagnosed with prostate cancer that had already spread to other parts of his body, including his skull (580). Instead of surgery and chemo, he chose hormonal therapy with Zoladex and began drinking Flor-Essence® Essiac tea. Within just two weeks of starting the tea, his PSA dropped dramatically, then reached normal a few weeks later (580). A second patient also wrote to the manufacturer of the tea in 1993 describing their dad's struggle with adenocarcinoma of the prostate. A month after the biopsy and diagnosis, the dad began drinking Flor-Essence® tea (2 ounces in the morning and 2 ounces in the evening). Three months later, he was cancer-free. He had received no surgery, no chemo, no radiation and no hormone therapy (580). You can find Flor-Essence® tea at most health food stores.

## Fenugreek for the Prostate

Triterpenes or plant saponins extracted from the herb, fenugreek, were found (in laboratory tests) to dramatically fight prostate cancer cells.

## Fish Oil & Vitamin E for Prostate Health

Fish Oils (DHA and EPA) protect the prostate. Those men who ingest at least 470 mg of fish oil daily cut their risk for this type cancer by 11%, and those taking vitamin E cut their risk by as much as 40% (73). A recent human study involving 20,000 men revealed that those who ate omega-3-rich oily fish at least three to five times per week, could increase their chances of surviving prostate cancer by nearly 50%. Since vitamin E in large amounts can thin the blood, be sure to check with your physician or Naturopath first, especially if you are already taking blood-thinners. Note that one of the richest and healthiest sources of omega-3 (besides flax oil, chia seeds, Lyprinol, avocado, salba, and oily fish) is KRILL oil.

## Flax Seed for Treating Prostate Cancer

Preventing cancer and maintaining health of the prostate gland is very dependent on balancing EFAs (essential fatty acids) and the body's hormone level. It has been suggested that flax seed, high in essential omega-3 oils for healthy prostate functioning, is an important dietary addition for men with prostate problems, or just those wishing to prevent them. It not only prevents cancer, but it should be considered a necessary adjunctive with any prostate cancer treatment program, as well as a colon cancer preventative (571).

See chapters 14 and 18 of this book for details on the Budwig flax oil diet, rich in omega-3, that has cured many ***incurable*** cancer cases, including ***inoperable*** brain tumors. Omega-3 is also one of nature's greatest pain relievers. Some people are able to get pain relief from enteric-coated fish oil capsules, which can also help colon disorders. As noted earlier, another excellent source for omega-3 is KRILL oil. Some studies indicate that krill oil could be many times more potent than fish oil. Use organic only.

## Fungus Cure Also Cures Cancer, Says Oncology Physician

See chapter 34 of this book for the amazing cancer cure that Italian Oncologist, Dr. Simoncini, is using to cure his cancer patients within just days! Cancerous growths are usually WHITE. He says that they are actually a fungus, which can be killed with a non-toxic soda bicarb solution that quickly alkalizes the tumor for destruction (582).

## Garlic Prevents Prostate Cancer

Multiple laboratory studies, as well as human research, has shown that garlic prevents cancer. Just eating a small amount of garlic every day will drastically cut the risk for prostate cancer. Fresh garlic also kills many forms of bacteria.

## Ginger & Prostate Cancer

The herb, ginger, not only has anti-inflammatory properties, but it stimulates the destruction of human prostate cancer cells, regardless of whether or not they are said to be dependent upon hormones (59).

## Ginseng & Prostate Cancer

Lab studies done by Laura Murphy, a physiologist and endocrinologist, showed that a compound from American ginseng could fight prostate and breast cancer (126).

When Dr. Murphy started to test ginseng in mice, she discovered that the herb reduced tumor growth by 50%; however, she does not promote ginseng used alone, stating that once the mice were taken off the herb, their cancers returned. She emphasized that the best results were not from an isolated extract of ginseng, but from using the entire root (439). Some ginseng is extracted using alcohol and some is extracted using water. She said that only water-extracted ginseng should be used by those having estrogen-sensitive type cancers (439).

Though it was American ginseng that they worked with, in an email to me on May 10, 2005, Dr. Murphy states that "all ginseng types have now been shown to elicit anti-cancer properties." The reason that she worked with American ginseng was "because…not much was known about the American variety." Though some herbal websites recommend that you avoid certain ginsengs, including American and Brazilian if you have prostate cancer, see Dr. Murphy's information (above) regarding the water-extracted ginseng as opposed to alcohol-based extracts.

Ginseng (especially the *Panax* variety) can raise blood pressure in some individuals (494).

## Grapes - Prevention for Prostate Cancer & Skin Cancers

Resveratrol in grapes has been touted as a potent protection against prostate cancer. Animal research has shown that it can fight off skin cancers as well (132).

## Green Tea & Black Tea Slow Prostate Cancers

Recent studies have shown that men who drink green tea and black tea can significantly cut their risk of prostate cancer, even inhibit the spread of the cancer. Researchers from the University of California have found the tea protective against prostate cancers (146). Green tea has also been shown, in animal testing by Israeli researchers, to actually regenerate brain cells, something hitherto thought impossible (169).

Studies of thousands of Japanese men with cancer of the prostate revealed that they could halt the spread of their cancer by 50%, simply by ingesting at least 5 cups a day of green tea. Some benefited from even more cups per day (135). If you drink large amounts of caffeinated tea, it can strip your body of vital nutrients, and also leave you dehydrated; however, when it comes to fighting plaque in the arteries, the caffeine-free tea may not be as effective.

## Guided Therapeutics Program – GTx – or Image-Guided Photothermal Therapy

This is a type of laser treatment being tested for treating localized prostate cancer. For details, see website: *http://www.ryerson.ca/physics/colloquia/colloquium/collweersink0809.html,* Ryerson University Department of Physics.

## Intensity Modulated Radiotherapy (IMRT)

This radiation treatment is currently under testing in Europe and is being used in the U.S as well. It uses targeted radiotherapy to help minimize damage to nearby normal cells. It is used for lung tumors, thyroid and breast cancers, as well as prostate, esophageal, nasal, head cancers, liver, brain, ovarian, cervical cancers and uterine growths. You may also see this treatment referred to as ***TOMO Therapy*** or *TOMO Treatment*—they are the same thing.

IMRT was first used at Memorial Sloan-Kettering Hospital for treating cancer of the prostate (163a). Rather than using one large radiation beam to target the tumor, this type radiation uses many beams to target cancer tumors more precisely, thus (hopefully) preventing excess damage to nearby normal cells (163a), though it is still considered radiation and will have some of the same side effects as any radiation would cause.

IMRT has been popular at treating tumors located around or near critical, vital organs (163a).

## IP-6 for Prostate Cancer Prevention

IP-6 is a substance regularly found in high fiber foods, such as *whole grain...beans*, [and] *nuts* (215). It was shown, in animal testing, to fight the progress of prostate tumors. When IP-6, also known as *inositol hexaphosphate*, was ingested by the animals, their tumors shrank by more than half (215).

## Isosilybin-B Fights Prostate Cancer

Isosilybin-B, a natural component found in the milk thistle plant, was recently discovered to have tremendous power for inhibiting prostate cancer, and those cancers already in progress, regardless of whether they are hormone-dependent cancers or non-hormone-dependent (445). Milk thistle also contains *silymarin* and *silibinin.* Don't expect to get large amounts of isosilybin-B in regular milk thistle preparations at your health food store; you have to hunt for it. Most regular milk thistle compounds contain very small amounts of isosilybin-B (445). Some websites, such as *Life Extension*™, do sell the milk thistle with this compound. Their supplement is called *Mega Silymarin with Isosilybin B.* See their main website, where you can do a search for isosilybin-B at: *http://www.lef.org* (445).

## Lycopene Cuts Prostate Cancer Risk

Lycopene can reduce the risk for prostatic cancers (119). When nearly 50,000 participating health care workers were followed in a research program conducted at Harvard, it was revealed that eating foods high in lycopene several times a week could cut their chances for prostate cancer in half (119). One of the best (and most popular) sources of lycopene can be found in tomatoes. Though most vegetables are more nutritious in their raw state (the way nature intended), cooked tomatoes may be one of the few exceptions when it comes to preventing cancer (579). It has been demonstrated that cooking tomatoes brings out more of the lycopene than raw (579). Research shows that prevention measures are most successful when cooked tomatoes are consumed at least twice a week *or more* (579). Even dehydrated tomatoes (that are rehydrated before use) have high concentrations of lycopene. Guavas are also rich in lycopene, as are watermelons and many other fruits and vegetables.

Dr. James Balch, author of *The Super Anti-Oxidants*, says that the Italians and Greeks, who are famous for their tomato-based recipes, have very low rates for this type cancer, and it isn't just prostate cancer that lycopene prevents, because scientists have also discovered that women who eat foods rich in lycopene can significantly reduce cervical cancer risk (337).

According to Dr. John W. Erdman of the University of Illinois in Chicago, to get the maximum dose of lycopene, you need to combine it with fat (337). This increases the absorption of lycopene in the colon (337). Good examples would be cooked or stewed tomatoes dressed with olive oil, tomato salad with an olive oil dressing, flax oil with your tomatoes, or fresh avocado mixed with tomatoes or salsa.

Hawaiians eat large amounts of tomatoes and they have fewer incidences of abdominal cancer (363). Other countries where tomato consumption is high enjoy lower rates for lung cancer. Another study showed that seniors who were tomato consumers, were 50% less apt to succumb to cancers as their counterparts who ate fewer tomatoes, and studies from Wales reveal that tomatoes may inhibit *acute appendicitis* (363).

Taking vitamin E supplements with lycopene could enhance its absorption power (243). A news release has stated that high levels of vitamin E could be harmful, contributing to overall mortality rates; however, what you were not told in this release was that most of the people involved in the study already had several other co-morbidities or illnesses affecting them, so of course they had higher death rates. Some nutritional food activists believe that vitamin E supplements in the gamma-tocopherol form (rather than the alpha form) are superior, while others support supplements that have both types.

Website *http://www.newstarget.com/001391.html* recommends eating your tomatoes with broccoli to conquer prostate cancer. Studies show this combo outperforms pharmaceutical drugs in preventing the disease (48).

## Magnesium Protects Against Prostate Cancer

Many people, women especially, are aggressively encouraged to take calcium for their bones as they age, but some health care professionals fail to emphasize the importance of magnesium, without which the cells cannot use calcium efficiently, and excess calcium can do more harm than good. Many of the most important nutrients in our cells must have magnesium to perform their anti-oxidant properties (566). Studies with animals prove that keeping them magnesium-deficient raises free radical activity and will result in malignant cancers. Stressors in the body (e.g., giving a person chemo and/or radiation) also decrease magnesium levels (566). According to Mark Sircus Ac., OMD, being deficient in magnesium raises the risk for prostate cancer (566). Be sure your calcium supplement also contains boron.

For information regarding a way of delivering magnesium chloride directly into the skin in an easily absorbable form (which also works as a pain reliever), see website: *http://www.ancient-minerals.com* (566b)

## Melatonin, Other Extracts, Herbs & Teas for Prostate Health

Doctor Ray Sahelian calls Melatonin **"Nature's Prostate-Shrinking Sleeping Pill"** (547). See his website at *www.raysahelian.com* for more information.

It is not recommended that patients with *leukemia, lymphoma and myeloma* take melatonin (507). There is a possibility that melatonin may accelerate the advancement of these type cancers (507). In addition to this precaution for melatonin, the supplement could cause depression and worsening of allergies in some individuals, and should not be taken by those on cortisone, nor those who are pregnant (192). It is also possible that the hormone can reduce blood flow, interfere with fertility, libido, reduce temperature and cause *retinal damage.* (192). Significant amounts of natural melatonin can be found simply in eating tart cherries (61).

## Milk Thistle Slows Growth of Prostate Cancer

Milk thistle, long known for its protective effects against liver damage, is discussed in great detail in chapter nine of this book because of its power to heal the liver. It is also important for prostate health, because it has been shown to help fight cancers that don't respond favorably to hormone treatment (243).

Be sure to read other notes in this book for those times when you should not take herbal preparations, even those as safe as milk thistle.

## Modified Citrus Pectin for Prostate Cancer

Discussed elsewhere in this book, this fruit pectin has been tested extensively in lab, animal, and human studies and proven helpful for sufferers of prostate cancer. It was found to be safe, effective, and non-toxic. There is a great deal of information on modified citrus pectin on the internet (198).

## Mushrooms That Kill Prostate Cancer Cells

According to Shari Lieberman, Ph.D., and Ken Babal, C.N., in their book, *Maitake Mushroom AND D-Fraction*, researchers found that Maitake D-fraction has the ability to cause cancer cells to self-destruct (469). Scientists conducting laboratory studies noted that D-fraction helped kill malignant prostate cells within one day of exposure (469).

Website *Herbs2000.com* recommends that you do not take maitake if you have *multiple sclerosis* (184). It was also discovered that taking vitamin C along with the Maitake D was more potent, allowing the dosage of maitake to be decreased, yet remain just as effective (184). Note that *Herbs2000.com* and most other such sites do not recommend herbs, mushrooms, and other nutrients as stand-alone cancer therapies. (When taking vitamin C, do not combine it with grape seed extract.)

## Myrrh - Biblical Herb for the Prostate

In laboratory testing, compounds from this biblical herb not only killed breast, brain and prostate cancer cells, it killed the drug-resistant cells without harming nearby healthy cells. Large scale human testing has not yet been done using this herb.

## Nanotechnology—*Lodamin*—Curing Prostate Cancer without Side Effects

A new drug, Lodamin, which works by halting the blood vessel growth that tumors need to survive, was shown (in animal testing) to be effective against many tumor types, including those of the breast, brain, ovaries, uterus, prostate, neuroblastoma and glioblastoma (401). It also worked very well in preventing cancer from going into the liver (401). The discovery of the drug, using *nanotechnology* and a derivative from a fungus, was quite accidental. Reports say that it can be taken orally without *side effects* (401). The drug also inhibited melanoma and lung cancer in mice (401). Lodamin is still in the testing phases, and is also being considered for treating macular degeneration and arthritis.

Shark cartilage and bindweed, also discussed in this book, work to starve tumors by cutting off blood supply to them, without adverse side effects to individuals using them. Note that many other targeted nanoparticles are being tested to fight prostate cancer. Some are being used as a delivery system to send chemo drugs right to the cancer cells only, bypassing healthy cells so that they are not damaged.

## Nexrutine® for Prostate Cancer Prevention

An ingredient that was developed by *Next Pharmaceuticals*, this compound has been found to be an inhibitor of prostate cancer (216). A human study on this natural anti-inflammatory found that it does not cause the stomach upset that is common in aspirin and NSAIDS. It is a derivative from an Asian tree's bark (216). Results of the laboratory study were published in 2006, showing that the bark extract was effective in blocking prostate cancer cell growth (216).

## Noscapine – Cough Medicine Ingredient for Prostate Cancer

A natural, common cough medicine ingredient, Noscapine, is already being used off-label to kill some forms of cancer, including prostate cancer, and without toxic side effects (323a).

## Onconase - New Non-Toxic Drug for Prostate Cancer

This drug (aka *Ranpirnase*) is a new pharmaceutical drug developed for treating mesothelioma. It is claimed to be *free* of the adverse effects that are normally seen in common chemo drugs (222). It is said to work on other cancers, such as those of the prostate. It was developed by a company known as *Alfacell* (222). The drug is also supposed to make it possible to give lower dosages of standard chemo drugs with the same cancer-killing effects. It is said to fight *solid tumor cancers,* such as *carcinomas*, as well as those of the *kidney, breast, lung, and prostate* (222). Just be aware that even though this new drug is said to be relatively free of toxic side effects, drugs such as this are sometimes combined with conventional chemo drugs that do have very toxic side effects. Human trials are currently underway.

## PSK Inhibits Prostate Cancers

A *kawaratake mushroom* extract known as *Polysaccharide kureha (PSK)* was discovered to be beneficial in slowing down the rate of prostate tumor growth and metastasis (236). PSK, sometimes referred to as *krestin,* from the *kawaratake,* has some very potent anti-oxidants and has been the focus of hundreds of research tests. There has been no toxicity when taken by mouth (236). It has also been very effective when combined with conventional treatments (236). You may see the karawatake mushroom referred to as the *coriolus versicolor* mushroom.

## Poly–MVA (Palladium Lipoic Complex)

See other chapters in this book on Poly-MVA, an amazing nutrient that many cancer patients are crediting with healing their cancers completely, including prostate cancers. For testimonials of people who used this substance to cure their prostate cancer (and many other types of cancer), see *http://www.polymvasurvivors.com/testimonials.html.* Many of these testimonials are given ten or more years ago, yet all survivors are still here as of March 2007. You may hear Poly-MVA referred to as *PolyDox.*

## Pomegranate Juice for Recurring Prostate Cancer

Pomegranate is the newest superstar among the anti-oxidants. A fruit that you rarely saw in stores ten years ago is appearing everywhere, and for good reason. This biblical fruit is packed with nutrients and anti-oxidants that fight free radicals in the body. It is now being touted as a deterrent for all types of cancer.

The seeds, and juice from the seeds, also promote heart health by fighting arterial plaque, lowering cholesterol, and preventing the type of inflammation in the colon that can lead to cancer (376). I would recommend that you juice fresh ripened pomegranate. I have tried some of the health food store juices that contain pomegranate only, and have found them to be extremely bitter-tasting.

Drinking pomegranate juice may end up as a helpful therapy to prevent and treat cancers of the prostate, especially those that return (359). You only need eight ounces of this powerful anti-oxidant drink daily (359). Not only is pomegranate juice full of anti-oxidants, but it also contains naturally-occurring estrogen (359). In a clinical trial, 48 men with prostate malignancies participated in drinking pomegranate juice. None reported side effects, nor did any of them experience further spread of the cancer, clearly showing that pomegranate could slow the spread of those already having this type cancer (359).

For a report on a phase II study of the benefits of pomegranate substances for men with prostate cancer, see website: *http://www.pomwonderful.com/pdf/Clinical_Cancer_Research.Pdf.*

## Pumpkin Seeds for Prostate Health

Human research in Stockholm on more than four dozen participants with enlarged prostates, who were given pumpkin seeds, then followed for a 90-day period, revealed that those eating the seeds had remarkable improvements without adverse reactions (394). Pumpkin seeds also help destroy parasites.

## Quercetin Fights Prostate Cancer

Quercetin is a powerful anti-oxidant that may help in the prevention of prostate cancer. This compound can be found in red onions and apples (440). It is also abundant in green tea, cayenne (551), berries, some nuts and seeds, broccoli, and in the herb, ginkgo biloba.

## Red Clover Destroys Prostate Cancer Cells

In a remarkable case described at *www.cancertutor.com/Other/Big_List.htm,* when an elderly physician with a high PSA (which was followed by a biopsy confirming adenocarcinoma) consumed a phytoestrogen from red clover one week before having surgery, post-surgical examination of the tumor cells (and comparing them with the biopsy) revealed results very much like that obtained with hormone treatment using estrogen; the cancerous growth had reversed (251). The physician used a popular form of natural plant hormone known as *Promensil.* He took *160 mg per day*; there were no undesirable reactions (251). Be aware that red clover can thin the blood, so check with your physician or Naturopath before using this or any other herb. You can find *Promensil* in health food stores and in vitamin sections of some grocery chains.

## Reduce Fat Intake—Cut Your Risk of Prostate Cancer

The cancer industry is finally admitting a definite risk for prostate cancer associated with high dietary fat intake. A vegetarian diet dramatically reduces the risk of prostate cancer. This is because fats in the diet raise testosterone levels, and testosterone feeds prostate cancer. It has been proven that lowering male hormone levels can restrict these cancerous growths, and research has revealed that the higher the fat in the diet, the higher the death rate from prostate cancer (550).

One really **big question** we should be asking ourselves is this: how in the world did we end up with such a deadly mixture of hormones in our meats and dairy products? It is because the FDA allows cancer-causing additives to be put into our food supply! The FDA's primary drive since its creation has been to protect the elite, billion dollar drug industries, rather than being concerned about the safety of U.S. citizens (550). We've seen evidence, just recently, of drug companies being dishonest about testing and research with their products, and covering up the truth about harmful side effects in their reports to the FDA. Much of this we have learned in news reports documenting fatalities among patients who were taking prescription medications (550). (Remember Vioxx®? Propulsid? Baycol? Rezulin?) The lure of wealth from the sale of billions in these drugs has warped the morals of many of the drug conglomerates. After all, why should they be worried about paying fines? A $300,000 fine is pennies for someone raking in billions of dollars in drug sales every year. It's a slap on the wrist!

The FDA spends a great deal of time trying to ostracize and eliminate those producing and promoting natural health products (550). All one has to do is read the history of antineoplastons and hydrazine sulfate to find this to be true.

## Resveratrol Halts Prostate Cancer Cells

Recall *The Grape Cure* diet in chapter three? In an article at *Life Extension* website, *www.lef.org,* Terri Mitchell lauds the powerful anti-cancer properties of resveratrol (500). Most amazing about this compound is that it seeks out and destroys the *cancer cells*, leaving normal cells alone, and promotes heart health as well (500). Resveratrol has proven that it can intervene and protect cells from the DNA defects caused by cancer (500).

Yet, another study looking at prostate cancer cells, emphasizes that resveratrol not only inhibits cancer from spreading, but also helps in restricting cancer cells that are hormone-dependent as well as those which are not dependent on hormones for survival (500). For an excellent 58-page study that was done on resveratrol's role in fighting cancer, including prostate cancer, see website at: *http://www.agrawal.org/PDF/ACR-Resveratrol1.pdf.* The study was conducted by M.D. Anderson Cancer Center and the UCLA Center for Human Nutrition (346). Resveratrol is also being touted as a way to fight obesity, since it keeps the body from storing fat.

My only question in all this is: **WHY ISN'T THIS BEING SHOUTED FROM THE ROOFTOPS?** How many men have been advised by their physicians (during their yearly physicals) to start eating grapes (resveratrol), tomatoes (along with a fat source, such as olive oil, flax seed oil, or avocado) (337), broccoli, pomegranates, vitamin E, vitamin D, and raspberries; to reduce their dairy consumption; to make sure that they are not deficient in other vitamins and minerals (e.g., chromium, zinc, magnesium, and boron), in order to drastically cut their chances of developing prostate cancer? (Especially since the studies are showing that resveratrol and raspberries could be useful in **halting prostate cancer once it has already been diagnosed!**) Though resveratrol and lycopene are now available in supplement form at most natural health food stores, whenever possible, it is best to obtain the nutrients from fresh, natural food sources.

## Rexin-G™ for Prostate Cancer & Other Spreading Cancers

Rexin-G™ has been undergoing clinical trials at Mayo Clinic, M.D. Anderson, and a few other facilities. It is a drug for cancers that have spread, and those types of cancer that conventional medicine says do not respond to chemo drugs (256). **Human** clinical studies, thus far, have had good results. In the very first human trial, 83% of the patients experienced tumor shrinkage. The patients all had spreading pancreatic cancer (256). Good responses were also achieved in **human** studies involving several other types of metastatic cancer. Due to the reports, this drug is now used for treating all forms of *solid tumors* in the Philippines that are resistant to conventional therapy (256). The U.S. FDA has given the drug its *orphan drug status* for use with pancreatic cancers in the U.S., as well as other types of cancer metastases, which means that trials will continue (256). It is given intravenously, so isn't exactly natural or painless, but could be considered gentler than older chemo drugs because it is said to be a non-chemo drug, showing itself in **human** clinical trials, not to have the adverse side effects normally associated with chemo drugs (256). You can get more information on this drug at *epeiusbiotech.com/rexin_g-factsheet.asp.* Epeius Biotechnologies are the producers of Rexin-G™ (257).

## Sagopilone Trials for Prostate Cancer

Although this is a synthetic chemo drug from Bayer Health Care and certainly not a natural substance, it is being mentioned in this chapter because you will find many internet and health journals talking about clinical trials in the U.S. and other countries using Sagopilone in combination with Prednisone for treating those prostate cancers that are not hormone-dependent. It is also being tested against other solid tumors.

## Saw Palmetto for Prostate Cancer

Saw Palmetto is a popular herb for prostate protection, but it works best in conjunction with stinging nettle root extract and other prostate-healthy herbs.

According to Ray Sahelian, M.D., author of the book, *Saw Palmetto Nature's Prostate Healer,* a study by Purdue University revealed substances from the berries that halted not only cancerous cells growing in the prostate, but those in the pancreas and kidneys as well (547). (This information is also available at Dr. Sahelian's website at *www.raysahelian.com/saw.html.)* Saw Palmetto has been used by many health care practitioners to treat problems with prostate inflammation and enlargement.

This herb is a best-selling prostate treatment in Europe. Many **human** studies show successful treatment of prostatic hypertrophy using this herb (364). Media reports recently came out with information denying the potency of saw palmetto for helping the prostate; however, saw palmetto by itself is rarely recommended by alternative physicians. It always works best with an adequate dietary regimen, and in combination with other herbs, like nettle root. It will do little to help your prostate to take herbs for prostate health if you are deficient in vital minerals, such as selenium, chromium, zinc, magnesium, and nutrients like vitamin C, lycopene, beta-carotene, CoQ10, B vitamins, and others.

## Selenium Cuts Risk for All Cancers

A *JAMA* article in 1996 stated that having sufficient selenium in the diet could prevent 69% of prostate cancer cases. Leafy greens are a good source of selenium as are Brazil nuts (507), wheat germ and eggs.

A **human** study (from the *British Journal of Urology*) involving 974 men taking selenium supplements, showed a 63% reduction in prostate cancer in those who were taking 200 **micrograms** of selenium daily for 4.5 years (266). There were also lower cancer deaths in the men taking selenium (from all types of cancer), and lower rates of colorectal and lung cancers. Further trials were planned (266). Some of these trials have been completed since my first book was released (reports from the latter part of 2008) denouncing the role of selenium in preventing prostate cancer. Please see the last chapter of this book for a discussion on that research.

## St. John's Wort

Italian scientists have recently discovered that this herb, in animal testing, can fight prostate cancer (477). Do not use it if you are on anti-depressant MAO inhibitors. As always, check with your physician or Naturopath first.

## Sunshine Prevents Prostate Cancer

Adequate exposure to sunlight can significantly prevent prostate cancer. Human studies in Great Britain on more than 200 participants with this type cancer (and nearly as many with hyperplasia), revealed that those having lower doses of sunlight were thrice as likely to have prostate cancer as men with greater sunshine exposure during their lifespan (280). If you have a hereditary tendency for melanoma, or other skin disorders, be sure to check with your physician or Naturopath before you attempt unprotected sunlight exposure.

## Testicular Cancers - Decreasing the Risks

Though this chapter deals mostly with prostate cancer, just realize that boosting the body's immune system will help prevent other cancers, such as testicular cancers, not just prostate cancers. Testicular cancers often appear at first as a small painless nodule that men will dismiss as insignificant. This form of "denial" can be fatal. If caught early, these cancers can be easily treated. Once they spread, treatment is much more difficult. Many of the alternative, non-toxic therapies given in this book will help boost the immune system, but there are two items to keep in mind that will increase the risk for this type cancer:

- In a male child who has a congenital malformation known as "undescended testis," if parents delay surgery, until "after the age of 13," to bring the testis down to the normal position, a study involving "nearly 17,000 men and boys from Sweden," revealed that this will increase the risk for *testicular cancer*, as noted in an article at *CancerConsultants.com* (525a).
- Firefighters, according to this same website, are "twice as likely to develop testicular cancer [and] roughly 50% more likely to develop multiple myeloma or non-Hodgkins lymphoma, and 28% more likely to develop prostate cancer" (466a). Research that involved *100,000 firefighters,* emphasized the importance of "protective gear" and always bathing completely when they are finished fire fighting (466a).

## Testicular Cancers – How Conventional Medicine Treats Them

Note that conventional medicine treats testicular cancer with chemo drugs and radiation. Recently, they are moving away from the radiation in those with **early** stages of the disease, and mostly recommending the drug, Carboplatin (171a). Sometimes just a single treatment is needed, which they say, evidenced from human studies involving hundreds of men, can bring about a cure. These patients usually undergo surgery as well, to remove the affected testicle (171a). Though a chemo drug, Carboplatin is being mentioned here because it is yet another choice for those fighting prostate cancer, if not choosing natural, less toxic therapy.

## Testosterone Levels & Prostate Health

High testosterone levels, and steroid injections containing testosterone, increase the risk for developing prostate cancer.

## Turmeric & Prostate Cancer

As described at the American Association for Cancer Research, the active ingredient in turmeric, *curcumin*, is effective at destroying cancer cells. (299). Turmeric triggers the work of a special gene, the *p53* gene, which fights cancer and the spread of cancer (180). Turmeric is safe when used as a spice; however, if you are taking turmeric in supplement form, do not use if pregnant, nor if you have gallstones, since it stimulates the gallbladder (571). Like garlic, turmeric can slow clotting time, so it should be used in caution by anyone taking blood-thinners (571), with blood disorders, or for anyone recovering from or contemplating surgery, or with ulcers and other gastric disorders. If you want a turmeric capsule that is free of magnesium stearate additive, see *Nature's Way®* brand. Yellow mustard is very high in turmeric. If you want your body to absorb turmeric more easily, eat it with pineapple or supplement with bromelain.

## Ukrain - Non-Toxic Cure for Prostate Cancer

Ukrain is a combination of two substances that, when given individually, are both toxic, but once combined, they are only toxic to cancer cells (287). Ukrain is only available through alternative health clinics in the U.S., Canada, and Europe. You will need to seek an alternative health physician in the United States for Ukrain therapy, or travel to Europe, Canada or Mexico where it is popular. (For pictures of how Ukrain works, see website: *http://www.ukrain-drug.net/webspeed/index.htm.)*

A **human** study that involved more than 200 advanced-stage cancer participants (who had failed all conventional treatments), showed remarkable results when they received Ukrain. They were given Ukrain, hyperthermia therapy, selenium, Tagamet, *Vitamin A*, and *thyme extract* (334). Several types of cancer were treated, but the best results were seen in prostate and seminoma cancers. 70% of the prostate cancer participants saw their cancers completely disappear! When all cancers were considered, more than 40% of all participants experienced *total remission.* This human study can be found at PubMed website PMID: 11345032 (334).

Another study with the use of Ukrain for prostate cancer in **humans** involved elderly participants who received dosages of "100 mg (10 mg intravenously every second day, 10 injections altogether...") Every single patient reported doing better after only "two to three injections of Ukrain." It was proven that their T-lymphocytes and T-helper cells had remarkably increased. See the full study at National Library of Medicine's PubMed website, NCBI PMID 11345026 (587).

Ukrain is sometimes combined with conventional medicine, such as radiation therapy. A patient who was diagnosed with *non-seminomatous germ-cell tumor of the testis*, who had received Ukrain after surgery and after *gamma-radiotherapy*, was observed for a two year period. He had no *recurrence* or spread of the disease. The case study can be read at National Library of Medicine's website *http://www.ncbi.nlm.nih.gov.* Refer to PMID 8899344 (548). Remember that Ukrain has no adverse effects—radiation often does—especially in large doses.

## Vitamin E & Selenium – Latest Controversy

Though prior human studies showing that having adequate selenium & vitamin E could cut the incidence of prostate cancer by at least *30 percent* (532), newer studies are saying that this may not be the case, but those studies do not say whether a natural or SYNTHETIC form of vitamin E was used. See the last chapter in this book for details on that research.

Apparently, keeping high levels of vitamin E in the body can protect against bladder cancer (524). In one particular study, vitamin E from alpha-tocopherol and gamma-tocopherol sources was used (524). Some researchers believe that the gamma form of vitamin E is superior to the alpha-tocopherol form in cancer prevention. If using the alpha, do not get vitamin E in the synthetic form which is called **dl**-alpha. Use the **d**-alpha. Some researchers believe that for best results, you need both: the vitamin E that is d-alpha with gamma-tocopherol and mixed tocotrienols.

Some good **natural sources** of vitamin E are: wheat germ oil, olive oil, sunflower oil (and seeds), dandelion greens, spinach, broccoli, turnip greens, almonds and other nuts, eggs (411) (492) (524), kiwi and mangoes, fortified cereals and fresh sprouts, especially wheat berry sprouts.

## Water (Adequate Hydration) Prevents Cancer

The late Dr. F. Batmanghelidj, M.D., in his book, *Your Body's Many Cries For Water*, said that cancer patients are dehydrated. It is important that you take sufficient water, depending on your body weight. Extra water also requires extra salt. "For every 10 glasses of water (about two quarts)," you need a "half teaspoon of salt per day" (341), unless your physician has you on a water-restricted or salt-restricted diet. Many people who go on long fasts drink large amounts of water, forgetting that they also need to increase their salt intake and other minerals.

## Soda Bicarb, Iodine, Magnesium & Invasive Prostate Cancer Cure

For an amazing study on the importance of alkalizing the body with a rapid, powerful ingredient as simple as sodium bicarbonate, see the book: *Sodium Bicarbonate Rich Man's Poor Man's Cancer Treatment* by Dr. Mark Sircus, Ac., OMD. He discusses a detailed step-by-step program that a man with prostate cancer (that had spread into his bones) used to alkalize his body with oral soda bicarb, curing his cancer within 11 days (566c). You can get *Arm & Hammer*® soda bicarb at your local grocers for about a dollar–a-pound. They do not advertise the product for cancer use, but it is used for alkalizing a "sour stomach." There has been some controversy about aluminum in baking soda, but *Arm & Hammer*® says that their product contains no aluminum. For a company that sells a soda bicarb that they guarantee to be aluminum-free, see Bob's Red Mill products at: *http://www.bobsredmill.com* (566c). Simply use pH testing strips that you can get at your local health food store to check your urine or saliva pH.

Dr. Sircus also has much to say about the pervasive lack of magnesium and iodine in the average diet, and why these deficiencies are causing heart disease, cancer, and many other diseases. These minerals are required in every single metabolic process of the body without which we cannot survive. See his amazing books, *Magnesium The Ultimate Heart Medicine* and *Magnesium Medicine The Lamp of Life*, available at: *http://www.magnesiumforlife.com* (566b). He also discusses a new transdermal form of magnesium that you simply spray onto your skin (or use as flakes in your bath or in a footbath), which can be found at website: *http://www. ancient-minerals.com* or *www.magneticclay.com*.(566b).

Also, see Dr. Sircus' book, *Iodine Bringing Back the Universal Medicine,* on the importance of iodine in fighting yeast (and killing cancer in the process), bacteria, malaria, flu, and many other ailments caused by a deficiency in this critical mineral (566a). You can find a food-grade, gentle form of superior iodine called *Magnascent* (or *Nascent* iodine) at *http://www.magnascent.com* and *http://www.magneticclay.com.* Also, see Appendix II. If you want a handy alkalizer that contains soda bicarb and potassium bicarb that you can carry with you, try *Alka-Seltzer*® *Gold.* It has no aspirin.

# CHAPTER 6

# GENTLE CURES FOR TOUGH COLON, COLORECTAL & ABDOMINAL CANCERS

*"My son, attend to my words, incline thine ear unto my sayings. Let them not depart from thine eyes; keep them in the midst of thine heart. For they are life unto those that find them, and health to all their flesh." (Proverbs 4:20-22)*

## I. Colon Cancer & Abdominal Cancer Vanish

### Case #1

George Malkmus had been a Baptist pastor for 20 years when he was diagnosed with colon cancer. He was 42-years-old and he refused to go the conventional medicine—cut, poison, and burn routine. He asked:

> What was I to do…? As a pastor of 20 years, I had sat at the bedside of so many people and watched the devastating effects of chemotherapy, radiation and surgery experienced by others in the treatment of their cancers, I had also conducted the funerals for many of them (147).

Reverend Malkmus cured himself completely of colon cancer, the same cancer that had killed his mother, who had been treated with conventional cancer therapy. He began a diet of raw fruits and vegetables that included large amounts of freshly-extracted juices. His diet is very similar to the one advocated by Eydie Mae Hunsberger and Ann Wigmore. His website at *www.hacres.com* gives details about his *Hallelujah Acres* diet (476). Reverend Malkmus believes that disease is caused when "mankind strays from the original Genesis 1:29 diet of raw fruits and vegetables [and], God intends us to earn this food by 'the sweat of thy face' (exercise)" (476). The *Hallelujah Acres* "diet and lifestyle not only cured his colon cancer," but Rev. Malkmus said it also "gave him relief from a variety of other ailments…high blood pressure, hemorrhoids, hypoglycemia, and severe sinus and allergy problems," and he insists that "He has not been to a doctor, or even taken an aspirin, for over twenty years, and is now in his mid-sixties with more energy than he had as a teenager" (476). You can find many health products at Hallelujah Acres website *http://www.hacres.com/products/productsasp* (476).

## Case #2

When a physician had part of his stomach removed due to cancer, and the cancer returned less than two years later, chemo was recommended. Few patients survive a year with this type of recurrence. Dr. E. refused chemo and opted instead to go on the Budwig diet (described below). The diet cured him, and that was over 18 years ago (100). Johanna Budwig, during a radio station program in September of 1967, discussed her success [using the Budwig diet] with a colon cancer patient who was 84-years-old. She was able to cure him within days, using her protocol (100).

The Budwig flax oil formula is given below. Please note, however, that the entire Budwig diet regimen includes many other specifics (for example restrictions on eating sugar and hydrogenated fats, etc.), which can be found in chapters 14 and 18 of this book, as well as website *www.healingcancernaturally.com/budwig_protocol.html,* and in Johanna's books:

> For each tablespoon of flaxseed oil, add 2 tablespoons of low-fat cottage cheese (or quark) or 6 tablespoons of yoghurt. The flaxoil/cottage cheese or flaxoil/yoghurt mixture should be fully blended until no traces of oil remain visible, proving that the highly unsaturated fatty acids have become water soluble (a hand-held mixer or a blender works well (100). [Quark is a pasty type of white cheese.]

This simple formula is eaten 3 - 4 times each day. See chapter 14 of this book for more details on the Budwig flax oil diet that many people have used to cure inoperable brain cancer. Chapter 14 and chapter 26 of this book will also tell you why you may wish to substitute organic yogurt, or use cottage cheese made from organic, raw milk. Note that yogurt (in **human** studies) protects the colon and wards off infections by increasing the body's immunity and supporting the liver.

Fermented soy products, such as Haelan, may help remove harmful estrogens from the body in estrogen receptor-positive cancers.

For information on Haelan, see the company's website at *www.haelan 951.com.* Information on Haelan's Research Foundation's website was accumulated from clinical studies performed on fermented soy beverages manufactured by Haelan Products, Inc. of Woodinville, Washington. The

Haelan fermented soy beverages are sold in the United States, without medical claims, and are available directly from the company or one of their distributors (143).

Recent studies show that flax seed can help slow the expansion of cancers in the breast and intestinal growths that do not depend on estrogen. Flax seed also reduces harmful cholesterol, elevates good cholesterol, and helps the body dump toxic estrogens (394). Flax oil can be found in natural health food stores and even some popular grocery chains. If you purchase flax oil, it should always be refrigerated and **never heated**. One of the best ways to take fresh flax is to purchase the organic flax seeds whole, grind them in a coffee grinder and mix in water, juice, or oatmeal. If putting it in a drink, you need to drink it quickly, because flax thickens very fast.

# II. Other Cancer Issues

## Abdominal Cancer & Gluten

Note that there are some types of cancer that can be caused by allergies. For example, it is believed that *gluten-sensitive-enteropathy,* sprue (or celiac disease) can lead to a type of t-cell lymphoma, an abdominal cancer that is actually a result of being allergic to the type gluten found in wheat, barley, rye and/or oats. People with this type allergy would also want to avoid any foods with the word ***couscous***, which is a ground semolina wheat. This gluten is not found in rice or corn. It is believed responsible for a type of dermatitis known as *dermatitis herpetiformis*. Most health food stores now sell breads and flours that are made without gluten.

## Abdominal Liposarcoma

Dr. Abram Hoffer, a medical doctor as well as a biochemist, well known for his use of Orthomolecular Medicine (megadose vitamin and/or mineral treatments), was able to extend the life of a patient with abdominal liposarcoma for six years with complementary medicine. The details can be found at his webpage: *http://www.islandnet.com/~hoffer/*. Complementary medicine is a combination of orthodox and alternative medicine (which includes orthomolecular medicine), also referred to as *CAM* (432).

## Fungus Cure Also Cures Cancer, Says Oncology Physician

See chapter 34 of this book for the amazing cancer cure that Italian Oncologist, Dr. Simoncini, is using to cure his cancer patients within just days! Cancerous growths are usually WHITE. He says that they are actually a fungus, which can be killed with a non-toxic soda bicarb solution that quickly alkalizes the tumor for destruction. He uses a soda bicarb wash for colon cancers (582).

## NEW Procedures for Finding Colorectal Cancers

**Scopes:** New, more precise diagnostic procedures are being used for early detection of colorectal cancers and for diagnosing other bowel diseases. The standard has been the colonoscopy, but colonoscopies may miss up to one third of cancers (330). You may hear these new procedures referred to as *optical coherence tomography*, light technology, endoscopies, spectroscopies, *autofluorescence, endocytoscopy, narrow band imaging (NBI), confocal endomicroscopy and endocytoscopy* (330), *and Third Eye Retroscope*™ (114). If you are undergoing diagnostics for bowel problems, or at high risk for colon cancer, you may want to bring these procedures to your physician's attention if they have not already suggested them (330).

**CD24**: This is a new blood test developed by Tel Aviv researchers, led by Professor Nadir Arber, that can screen for colon cancer with special *biomarkers* which detect the presence of polyps in the colon (82a) It is a simple, gentle, *non-invasive* procedure that is said to have a greater than 80% accuracy rate (82a). It is not yet available in the U.S.

**CCSA-2:** This is a new blood test that spots a protein called *Colon Cancer-specific Antigen-2* and helps identify colon growths that are most likely to end up malignant.

**ColoSure:** is a new test produced by *LabCorp* to *test for cancer-related genes* in *stool samples* (175). More and more studies are showing genetic traits for some colon cancers.

**FIT Testing:** (*fecal immunochemical testing*) is a test that may help detect *colorectal cancers earlier*, even using them in between routine colonoscopies, especially for people who are at high risk for colon cancer (115). FIT testing is done at home and is non-invasive. Two types of FIT tests developed by *Quest Diagnostics* are *InSure FIT* and *Insure Quik FIT*. See more details at: *http:///www.emaxhealth.com/100/22493.html*, and also check with your physician or Naturopath about diagnostic testing devices, especially if you are at high risk for colon cancer (115), e.g., you have a familial history of colon polyps, colon cancer, or have already had colon polyps or colon cancer yourself.

**iFOBT**: is an at-home colon cancer screening test for occult blood.

**Virtual Colonoscopy & Optical Technology:** Though there are some new advances in virtual colonoscopy, the procedure has been around a few years. It involves insertion of a tube into the rectum, putting air into the colon, then taking pictures of the colon. The downside is that a physician cannot always see smaller polyps, and if polyps are seen, they can't be removed this way. Also, the pictures are not usually as clear as those in a routine colonoscopy which uses imaging to assist the doctor. The upside is that no sedatives are needed, and the procedure only takes about ten minutes, and it has recently been reported that this test can also check for bone density.

Northwestern University is testing a new type of *optical technology* for finding early cancers of the colon, which will be less invasive than current colonoscopy procedures (210).

## OncoVAX-Immunotherapy Treatment for Colon Cancer

OncoVAX may be the new kid on the block when it comes to helping the body fight cancer; however, it has been around for more than thirty years with many millions of dollars spent on its research (594). Developed by a company known as *Vaccinogen,* OncoVAX is being studied and used in Switzerland (594). The Swiss consider it a *transplant.* It may still be some time before the treatment is sanctioned in the U.S. In this therapy, the patient first has surgery for colon cancer. The tumor cells are taken from the patient and used to make a vaccine from the patient's own cells. The vaccine is then given to the patient over a period of *six months* in a series of four injections (594). The vaccine then works to help the patient fight the disease with his or her own immune cells. The Vaccinogen company has just recently opened a center in Frederick, Maryland. More information can be found about OncoVAX on the internet and at website: *http://www.fredericknewspost.com/sections/news/display.htm?StoryID=70291* (594).

## Radio-immunotherapy (131-I Labetuzumab) for Colorectal Cancer which has Spread

Though by no means a *natural* treatment, this drug, developed by Immunomedics, Inc., is being mentioned because proponents say that in a Phase II study involving 40 patients (with colorectal cancer that had spread to the liver), there were some positive results, with the only side effect being "transient myelosuppression," as noted by Dr. Johannes Meller of the University of Gottingen, Germany (254). In other words, the patients experienced only mild immune system (bone marrow) suppression (254). Further testing is planned.

## Rexin-G™ for Colon, Pancreatic Cancer & Other Advanced Cancers

Rexin-G™ has been undergoing clinical trials at Mayo Clinic, M.D. Anderson, and a few other facilities. It is a drug for cancers that have spread, and those types of cancer that conventional medicine says do not respond to chemo drugs (256). Human clinical studies, thus far, have had good results. In the very first human trial, 83% of the patients experienced tumor shrinkage. The patients all had spreading pancreatic cancer (256). Good responses were also achieved in **human** studies involving several other types of metastatic cancer. Due to the reports, this drug is now used for treating all forms of *solid tumors* in the Philippines that are resistant to conventional therapy (256). The U.S. FDA has given the drug its *orphan drug status* for use with pancreatic cancers in the US, as well as other types of cancer metastases, which means that trials will continue (256). It is given intravenously, so isn't exactly natural or painless, but could be considered gentler than older chemo drugs. Actually, it is said to be a non-chemo drug, showing itself in human clinical trials, not to have the adverse side effects normally associated with chemo drugs (256). You can get more information on this drug at *epeiusbiotech.com/rexin_g-factsheet.asp.* Epeius Biotechnologies are the producers of Rexin-G™ (257).

# III. Fighting Colon, Rectal & Abdominal Cancers With Nutrients & Non-Toxic Substances

## AHCC—Mushroom Combo Enhances Immunity

AHCC *(Active hexose correlated compound)* is actually a complex compound from the mycelia of many mushrooms (206). In **human** testing, it was found, when given to patients by mouth for a period of two to six months, to significantly increase the body's natural immunity, thus enabling the death of stomach cancer cells and several other types of cancerous cells. The patients received three grams per day of AHCC (206). This compound is found in many natural health food stores and through online supplement providers, such as *www.discount-vitamins-herbs .net.*

## Apples, Apple Juice & Unfiltered Apple Juice Help Prevent Colon Cancer

Eating apples, which are rich in pectin, and drinking apple juice keep the colon healthy (23). A substance known as *butyrate* is found in apple juice and pectin which thwarts cancerous growths in the colon (23). Another report from *sciencedaily.com* says that scientists in Germany have recommended ingesting 8 to 24 *ounces per day of cloudy apple juice (unfiltered)* for preventing colon cancer. This drink, in animal studies, decreased *small intestine* tumors by *38* and *40 percent* (212). Researchers in Poland said that the unfiltered juice has four times the anti-oxidants of filtered juice (212). Apples are also important in preventing osteoporosis, reducing the incidence of asthma in children, helping to prevent lung, liver, and breast cancer, and reducing cellular need for insulin.

## Aronia Berries for the Colon

Aronia berries have gained the reputation of being higher in plant anti-oxidants (known as *proanthocyanidins*) than any other berry found in nature, and may help in fighting cancer of the colon (13). They are also useful in maintaining a healthy urinary system (13).

## Avanex 7-1037 for Colorectal Cancer & Other Tumors

A new drug that, in animal testing, was able to destroy colorectal and other tumors without the harmful effects that most chemo drugs cause, Avanex 7-1037, is undergoing further testing (29). More information on this drug can be found at *anavex.com* website. Additional studies are being done in France. Also, see website *pr.com/press-release/67828,* for more information (29).

## Beta-Carotene Cuts Colorectal Cancer Risk in Human Study

A scientific, randomized, clinical trial involving over 700 people showed that consuming beta-carotene supplements cut the risk for colorectal cancer recurrence by 44% in non-smoking participants, as long as they did not consume alcoholic beverages (339).

## Bindweed May Fight Cancer Better Than Shark Cartilage

For more information on a common field weed that is touted to be effective at fighting cancer, see chapter 34 in this book (150) (301a). It is also discussed in the chapters in this book that deal with breast cancer, ovarian cancer, and pancreatic cancer.

## Black Raspberries for Colon Cancer Prevention

Scientists from Ohio State University found that rodents ingesting black raspberries had *60 percent* fewer esophageal tumors and *80 percent* fewer colon tumors. Clinical trials on humans are currently in progress (213).

## Blueberries for Colon Cancer Prevention

An ingredient in blueberries, known as *pterostilbene* (mentioned elsewhere in this book), was found by researchers at the U.S. Department of Agriculture and Rutgers University to prevent colon cancer in animal studies (37). It also helps lower cholesterol "as effective as a drug," with possibly "fewer side effects," according to lab research (37), and it fights heart disease, enhances memory and inhibits liver cancer (38). (When was the last time you ate blueberries?)

## Burzynski's Antineoplastons for Curing Colon Cancer

I discussed this non-toxic treatment in several other chapters of this book (e.g., see chapter 14 on brain cancer). Antineoplastons are a non-toxic treatment for cancer developed by Dr. Stanislaw Burzynski. The only place that the FDA will allow him to operate his clinic is in Houston, Texas.

June H. was diagnosed at age 78 with *adenocarcinoma* of the colon that had spread to her lymph nodes. This was in June of 2002. She chose not to have the chemo and radiation her physician recommended and instead, went to see Dr. Burzynski and underwent his PB (oral antineoplaston) non-toxic cancer treatment. By April of 2003, her cancer had disappeared and she is now considered cancer-free. For details about her case, see website: *http://burzynskipatientgroup.org/juneh.htm.* For the main Burzynski website, go to: *http://www.burzynskiclinic.com.* The FDA has finally approved the use of PBs (sodium phenylbutrates), which you can obtain by prescription from your physician, and the use of antineoplastons as *orphan drug status* for gliomas. (PBs, taken orally, are converted by the liver into antineoplastons.)

## Chicory Root

*Chicory Root,* commonly put in popular coffee recipes, has a cancer-fighting substance called *inulin,* not to be confused with insulin (74). According to *cancertutor.com,* researchers (in animal testing) have found that this compound helps block cancerous colon cells. Their findings were recently described in the *British Journal of Nutrition* (74).

## Cholesterol Drug for Colon Cancer - No Toxic Side Effects

For detailed information on a new cancer-treatment regimen that includes combining "low-dose interferon with lovastatin," so far used in melanoma (but also being considered for other cancers like colon cancer—doctors saw tumors start to regress—often in a mere *few weeks*) (76a), see website *www.neoplas.org,* and chapter 34 in this book. The treatment has no toxic side effects as found in chemo and *radiation* (76a). Just be aware that statin drugs can strip CoQ10 out of your body. If you choose this treatment, let your doctor know this so that he or she can advise you on CoQ10 supplementation. Some physicians are not yet aware of this downside to statin drugs.

## Citrus Fights Colon Cancer

New research from Texas A & M University and Japan's Kanazawa Medical University has proven that citrus fruits fight not only cancer, but *high cholesterol and obesity* as well (535). In animal testing, *freeze-dried grapefruit* reduced the formation of *early* cancers of the colon. Cancer-fighting properties were also found in a tangerine extract known as *nobiletin.* Scientists from the University of Hawaii discovered that *6 ounces of grapefruit a day* helps fight the toxins in cigarette smoke, thus, may also fight cancer risk in smokers (535). Be aware that you cannot drink grapefruit juice when you are on certain medicines. Always check with your physician or Naturopathic doctor.

## Coffee Drinking Helps in Prevention of Colon Cancer

Scientists in Germany have discovered, in animal testing, that coffee—rich in an anti-oxidant known as *methylpyridinium*—produces *enzymes* in the body capable of fighting colon cancer; however, don't look for the substance in the raw beans, it isn't there (154). It forms when the coffee goes through the *roasting process*, and you get the substance whether you drink *caffeinated* or *decaffeinated coffee*. Stronger coffee worked better. Further research is planned (154). Coffee also helps in other cancers (discussed elsewhere in this book), and it may even help decrease the risk for type II diabetes (80), but beware, because *four or more cups* (daily) can also double your risk for *rheumatoid arthritis* (81).

## Cranberries Halt Colon Tumors

Cranberries (high in proanthocyanidins), in research studies, halted the progression and formation of cancerous colon growths. (Cranberries also fight leukemia and cut the risk for ulcers and bladder infections (22.)

In a clinical trial with hundreds of children with the *H-pylori infection,* cranberry juice was able to kill H-pylori when they drank the juice for *three weeks* (*200 ml—daily*). This bacteria can also cause ulcers, gastritis, and increases the risk for a type of lymphoma and stomach cancer (102).

## Curcumin (Turmeric) & Colon Cancer

There have been more than a thousand articles published in scientific and medical magazines and journals on the importance of curcumin (turmeric) in fighting cancer of the colon, liver, lungs, and other cancers and ailments. 400 or more articles can be found in the National Library of Medicine PubMed. This ingredient may be the world's next wonder drug. It is the main ingredient in the common table spice, turmeric. Be sure to discuss curcumin or turmeric with your physician before taking supplements. It can stimulate bile production (571) and cause problems for those who have ulcers or other gastric disorders. If you want a turmeric capsule that is free of magnesium stearate additive, see *Nature's Way*® brand. The best way to get curcumin is not in curry powder, but in organic turmeric. Curcumin is a natural anti-inflammatory. This is important, because many scientists believe that cancer starts as an inflammatory process. Turmeric has been shown to activate gene *p53,* which helps in the destruction of cancer cells (83). Note that turmeric is also being studied for its potential ability to help in the treatment of cystic fibrosis, and research has shown that it may help prevent diseases like Crohn's and colitis. Yellow mustard is very high in turmeric. If you want your body to absorb turmeric more easily, eat it with pineapple or supplement with bromelain.

## Cytotron Therapy

See chapter 34 in this book for more details on this gentle, painless, non-invasive cancer therapy that many people are also using to restore cartilage in their joints, making joint-replacement surgeries completely unnecessary (90). You may hear this referred to as *QMR* or *Quantum Magnetic Resonance*—they are the same thing.

## ECT—ElectroChemical Therapy for Gastric Cancer

Also described as *direct-current* ECT, this therapy originated in China (474). Widespread human testing has not yet been carried out in the U.S. In animals, *platinum electrodes* are placed on the tumor and treated with direct current (474). Animals with *colorectal carcinomas* that had spread to the liver had *significant* tumor shrinkage (474). More studies are planned in the U.S.

Currently, an ECT machine developed by *Solco Biomedical* (known as the "Solco SET-C21" by Swedish Professor, Nordenstrom), is claimed to have minimal side effects, boosts the immunity, and changes the pH of cells via electrochemical reaction. It is available from Korea. The therapy is being used for most cancers including gastric, breast, lung, skin, and liver (275). It is widely used in Chinese hospitals, Korea, Germany and some cancer treatment centers in the U.S.

## Flavenols & Colon Cancer

Flavenols are merely anti-oxidants that occur in all fruits and vegetables given to us by our Creator. Researchers are experimenting with many types of food flavenols, even trying to produce synthetic versions for fighting cancer. Substances like cocoa bean (from where we get chocolate) are being tested. Nutritionists say that dark chocolate is best, but beware, because some chocolate processors remove the flavenols and add fat and sugar, making them unhealthy. Some excellent flavenols are the pine bark extracts, OPC's, pycnogenols, and quercetin (discussed elsewhere in this book).

According to a new study involving 2000 **human** participants, other flavenols, such as those found in *tea, onions, beans, and apples,* can dramatically cut your risk for colon cancer by as much as *76 percent* (378). Research was led by Gerd Bobe from the *National Cancer Institute.* After the study, the researchers said that these flavonols could dramatically decrease "advanced adenoma recurrence" (378). In 2006, scientists in Italy reached similar conclusions—that some flavonols could cut in half a person's risk for intestinal cancers (rectal and colon) (378). Other flavenol sources include some types of wine, nuts, and other fruits and vegetables (378).

## Flax Seed Prevents Colon Cancer

Animal testing has shown that ingesting ground flax seed can inhibit cancers of the colon. Ground flax meal is much better than using flax oil for this purpose, because the flax meal is so much higher in disease-fighting lignans than the oil (374).

## Magnesium for Gastric Cancer Prevention

This is one of the most important cancer-fighting minerals in the body. Studies with animals have proven that keeping them magnesium-deficient will result in malignant cancers. Adequate levels of magnesium in the body can protect against gastric cancer (566). To find out more, including details for a way of delivering magnesium chloride directly into the skin in an easily absorbable form (which also works as a pain reliever), see website: *http://www.ancient-minerals.com* (566b). Epsom salts, that some people use in their bathwater, contain magnesium, but it is magnesium sulfate and is inferior to the magnesium chloride at above website.

## *The Maker's Diet*

Jordan S. Rubin, N.M.D., Ph.D., in his book, *The Maker's Diet*, documents a determined struggle of trying to regain his health when he rapidly deteriorated and almost died, not from cancer, but from Crohn's Disease. He wasn't sure whether the MMR (measles, mumps, rubella) vaccine he received at age 15 (which has been implicated in causing digestive disorders like Crohn's and autism) may or may not have been a factor leading to his disease, but he realized that his unhealthy diet and lifestyle certainly contributed to his illness (539). Near death, he finally met a nutritionist who recommended a biblical diet to him that he followed and regained his health (539). He advocates similar dietary restrictions as those of the Old Testament in Deuteronomy 14 and Leviticus 11 (539).

As far as the admonition regarding clean and unclean animals, much later in the Bible (in the New Testament), the apostle Peter was given a vision from heaven revealing a change in dietary restrictions in Acts chapter 10, allowing for the consumption of animals previously banned from the *kosher* diet; however, in spite of all this, our meat supply has become polluted with hormones, herbicides, and pesticides. As for fish and seafood, it is widely known that mercury poisoning and other health issues with fish and seafood have existed for years. If you include dairy products, seafood, and meats in your diet, buy certified ORGANIC only so that you are assured you will not be consuming hormones and other toxins that may take you longer to recover and make you more ill than you already are. Regardless of all this, I believe the evidence is overwhelmingly in favor of a raw foods vegan diet for those interested in cancer prevention, treatment and recovery, as opposed to one that allows meats and dairy.

See chapter 26 on dairy, later in this book, before you decide to keep dairy products in your diet, organic or not. Realize too that researchers believe that some cancers have a genetic tendency.

## Olive Oil & Olive-Skin Pomace for Colon Cancer Prevention

Scientists in Ireland have recently discovered, in laboratory testing, that the anti-oxidant effects from consuming extra virgin olive oil may help in colon cancer prevention (595). Scientists from the University of Granada and the University of Barcelona recently discovered a triterpene known as *maslinic acid* in olive-skin pomace, capable of killing colon cancer cells (85a).

## Proteolytic Enzymes for Gastric Cancer

Proteolytic enzymes are enzymes made by the pancreas. Papain (found in pineapples) and enzymes found in papaya are also considered proteolytic enzymes. You can find these enzyme supplements in health food stores.

Human trials showed that proteolytic enzymes—combined with chemo—could increase the lifespan by 3.5 years in dozens of stage III stomach cancer patients, as well as help to decrease the side effects of the chemo (514). Be sure to read the rest of this book before starting chemo.

## Raisins Help Prevent Colon Cancer

Raisins are very high in fiber, but they also contain a wonderful substance that keeps the colon cleaned out, making it more healthy and less susceptible to disease. Eat organic raisins. Avoid raisins which have sulfide and other preservatives. Sunview® has delicious organic raisins.

## Vegetables Help Fight Colon Cancer with Quercetin & Curcumin

One of your best defenses in fighting colon cancer is ordinary vegetables, specifically those containing two powerful anti-oxidants, quercetin and curcumin, such as *onions and curry* (252a). A small human study involving patients with the hereditary disorder, *familial adenomatous polyposis,* which causes massive numbers of polyps to grow in the colon and rectum, which in turn leads to colon cancer, showed that including high amounts of onion and curry worked very much like NSAIDS, anti-inflammatory drugs at fighting the overgrowth of the polyps, except these natural foods do not have the adverse side effects that are associated with NSAIDS

(252a). There was a dramatic drop in the *colorectal cancer cells*, as well as a decrease in the *number of polyps…by 60 percent* (252a) in this study. Even the polyps themselves shrank in size by *51 percent.* The volunteers were given "…20 mg of quercetin (…from onions) and 480 mg of curcumin (…from curry)" during a six month study (252a). Those involved in the study said you could get the same results by adding onions to your diet every day, but not so with the curry – you would have to use supplements to get the amount of curry needed (252a). More studies will be needed on both substances. (If using curry, I recommend organic turmeric as your curry source, since some of the curry found on supermarket shelves may be mixed with undesirable dyes and additives.)

## IV. How Resveratrol Cured Abdominal Cancer

Resveratrol has proven so potent against cancer that an entire chapter in this book has been devoted to it. Please see chapter three for more information on this amazing ingredient found in common table grapes. Chapter three also tells the story of Johanna Brandt, author of *The Grape Cure*, who completely cured her own abdominal cancer without surgery, chemo, or radiation. If you go to the U.S. National Library of Medicine (which is also a service of the National Institutes of Health) on the internet, you can type in *resveratrol* and immediately find more than **2000 scientific studies conducted on resveratrol.** Resveratrol is found in wine and grapes. A very similar plant phenolic acid known as *piceatannol,* also found in wine and grapes, is a popular component of many folk remedies, and has been found, in laboratory tests, to inhibit colorectal cancer cells (403). Since excess use of fermented wines can cause liver damage, your safest source is natural products, such as grapes and unfermented grape juice.

For an excellent 58-page study that was done on resveratrol's role in fighting cancer, including stomach cancer, see website: *http://www.agrawal.org/PDF/ACR-Resveratrol1.pdf.* The study was conducted by M.D. Anderson Cancer Center and the UCLA Center for Human Nutrition (346). Resveratrol is also being touted as a way to fight obesity, since it keeps the body from storing fat.

In 1989, Johanna Brandt's *Grape Cure* book was published under the title: *How to Conquer Cancer, Naturally,* by Tree of Life Publications, Joshua Tree, California. This edition included several pages of testimonials, including a brain cancer patient who had been sent home to die, cured on the grape diet, and a woman who was given up as terminal when it was discovered she had aggressive abdominal cancer. The physician taking care of her testified to her astounding and complete recovery while using only *The Grape Cure* diet (356).

## V. Herbs Effective Against Colon & Stomach Cancers

### Abajeru (*Chrysobalanus icaco*) for Colon Cancer & Other Cancers

Isolated from a tropical plant of the Brazilian Rain Forest (aka as *coco-plum*), abajeru was once used by locals for fighting arthritic pain and for diabetes (145a). When researchers first conducted lab testing, they found that the bush extract killed not only cancerous *breast-brain-lung-bowel-larynx and pancreas tumors*, but even difficult-to-treat leukemia cells died. In testing **humans,** they were surprised to see that it was effective in 90% of the cases. You can find this substance in health food stores and on the internet at many websites (145a).

### Artemisinin for Fighting Cancer

Artemisinin (also called *wormwood)* has been very popular in killing parasites; however, in experimental studies, this herb worked against many cancers, especially colon and leukemia, and the herb is capable of traveling through the bloodstream and into the brain, which may help the body fight tumors of the brain. Poly-MVA does this as well (322) as antineoplastons. The problem with some cancer-fighting remedies and chemo drugs is that they cannot cross-over into the brain.

This herb should not be taken on an empty stomach. Be sure to consult with your physician before taking artemisinin if you are on radiation or have recently been treated with radiation therapy. See chapter 14 on brain cancer (and other sections of this book) for more information on poly-MVA. For testimonials on Poly-MVA, see website: *http://www.polymvasurvivors.com/testimonials.html.* Many of these testimonials are given ten or more years ago, yet all survivors are still here as of March 2007. Do not use wormwood without consulting with your physician or Naturopath. Excessive dosing can be harmful.

## Astragalus for Enhancing the Immunity

Astragalus is an herb which boosts the immune system in fighting cancer. Check with your physician or Naturopath about using this herb, especially if you have an infection or are running a temperature (107).

## Chlorophyll & Chlorophyllin for Colon Cancer & Liver Cancer Prevention

Scientists have discovered that eating green foods, which are high in natural chlorophyll, could protect from all cancers, but especially those of the colon and liver (76). Animal studies have shown that natural chlorophyll and chlorophyllin (an extract made from chlorophyll) fight cancer. This substance can also protect against the dangerous fungus that often affects nuts and cereals known as *aflatoxin,* a source of liver cancer, especially in nations that do not have adequate safety measures for storing grains (76). Chlorophyll and chlorophyllin also protect against DNA damage from other cancer-causing substances, especially those found in *grilled meats* and *diesel exhaust* (76). Dr. George S. Bailey discussed the protective effects of this green substance in the LPI Research Newsletter "Chlorophylls and Cancer Prevention: passing the First Hurdle." They described a **human** study using chlorophyllin (conducted in Eastern China) on a group of people who were at risk for liver cancer from *aflatoxin exposure* (76). They were given the chlorophyllin *thrice daily* in 100 mg pills for a total of *300 mg.* The participants in the clinical trial experienced a 55% decrease in urinary output of the aflatoxin compounds (76), indicating that the green extract was neutralizing the fungus.

A new 20 year clinical trial is being done in China for testing chlorophyllin. They explained that eating a *moderate-to-high* amount *of green vegetables* would be necessary to obtain the same dosage *of chlorophyllin* given in the clinical trial (*300 mg*) (76). High amounts of chlorophyll in the diet via green vegetables could also help prevent the type of colon cancer caused by an iron found in red meats (76). There is no toxicity in natural chlorophyll and chlorophyllin, however, do check with your physician before supplementing, especially if you are taking blood-thinning medications, are nursing, pregnant, or have a chronic illness.

## Echinacea Herb for Cancer Prevention & Health

See chapter 19 for more information on this important herb that many people use for fighting colon cancer and other health problems.

## Essiac Tea & The Nurse Who Cured Hundreds, Perhaps Thousands of Cancer Patients with Four Herbs

In 1924 Rene Caisse's aunt was diagnosed with advanced cancer of the stomach and liver and told that she was terminal. Rene, a Canadian nurse, asked her aunt's physician about using an herbal formula that she had obtained from another patient who used the tea to cure her breast cancer. The story is described in Reese Dubin's book, *Miracle Food Cures From the Bible* (386). The patient told Rene that she had been given the tea recipe by an Indian friend of her husband's. The physician approved for Rene's aunt to try the same herbal blend. It contained four herbs: *slippery-elm bark, sheep sorrel, Turkish rhubarb, and burdock root* (386). Rene's aunt used the herbal remedy for only 60 days. She was completely cured and outlived her ordeal by more than 20 *years* (386).

When Dr. A.F. Bastedo of Bracebridge, Ontario, allowed Rene to use her formula on a terminally ill bowel cancer patient of his, the patient's recovery was so dramatic that he talked the authorities into letting Rene use one of their hotels as a cancer clinic, to which they agreed (580). Shortly thereafter, Rene's 72 year-old mother was discovered to have terminal liver cancer and given just days to live. Rene treated her own mother with the formula she named *Essiac.* Her mother not only recovered, but she lived a normal life for another 18 years, dying at the age of 90 from cardiac problems (580).

The physician, R.O. Fisher, M.D., was so completely amazed with the results of the remedy, he began working with Rene on researching with animals, then used the concoction on several of his own terminal cancer patients with excellent results (386). Other physicians began referring their terminally ill patients to Rene. A short while later, a physician asked Rene to use her herbal tea remedy on a diabetic colon cancer patient. To their astonishment, not only did the tea and the injections made from the tea cure the bowel cancer, but the diabetes as well! Only three of the herbs were used in the injections. The exact *injectable* formula that was developed was said to have been lost (386); however, long before Rene's death, Dr. Brusch, who worked closely with Rene, found that the injectable form of the tea was no longer needed, because the drinkable form was found to be just as effective (580).

One of the most amazing books describing the effectiveness of this tea and how it was suppressed by the health industry in Canada is *The Essiac Report Canada's Remarkable Unknown Cancer Remedy,* by Richard Thomas, who claims that Flor-Essence® is the original (drinkable) formula that Rene Caisse used. The book says that Rene gave her original recipe to Dr. Brusch, and it is now marketed as *Flor-Essence*® (580).

Note that there is some competition between the tea produced by Resperin of Canada, known as Resperin Canada Essiac®, and Flor-Essence® Essiac tea. Both companies claim that they have the original Essiac formula (the drinkable formula, not the injectable) that Rene Caisse used in treating her cancer patients.

Dr. J. A. Faulkner, who was provincial Minister of Health in Canada at the time Rene was treating patients, was supportive of the Essiac formula. He discussed the formula with Sr. Frederick Banting, M.D., who is considered a co-discoverer of insulin and who at that time, was one of the most highly acclaimed doctors in the world (580). He was so impressed with the formula, that he tried to talk Rene into coming to work with him at the Banting Institute in Toronto. She refused, because she had already tested her formula many times on mice and felt that her human patients needed her more (580).

Richard Thomas' book will show you many of the original letters written by physicians and patients who used this amazing tea. Unbelievable as it sounds, the only way that the tea was finally able to make it into health food stores was to change the name and remove all claims, so that it could not be considered a drug. Mr. Thomas, in one chapter of his book, refers to Rene as *St. Rene* (580).

Several Canadian physicians were so amazed at the results of Essiac tea, that in 1926, they petitioned the Canadian government to let Rene conduct further studies on the formula, insisting that she be allowed the proper equipment for doing so (386). Instead, Ottawa officials came to arrest Rene for practicing medicine. When it was discovered that she was working under the supervision of several very distinguished Canadian physicians, they backed down (386). Over many decades, Rene ultimately went on to treat multiple hundreds of terminally ill cancer patients with her herbal tea remedy, many of whom recovered completely. She did not charge for her services and always worked with prominent physicians. She accepted countless Canadian and American patients (386).

Cynthia Olsen, in her book, *Essiac A Native Herbal Cancer Remedy*, says that, in 1932, a story in the *Toronto Star* credited Rene with a "Notable Discovery Against Cancer," but because of this article, Rene Caisse was again threatened with legal action, including prison (521). Ms. Olson further explains that in 1938, Rene's supporters, including many physicians, again petitioned the government of Ontario to pass a bill giving Rene permission to use her formula for cancer patients unharrassed (521). Thousands of people signed the petition, but it fell three votes short of being passed, mostly because the Cancer Commission and the CMA (Canadian Medical Association) were in bed together (521). A few months later, 387 of Rene's patients came forward to testify in her behalf. For some never revealed reason, the Cancer Commission allowed just 49 to testify (521). One patient in particular, Herbert Rawson, was pushing fifty when two physicians diagnosed him with rectal cancer. He declined surgery and came to Rene Caisse with a note from his physician giving Rene the green light to allow him to use her formula (521). He started Essiac and received the *last of 30* treatments slightly more than a year later. Examinations shortly thereafter revealed no cancer whatsoever, and he outlived his ordeal another 25 years, his cancer never returning (521).

Because of continual threats of arrest, Rene finally shut her clinic doors, but covertly continued to see patients over the next three decades; however, she was constantly observed and faced years of imprisonment if it was found that she was using her formula (521). Rene's fame came to the attention of publishing editor, Ralph Daigh, who was suspicious of the medical establishment. Daigh's support of Rene and her herbal formula resulted in her being able to work with then President John F. Kennedy's private doctor, Charles Brusch, M.D; however, the president was killed before he was able to bring about any change in the way Rene Caisse and her formula were treated by the Canadian health system (521).

Dr. Brusch gave Essiac tea his total endorsement, firmly stating that Essiac was curing cancer patients. He admitted that the formula had been tested in several laboratories and said (in 1990) that he had even cured his own colon cancer using only Essiac (580). He had been diagnosed in 1984. He said that before Rene died in 1978, she *confided* to him the Essiac formula (580).

Rene wanted nothing more than to selflessly help cancer patients with her herbal tea remedy, yet she endured years of incessant and needless harassment from the Canadian Ministry of Health. She died from problems related to hip surgery when she was 90-years-old, and she had credited her own lifetime of excellent health and lack of illness to the fact that she had taken Essiac tea for half a century (386). She shared the formula with Dr. Brusch, whom she worked with for years.

See chapter sixteen in my book for the story of a young boy who was cured of lymphoma using a natural program that included Resperin Canada's Essiac® tea formula and 714X injections. A website that has Essiac® Resperin Canada is also given in that chapter. Do not use the tea if you are pregnant or nursing, and always check with your physician before ingesting herbs and other supplements. You can find this tea in both brands (and others) in health food stores and on the internet.

## Fenugreek for Cancer

Triterpenes, or plant saponins extracted from fenugreek were found, in laboratory tests, to have amazing anti-cancer properties against breast and prostate cancer cells. They may also inhibit other cancers, such as abdominal cancers.

## G.I.S.T.

These are gastro-intestinal stromal tumors (sarcomas), usually having a genetic tendency, but smaller ones can be benign, rather than malignant. They are usually found in the stomach or intestines, and can rarely occur in the throat. They are often surgically removed. Just be aware that if your physician uses a chemo drug known as Sutent® for this type cancer, the drug can cause cardiac complications in some individuals. (Many items I have discussed in this book have no side effects.) Some physicians are using the drug, Glivec, after surgery in those with GIST tumors, but Glivec can have some potentially life-threatening side effects!

## Garlic Against Abdominal Cancer

Garlic is also important in cancer prevention. A human study was done in China testing the potency of garlic in cancer prevention. At the conclusion of the study, data showed that people who did not eat garlic had a much higher risk for developing cancer. Those who ate garlic had a drastically lower rate of abdominal cancers in comparison to the county where garlic was not eaten. It was found that those who had the lower cancer rates, ate not only a serving of garlic per day, but similar vegetables, such as onions and leeks (549).

Scientists were surprised to find that the garlic-eaters could also protect themselves against cancer of the esophagus by including leafy greens, yellow vegetables, and fruits in their diet (549). One does not necessarily need to consume large quantities of garlic to benefit from its protective action. Apparently, it takes a very small amount of garlic every day to drastically decrease your risks for cancer. Less than one clove per day boosts the immune system (591). (Garlic has blood-thinning properties, so be sure to clear usage with your physician or Naturopath.)

## Goldenseal (Berberine) Suppresses Colon Cancer

An ingredient in goldenseal known as *berberine,* can suppress the formation of colon cancer (59). As noted at website *lef.org,* It also helps in preventing cancer of the bladder, and (in laboratory testing) kills skin cancers, leukemia, and brain tumors (59). If taking this herb, use a standard preparation that contains at least *5% hydrastine.* Some *herbalists* will tell you to rotate *goldenseal…rather than* using it continuously (59).

Do not take goldenseal or other herbs that have berberine (or similar herbs) longer than two weeks, nor should it be used for those who have bile disorders or may be pregnant (83). It is also advised not to use this herb in combo with *vitamin B6* or with *histidine,* nor for those with *glaucoma,* heart problems, lung problems, or hypertension (83).

## Graviola for the Colon

According to website *www.mnwelldir.org,* graviola is an herb found in the rain forest that South Americans use for treating liver and heart disease, as well as chronic conditions like asthma and arthritis (133).

Some remarkable cancer cures are being credited to this herb. For example, a popular Christian T.V. talk show host, who had surgery for colon cancer (then refused chemo and radiation afterwards), credits her complete healing from cancer to *graviola* and her faith in God.

Lab research that was apparently never published, indicated that Graviola may be comparable in potency to the chemo drug Adriamycin, but without the toxicity (133). As noted at *www.mnwelldir.org,* this herb, in lab testing, destroyed cancer cells without harming healthy cells, including those of the breast, prostate, lung, colon, and pancreatic cancer (133). Health Sciences Institute website says that the National Cancer Institute knew over 30 years ago that this plant could significantly fight cancer cells, yet the information was apparently suppressed (34). Though clinical trials on humans have not yet been done, obviously some humans are already using the herb. Check with your physician before using this herb.

Raintree puts graviola in their herbal formula known as *N-Tense*, which is available at their website *www.rain-tree.com*. The company reports that the herb could cause some people to have abdominal discomfort if they take large amounts (more than *five grams*), especially without food (34); however, as noted above, extensive human testing has yet to be done. (*N-Tense* is composed of 50% graviola along with other rain forest cancer-fighting botanicals.)

## Green Tea Protects Against Stomach Cancer, Bladder Cancer & Regenerates Brain Cells

Researchers have known for many years of the anti-cancer properties of green tea. Studies show that stomach cancer rates dropped dramatically in humans drinking *7 cups or more a day* (83). Scientists in China found that regularly drinking green tea cuts stomach cancer risk by as much as 50%. Green tea has also been found, in animal testing by Israeli researchers, to actually regenerate brain cells, something hitherto thought impossible (169). See chapter thirteen for green tea's ability at blocking bladder cancer in animal studies (134). A **human** study (from Japan) shows that this tea can reduce a woman's risk for getting stomach cancer by a whopping *75%* (136).

## Milk Thistle Fights Colon Cancer

Though milk thistle (not to be confused with *blessed thistle*, a different herb) is most popular for its effectiveness at rejuvenating the liver, compounds (like silymarin) from the herb may also help in the prevention of colon cancer (271). See chapter nine for more information on milk thistle, and instances when it should not be used.

## Other Herbs Effective Against Colon Cancer

Cat's claw has long been important in colon cancer prevention. It helps promote the proliferation of good bacteria within the gut (409). This herb is an excellent source of pycnogenols. You can find it in tea bags and in supplements. See chapter 20 for instances when you should not take this herb. Besides the herbs found in Essiac tea and herbs and spices, such as astragalus, garlic, and turmeric (discussed elsewhere in this book), see chapters 19 and 20 for other anti-cancer herbs and anti-oxidants.

## PC-SPES & Snow Rose for Colon Cancer

The herbal combo, PC-SPES, was once used for prostate cancer, but was removed from the market when hit with a contamination problem; however, new research has found that PC-SPES can help fight colon cancer, and it was found (in animal testing) to be helpful at fighting intestinal tumors (73).

Longevity of life is not uncommon in the country of Georgia (once part of the old U.S.S.R). The population at last count was 3.2 million people with more than twenty thousand that are 100-years-old or older (332)! These people have been the subject of much research due to their longevity, and it has been surmised that their long and healthy life spans are due to their diets (332). They consume large amounts of Alpine Tea along with a type of kefir made from grain that is exceptionally high in probiotics. They drink plenty of mineral-rich glacial water and consume a diet that includes honey and wine (332). Alpine Tea's main ingredient is *Rhododendron caucasian*, an herb harvested high in the Caucasian Mountains (332). This herb, also known as ***snow rose,*** decreases an enzyme in the body that may produce colon cancer (332). Snow rose has been studied for its effectiveness in treating coronary artery disease, unhealthy blood fats, mental disorders (e.g., depression and psychotic problems), as well as high blood pressure, gout, and arthritic disorders (332). The herb was also able to completely kill thousands of *staphylococcus aureus bacteria* in test tube experiments, outperforming both pine bark and grape seed (332).

*Rhododendron caucasicum* is often combined with other herbs for increased potency. (Be aware that you cannot harvest the rhododendron in your flower bed thinking it is the same herb. They are not the same.) If you are purchasing Alpine Tea, be sure that it is the tea containing *Rhododendron caucasicum.*

## Suma (*Pfaffia*) for Abdominal Cancer

Suma or *Pfaffia paniculata* (often called *Brazilian ginseng)*, in animal studies, was able to fight abdominal malignancies (279). It has also been referred to as *the Russian secret,* as their athletes often take it for stamina and weight-lifting without the side effects associated with steroids (279). The powdered root can cause a severe allergy *if inhaled*, and consuming excessive amounts of the tea may cause stomach upset (279). Check with your physician or Naturopath first. For more information on suma, contact *www.rain-tree.com* (279).

## Tian Xian for Gastrointestinal Cancer

When a patient was diagnosed with colon cancer and he failed to respond to chemo or surgery, he was given less than 60 days to live. A family member bought some Tian Xian for him. He began taking the herb and survived his ordeal, living on for several more years (293). Tian Xian is a Chinese herb ("pronounced *Dianne Sean*") that has been used in China to control, inhibit, and destroy cancer cells. See website: *tianxian.com* (293).

## ZoonCan for Colorectal Cancers

ZoonCan (also known by its Chinese name of *Zhongjiefeng Pian)* is an herbal remedy which may be important in helping the body fight cancers, especially those of the pancreas, colon, and rectal area (84). It has also been used in **human** studies for other cancers. See website: *4uherb.com/ cancer/ colorectal / treat.htm* for more details (84).

# VI. Minerals, Vitamins & Other Nutrients for Colon & Abdominal Cancers

## B6 for Colorectal Cancer Prevention

A huge health study involving more than 81,000 patients in Japan (described in the *Journal of Nutrition),* revealed that men with low amounts of vitamin B6 had a 30% greater risk for developing colorectal cancer (380). Some good natural sources of B6 include: avocado, onions, salmon, leafy green vegetables, tuna, cabbage (and other cruciferous vegetables), bananas, garlic, and blackstrap molasses.

## Calcium Prevents Colon Cancer

Current research has shown that calcium can help prevent some cancers (such as colon cancer) so dramatically that some physicians are even recommending it to all their patients (83). This is because calcium accelerates the removal of toxins from the digestive tract. If you decide on calcium supplements, you should find one that is combined with magnesium. Magnesium enables calcium to be utilized properly by the body (83). Calcium and magnesium are also important in the prevention of osteoporosis. In taking calcium and magnesium supplements for bone health, be sure that boron is included, and try to get most of your vitamin D from natural sunlight. You may also want to consider the supplement, **ipriflavone,** for osteoporosis prevention and bone rebuilding. (If you have a history or genetic disposition toward melanoma, consult with your physician before prolonged sun exposure.) Studies have shown that patients who use some conventional chemo drugs for colon cancer, can significantly reduce the side effects of the drugs by receiving calcium and magnesium intravenously before and after treatment.

## Carctol for Digestive Tract Cancers

This is an herbal remedy discussed more extensively in chapter 34 of this book. Those who use Carctol claim that it is particularly helpful for fighting digestive cancers.

## CoQ10 - A Curative & Preventative

You may want to consider adding CoQ10 supplements to your daily diet if you are fighting cancer. This amazing nutrient has even helped those with cancer of the breast to experience total regression (564). CoQ10 is also known as *ubiquinone.* The late Dr Karl Folkers, a primary researcher of CoQ10, believed that insufficient amounts of CoQ10 and B6 could induce cancer in humans. He tested 83 people who had many different types of cancer. They were all deficient in CoQ10 (564).

Another study found an alarming rise in breast cancer cases in women taking meds for cholesterol-lowering effects. Apparently, they lowered cholesterol, but increased their risk for breast cancer (564). Recent news reports say that statins (cholesterol-lowering drugs) do not prevent plaque build-up in arterial walls. Much research has been done showing that cholesterol-lowering drugs strip CoQ10 out of the body! (Are you taking cholesterol-lowering drugs? Does your physician have you on CoQ10?) There are many natural, safe ingredients discussed in this book that lower cholesterol without side effects (e.g., policosanol, niacin, *Ecklonia Cava,* Calcium D-Glucarate, krill oil, ginseng, barley, celery, shiitake, red grapes, resveratrol, cernitin, and Chinese red yeast rice with guggal). Some reports are saying that certain statin drugs (e.g., Vytorin), could increase your risk for cancer by 50%, and that the statin drug, Zetia, could cause liver damage. Reports are already filing in that Vytorin can cause strokes, liver damage, and heart attacks. Let your physician know of your concerns if you are taking statin drugs. Do not take red yeast rice or red yeast rice products if you have liver disease, or if you are already taking cholesterol-lowering drugs.

Current research revealed that CoQ10 can help kill cancer cells without damage to healthy cells (290). Not only that, but the National Cancer Institute acknowledged in 2005 that CoQ10 can extend the lives of those with colorectal cancers and other cancers. Issels Treatment Centers use CoQ10. Their phone #888-447-7357 (290).

## CoQ10 & Multiple Sclerosis

There are other reasons that you may want to supplement with CoQ10 besides its cancer-fighting properties. Dr. Ray D. Strand, M.D., gives an amazing account of his experience treating a patient who came to him with M.S. (multiple sclerosis) in his book, *What Your Doctor Doesn't Know About Nutritional Medicine May Be Killing You* (573). When a young man suddenly developed unexplainable weakness and numbness in his extremities, and was subsequently diagnosed with multiple sclerosis, he was fortunate enough to hear a lecture by Dr. Strand, and receive treatment that eventually resulted in complete remission (573). Dr. Strand's nutritional program included more than just using CoQ10. He also used minerals, many anti-oxidants, essential fatty acids, and grape seed extract, which he discusses in detail in his book (573).

Vegetarian diets and low fat diets significantly reduce the risk for multiple sclerosis. Research shows that curcumin may be beneficial in fighting M.S. It appears to have a protective effect on nerve cells. See chapters 19 and 20 for instances when you should not use curcumin (turmeric), and p. 488 for the link between MS & vitamin D deficiencies.

## Ellagic Acid Fights Colon Cancer

Research has shown that ellagic acid (abundant in berries and cherries) is important in fighting colon cancer. One of the best sources is red or black raspberries. Other foods that contain this nutrient (besides cherries) are walnuts, grapes, cranberries, pecans, pomegranates, strawberries, and most other berries. (Cranberries also cut the risk for ulcers and bladder infections and they help fight leukemia (22.)

## Folic Acid & Colorectal Cancers

Folic acid (folate) is critically important in the prevention of colon cancer. At his website, *www.newmediaexplorer.org*, Chris Gupta discusses the fact that it was three decades before the FDA finally admitted that this vitamin could prevent severe spinal cord birth defects (296). In the meantime, many countless birth defects occurred, because the FDA refused to allow vitamin manufacturers to recommend that women use folic acid during pregnancy (296)! Chris also describes the results from the *Nurses Health Study* at Harvard, which involved thousands of nurses, and revealed that those nurses who had taken the vitamin over a long period of time (at least *15 years*), dramatically reduced their chances of intestinal cancers (296). Doses given were *400 mcg.* Apparently, this is one time that supplementing the diet with folic acid worked better and proved more effective than ingestion of the vitamin via dietary means (296). It is also important to note that the many thousands of women who took part in this study had greater protection the longer they used folic acid. Those using the vitamin briefly had less protective results. Women who supplement with this vitamin can slash their risk for colon cancer by as much as *75%* (296).

Why is the FDA trying to take away your right to choose supplements and vitamins? Why are they trying to put vitamin and supplement retailers out of business? Because, as stated by Richard Thomas in his book, *The Essiac Report Canada's Remarkable Unknown Cancer Remedy,* "The FDA has admitted in print that **'they do not want the presence of dietary supplements in the market to act as a disincentive to the development of drugs'"** (580). They are working relentlessly to try to eliminate competition for the drug industry!

## Ginger Extract Inhibits Colorectal Cancer

A compound found in ginger (gingerol) which gives it that wonderful, zesty flavor, was found, in animal testing, to prevent colorectal tumors from growing. The study was conducted by the University of Minnesota (123).

## Grape Seed Extract

See chapter three for more information about the powerful ingredient in grapes (resveratrol) that has demonstrated amazing curative properties for helping to prevent and fight nearly all cancers.

For an excellent 58-page study that was done on resveratrol's role in fighting cancer, including colon cancer, see website: *http://www.agrawal.org/PDF/ACR-Resveratrol1.pdf.* The study was conducted by M.D. Anderson Cancer Center and the UCLA Center for Human Nutrition (346).

Grapes also contain important pycnogenols (507). These plant bioflavonoids are found in certain tree bark, the seeds of grapes, and are sold as supplements (507). They are super anti-oxidants, important in preventing disease and boosting the immune system. These extracts are said to be many times more powerful than vitamin C and vitamin E (507). Apparently, the only substance that can outperform pycnogenol's anti-oxidant ability is green tea (507). Green tea has also been found (in animal testing by Israeli researchers) to actually regenerate brain cells, something hitherto thought impossible (169). Do not take grape seed extracts with Vitamin C. Research suggests that taking them at the same time may raise blood pressure in some individuals.

## Modified Citrus Pectin Cuts Cancer Risk

In the *Journal of the National Cancer Institute,* animal studies showed that citrus fiber helps fight against colon cancer and breast tumors (383).

## Quercetin Prevents Colon Cancer

One of the most popular newcomers in the natural anti-cancer arsenal is a potent bioflavonoid known as *quercetin.* It is a very powerful cancer fighter, not only preventing the DNA abnormalities that can result in cancer, but—once a tumor is already forming—can help stop its progression. Vegetables high in this nutrient include most onions, except the white variety (551). In animal studies, quercetin inhibits the formation of intestinal cancers (571). It is a super anti-oxidant, able to neutralize enzymes known to accelerate the spread of cancer (571).

Taking bromelain tablets will increase the body's ability to assimilate this powerful substance. Bromelain is an extract from pineapples, so if you are allergic to pineapples, this substance is not for you, nor if you are on blood thinners, since it can thin the blood. Quercetin is not recommended for those who may be taking certain immunosuppressant drugs and/or calcium channel blockers (83). Always check with your physician or Naturopath about supplements, especially if you are already on prescription medications, to rule out any incompatibilities.

Scientists at Cornell have confirmed that onions containing the most concentrated amounts of these cancer-fighting compounds are the *western yellow...pungent yellow and northern red onions* (471). These chemicals can effectively inhibit the proliferation of intestinal and liver cancers (471). Quercetin is also found in *teas...beans, and apples* (378), in black and purple berries, and leafy greens. It is a wonderful anti-inflammatory and one of the best **natural** anti-histamines known.

## Selenium May Reduce Colorectal Cancer Risk

Insuring that you ingest adequate amounts of a common mineral known as selenium could reduce your risk for colorectal cancer (266a). Most health advocates recommend about 100 micrograms per day, though this is higher than the RDA. Those already fighting cancer often use more (see other places in this book), but beware, because too much in supplement form can be harmful.

## Zinc Combo Stops Abdominal & Esophageal Cancers

Although we need only small amounts of zinc, a deficiency has been connected to many cancers, especially those of the esophagus and upper abdomen (507). Remarkable evidence of the link between cancer and zinc was revealed in data from a research study conducted in Linxian, China in the 1990s (507). This province holds the infamous reputation for having more throat cancer than any other region of the world (507). It was theorized that the area lacked adequate amounts of important minerals, such as selenium and zinc in their soil (507). Chinese researchers collaborated with those in the U.S. to try to determine the exact cause. Zinc, selenium, and beta-carotene studies were done over a period of nine years involving thousands of Chinese participants. The human subjects, as described by Dr. Ralph Moss, author of *Anti-oxidants against Cancer*, were given larger doses than the RDA. He says that those participants receiving the supplements cut their gastric cancer rates more than half (507), and those "taking beta-carotene, vitamin E, and selenium [had] a 42 percent reduction in esophageal cancer" (507).

# VII. Vegetables for Healing

## Fiber, Cruciferous Sulfur Veggies & Colon Cancers

Many prestigious medical journals have touted the importance of fiber in preventing colon and other cancers. Perhaps no other source of fiber has become more prominent lately than cruciferous vegetables like *cabbage, kale, broccoli*, and others (430). The compounds in these powerful veggies help fight colorectal cancers, remove dangerous toxins, and boost the body's ability to fight carcinogens (430). Other vital nutrients found in cruciferous vegetables are called *indoles*.

Recent studies have shown that indoles are critically important in preventing and treating colon and abdominal cancers. It is best to eat cruciferous vegetables raw, as cooking destroys much of their vitamin and enzyme content. Consuming them with *cloves* and a spice known as *jambul* has been associated with decreasing the risk for stomach cancer (278). Another good source of high fiber is steel-cut oats. They also help lower insulin levels in the body. Most health food stores carry steel-cut oats.

When the National Cancer Institute researched the dietary habits of nearly half a million participants, they discovered that those people who include generous amounts of fruits and vegetables, heart-healthy fats, whole grains, and important vitamins and minerals (e.g., vitamin D and calcium) in their diet, along with very little amounts of saturated fat, red meat and sugar, had a much greater chance for avoiding cancers of the colon and rectum (532a).

## Lutein & Lycopene Inhibit Colon Cancer

Lutein is a carotenoid found in many fruits and vegetables. Research has documented that people who regularly eat dark leafy greens and other foods high in lutein could dramatically reduce their risk for cancer of the colon. Statistics have proven that lutein-rich diets are colon-healthy. (Lutein is also critical for healthy eyes.) Avocados and egg yolks are lutein-rich. Lycopene, discussed in other chapters of this book, has been the subject of thousands of research studies and shown to be a powerful preventative for colon cancer. Tomatoes and watermelon are rich in lycopene, as are most red and pink vegetables and fruits.

## Mushrooms that Inhibit Colorectal Cancers & Prevent Their Spread – Maitake, Karawatake, Reishi & Shiitake

**Maitake** mushroom is an important stimulant for the immune system. An extract from this mushroom, ***Maitake-D*** (sometimes called *Maitake-D-Fraction*), has shown impressive anti-cancer properties (83). As noted by *herbs2000.com*, this mushroom is also known as the *Grifola frondosa, dancing mushroom*, and *hen-of-the-woods*. Combine it with *vitamin C* for more efficient absorption, but do not take maitake if you have multiple sclerosis (184) (469). The website says that PSK or *Polysaccharide kureha,* also commonly referred to as *krestin,* comes *from the kawaratake mushroom* (236), or **coriolus versicolor**. PSK (krestin) is the subject of hundreds of research studies since it appears to prevent the spread of tumors (236). Outside of the United States, PSK is sometimes a cancer therapy of choice, often given as an adjunctive with other cancer treatments (469).

For colorectal cancers, **Reishi mushroom** tablets are also recommended for their ability to boost the immune system (83).

**Lentinan** is an extract of the **Shiitake** mushroom. Deanne Tenney, in her book, *Medicinal Mushrooms*, reports that this extract triggers the body's manufacture of immune cells that destroy cancer cells (576). Lentinan injections are popular for fighting abdominal cancers, but they are considered *alternative therapy*, so you will have to seek an alternative practitioner to administer them (202). Research revealed that shiitake can increase survival time for terminal cancer patients without major adverse reactions. Also, if you have already had surgery to remove cancer, it is believed that this mushroom may help keep it from returning (576).

# VIII. Fruits That Can Save Your Life

## Cherries Prevent & Treat Stomach Cancer

According to tests conducted at Indiana University School of Medicine in Indianapolis, in animal testing, an ingredient found in cherries (known as *perillyl alcohol)* was effective at preventing many types of cancer, including those of the stomach (604). This is described in Selene Yeager's book, the *Doctors Book of FOOD REMEDIES*. She reported that the substance not only works in the cancer prevention stage, but in fighting cells that have already formed (604). Cherries are a natural anti-inflammatory. They can also help fight arthritis pain.

## Papaya - Healing Fruit for Colon Cancer

See Chapter 20 for examples of papaya extract's ability to shrink colon cancer and even put metastatic cancer into remission.

# IX. Other Supplements & Treatments for Abdominal & Colon Cancers

## Bacteria & Colon Cancer

Scientists have recently begun, in animal studies, to experiment with genetically-modified strains of bacteria, such as salmonella, to use them for fighting cancer of the colon and other cancers (382a). Only time will tell how this altered bacteria will work in humans.

## Beta-Sitosterol Inhibits the Spread of Colon Cancer

Beta-sitosterol is a *naturally-occurring* plant nutrient (20). Most diets have deficient levels of beta-sitosterol. It has been found to inhibit the growth of colon cancer cells and it can treat ulcers, unstable blood sugars, boost the immune system, and help fight prostate cancer and *lymphocytic leukemia* (20). This compound should not be taken by those with any type of disorder that interferes with their ability to properly assimilate fats (e.g., *beta sitosterolemia* or *adrenal leukodystrophy*) (249) (315). This supplement is available at natural health food stores in tablet or capsule form, and you may find it combined with herbs or other nutrients.

## Burzynski's Antineoplastons

See chapter 14 of this book for amazing cases of cancer patients completely cured of *terminal* cancers, people who were basically sent home to die, then chose non-toxic antineoplastons from the Burzynski Clinic in Houston, Texas, to cure their cancer. See many of the patient's own stories about their success in fighting cancer with antineoplastons at this website: *http://burzynskipatientgroup.org/stories.html.* The main Burzynski Clinic website can be found at *www.burzynskiclinic.com.* Also, see this site: *http://burzynskipatientgroup.org/juneh.htm* for a 78 year-old woman's amazing testimonial of her successful use of Burzynski's PBs (sodium phenylbutrates) to cure her colon cancer. When surgery revealed that her cancer had spread, she refused radiation and chemo and was completely cured using non-toxic PB treatment from Dr. Burzynski's clinic. The difference between antineoplastons and PBs is that antineoplastons are given intravenously and PBs are taken orally. PBs are converted by the liver into antineoplastons. The FDA has finally approved the oral form of antineoplastons (PBs) for off-label use, and certain antineoplastons were recently given *orphan drug status* by the FDA for use on gliomas. Some individuals can have side effects from antineoplastons, but they are quickly reversible, unlike toxic chemo drugs that often cause fatal adverse reactions.

## CyberKnife® Therapy for Tumors

See chapter 34 in this book for details on CyberKnife® therapy, which is being used successfully for many cancers, including hard-to-reach brain tumors. It is a gentle, painless procedure that does not require an incision, surgery, sedation, or inpatient stay. It takes very little time, and as soon as the procedure is over, the patient is able to walk out and return home. There are very few risks and side effects, though it does involve some radiation (89a), and it can damage nearby healthy cells. Also, look under NanoKnife™, chapter 34.

## Poly–MVA (Palladium Lipoic Complex)

See chapter 10 and 14 for more information on the amazing nutritional formula, known as Poly-MVA, that many *terminal* cancer patients have credited to bringing their cancers into total remission. The main Poly-MVA website is located at *www.polymva.net.* For testimonials of people who used this substance to cure many types of cancer, see website *http:/ /www.polymvasurvivors.com/testimonials.html.*

## Shark Cartilage Halts Abdominal Tumor

When scientists discovered that sharks rarely get cancer, regardless of how contaminated their environment, investigators began looking into the secret of their resistance to this disease. Dr. William Lane, Ph.D., wrote in his book, *Sharks Don't Get Cancer,* that it is the *cartilage* that protects, because cartilage keeps blood vessels from spreading (550). Cancer cells must be fed via a blood vessel system in order to survive. Within two weeks of growth, cancer cells flourish with their own vascular system, which is blocked by shark cartilage, and this eventually shrivels the tumor (550).

A physician from Central America successfully used shark cartilage to treat a patient with a large stomach tumor. Within 30 days the growth halted. Another six months, and the once enormous tumor was the size of a *walnut* (550). This extract has also been used against ovarian, cervical, and uterine cancers. See chapter seven for more details.

Shark cartilage is not for use with children, nor during pregnancy, or if you have recently had a heart attack, transplant, surgery, chemo or radiation. It is not for those with high blood pressure, pheochromocytoma (adrenal tumor which can cause excessively high blood pressure), ulcers, allergies to seafood, or circulatory diseases. It is not for those with liver disease, except it has been used successfully against liver cancer. More information can be found in chapter seven of this book. Be aware that you should always consult with your health care practitioner for specific dosing for your own individual needs.

See chapter 34 of this book for information on a non-toxic herb, known as *bindweed*, that is said to have *100 times* the ability at blocking blood vessel formation as that found in shark cartilage (150) (301a). There are also some newer, safer drugs coming on the market which fight blood vessel formation in tumors. In its wild state, bindweed could be toxic. Consult with your physician or Naturopath before using.

## SIRT - Sir-Spheres® - Therapy for Inoperable Colorectal Cancers that Have Spread to the Liver

See chapter nine in this book on LIVER CANCER (under Section IV, which discusses bland embolization (or chemoembolization) and SIRT or Sir-Spheres®, a new therapy being used to treat inoperable liver tumors (some of which have spread from the colorectal area) (265a).

## Soy Supplements

There is a great deal of controversy about soy products, but fermented soy is fine. Research has shown that soy (unfermented) may harm the functioning of the thyroid gland, as well as other problems in some individuals. The harmful substances are not found in fermented soy.

Haelan is nothing more than a drink that is made from fermented soy and used by some cancer patients to fight their disease. Its origin goes back to China where it was produced in the 1980s as a nutritional drink (541). Haelan has anti-oxidants, including *protease inhibitors*, which are known to be DNA protective. Fermented soy is also very high in vitamins and minerals (541). See chapter four in this book for more details about Haelan.

Also, for information on Haelan, see the company's website at *www.haelan951.com.* Information on Haelan's Research Foundation's website was accumulated from clinical studies performed on fermented soy beverages manufactured by Haelan Products, Inc. of Woodinville, Washington. The Haelan fermented soy beverages are sold in the United States, without medical claims, and are available directly from the company or one of their distributors (143).

## Sunshine, Vitamin D & Exercise Prevent Colon Cancer

Is it any wonder that more and more research is showing that adequate sunshine prevents the development of colon and rectal cancers? This is mostly because sunshine supplies natural Vitamin D, something we cannot live without. Natural sunshine boosts the immune system. It also accounts for the reason why we have a **flu season** in the Winter months. Most people do NOT get enough natural sunshine (and vitamin D) in the Winter, their immunity suffers and makes them more susceptible to viruses, bacteria, and all manner of infection. Most people need ten to twenty minutes of natural sunshine daily (without using sunscreen), or at least thrice weekly, to manufacture vitamin D. Those who have had a history of melanoma need to consult with their physician about sun exposure. There are also some medications that caution you to avoid sunlight while you are taking them. Regular physical exercise has also been shown to inhibit all forms of cancer, especially colon cancer and colorectal cancers. It is best to get both anerobic exercise (e.g., walking or biking) and aerobic exercise, such as weight-lifting, for optimal results.

## Ukrain Effective Against Colorectal Cancer Without Toxic Side Effects

Ukrain, discussed in previous chapters, was named after the country of the physician who developed it (without the "e"). It is a merger of two compounds, both highly toxic; however, it was found that when these two ingredients were combined, they were only toxic to cancer cells, making Ukrain a completely non-toxic substance (287)(506).

A study involving 96 people (with colorectal cancer) who were treated—half with Ukrain and half with 5FU chemo drug and radiation—showed dramatic results. Within less than two years, more than 75% of those who received the Ukrain were still alive, but only 33% of those on the conventional chemo and radiation were still alive (574). You can read this **human** case study at the National Library of Medicine's website NCBI PubMed, PMID 8899313 at *http://www.ncbi.nlm.nih.gov/pubmed/8899313* (574). Ukrain has not yet received approval by the FDA. Call Issels regarding Ukrain therapy at #1-888-447-7357. Also, Advanced Alternatives Cancer Centers do use Ukrain therapy. See testimonials from their patients at *www.aacancer.com/sitemap.html.* They have a treatment center in Freeport, Bahamas.

Another human study was done on 48 people with cancer of the rectum (353). Half of them received chemo and radiation and the other half received only *one series* of Ukrain before having surgery ("10 mg every second day, to a total of 60 mg) and one series after the operation (to a total of 40 mg)" (353). They received another course six months post-op. Within 14 months, one fourth of those on the chemo and radiation relapsed, however just "8.3%" of the participants getting Ukrain relapsed. (353). The Ukrain repeatedly outperformed both chemo drugs and radiation therapy. In spite of all this, if you are diagnosed with cancer, your physician usually will not volunteer information about Ukrain unless he or she is an alternative medicine doctor or keeps current with them. You will have to seek an alternative health physician in the United States, Europe, Canada or the Ukraine, where it is popular therapy.

Also, for one of America's largest alternative health care centers, the Whitaker Wellness Center, which is in Newport Beach (4321 Birch Street), California, see this link: ***http://whitakerwellness.com/about_us/medical_team.*** Dr. Julian Whitaker, who runs this health care center, has written many books on alternative healing. They use many of the alternative health treatments that I have mentioned in my books, including chelation, hyperbaric oxygen, and different IV therapies.

## Vitamin Eliminates Rectal Polyps

One of the most publicized reports on the efficacy of using vitamin C (the ascorbic acid oral form) for eliminating rectal polyps, was written in the November 1975 issue of *Surgery* (571a). A mere "3000 mg of ascorbic acid, as a time-release preparation, were given each day," and it "reduced the number of rectal polyps in five of…eight patients and caused a major reduction of polyps in three others..." Polyps in three of the participants were not affected. Those conducting the test attributed the positive results to the ascorbic acid, and felt that the three unaffected by the oral ascorbic acid should either have higher doses, or "3 percent sodium ascorbate enemas in addition to the oral intake" (571a).

## Vitamin Supplements

A good balanced vitamin-mineral supplement is recommended for anyone fighting cancer or any other serious illness.

Many foods that you juice will have natural forms of vitamins and minerals, such as beta-carotene and calcium in carrot juice. All vitamins and minerals are important in cancer prevention and treatment. For example, once in the body, **vitamin D** is turned into a hormone that can cling to and neutralize colon cancer cells. Adequate vitamin D can cut your threat of colon cancer in half (83). One of the best ways to get adequate amounts of vitamin D is ten to twenty minutes a day of full sun exposure without using sunscreen. This may be the most critical vitamin for those who have a history of stage I cancers of the colon. You need at least *500-1000 mg* of vitamin D (83) each day. Some naturopaths are even suggesting 1500-5000 mg of vitamin D per day. Always check with your physician about sun exposure, especially if you have a prior history of skin cancer, or are taking medications that may cause sun sensitivity, or have a hereditary predisposition to melanoma.

Avoid taking iron supplements unless ordered by your physician for anemia or other blood disorders, because they may injure cells in the colon (83).

## Water (Adequate Hydration) Can Prevent Cancer

So important to our survival (it isn't actually considered a supplement), water, in recent studies, has been shown to decrease the risk of developing cancer. To benefit from water, be sure that you drink it chlorine-free and fluoride-free. According to website *www.herbs2000.com,* research in Taiwan found that drinking adequate water—*8 glasses a day* for the men studied—dramatically decreased their chances of getting colon cancer. According to the late Dr. F. Batmanghelidg, M.D., author of *Your Body's Many Cries For Water,* cancer patients are usually dehydrated. Lack of sufficient water has been linked to the cause of asthma, lupus, Crohn's Disease, diabetes, irritable bowel syndrome, degenerative disc disease, arthritis, migraines, cancer, and all auto-immune disorders. When drinking water, you need to increase your salt intake. Dr. Batmanghelidg recommended that "for every 10 glasses of water (about two quarts)..." you need a "half teaspoon of salt per day" (341). See website at: *www.watercure2.org*. Always check with your physician if you are on a water-restricted or salt-restricted diet, and be sure to read chapter 23, later in this book, for more information on hydration.

## Wheat Grass Juice & Other Green Drinks for Cancer

Green drinks are very detoxifying. There have been many cases of people using several glasses of green drinks a day to detoxify their body and cure their cancers. These drinks contain chlorophyll which alkalizes the body and increases oxygenation. They are rich in magnesium and other vital minerals and vitamins. See chapter 17 for more information on God's wonderful grasses and green foods.

## Zapping Cancer with Iodine & Magnesium

Dr. Mark Sircus has much to say about the pervasive lack of magnesium and iodine in the average diet, and why these deficiencies are causing heart disease, cancer, and many other diseases. See his books, *Magnesium The Ultimate Heart Medicine* and *Magnesium Medicine The Lamp of Life,* available at: *http://www.magnesiumforlife.com,* and *Iodine Bringing Back the Universal Medicine* (566b). For more details on his books and resources for finding the best forms of transdermal magnesium oil and a superior form of gentle, food-grade iodine, see page 129, 400, and chapter 34.

# CHAPTER 7

# GENTLE CURES FOR TOUGH CERVICAL, UTERINE, OVARIAN & VULVA CANCERS

*"But unto you that fear my name shall the SUN of righteousness arise with healing in his wings, and ye shall go forth and grow up as calves of the stall." (Malachi 4:2)*

## I. New Diagnostic Testing

### OvaSure™ - for Early Detection of Ovarian Cancer

In spite of being told for many decades, that there are no symptoms of ovarian cancer, researchers now say that there are at least four symptoms women need to watch for. Not only that, but a new test that claims *nearly 100 percent* reliability at detecting early ovarian cancer, just came out in June of 2008.

* First for the symptoms: women are being told that they must be in tune with changes in their body, regardless of how subtle or insignificant they think them to be, and regardless of physicians who ignore their complaints. These four main symptoms are: (1.) feelings of pain in the pelvic or abdominal area (2.) bloating (3.) *difficulty eating* due to *feeling full* after just a few bites of food, and (4.) urinary problems, such as feeling an urgent need to urinate, or going too often (329).

* This same article discusses the CA-125 test and combining it with the symptoms for early detection (329); however, there is a new screening test that has been made available through LabCorp, which claimed that it was "nearly 100 percent effective in detecting the cancer in its early stage" (325). Per an article at *TheTimesNews.com* by Michael Abernathy, the test is known as **OvaSure™** (325). The blood test "uses six markers in the blood to detect the cancer and has more than 99 percent certainty in differentiating between women with and without ovarian cancer" (325). It was removed from availability near the end of 2008 since it has not been given FDA approval. This test, or one like it, could end up saving many lives. The FDA is reviewing the records from LabCorp. They are not certain that enough testing went into proving the efficacy of OvaSure™. You will hear more about this in the coming weeks and months ahead. A

next step your physician may order is a diagnostic test known as the trans-vaginal ultrasound. Also, see below in this chapter, on using the PET/CT for staging ovarian cancer non-invasively.

## Other Diagnostic Tests: CA-125, AFP, HcG, BRCA-1, BRCA-2, Oncotype, Amplichip, Mammaprint, AMAS & Microvascular Ultrasonography Imaging (Microvascular Ultrasound)

Other tests used in conjunction with **CA-125** to aid in diagnosing diseases, such as ovarian cancer (besides the new ovarian cancer test from LabCorp noted above), include ***AFP*** *(alpha feto protein*) and ***hCG*** *(human chorionic gonadotropin*, levels of which are sometimes high in those with ovarian cancers, however, they can also be abnormally high during a woman's pregnancy (169). If you happen to have a genetic background for ovarian and/or breast cancer, your physician may order tests to verify this. They are known as the **BRCA-1 and BRCA-2** test, and will determine if you have a genetic trait that increases your risk for these type cancers (169).

A BRCA-2 mutation in men can result in a very lethal form of prostate cancer. Your physician may choose any or all of these tests to diagnose or rule out disease. Note that many physicians consider some types of cancer hereditary, but there is disagreement and controversy about this. Some do not consider the BRCA-1 and BRCA-2 tests as thoroughly reliable. Oncotype (genetic) diagnostics are still controversial. **Amplichip** is a DNA blood enzyme test. **Mammaprint** is a genetic test that looks at 70 different breast genes and tells a physician how likely it is that a breast cancer will spread. Another test (that has a greater than 95% accuracy) for detecting all cancers is known as the **AMAS** or "Anti-Malignin Antibody in Serum" test. It will detect cancer anywhere in the body, even tiny amounts, yet some physicians are not familiar with it, or never use it. The test can be found under the name of *Target Reagent,* and if you need to get this lab test and see if your insurance covers it, the CPT code for the test is 86-317.

A report from the U.S. National Institutes of Health at *ClinicalTrials.gov,* describes the use of **microvascular ultrasound** for detecting *Early Stage Epithelian Ovarian Carcinoma* (194). The New York University School of Medicine has sponsored a study on this diagnostic tool under the *ClinicalTrials.govIdentifier NCT00531570* (194), or go to *http://www.cancer.gov/clinicaltrials/search.* It is hoped that this tool will help physicians differentiate between non-malignant tumors and those that are malignant (194). Also, see the rest of this chapter.

## More Screening Tests

Note that there are other new screening tests for early ovarian cancer detection that are coming on the market. Another such test is known as *OvPlex,* from an Australian company *(Melbourne biotech company HealthLinx),* which says it has a *94 per cent accuracy* thus far in *clinical trials* (479). Be aware that if your physician has ordered a **ChemoFX** lab test for you, they are checking to see how well the type ovarian cancer you have will respond to their chemo drugs.

# II. Treatment & Risks

## Cytotron Therapy

A new cancer (and arthritis) treatment developed and available in India that you will not yet be able to get in the U.S., is being successfully used on humans and is known as *Cytotron Therapy.* It is gentle, completely painless, and non-toxic. See chapter 34 in this book for more details on what is also called *QMR* or *Quantum Magnetic Resonance* (90).

## Fungus Cure Also Cures Cancer, Says Oncology Physician

See chapter 34 of this book for the amazing cancer cure that Italian Oncologist, Dr. Simoncini, is using to cure his cancer patients within just days! Cancerous growths are usually WHITE. He says that they are actually a fungus, which can be killed with a non-toxic soda bicarb solution that quickly alkalizes the tumor for destruction (582).

## Grilling & Frying Foods Increase Risk of Ovarian Cancer

According to *NaturalNews.com*, women who consume fried foods, even small servings of chips, will double their risk for *ovarian or endometrial cancer* due to a substance in the food known as *acrylamides* (417). In testing 62,000 women over an eleven-year time frame, scientists found that the cancer-causing substance aggregates in foods that are high in starch to begin with, then "fried, baked, grilled or roasted" (417). Testing with acrylamides uncovered some amazing results. Using the herb **rosemary** in baking wheat bread, for example, slashed the acrylamides by greater than half (361). Even very minute amounts of rosemary, as low as *one per cent of the dough*, was able to cut acrylamides (361).

## Non-Toxic Immunotherapy – Global First Of a Kind Miracle Cure for Acute Myeloid Leukemia – Breast & Ovarian Cancer Next?

See chapter 34 under this title for a new immunotherapy treatment, where a woman was put into total remission from *acute myeloid leukemia* by *natural killer cells* taken from her own daughter, treated, then injected into her mom (568a). It is hoped that this treatment (a first in the world - in London) is on its way to all other nations of the world), and that it will be just as successful against other cancers, such as breast and ovarian cancer (568a).

## Intensity Modulated Radiotherapy (IMRT) for Ovarian, Cervical & Uterine Cancers

This radiation treatment is currently under testing in Europe and is being used in the U.S as well. It uses targeted radiotherapy to help minimize damage to nearby normal cells. It is used for lung tumors, thyroid, and breast cancers as well as prostate, esophageal, nasal, head cancers, liver, brain, ovarian, cervical cancers, and uterine growths. You may also see this treatment referred to as ***TOMO Therapy*** or *TOMO Treatment.*

IMRT was first used at Memorial Sloan-Kettering Hospital for treating cancer of the prostate (163a). Rather than using one large radiation beam to target the tumor, this type radiation uses many beams to target cancer tumors more precisely, thus (hopefully) preventing excess damage to nearby normal cells (163a), though it is still considered radiation and will have some of the same side effects as any radiation would cause.

## Kamunggay (Moringa) for Epithelial Ovarian Cancers

This plant (also referred to as *moringa, mulunggay,* the *drumstick tree,* or *horseradish tree)* is said to be an important herb for fighting ovarian cancers which start in the *epithelial* cells (232). This type of ovarian cancer is often called the *silent killer*, since the disease has usually progressed before symptoms occur. Extracts from the plant's bark and root have anti-cancer and hormone benefits (232). In the green leaves of this plant are found important plant chemicals that help fight the formation of cancerous cells (232). The healing abilities of moringa have resulted in the determination to promote its use in alternative medicine (232).

## Magnesium for Cancer Prevention

This mineral is critical for the prevention of all types of cancer, including leukemia, and those involving the stomach, prostate, breast, and bones (566). See page 400 for more details on using transdermal magnesium.

## PET/CT Scan Used to Stage Ovarian Cancer Non-Invasively

Combining a PET (*positron emission tomography* with a CT (*computed tomography*) for those who are diagnosed with ovarian cancer before it has advanced, may help physicians more successfully stage the cancer (and determine whether or not it has spread) without subjecting the patient to risky surgeries (226).

## Plant-Based Diets Decrease Risk for Ovarian Cancer by 50% - Dietary Flavonoids at Top

It's true—vegetarians are at much lower risk for ovarian cancer (538a). According to findings published in the *International Journal of Cancer*, from studies done in *Italy* on "1031 women with ovarian cancer" and "2411 women with non-cancerous conditions requiring hospital admission," the women "who consumed the greatest amounts of flavonols and/or isoflavones" (nutrients found in fruits and vegetables), had *50%* fewer cases of *ovarian cancer* (538a).

## RM-10 & Advanced Ovarian Cancer

When Jordan Rubin (author of The *Maker's Diet* and other health books) found that his own 80 year-old grandmother had an advanced form of ovarian cancer, he began to look at ways that her immune system could be activated to kill the cancer cells (30). He studied *polysaccharides* or *glyconutrients* as well as mushrooms, cat's claw, and aloe vera. He used a *fermentation process* with many of the *homeostatic soil organisms,* that had gotten him well from Crohn's, to *predigest the 10 mushrooms, aloe vera and cat's claw* in a compound that would enable his grandmother to easily absorb the nutrients (30). The formula, known as *RM-10*, is sold through *Garden of Life* products. Using RM-10, Rubin's grandmother completely recovered from ovarian cancer, and it also healed a *fatty liver.* (30). You can read more about her remarkable recovery and where to get *Garden of Life* RM-10 and other products at website *http://www.crohns.net/Miva/education/testimonial_rosemenlowe.shtml* (30). I also discuss glyco-nutrition in chapter 34 of this book.

## Rexin-G™ for All Cancers

Rexin-G™ has been undergoing clinical trials at Mayo Clinic, M.D. Anderson, and a few other facilities. It is a drug for cancers that have spread, and cancers that conventional medicine says do not respond to chemo (256). **Human** clinical studies, thus far, have had good results. In the very first human trial, 83% of the patients experienced tumor shrinkage. The patients all had spreading pancreatic cancer (256). Good responses were also achieved (in **human** studies) involving several other types of metastatic cancer. Due to the reports, this drug is now used for treating all forms of *solid tumors* in the Philippines that are resistant to conventional therapy (256). The U.S. FDA has given the drug its *orphan drug status* for use with pancreatic cancers in the US, as well as other types of cancer metastases, which means that trials will continue (256). It is given intravenously, so isn't exactly natural or painless, but could be considered gentler than older chemo drugs because it is said to be a non-chemo drug, showing itself in **human** clinical trials, not to have the adverse side effects normally associated with chemo drugs (256). You can get more information on this drug at *epeiusbiotech.com/rexin_g-factsheet.asp.* Epeius Biotechnologies are the producers of Rexin-G™ (257).

## TAP—Tumor-Activated Prodrug or TAP Technology for Ovarian Cancer

Researcher, Dr. Anne Kellogg, a pathologist from East Carolina University, is the developer of a new type of monoclonal antibody that may pave the way for treating breast, ovarian, and *other cancers* more effectively and perhaps with fewer side effects than mainstream chemo

(207). She called the new antibody *DS-6* and describes it as a *delivery vehicle* for a cancer-killing agent that was produced by a company known as *ImmunoGen.* The antibody works by sticking onto tumor cells and allowing itself (as well as the cancer-killing agent) to get inside the cell where it then destroys the cell (207). Before the antibody and its cancer-killing agent actually reach the tumor cell, it is in an inactive state within the body, and is only *activated* once it gets into the abnormal cell (207).

# III. Natural Foods That Prevent & Kill Cervical, Ovarian & Uterine Cancer Cells

## AHCC—Mushroom Compound (*Active hexose correlated compound)* Helps Immune System Kill Ovarian Cancer Cells

AHCC is a complex compound from the mycelia of many mushrooms. In human testing, it was found (when given to patients in doses of "3g/day orally for 2-6 months") to significantly increase the body's natural immunity, enabling the death of cancerous ovarian cells and several other types of malignant cells (206). This compound is found at many natural health food stores and online supplement providers.

## Berry Extract Kills Cervical Cancer Cells

Researchers have discovered that compounds from blueberries and strawberries fight cervical and breast cancer cells.

## Beta-Carotene Helps Prevent Cervical & Endometrial Cancer

Studies show that lacking this important nutrient is the most vital indicator (among nearly a dozen that were tested) for an increased risk of developing cervical cancer (366). According to Jack Challem, author of *All About Carotenoids Beta-carotene, Lutein & Lycopene,* this holds true for dysplasia and cervical cancer (366). It was also discovered that *synthetic* beta-carotene did not offer the same protection as that supplied by nature (366). (Surprised?) One of the best ways to get beta-carotene naturally is to juice raw carrots and other foods rich in beta-carotene. The body then converts beta-carotene into natural vitamin A.

Mr. Challem has a new book out: *Stop Prediabetes Now,* with co-author Ron Hunninghake, M.D. Also see his new book*: The Food-Mood Solution.* For more information on both books, see website*: http://www.thenutrition reporter.com.*

In *Earl Mindell's Food as Medicine*, Dr. Mindell suggests many foods for fighting cervical cancer—those rich in beta-carotene, including not only carrots, but leafy green vegetables, deep yellow vegetables (e.g., sweet potatoes and squash), lycopene-rich foods, vitamin C, and folic acid (493). These same foods also fight other cancers (e.g., oral and pancreatic).

When Swiss and Italian researchers checked the dietary trends of hundreds of their citizens, they discovered that women could slash the occurrence of endometrial cancers in half by eating very small quantities of beta-carotene daily (e.g., *one-half cup* of *yellow squash*) (604).

## Broccoli Prevents Cervical Cancer

Studies have shown that women could dramatically reduce their risks of developing cervical cancer by eating more broccoli (363).

## Carrageenan (Seaweed Extract) Fights Cervical Cancer

A substance derived from *red algae* seaweed (*carrageenan*) can actually halt the spread of the *HPV virus*, one of the many viruses believed to be responsible for cervical cancer (265). Testing by the NCI also showed that the extract had some inhibition against *HIV and herpes, but was 1000 times* stronger against HPV (265). Carrageenan is completely safe and is a common *thickener* found *in baby formula.* Those working with this substance are hoping to develop a *gel* from carrageenan that women could use to aid in blocking the HPV virus (265).

## Cherries Inhibit Ovarian Cancer

Dr. Raymond Hohl, M.D., from the University of Iowa, revealed that eating cherries can fight the incidence of all types of cancer. It is the *perillyl alcohol* in cherries that stunt cancer growth (61).

## Citrus Pectin Prevents Cancer Metastasis

Modified citrus pectin is found in all plants. In animal studies, it fights the metastasis or spread of cancer cells (351). It also lowers unhealthy cholesterol levels. Some very good natural sources of pectin include citrus and apples (342). Of course, anything containing these ingredients, such as jams and jellies (e.g., apple jam and marmalade), would also be very high in pectin.

## Cryo Treatment

Usually guided by doppler imagery, cryo treatment involves freezing cancerous growths with a controlled method that seeks to leave healthy tissue undamaged. It has been used effectively in many types of cancer. It usually causes less damage to the body than radiation or chemo and is less invasive. It can't be considered gentle, painless or natural, but is being mentioned here simply because it may be a more favorable choice than chemo or radiation, depending on the type cancer. It has been successfully used for abnormal cells of the cervix, retinoblastoma, skin cancers (before they become malignant), prostate cancer, liver growths and others, and is sometimes used in combination with other cancer therapies. See chapter 34 for a new retinoblastoma treatment that often saves a child's eyesight.

## Cryptoxanthin & Cancer

See chapter 21 for more information on this important carotenoid.

## Ellagic Acid Fights Cervical & Other Cancers

Dr. Daniel Nixon, from MUSC, revealed that ellagic acid, in laboratory testing, could destroy abnormal cells of the cervix and the HPV or human papilloma virus (104). The anti-oxidant also prevented proliferation of the abnormal cells and kept them from harming the p53 gene, a gene that prevents normal cells from mutating. Other cancers also responded (104). One of the richest natural sources of ellagic acid is raspberries. Cherries, berries, pomegranates, strawberries, walnuts, cranberries, and pecans also contain this nutrient. (Cranberries also fight leukemia, and they lower the risk for ulcers and bladder infections (22.)

## Flax Seed Reduces Uterine & Cervical Cancers

A research study involving flax seed revealed that women who consume flax seed supplements can reduce their risk for several types of cancer. The main gist of this research emphasized that using flax seed may prevent and *treat* many types of cancer, including those involving the *breast, uterus, and cervix* (571). An excellent way to incorporate flax oil into the diet is to use fresh organic whole flax seed (either the golden or the brown). Put 2 tablespoons in a coffee grinder. Grind until powdery, add to 8 ounces of water (shake well) and drink. Just be sure to drink it immediately. If you let it sit—even for a few seconds—it will thicken too much. Drink additional water, or juice, if needed. It can be used as a breakfast drink, then again later in the day (Each tablespoon of flax gives you about one teaspoon of flax oil). Try adding one tablespoon of flax oil to a baked potato or your favorite salad dressing, fruit smoothie, or juice. (Most of us need 2 or 3 tablespoons of flax seed oil per day.) Flax is very rich in omega-3 oil.

## Ginger & Ovarian Cancer

Recent studies show that ginger may help protect against ovarian cancer. Though human testing has not yet been widely conducted, it is known that ginger does have anti-inflammatory and anti-nausea properties (124). Research from China indicates that including ginger in your diet can help prevent and treat ovarian cancer (124).

## Grapes Toxic to Cancer Cells

In a laboratory study recently completed, it was noted that resveratrol (found in common table grapes) could halt the growth of human ovarian cancer cells. Resveratrol, even in **large doses,** is not toxic. Animal research revealed that there were no adverse side effects. Even when they were given massive doses—many times greater than you or I would ever ingest in comparable amounts—there were no ill effects.

See Chapter three in this book for ovarian and cervical cancers that were completely healed using resveratrol (in grape juice). Also, for an excellent 58-page study that was done on resveratrol's role in fighting cancer, including ovarian cancer, see website: *http://www.agrawal.org/PDF/ACR-Resveratrol1.pdf.* The study was conducted by M.D. Anderson Cancer Center and the UCLA Center for Human Nutrition (346).

Resveratrol is also being touted as a way to fight obesity, since it keeps the body from storing fat. You can find resveratrol in many foods, including fresh grapes, red wine, and pomegranates, as well as resveratrol supplements in health food stores.

## Green Tea (& Black Tea) for Ovarian Cancer Prevention

When more than 60,000 women were studied for green tea consumption, it was found that those women who consumed more green and black tea cut their risk of ovarian cancer by 24% just by drinking one cup per day, and 50% if they drank *two or more cups per day* (139). A **human** study was done from 1999-2000 on hundreds of people in China to find out the effect tea had on ovarian cancer. At the conclusion of the study, it was determined that the more green tea women consumed, the greater it reduced their risks for ovarian cancer (612). If you consume caffeinated tea, it can strip your body of essential vitamins and minerals since caffeine acts as a diuretic, however, the decaff tea will not help remove arterial plaque as well.

## Lycopene & Endometrial Cancers

Lycopene, discussed earlier, is a potent anti-oxidant and, in laboratory studies, was effective against endometrial cancer. When lycopene was tested against human endometrial cancer cells, it was found to be considerably stronger at halting tumor growth than alpha-carotene or beta-carotene. The same results were found in fighting lung and breast cancer cells (507). High levels of lycopene were also linked to dramatic reductions in other cancers, especially those of the abdomen, colorectal, head-and-neck (507). Look for this nutrient in veggies and fruits (e.g., watermelon, guavas, carrots, and red tomatoes).

## Mushrooms that Inhibit Cancer

Mushrooms (reishi, maitake, shiitake, and several others) can fight cancer. According to the *Wellness Directory of Minnesota's*™ website, *http://www.mn welldirorg,* one mushroom in particular that is effective in helping the body fight ovarian cancer, is the agaricus mushroom (*Agaricus Blazei Murill or ABM*) (11). Use as with any other mushroom. It contains a compound that stunts solid tumors, as well as cancer cells of the sigmoid, breast, ovaries, liver and lungs (11). Do not take maitake products if you have multiple sclerosis (184).

The School of Medicine at Ehime University in Japan found, in animal studies, that Agaricus Blazei Murill can prevent cancer, even when the animals were given LLC or *Lewis Lung Carcinoma* cells (447). Not only did the mushroom prevent the growth of tumors, but kept them from spreading as well. The report also showed that the mushroom increased *natural killer cells* in the immune system (447). The substance that was extracted from the Agaricus mushroom was *sodium pyroglutamate* (447). There are many websites that provide agaricus or ABM mushroom, some in dried form, some fresh. (See chapter 25 of this book for more information about the amazing healing and curative powers of mushrooms and their extracts.) Other mushrooms important in fighting cancer have been mentioned in several chapters of this book.

Other cancer-fighting mushrooms are the reishi, mesima, chaga, tinder polypore, and split-gill mushroom (15).

## Polysaccharide Kureha (PSK)

PSK is an important supplement for preventing the spread of tumors. You will sometimes hear or see it called *krestin.* It comes from the *kawaratake* mushroom (236), also known as the *coriolus versicolor* mushroom, though some people refer to the extract by this name.

PSK is a potent anti-oxidant that boosts the immune system. The Japanese have been using the complex polysaccharides in this mushroom for more than 20 years (236). It is non-toxic and easily absorbed by the body at the cellular level, when swallowed. It is often used with other cancer therapies (236) and can be found in tablet form. Consult your physician if you intend to use PSK (236). Outside of the U.S., PSK is the most popular cancer treatment world-wide (11). Many U.S. physicians do not know that this supplement exists. This is because when you are diagnosed with cancer in Japan (for example), they start using the **least toxic** treatments **first**—then progress to the most toxic (11).

We do things backwards in America. Cancer patients are given the deadliest treatments first, and if the cancer is still there, they are either zapped with more chemo until it sucks out what little life they have left in them, or else they are told they are *terminal*, and nothing else can be done for them. They are rarely told about safer, gentler, alternative treatments available. Patients only hear about them from a relative or a friend who has researched them, or from reading a book, such as this one. Often, their immune system has already been irreversibly obliterated by chemo and radiation; however, remember this, as long as you are still alive, it is NEVER too late, regardless of what your diagnosis is. There are many cases in this book of *terminally ill* cancer patients, completely cured of cancer, using natural, non-toxic therapies (e.g., see chapter 14).

## Vitamin C for Ovarian Cancer

There has been much controversy about megadosing with vitamin C for cancer, but most researchers agree that giving vitamin C directly into the bloodstream (intravenously), gets best results. Linus Pauling, Dr. Abram Hoffer, Dr. Irwin Stone, and many other chemists and researchers have believed and taught this for years. It seems that the modern medical community may finally be taking them seriously.

*The National Institute of Diabetes and Digestive and Kidney Diseases* in Bethesda, Maryland, discovered recently, that giving large amounts of this vitamin intravenously to mice with ovarian cancers, glioblastoma, and cancers of the pancreas, halted the cancer *growth by up to 53%* (329a). The study was headed up by Mark Levine, who said that the vitamin C worked by forming *hydrogen peroxide* which destroyed the *cancer cells* (329a). Cancer Treatment Centers of America *(CTCA)* in Zion, Illinois, is also testing IV Vitamin C on patients with advanced cancer (329a). Recent studies reveal that adequate vitamin C levels can cut your risk for developing diabetes in half.

## Zhu Ling, Chicken-of-the-Woods, Enokitake, Mesima, Chaga, Ice Man, Polypore, Pearl Oyster (Hiratake)

These are other medicinal mushrooms you will see in supplement form that have anti-oxidant, anti-cancer, or anti-viral properties. (This does not include their scientific names and some of the many indigenous names.)

# IV. Hormones Against Cancer - How Excess Estrogen Increases the Risk for Ovarian Cancer

See chapter 22 in this book (on hormone replacement therapy) for information on the dangers of excess estrogen and how it contributes to uterine cancer, breast cancer, ovarian cancer, excess weight, mood swings, infertility, cystic breasts, uterine fibroids, and a host of other ailments. In *What Your Doctor May Not Tell You About Menopause*, Virginia Hopkins and the late Dr. John Lee discuss the dangers of excess estrogen found in the West and how it may account for the rampant increase in ovarian and breast cancers in women. Lack of exercise and excessive calories were also contributing factors (466). Studies have shown that women who never have children are at increased risk for this type cancer.

The higher the dietary fat, the more estrogen is produced by the fat cells. Fat cells produce more estrogen, thus you have a vicious cycle, and the increased risk for women's cancers (466) and prostate cancer in men. Besides controlling high estrogen levels by eating less and exercising more, see chapter 22 for information on how natural progesterone can help play a part in the prevention (and reversal) of estrogen dominance, cancer, and all of the health ailments noted above.

## V. Vitamins & Minerals That Fight Cervical Cancer

### Folate & Vitamin C Prevent Cervical Cancer

Insufficient amounts of folic acid and vitamin C can drastically increase a woman's risk for this type cancer (351). Some good natural sources of folate are oranges, leafy greens (spinach, kale, turnip greens), and cruciferous vegetables, such as cabbage and broccoli (411). It comes as no surprise that physicians tell women with abnormal pap tests (besides needing further testing), that they should be sure they are getting adequate folic acid and vitamin C in their diet. Cigarette smoking also increases the risk for cervical cancer and most other cancers. Natural sources of vitamin C are cherries, oranges, currants, papaya, cantaloupe, peppers, leafy green vegetables, rose hips, pomegranate, watermelon, berries, and many other fruits and vegetables.

### Selenium Fights Cervical & Ovarian Cancer

Selenium, discussed earlier in this book, is gaining much attention for its ability to fight cancer. Selenium, combined with vitamin E, has anti-inflammatory properties (288). When two different universities conducted research over several years on this mineral, they discovered that it only took *200 mcg [micrograms] of selenium daily* to slash all incidences of lung, prostate, intestinal, and rectal cancers (288). Selenium helps prevent just about every other cancer imaginable, and insufficient levels of this mineral increased the risks for malignancies, metastases, and death (288).

## Vitamin C & Poly–MVA

Apparently, even in small amounts, vitamin C can prevent cancer. When researchers were looking for an explanation as to why Latin-American women have excessively high rates for cervical cancers, as compared to the rest of the world, they discovered that if women there would supplement with even small amounts of vitamin C on a daily basis, they could slash their risk of this cancer by greater than one-third—and it did not require much—slightly more than 300 milligrams daily (148).

See chapters 10 and 14 for info on Poly-MVA.

## Vitamin E & Glutathione Prevent Cervical Cancer

The risk for invasive cancers can be greatly decreased by simply supplementing with 200-400 IU per day of mixed tocopherols (vitamin E) (70). Also, insufficient levels of *glutathione* can mean an increased incidence for cervical cancer (70). Having a pap test with abnormal cells, however, does not necessarily mean a cancerous condition. Lesions that are suspicious in the cervix will lighten in color or whiten if coming into contact with *vinegar* (a way that they can be tested) (70). An excellent natural source of glutathione is asparagus. Some researchers believe that the gamma form of vitamin E is superior to the alpha-tocopherol form, however, it is best to have mixed tocopherols and tocotrienols. Do not purchase vitamin E unless you see **tocotrienols** on the list of ingredients! If you decide on the alpha-tocopherol vitamin E, use the **d**-alpha (which is natural), not the **dl**-alpha (which is synthetic), and be sure it is mixed with tocotrienols! (Avocados are also high in glutathione.)

Some good **natural sources** of vitamin E are: wheat germ oil, olive oil, sunflower oil (and seeds), dandelion greens, spinach, broccoli, turnip greens, almonds and other nuts, eggs (411) (492) (524), kiwi, mangoes, fortified cereals, and fresh sprouts (especially wheat berry sprouts).

## VI. Herbs That Help Prevent & Treat Ovarian, Cervical & Uterine Cancers

### Andiroba Helps Prevent Cervical Cancers

According to *www.rain-tree.com*, andiroba is a very tall tree found deep in the rain forest, as well as other areas (19). Oil from the tree has been used for a multitude of purposes, including pain relief (19). Scientists have discovered that this tree has anti-cancerous effects. As recently as 2002, scientists noted that the oil from the seeds of the plant may help restore normal cells in those with *cervical dysplasia* (19). Other parts of the tree have been successfully tested (lab studies) against sarcoma. The oil is used to treat skin disorders, skin cancers, parasites, rashes, and fungi (19).

### Astragalus Tincture or Capsules

Astragalus is important in slowing the progression of abnormal cells and triggering the body's immunity. Check with your physician or Naturopath about using this herb, especially if you have any type of infection or are running a temperature (107).

### Bindweed (*Convolvulus arvensis*) for Ovarian Cancer

Bindweed is a common field weed that you may find sold as *VascuStatin/Angioblock*, or under the name *PGM proteoglycan mixture*, "the active ingredient of VascuStatin, or *MPGC*" (301a). It is a supplement from *Allergy Research Group*®. VascuStatin supplement has a significant amount of *leaf extract of bindweed* (301a). Bindweed is being used successfully by some health practitioners for fighting cancer, including ovarian and pancreatic cancers. It is said to be non-toxic and "100 times stronger than shark cartilage powder" at preventing the growth of new blood vessels (301a). See chapter 34 for more details on bindweed. Also, see page 3 of their website *(http://organicpharmacy.org/products/VascuStatin)*, for the case of a woman with ovarian cancer who was given a year to live, then started taking bindweed *tincture*. Seven years later, she is still very much alive and doing well. (301a). On page 2 of their website, you will be given warnings about when this substance should not be taken. For *maximum positive effect*, it is supposed to work best when combined with *Imm-Kine* (muramyl polysaccharide glycan complex or MPGC), a patented formula containing muramic acid (and other ingredients) that stimulate the immune system. As always, be sure your physician is directing your care while on this or any other supplement (301a). Apparently, in animal tests, the PGM worked whether it was given by mouth, intravenously, *subcutaneous*, or by *intraperitoneal* route (through the abdomen) (301a). PGM works by several methods, including boosting the body's natural immunity. Bindweed has been used in many human cancer cases (e.g., see chapter four and its success against a stage IV breast cancer (301a), and chapter 12 for its effect on a patient with pancreatic cancer) (150). Also, see chapter 34 for more details on bindweed.

## Cancer Bush—*Sutherlandia frutescens*—Fights Cervical Carcinoma & Ovarian Cancer

*Sutherlandia frutescens*, known as the *cancer bush*, grows in Southern Africa and is used there to treat cancer (368). When the plant was tested at the University of the Western Cape in Cape Town, South Africa, researchers discovered (in animal testing) that it killed *cervical carcinoma* cells, as well as ovarian cancer cells. They are planning further research (368).

## Cat's Claw for All Cancers

Cat's claw raises levels of white blood cells that fight cancer cells. Do not use this herb if you are breast feeding or pregnant. Do not combine it with hormones or diabetic medications, including insulin (107). See chapter 20 for other times when you should not take cat's claw.

## Chinese Skullcap for Inflammation

Chinese Skullcap (*Scutellaria baicalensis*) is said to help the body fight viruses (such as HIV) that can induce cancer. It exerts a natural anti-inflammatory action on the body (375). Do not use without consulting your physician or Naturopath.

## Emodin & Cervical Cancer

Emodin has been an herb of choice in Chinese medicine for years. It has anti-cancer properties against many types of cancer, including those of the cervix in human cells (569). In laboratory testing, it has been able to kill cancer cells (569).

## Essiac Tea & Advanced Ovarian Cancer

Chapter six of this book has more details on the herbal remedy, Essiac tea, and the story of the Canadian nurse who used the tea to cure many of her cancer patients. In an article at *www.1001herbs.com,* a case history is given of Myrna, a patient diagnosed with an aggressive metastasizing cancer of her ovaries that was already in her lungs and lymphatic system (496). Physicians told her that surgery to remove all of her cancer was not possible due to the large amount of tumors. They did perform a hysterectomy, gave her only months to live, and she was basically sent home to die (496). When Myrna asked her doctors if anything else could be done from an alternative approach—such as using nutrition to extend her life and retard the disease—she was told that nothing could be done. She was, however, placed on hormone therapy, and she obtained the herbs for Essiac tea, which her grandmother brewed for her (496). She went to her physician on a weekly basis, and x-rays showed that the tumors were slowly shrinking. Not only were the tumors disappearing, but her labs were normal (496). Within one year after starting the Essiac, Myrna's physician called to inform her that all her diagnostic studies showed her to be totally cancer-free. She has been without recurrence in the past several years (496). The *hormonal therapy* was not identified.

Note that there is some competition between the tea produced by Resperin of Canada Essiac® and Flor-Essence® Essiac tea. Both companies claim that they have the original Essiac formula (the drinkable formula, not the injectable) that Rene Caisse used in treating her cancer patients. You can obtain Flor-Essence® at many natural health food stores in an already prepared drinkable form, or a powdered form that you brew yourself.

## Essiac Tea & Uterine Cancer

An informative book describing the effectiveness of this tea and how it was suppressed by the health industry in Canada is called *The Essiac Report Canada's Remarkable Unknown Cancer Remedy,* by Richard Thomas, who claims that Flor-Essence® is the original (drinkable) formula that Rene Caisse used. In his book, he says that Rene shared the original recipe with Dr. Brusch. It was perfected to the point that injections no longer needed to be given, because the oral formula was effective. Mr. Thomas claims that the original formula was developed into Flor-Essence® tea, which can be found at most health food stores (580).

Richard Thomas describes the case of a woman who came to Rene with uterine cancer and weighing less than 90 lbs. She received the Essiac formula and gave her testimony **45 years** later to *Homemakers*. She was still living a normal life and doing well more than four decades after receiving the Essiac treatment (580). Another woman, discussed by Mr. Thomas, was treated with the Essiac formula for bilateral breast cancer and uterine cancer. She had been sent to Rene by her physician as terminal. Three months later, she had returned to work. **40 years** later, she was still alive and well, without ever having cancer again (580).

## Espinheira Santa Inhibits Ovarian Cancer

Espinheira santa is an herb often referred to as *South American holly*, and used medicinally for many ailments (109). Lab studies show that this herb may help fight lung and ovarian cancers. (109). It can be purchased in tincture form and is also sold in bulk-tea format.

## German Chamomile

Chamomile is commonly prepared in tea bags. It contains compounds that fight the ability of cancer cells to spread (107).

## Graviola

See Chapters five and six for more information on how a common herb, *graviola,* from the Amazonian Rain Forest has been used to fight cancer.

## Green Tea & Ovarian Cancer

Green tea is an excellent source of very powerful anti-oxidants that inhibit the ability of estrogen to be absorbed by tumor cells. It is best to wait at least 60 minutes after drinking green tea before taking any type of prescription medicine (107). Green tea has also been found—in animal testing by Israeli researchers—to actually regenerate brain cells, something hitherto thought impossible (169).

## Inflammation & the Cancer Process - Ovarian Cancer

There appears to be a close connection between an underlying infection and the subsequent development of cancer. This is probably the reason that the media recently publicized that following an aspirin regimen could help reduce *lung cancer* in *women* by 50% over those not on aspirin (351). They claimed the same protection against other cancers, such as those of the breast and intestines (351). Aspirin usage, however, has some very unpopular side effects. Many people are hospitalized yearly with fatal complications (e.g., hemorrhage) from using aspirin and NSAIDS. There are natural plant flavonoids that can block the enzymes responsible for inflammation (351). These substances can be found in leafy greens, some cruciferous vegetables, berries, tea, citrus, other fruits like apples, and in the herb *ginkgo biloba* (351).

## Iscador Extends Life Span of Cancer Patients

Human studies, reported as recently as December of 2008, show that Iscador can help extend the life span of those with cancer, most notably, those with ovarian and cervical cancers (197a). See chapter 4 for more information on Iscador, also known as *mistletoe.*

## Snow Fungus Inhibits Cervical Cancer

Snow fungus *(Tremella fuciformis),* also called *white jelly leaf*… [and] *white tree-ear*, has been used for many centuries in Asia for medicinal purposes (273). The fungus has been identified as an important stimulant for the immune system, having the ability to fight cancer, blood fats, infection, and enhance liver function (273). This herb also helps the body kill cancer (273). In laboratory studies, extracts have been able to destroy various types of cancer cells, including those of the cervix (273).

## Turmeric & Cervical Cancer

Turmeric is a popular spice used throughout the world. It contains a very impressive anti-oxidant known as *curcumin* that triggers immunity for suppressing cancer (70) (89). Excessive levels of estrogen inhibit the immune system from doing its job adequately, as do toxins. It is the curcumin in turmeric that motivates the main gene that fights cancer and abnormal cells like those of cervical dysplasia (70) (89). See chapter 20 for instances when you should not use curcumin (turmeric).

## VII. Other Anti-Cancer Supplements & Treatments

### BSI-201

This is a new drug, still in testing phases, developed by BiPar Sciences, Inc., that is said to have no toxic side effects (561a). Tests thus far involve those cancers (e.g., breast and ovarian) that are fast-growing (561a).

### Burzynski's Antineoplastons

See chapter 14 of this book for amazing cases of cancer patients completely cured of *terminal* cancers, people who were basically sent home to die, then chose non-toxic antineoplastons from the Burzynski Clinic in Texas. Antineoplastons are also used to treat ovarian, uterine, and cervical cancers and nearly every other cancer. Also, see the patient's own stories about their success in fighting cancer with antineoplastons at website: *http://burzynskipatientgroup.org/stories.html.* Many of these cancers were very aggressive, terminal tumors. The FDA has finally approved the oral form of antineoplastons, known as *sodium phenylbutrates* (PBs). Note that antineoplastons A10 and AS2-1 were recently given orphan drug status by the FDA for use on human brainstem gliomas.

### CyberKnife® Therapy for Tumors

See chapter 34 in this book for details on painless CyberKnife® therapy, which is being used successfully for many cancers, including hard-to-reach brain tumors. It does not require an incision, surgery, sedation or inpatient stay. It takes very little time, and as soon as the procedure is over, the patient is able to walk out and return home. There are very few risks and side effects, though it does involve some radiation (89a), and it can damage nearby healthy cells. Also, read about the new painless therapy, NanoKnife™, on page 630.

## Hydrazine Sulfate Inhibits Cervical Cancer

See Chapter 16 for details on hydrazine sulfate, a therapy developed and used by Joseph Gold, M.D. for treating many forms of cancer, including cervical cancer.

## Natural Treatments for Curing Uterine, Cervical & Peritoneal Cancers

When a biochemical researcher began experimenting on sharks to find out why they rarely develop cancer, regardless of how polluted their environment, the next step was human testing (386). Three physicians treated ten cancer victims without charge, all of them having advanced cancer and given just a few months survival time (386). One patient left the study and one died, leaving eight to participate. Though these were all terminal cases, in seven patients tumors decreased and some were considered *miracle cures* (386). One was a middle-aged woman with stage III endometrial and cervical cancer that had gone into her bladder. She had no response from radiation; however, 49 days after she began using shark cartilage, she was pain-free, with massive tumor-shrinkage. Eleven weeks into this therapy, and her tumor was completely gone (386).

Another woman, in her sixties, with the same type cancer (which spread AFTER she received radiation), was **nearly three months into shark cartilage treatment, when she was told that the tumor had completely disappeared** (386).

A patient, in her thirties, with stage IV colon cancer that had metastasized to her peritoneal area, was told she was terminal. After using shark cartilage for 60 days and undergoing surgery for an abscess, it was discovered that her tumor had nearly disappeared. Less than one month later, she was found to be completely cancer-free, and was described as a *miracle cure* (386).

It is remarkable that one of the first benefits of shark cartilage was its ability to reduce pain, and in all of the clinical trials done, though some of the patients had no change (some did better, then relapsed), it was found that the therapy had no adverse effects whatsoever, regardless of the dosages used. For the testing, the substance used was *pure*. Patients having advanced tumors (*Stage III and Stage IV*) were given the shark cartilage based on body weight. For example, a person weighing 200 lbs would receive 100 grams of the pure shark cartilage; a 180 lb person would receive 90 grams; a 100 lb person would receive 50 grams. The substance was given every day and administered either orally or as a *retention enema* (386). Pure shark cartilage can be found at most health food stores. Even some pharmacies now carry the capsules.

It appears that giving shark cartilage has not only helped many cancer patients, but those suffering from arthritis, psoriasis, and enteritis as well (386). One particular case involved a patient bedridden with *rheumatoid arthritis* (386). The patient opted for shark cartilage treatment. He suffered for more than two decades with no relief from conventional therapy. Less than a month later, he was completely pain-free, and it was reported that his misshapen spine was improving and re-aligning (386).

Since shark cartilage works by preventing new blood vessels from growing (which tumors depend on to survive), it is not recommended during pregnancy, for children, or for patients recovering from surgical procedures, heart attacks (because after a heart attack, the body often grows secondary blood vessels on its own to circumvent clogged vessels), transplants, during chemo or radiation, or for those contemplating surgery. It is not for those with high blood pressure, pheochromocytoma (adrenal tumor which can cause excessively high blood pressure), seafood allergies, liver disease (although it has been used successfully in treating liver cancer), ulcers, or circulatory diseases. You should be consulting with your natural health physician for specific dosing for your own individual needs before taking this supplement.

According to Harvard Medical School, when blood vessels branch out within the body, this process is known as *angiogenesis*, a condition without which tumors cannot grow. These researchers recommended *2,000 mg a day* (278) of the substance. Shark cartilage is available at most health food stores and even some pharmacies, as noted earlier.

Conventional medicine has never recognized shark cartilage as a remedy for cancer in spite of its anti-angiogenesis factors, but you will never guess what a pharmaceutical company began pushing eight years ago to target tumors—a chemo drug described as having the ability to inhibit the formation of new arteries and veins to prevent tumors from being supplied with the nutrients that they need to survive—something that shark cartilage already does. This ability to cut off circulation to tumors is not really new. The only catch is this: the chemo drug has some potentially toxic side effects, some of them fatal (e.g., intestinal rupture and hemorrhage). Do you know how many potentially toxic side effects shark cartilage has? Thus far, there have been no serious side effects associated with the use of shark cartilage. Shark cartilage, a natural product **cannot be patented**. Better to CREATE a synthetic drug (with two dozen or more potentially deadly side effects) that can be patented and sold for millions of dollars, than to tell the public that a NATURAL substance that inhibits new blood vessel formation (without **TOXIC side effects)** is already available.

Tumors must have a reliable system of blood vessels, without which they will shrivel up and die. Without this network of blood vessels, tumors will grow no larger than a few millimeters in size (268).

See chapter 34 of this book for more information on an herb known as *bindweed* that is said to have *100 times* the ability at blocking blood vessel formation as that found in shark cartilage (301a), and bindweed is non-toxic. (It can be toxic when it is gathered and used wild.) A woman with advanced ovarian cancer, who was told that she had *only one year to live,* began taking *tincture of bindweed.* That was seven years ago (301a).

Also, see information on a new, safer drug below (Lodamin), which works by cutting off blood supply to tumors.

For an amazing case study from Guisseppi A. Forgionne Ph.D., about an 89 year-old woman who experienced total remission from advanced peritoneal cancer using an alternative nutritional approach, see website *http://www.cancerlynx.com/peritonealcase.html* (400). After having surgery, she refused chemo. According to the article, her nutritional regimen included *2 grams of wheat grass* per day (a week after her surgery), then *100 mg* of *CoQ10* daily a week after that, and within 2 more weeks, the addition of *9 grams of bovine cartilage/*day. *Nine months* later, her CoQ10 was changed to *150 mg per day* (400).

## PARP Inhibitors - New, Safer Drug for Women with BRCA1-BRCA2 Mutations for Breast & Ovarian Cancers

A new drug undergoing clinical trials in "Europe, the United States and Australia by…pharmaceutical giant, AstroZeneca, involved women who were at death's door with end-stage cancer" (348a). Most had failed standard treatments of "surgery, chemotherapy and radiotherapy," as noted by William Birnbauer in an article at *theage.com.au* website 08/17/2008 (348a). The drug, known as a *PARP inhibitor,* was able to "reduce tumour sizes in 46% of the cases" and 59% of the" women experienced either "tumour shrinkage or stabilization" (348a). Though the "international trials involved just 63 people with advanced breast cancer" and 63 "with advanced ovarian cancer," results are encouraging and trials are continuing. This drug zeroes in on cancer cells, so the usual side effects seen by standard chemo (e.g., "hair loss and nausea") don't occur, because chemo attacks both cancer cells and healthy cells (348a).

## Soy (Fermented) & Endometrial Cancer

Studies are showing that soy can harm the thyroid, and many people cannot tolerate soy. When choosing soy, fermented soy products are fine. (Fermented soy products, such as Haelan, may help remove harmful estrogen from the body in estrogen receptor-positive cancers.) Genistein (found in soy) can also help lower blood pressure. For information on Haelan see the company's website at *www.haelan 951.com.* Information on Haelan's Research Foundation's website was accumulated from clinical studies performed on fermented soy beverages manufactured by Haelan Products, Inc. of Woodinville, Washington. The Haelan fermented soy beverages are sold in the United States, without medical claims, and are available directly from the company or one of their distributors. (143).

Website, *herbs2000.com,* recommends that those with endometrial cancer avoid certain herbs, including peony and fennel seed (107).

## Ukrain for Cervical Cancer

A woman with Grade IV cancer of the cervix, who received Ukrain, showed no cancer a year later. Within three years she had a healthy baby. That was eight years ago and she has remained cancer-free. For the case report, see the National Library of Medicine NCBI PubMed website: PMID 8899342 (456).

## Ukrain for Retroperitoneal Sarcoma

A young woman, who underwent surgery to remove a *synovial sarcoma*, went into complete remission after receiving 10 injections of Ukrain (10 mg. per day on *alternate days*) post-operatively, and was still cancer-free four years later. She experienced no adverse effects (530).

# VIII. Miscellaneous Risk Factors & Treatments

## Drinking Coffee May Reduce Risk for Ovarian Cancer

A **human** study involving 80,000 participants showed that consuming a minimum of *three cups of coffee a day* could decrease the risk for ovarian cancer; however, caffeine can contribute toward the incidence of miscarriage (384). It also acts like a diuretic and can dehydrate the body.

## Fiber Lowers Risk of Endometrial Cancers

Research shows that women can reduce their risk of endometrial cancer by nearly half, simply by eating more fiber. This lowered their incidence of endometrial cancer (275). There are many excellent sources of fiber, including fruits and vegetables. Cereals, such as steel-cut oats, are very high in fiber. Steel-cut oats also help lower insulin levels in the blood, as does cinnamon.

## Low Fat Diet Reduces Risk for Ovarian Cancer

Reducing the amount of dietary fat in your diet will improve your overall health and prevent chronic diseases and cancer. Scientists found that the incidence of ovarian cancer could be dramatically decreased by having women limit their fat intake by a mere *ten grams per day* (604).

## Milk & Dairy Products Increase Risk for Ovarian Cancer

The type of sugar found naturally in milk, *galactose,* has been linked with an above average occurrence for ovarian cancers (551). Since those studies were done, other **human** studies have shown that milk (especially lactose) consumption increases a woman's risk for ovarian cancer.

## Nanotechnology—Lodamin—Curing Ovarian & Uterine Cancer Without Toxic Side Effects

A new drug, Lodamin, which works by halting the blood vessel growth that tumors need to survive, was shown in animal testing, to be effective against many tumor types, including those of the breast, brain, ovaries, uterus, prostate, neuroblastoma, and glioblastoma (401). It also worked very well in preventing cancer from going into the liver (401). The discovery of the drug, using *nanotechnology* and a derivative from a fungus, was quite accidental. Reports say that it can be taken orally without *side effects* (401). The drug also inhibited melanoma and lung cancer in mice (401). Lodamin is still in the testing phases, and is also being considered for treating macular degeneration and arthritis.

Note that shark cartilage and bindweed, also discussed in this book, work to starve tumors by cutting off blood supply to them, without adverse side effects.

## Radiation & Pelvic Lymph Node Removal No Longer Recommended for Early Endometrial Cancer

Conventional medicine has routinely treated **early** endometrial cancer with hysterectomy and removal of the ovaries and tubes, along with radiation and removal of the pelvic lymph nodes (299a). Now, scientists are saying, after the results of **human** studies, that they are no longer recommending that these women undergo the radiation and pelvic lymph node removal, indicating that it does not affect recurrence or survival rates. The study spanned four countries (299a).

## TGFBI Protein & Ovarian Cancer Treatment

Conventional medicine often uses Paclitaxel chemo for ovarian cancer, but they admit a response rate of only 50%. Recently, they have announced that patients who lack a certain protein in their body, known as *TGFBI,* are the ones who are not responding to conventional treatment (444). If your physician decides to test you for this protein, they will be checking to see whether or not you are a good candidate for Paclitaxel, based on whether or not you have TGFBI. Paclitaxel, like most chemo drugs, can have some very serious side effects.

## Talc & Ovarian Cancer

Do not use talc powder, especially in the genital area; it has been linked to causing ovarian cancer and may be as harmful as asbestos!

## Targeted Nanoparticles for Ovarian Cancer & Implanted Magnetic Sensing

A company by the name of *Carigent Therapeutics, Inc.*, was recently awarded a grant for research on *targeted nanoparticles* to treat ovarian cancer. Paclitaxel or Taxol®, a chemo drug that goes by several different names, is widely used by conventional medicine to treat many types of cancer, including ovarian tumors (66). Nanoparticle therapy's ultimate goal is to be able to develop a way that this drug can be sent to cancer cells in a concentrated and controlled fashion, hoping to make it more efficient at killing cancer cells and less toxic to normal cells (66). Nanoparticles are also used as a way to monitor the effectiveness of chemo drugs, and for checking on cancer growth in a procedure known as *implanted magnetic sensing* (204). Some of the adverse effects of Paclitaxel are from its current delivery system, which requires it to be mixed with ingredients that would not be needed in the nanoparticle delivery system (204). Only time will tell whether the nanoparticle system is safer. One of the problems with the current use of Taxol®, which is often given for breast cancer, is that it can cause uterine cancer. There are other potentially adverse side effects as well.

## Vaccinations & Cancer

According to Robert Morse, M.D., in *The Detox Miracle Sourcebook*, think carefully before choosing vaccinations (503). They may be the culprit in such diseases as *cancer*, *multiple sclerosis*, *arthritis*, Crohn's, *diabetes*, and many other conditions (503). They have also been implicated in auto-immune disorders, digestive disorders, SIDS, Guillain-Barre syndrome, Alzheimer's, and autism. There is a possibility that physicians are going to recommend that children's vaccines be spaced out over a longer period of time and giving them fewer vaccines at a time to cut the risk for autism. This, ONLY after many lawsuits against vaccine companies from parents who sued them after their children developed post-vaccination autism! (Also, see p. 488 for the link between MS & vitamin D deficiency.)

## Water – Adequate Hydration to Prevent Cancer

See chapter 23 for more information on how adequate water intake can dramatically reduce the risk for cancer and chronic diseases.

# IX. Vulva Cancers - New Topical Drug Shrinks Cancer Cells

Cancers of the vulva are usually treated with laser or surgery, depending on the depth of the cancer and staging (588a). Some of these type cancers may extend down into the vaginal wall. The New *England Journal of Medicine,* however, has just publicized a report on a new topical drug Aldara™ (Imiquimod), which "may be an effective alternative to surgery for the treatment of precancerous changes to the vulva called vulva intraepithelial neoplasia" (588a). Aldara™ works by boosting the body's immune system in order to kill the cancer (588a).

The topical medication was tested on nearly two dozen women with either *grade 2 or 3 VIN.* Within 20 weeks "21 of the 26 women" using the topical medication had a *25%* decrease in the size of their *lesion* (588a). Women using the Aldara™ had "tissue samples" showing a "significant increase in the number of immune cells at the site," after application of the Aldara™ (588a). This did not happen in the *placebo group.* "After 20 weeks nine patients" using the Aldara™ "had a complete response and were still free from disease at 12 months" (588a). Treatment of VIN is considered "critical as it can progress to cancer." For further details on this trial, see website: *http://patient.cancerconsultants.com/CancerNews_Cancer.aspx?DocumentId=41797* (588a). As with most topical drugs, this one can cause skin reactions in some individuals.

# X. Iodine & Women's Cancers

There is a silent epidemic in America and many parts of the world, an epidemic of iodine deficiency. Dr. Mark Sircus, Ac., OMD, has much to say about the pervasive lack of iodine in the average diet, and why this deficiency is causing many illnesses and diseases, including breast cancer, thyroid cancer, and many other cancers (566a). See his book, *Iodine Bringing Back the Universal Medicine,* on the importance of iodine in fighting yeast (and killing cancer in the process), killing bacteria, parasites, malaria, flu viruses, and many other ailments caused by a deficiency in this critical mineral (566a). You can find a food-grade, gentle form of superior iodine called *Magnascent* (or *Nascent* iodine) at *http://www.magnascent.com* and *http:// www. magneticclay.com.* Also, see chapter 34 for more details on Dr. Sircus' books on magnesium and using soda bicarb for fighting all forms of cancer gently, rapidly and inexpensively.

# CHAPTER 8

# GENTLE CURES FOR TOUGH LEUKEMIAS & MULTIPLE MYELOMAS

*"O' Lord my God, I cried unto thee, and thou hast healed me." (Psalm 30:2)*

## I. Leukemia, Myelomas & Bone Marrow Transplants

Leukemia is sometimes referred to as a *blood cancer*. When a person is diagnosed with leukemia, usually what occurs is a dramatic elevation in their white blood cell count because immature, cancerous, white blood cells (called *blasts*) are multiplying so rapidly that they crowd out normal blood cells, causing hemorrhage. There may not be enough platelets for proper clotting. Infections occur since there are not enough normal, mature white blood cells to fight viruses and bacteria, etc., and severe weakness and anemia (and many other symptoms), because normal red blood cells may be crowded out. (The cells in *hairy cell* leukemia actually develop tiny hairy-looking little outgrowths from the cellular wall that are obvious under a microscope, hence its name.)

Every year, many thousands of people in the U.S. are diagnosed with various leukemias. In acute leukemia (as opposed to chronic leukemia), the cancerous blood cells that develop are immature and unable to function and they multiply rapidly, crowding out normal, healthier cells. The disease progresses quickly. In chronic leukemia, the cells are more mature, thus slightly more efficient (than the more immature cells of acute leukemia), and they divide and multiply much more slowly, thus, the progression of the disease is less rapid. There are many subclasses of leukemia. Most of our blood cells form in the body's bone marrow, though some do form in the spleen. Leukemia that forms from cells of the bone marrow is called *myeloid* leukemia. If forming in the lymphatic system, it is called *lymphocytic* leukemia. We depend on red blood cells for vital functions, such as carrying oxygen and other nutrients to and from the cells, while white blood cells are the body's immune system policemen, protecting us from outside invaders and inside mutants.

When the immune system becomes compromised, such as during times of acute and chronic stress; through exposure and ingestion of harmful chemicals, toxins, radiation, medications; lack of proper rest, diet, exercise, and fluids; the result can be the overgrowth of cancerous blood cells. These malignancies then crowd out the healthy cells, causing serious complications, hemorrhage, and nutritional starvation, which results in death (if left untreated), and sometimes results in death even IF treated, as some people do not respond to treatment.

There are also some circumstances where people may be genetically predisposed to developing certain types of leukemia, and it is a fact that radiation, toxins, chemo drugs, and nuclear fallout can cause leukemia. Unfortunately, many people who undergo radiation or chemotherapy treatment for one type of cancer, often develop leukemia later as a result of the radiation (or chemo) that they received for the prior cancer. This is a well-known (but often not discussed) *side effect* of radiation and chemotherapy treatment. A cruel twist. Just as other cancers can be prevented and often cured by immunotherapy (boosting the immune system by natural means to help the body heal itself), the same can be said of some leukemias. Some of the more rare types of leukemia, the chronic myeloproliferative disorders, such as chronic eosinophilic leukemia (CEL) and chronic neutrophilic leukemia (CNL), are not discussed in detail in this book.

## Myelomas

Myelomas are tumors that have their origin in the body's *bone marrow*. When these cancerous cells multiply and invade the bone and bone marrow, forming multiple tumors, the disease is known as *multiple myeloma*. This abnormal process crowds out the natural antibodies, wreaking havoc in the immune system and increasing the odds for life-threatening infections (283). As for multiple myeloma, many Oncologists believe that this disease cannot be cured, though there are treatments available. They also say that one cannot prevent the disease, and usually by the time a person is symptomatic, their cancer has severely progressed; however, is it true that multiple myeloma cannot be prevented?

Cancers, including myeloma and leukemia, are the result of an immune system gone berserk. Though many cancers can be hereditary or caused by environmental conditions out of our control, are there other types of cancer that we can prevent by boosting the immune system, much as we try to prevent the flu and common cold ? (For example, with juicing and proper nutrition, exercise, getting plenty of rest, fresh air, prayer, positive mental attitude, etc.) Is it not reasonable to assume that we can sometimes prevent leukemia and myeloma by strengthening the immune system? Not only that, but it has been proven that excellent nutrition can cancel out some of the risks of genetically-caused cancers.

## Mini-Transplants

You may often hear other patients, or your physician, speaking of a "mini-transplant," as opposed to a standard transplant. The mini-transplant is being used for leukemias, metastasizing melanomas, myelodysplasia, multiple myelomas, kidney cancers, lymphomas, and others (339a). Patients may not be subjected to the total body irradiation and intensive chemo rounds that are found in a routine bone marrow transplant (339a). They are still, however, given some immunosuppressive drugs. They claim that this type transplant, where the patients are subjected to less intensive chemo and radiation, is "Less Toxic," and results in fewer deaths (339a). For example, instead of 25% of the patients dying from the main transplant procedure, only 10% die with the mini-transplant (339a). How do these odds sound to you? If they sound great to you - it's your choice. You may wish to read the rest of this book to see what other choices cancer patients have made.

## Bone Marrow Transplants (BMT)

Before you decide for certain on a bone marrow transplant for cancer, see chapter 16 in this book for the most amazing story of Maryjo Seigel, who opted out of a recommended bone marrow transplant when she was diagnosed with deadly non-Hodgkins lymphoma in 1991. She chose a non-toxic treatment known as Burzynski's antineoplastons (562). Maryjo testified about her amazing non-toxic cancer cure before the U.S. House of Representatives Government Reform and Oversight Committee on February 02, 1998 (562). That testimony is discussed in detail in chapter 16 of this book. She is still doing great and has never had a reoccurrence of the lymphoma! If you would like to contact her, you can write her at her email address: *maryjo@siegel.net,* and she will be happy to tell you all about her experience with antineoplastons. She also sent a letter to Ted Kennedy after he had been diagnosed with a brain tumor, telling him about the many people who have been cured of deadly brain cancers and other cancers (like hers) by the Burzynski clinic without using toxic drugs and radiation. You can read part of her testimony in chapter 16 of this book, and complete details of her experience at the Burzynski group website: *http://burzynski patientgroup.org/maryjo.htm* (562). Many high profile people have died recently from conventional cancer treatment. It is a shame that more of them did not research non-toxic treatments, such as Dr. Burzynski's antineoplastons, before allowing themselves to be poisoned with drugs and radiation that destroy the immune system.

Conventional medicine attempts to treat some forms of leukemia and myeloma with chemotherapy drugs in a procedure known as a bone marrow (or stem cell) transplant. Acute lymphocytic and non-lymphocytic leukemias, brain tumors, Ewing's sarcoma, breast cancer, Hodgkins and non-Hodgkins lymphoma, neuroblastoma, ovarian cancer, and small cell lung cancers are often treated by conventional medicine with BMTs.

There are three different kinds of bone marrow transplant, depending where the cells are taken from: *Allogeneic,* where a donor (other than an identical twin) provides the cells; *Autologous,* where cells are taken from the patient, stored, then reinfused following high-dose chemotherapy; and *Syngeneic,* using an identical twin (42).

Note that some bone marrow transplants may involve the use of stem cells taken from cord blood. Many people are objecting to the use of unethical stem cell experimentation on embryos, and this should not even be considered, especially since there are other stem cell resources. Stem cells can even be extracted from wisdom teeth for research and scientific study. Many parents are now using blood banks to store their newborn's cord blood, hoping that they will never need it, but as an insurance in case they do!

Part of the bone marrow transplant may involve what is known as TBI or **total body irradiation**. The goal during this time is the destruction of your own bone marrow and the complete disablement of your immune system. Make no mistake—this is a deliberate and total **destruction of your immune system**—there is nothing accidental about it. During many of the actual phases of the bone marrow transplant, patients are subjected to multiple rounds of chemotherapy. Right before the transplant, they are usually given very high dose chemotherapy (depending on the type transplant), which suppresses the body's immune system.

During much of the time, those undergoing the procedure will be very susceptible to infection, disease, and excess bleeding, hence the reason for reverse isolation. Patients are often given very high doses of antibiotics, which in themselves may cause toxic side effects (e.g., massive yeast infections, allergic reactions, or kidney damage). They may also be given blood products to help fend off infections. (Keep in mind that after destroying the entire immune system, the Oncologist now attempts everything possible to ***fix* the damage** that was done in hopes that the immune system will accept the transplant, rather than reject it, and begin to repair itself.) Other side effects of the bone marrow transplant can be pneumonia, liver problems, open skin sores, gastric problems, and many others. The newly implanted bone marrow cells begin growing and dividing in a process known as *engraftment,* usually around the 14th day or so after the BMT. Nurses working with bone marrow transplant patients know that engraftment is a critical stage.

If all goes as planned, the patient should eventually start producing their own white blood cells, platelets, and red blood cells, and will be sent home from the hospital. The entire hospital stay could be a two month process. It may take another six months (to a year) before their lives will ever resume a semblance of normalcy. Those who receive their own cells are generally at a lower risk for complications and may return to usual routines quicker than patients receiving allogeneic transplants. Patients who undergo bone marrow transplant from a donor often experience a serious problem known as GVHD or *graft-versus-host-disease.* Their body actually begins to reject the transplanted blood cells, much like someone getting a kidney transplant will reject a donor kidney. If the rejection is mild, prognosis is good. GVHD is fatal without treatment.

Sometimes antibodies are given to help remove t-lymphocytes, which may be the culprit in causing the rejection, especially if physicians believe there is a high possibility of rejection (e.g., a match that is far from perfect) (314).

It is a sad irony that one of the many possible adverse effects of getting a bone marrow transplant for multiple myeloma (and other cancers) is *leukemia.* Patients may survive the BMT, return to their normal routines, then a year or two later, be diagnosed with leukemia from all the chemotherapy and total body irradiation. It is not at all unusual to come down with secondary cancers after taking chemotherapy or radiation. Chemo and radiation patients can be lulled into a false sense of security (believing that they have beaten their cancer odds), because they go along for a year or two living out their normal routine, only to end up with a worse cancer than the one they started with! I saw this happen over and over again in my own experience while following these patients in case management.

According to *Taber's Cyclopedic Medical Dictionary*, once a person has received chemo or radiation, their risk for developing non-Hodgkin's lymphoma is greater than *100 times* over those who do not receive such treatment (283). It is believed that the therapies used to depress the immunity may stimulate viruses that cause cancer (283). Do you realize what they are SAYING here? They are telling you that if you take chemo or radiation, your chances of getting this OTHER cancer (NHL) is *100 times* greater as opposed to those NOT taking chemo and radiation. How do you like those odds? When your physician tries to push chemo and radiation onto you or your loved ones, ask them about these odds.

During the time that I worked as a Transplant Coordinator R.N. for an insurance company, I telephonically followed the cases of hundreds of transplant patients from beginning to end. I recall that the BMT patients were often miserable. In anguish, they would tearfully cry to me about all the horrible side effects they were experiencing from the toxic chemo drugs or radiation they had received. I could understand their terrible desperation, and though I would try to reassure them that they were doing well and stood a good chance of recovery, in my innermost being, my heart was sinking because I knew that many of them were dying. I knew that the BMT process had inflicted upon their immune system a fatal blow from which they might never recover. It was discouraging (but I knew very little about alternative therapies at that time), and one of the many reasons why I began researching alternative cancer therapies, which led to this book. The remainder of this chapter deals with natural ways to prevent and fight leukemia and multiple myeloma, many of which have even cured those already with the active disease.

## Chemo Combo for Multiple Myeloma Patients

Conventional medicine is now treating relapsing multiple myeloma patients (which means that they had the cancer, then it returned in spite of chemo) with a combination of the drugs *pomalidomide and dexamethasone (pom/dex)* (84a). The ongoing human study on this treatment is being conducted by the Mayo Clinic. Dexamethasone, of course, is a steroid, and Pomalidomide is considered an *immunomodulatory drug IMiD* (84a), a thalidomide-type drug that boosts the immune system, though it does have the potential for adverse effects (e.g., thrombocytopenia and neutropenia). They are being mentioned here, because, if you know someone being treated for recurring multiple myeloma, you may hear them mention these drugs. (Be sure to read the rest of the material in this chapter on the many non-toxic treatments for multiple myeloma.)

## Chemo Pill for Advanced Leukemia & Lymphoma

A new chemo pill that developers claim does not have the adverse side effects normally seen with usual chemo drugs, is being touted as a way to fight several types of lymphoma and leukemia. It is known as *fostamatinib disodium* and thus far, in **human** trials, is showing great promise for aggressive lymphomas and leukemia. For details, see website: *http://insciences.org/article.php?article_id=570*, and the research information from the University of Rochester Medical Center (72a).

## Cord Stem Cells - Recent Studies

Italian scientists discovered that *directly* injecting *stem cells* taken from *umbilical* cords into the *bone marrow* of leukemia patients, brought dramatic results in many of those with advanced disease (402a). *32 participants were suffering with AML* or *acute myeloid leukemia* and *12* had *ALL* or *acute lymphoblastic leukemia.* Their *median* age was 36. There were no other qualified donors, and at least 14 of them had failed other conventional treatment. None of the patients experienced rejection of the cells, or GVHD. At *13 months,* 16 of the participants were in *remission.* Four had *relapsed* and *died. Infection* killed *seven* and *five* expired from *complications* (402a).

## Depressed Immunity in Cancer Patients & MRSA

Cancer patients, especially those who have undergone chemo or radiation, will find that their immune systems are severely depressed. They often succumb to ravaging infections, such as MRSA (*Methicillin-Resistant Staphylococcus Aureus*), and other diseases that normally would not have overwhelmed their immune system.

Researchers have discovered a volcanic ash clay from central France, called **agricur** (also known as *bentonite clay*), that can kill the MRSA bug, as well as E-coli bacteria, salmonella and buruli (flesh-eating bacteria). For more details, see the article at *http://www.naturalnews.com/z023022.html* by David Gutierrez (419). There are several internet sites that sell this clay; some by the pound, some in capsules. You may want to stay away from pork, because recent reports reveal that MRSA is common in swine herds! Also, grapefruit seed extract is very powerful at killing bacteria and viruses. It is so potent at killing pathogens, that some hospitals actually use it in their respirator equipment.

# II. New Treatments

## CyberKnife® Therapy for Solid Tumors

See chapter 34 in this book for details on CyberKnife® therapy, which is being used successfully for cancer, but is generally for solid tumors, including hard-to-reach brain tumors. It is a gentle, painless procedure that does not require an incision, surgery, sedation or inpatient stay. It is very quick, and there are few risks and side effects, though it does involve some radiation (89a), and it can damage nearby healthy cells. Also, see NanoKnife™, chapter 34.

## Cytotron Therapy

See chapter 34 for more information on this new cancer (and arthritis) treatment, which was developed in India. It is gentle, completely painless, and non-toxic (90).

## Fungus Cure Also Cures Cancer, Says Oncology Doc

Italian Oncologist, Dr. Simoncini, is using soda bicarb to cure his cancer patients within just days! He says that cancer is a fungus, which can be killed with a non-toxic soda bicarb solution that quickly alkalizes and kills cancer (582). The very first person Dr. Simoncini cured was an 11-year-old comatose **leukemia** patient! He uses mostly intravenous soda bicarb; however, Dr. Mark Sircus, in his book, *Sodium Bicarbonate Rich Man's Poor Man's Cancer Treatment,* says you don't need to travel to a European clinic to cure your cancer. Oral soda bicarb is just as efficient at killing cancer, and your local grocery store has soda bicarb for pennies on the pound (566c). Is cancer a fungus? Well if it isn't, then why do some children and adults with leukemia suddenly and fully recover when they are given anti-fungals, and soda bicarb is a very inexpensive ANFI-FUNGAL (566c)! See chapter 34 for more details.

## Non-Toxic Immunotherapy - Global First Of a Kind Miracle Cure for Acute Myeloid Leukemia

In a history-making event by physicians at the Royal Free Hospital in London, a woman suffering from *acute myeloid leukaemia*, who had already failed chemo and three routine transplants, was put into total remission with *natural killer* cells taken from her 21 year-old daughter (568a). The cells were removed from the daughter, treated, then *injected* into the mother. Just *two days* after receiving *57 million* of the treated *natural killer cells*, they had multiplied into *137 million*…(568a) Within one week, the procedure was a success, making the event a *world first!* A dozen more patients are lined up for this procedure, and it is hoped that the *same technique* will be successful against other cancers, such as those of the ovaries and breast. If the patient relapses, the procedure can be repeated (568a). For many years, alternative health advocates have been promoting products that boost the body's immunity. They have been telling the public that it is the body's own **IMMUNITY** that will heal disease.

## Onconase for Leukemia

See other chapters in this book for more info on Onconase *(Ranpirnase)*. It is a new drug claimed not to have the toxic side effects normally found in chemo drugs. It has helped in treating T-cell leukemias, CLL, and AML.

## Rexin-G™ for Metastatic Cancers

Rexin-G™ has been undergoing clinical trials at Mayo Clinic, M.D. Anderson, and a few other facilities. It is a drug for cancers that have spread, and those types of cancer that conventional medicine says do not respond to chemo drugs (256). **Human** clinical studies, thus far, have had good results. In the very first human trial, 83% of the patients experienced tumor shrinkage. The patients all had spreading pancreatic cancer (256). Good responses were also achieved in **human** studies involving several other types of metastatic cancer. Due to the reports, this drug is now used for treating all forms of *solid tumors* in the Philippines that are resistant to conventional therapy (256). The FDA has given the drug its *orphan drug status* for use with pancreatic cancers in the U.S., as well as other types of cancer metastases, which means that trials will continue (256). It is given intravenously, so isn't exactly natural or painless, but could be considered gentler than older chemo drugs, because it is said to be a non-chemo drug, showing itself in **human** clinical trials, not to have the adverse side effects normally associated with chemo drugs (256). You can get more information on this drug at *epeiusbiotech.com/rexin_g-factsheet.asp*. They are the producers of Rexin-G™ (257).

## Salinosporamide-A—for Multiple Myeloma

Salinosporamide-A is a cancer-fighting bacteria (straight from the ocean) which may be the next greatest healer for *multiple myeloma* patients (64). Bradley Moore, Ph.D., a marine biochemist in San Diego, said that the discovery of the bacteria was made in 1991, but they are just now unlocking the *genomic sequence* of the bacteria, and it is being used in clinical trials on **humans**—not only for multiple myeloma—*but solid tumors* as well (64).

## Sprycel® - Milder Drug for Chronic Myeloid Leukemia

Sprycel® is still undergoing testing for chronic myeloid leukemia (CML). It is usually given to those who have not been helped by Gleevec®; however, I did read one report that said it was more effective than Gleevec® in some individuals, and tests are still ongoing. It is claimed that side effects, thus far are **mild** (bone and muscular aches and pains). More will be known when further tests are complete. Just be aware that some chemo drugs that have "mild" effects are often combined with chemo drugs that have devastating and very toxic side effects. Be informed. Ask questions. Don't be a guinea pig!

# III. How Vitamins, Minerals & Nutrients Have Prevented & Cured Cancer

## High Dose Vitamin C Cures Teenager's Cancer

Have you or someone you love been diagnosed with leukemia? Be sure that what you (or they) have really **is leukemia** and not a vitamin C deficiency, or even a *folic acid* or *B12 deficiency* (550). Those words of warning from Maureen Kennedy Salaman, author of *Nutrition: The Cancer Answer II.* A *vitamin C* deficiency (scurvy) can resemble leukemia, as can *folic acid* and *B12* deficiencies (550).

In a report by Irwin Stone, he describes what happened when Dr. Bernard Rimland (their *Program* Chairman) had a *daughter* who was diagnosed with terminal *Hodgkin's disease* (571a). She was admitted to the hospital *in acute renal failure*, with the *worst gallium scan* they had ever *seen.* She was graded as "the most severe Stage IV-B, with" spread into "the kidneys and liver" (571a). Dr. Rimland began her on a high dose vitamin C regimen. Her physicians "gave her less than one year to live" (550). She received chemo, which made her much sicker, and she became severely depressed. Once back home, her father immediately started her on a regimen that included *1000 mg/day* of *niacinamide* and *40 grams* per day of *vitamin C*. He divided the dose throughout the day (550) (571a). Dr. Rimland believed in high-dose vitamin C for leukemia. He noted that Irwin Stone had documented many cases of people who recovered from leukemia using this treatment. The high dose nutritional program saved his daughter's life and he feels might have spared other children, but he could not convince the Oncologists (550) (571a). Also, see internet site: *ht tp://www.seanet.com/~alexs/ascorbate/197x/stone-i-orthomol_psych-1976-v5-n3-p183.htm,* for reports on other cancer cases treated successfully with vitamin C (571a).

Not only did Rimland give his daughter megadoses of vitamin C throughout the day in divided doses, but he himself takes these megadoses. They also included vitamins E, A, and the minerals selenium and calcium (550). (Note: Since vitamin A can be toxic when taken in large doses and natural beta-carotene is not, I would recommend taking the vitamin A in beta-carotene form by juicing fresh carrot juice daily. The body converts natural beta-carotene into vitamin A.) For those who are concerned about stomach upset from high dose (oral) vitamin C (ascorbic acid), get the buffered C powder or crystals in health food stores, use the sodium ascorbate (rather than the ascorbic acid form), or purchase *Ester-C®*, which is buffered vitamin C with calcium ascorbate. High dose vitamin C is also given intravenously (sodium ascorbate form) by many alternative health physicians. It is a non-acidic form and bypasses the stomach, so does not usually cause gastric upset.

## How to Prevent Leukemia in Your Children Before They Are Born

Seven studies by researchers at the University of Toronto from 1960-2005, looking at how a mother's vitamin intake could affect her child's later development of cancer, had some surprising results (407a). As noted by *CancerConsultants.com* website, all vitamins were studied, including *folic acid*. Mothers who took vitamin supplements (that included folic acid) had children with *36%* fewer cases of *pediatric leukemia*; *18% reduction in pediatric brain tumors*, and *47% reduction in neuroblastoma* in their children. Authors of the study theorized that folic acid might have been the most important of the vitamins (407a), and it is already a well-known fact that women who take folic-acid can prevent neural-tube birth defects in their babies.

This study is described in the Journal *Clinical Pharmacology and Therapeutics* retrieved from website article: "Vitamins During Pregnancy Decrease Childhood Cancer Risk" at: *http://patient.cancerconsultants.com/CancerNews_Neuroblastoma.aspx?DocumentId=39373* (407a). More proof that nutrition plays a critical role in disease prevention, even in the womb!

## How Vitamin C Deficiency is Linked to CSS Syndrome

Dr. Irwin Stone presented much of his work on the connection between ***CSS Syndrome*** (*Chronic Subclinical Scurvy*) and ascorbate deficiency in his book, *The Healing Factor*, 1972 (571a). He believed that the disease we refer to as "scurvy," is actually the result of "…a potentially fatal genetic liver-enzyme disease called 'hypoascorbemia," and that this disease "affects 100 percent of the population," due to a "defective gene" that we carry (571a). He says that taking the very small amounts of vitamin C we humans take each day will simply "avoid the terminal signs" of CSS, but if you want to actually "correct this human genetic defect," you must be concerned about taking much larger daily doses of ascorbate. Animals are able to produce thousands of milligrams of their own ascorbate daily, something we humans are not capable of doing. Leukemia is caused by CSS (571a). If you wish to get a test strip that can check your urine (or saliva) to determine if you have sufficient vitamin C in your body, you can order them at website: *http://www.nutri.com/strips/index.html*. This is for informational purposes only. I am not affiliated with them, so I cannot vouch for the integrity of their products.

- **Proof that Vitamin C Cures Myelogenous Leukemia & CSS**

As discussed by Irwin Stone, a "case history published in the *Medical Times* 22 years ago (Greer 1954)," showed that *ascorbate* could be used to bring about a total *remission* in "myelogenous leukemia" (571a). The patient was given "24,500 mg to 42,000 mg of ascorbate…giving complete remission" (571a). Whenever the ascorbate was deliberately stopped (twice) *as an experiment,* all symptoms returned. As soon as "the ascorbic acid was resumed, the temperature returned to normal within six hours…and the remission reoccurred." For some reason this research was mysteriously discontinued (571a). Dr. Stone believed that the puny 45 mg of ascorbate that is recommended daily, known as the RDA, is terribly inadequate at preventing lifelong CSS, which brings with it all manner of chronic disease, leukemia, "heart disease, cancer, the collagen diseases, kidney diseases, and the many infirmities found in the senior citizens" (571a).

## Magnesium Deficiency Seen in Many Children with Leukemia

Many people, women especially, are aggressively encouraged to take calcium for their bones as they age, but health care professionals do not always emphasize the importance of magnesium, without which the cells cannot use calcium efficiently. Many of the most important nutrients in our cells must have magnesium to perform their anti-oxidant properties (566). Studies with animals have shown that keeping them magnesium-deficient will cause malignant cancers. Many women are also warned against drinking alcohol, due to the increased risk for breast cancer; however, alcohol consumption uses up magnesium in the body, so is it possible that the magnesium deficiency, thus created, is the real culprit in causing the cancer (566)? Stressors (e.g., giving a person chemo and/or radiation) also decrease magnesium levels in the body (566). Why is it that, according to Mark Sircus Ac., OMD, a whopping *78%* of children diagnosed with leukemia have a past record of *anorexia*, and these same children are also very deficient in magnesium? Human studies have also shown that high magnesium amounts in the body can help prevent stomach cancer (566). Many chronic illnesses are attributable to magnesium deficiencies, including migraine headaches. Natural sources of magnesium include: sunflower seeds, pumpkin seeds, almonds, walnuts, cashews, Brazil nuts, peanuts, and whole grains. See pp. 129 and 400 for info on a new form of magnesium that you put on the body like lotion.

To find out more, including information about a way of delivering magnesium chloride directly into the skin in an easily absorbable form, see website: *http://www.ancient-minerals.com* (566b). Some people use Epsom salts in their bath water, but it is magnesium sulfate, an inferior form.

## More Evidence for Vitamin C

Linus Pauling was an early advocate for high dose vitamin C therapy. He won the Nobel Prize twice, once in 1954 for chemistry, and then in 1962, the Nobel Peace Prize. He authored several books on chemistry, quantum mechanics, vitamin C, and cancer. He has been followed by others who have taken up the banner in favor of megadosing with vitamin C, including Dr. Abram Hoffer and Dr. Robert Cathcart. Dr. Cathcart's website at *www.orthomed.com* gives startling revelations about diseases, such as "Ebola…and West Nile," as well as many others that he says could possibly be "cured or ameliorated by massive doses of vitamin C" (365). I spoke at length with Dr. Cathcart by phone on July 5, 2005 regarding many of these issues. If you look at a table of the U.S. RDA (Recommended Daily Allowance or sometimes referred to as the Recommended Dietary Allowance) for vitamin C, it is very low at only 60 milligrams. (Most people could probably burn this much up during two minutes of stress.)

Did you know that scientists are very concerned about the health of their laboratory monkeys? They have to keep them on healthy diets so that they stay well (433). It is amazing that monkeys, used in animal experiments, require many times the vitamin C that is recommended for humans, yet studies show that their nutritional requirements are very similar to that of humans (433).

If you still have doubts about the way that natural cancer cures are being suppressed, consider the scientific findings on vitamin C, which show it is lethal to certain cancer cells (433). Thousands of grams of vitamin C per day have been ingested by humans, as well as given intravenously, without noxious side effects. Just be sure to use the buffered form of vitamin C if you are taking large amounts, or are concerned about stomach upset or diarrhea.

## Polyporus Umbellatus Mushroom for Leukemia

This immune-boosting mushroom is one of ten mushrooms found in *Garden of Life's* RM-10 product developed by Jordan Rubin (317). His 80 year-old grandmother used the product to heal her advanced ovarian cancer. See chapter six and website: *http://www.crohns.net/Miva/education/testimonial_rosemenlowe.shtml* (30). It has also been helpful for those with urinary tract infections and may help the body's immunity in halting the spread of leukemia (317). For information and resources where you can obtain RM-10, see website: *http://www.crohns.net/Miva/productinfo/whatsinRM10.shtml* (317). In a **human** study involving 146 people, this mushroom was helpful in cutting in half the reoccurrence of bladder cancer in the participants (317).

## Treating Leukemia with Vitamin A & Zinc

Research shows that the lifespan of *chronic myeloid leukemia* patients could be extended by minimal supplementation with vitamin A (551). It appears that Vitamin A also plays an important role in tumor prevention. Even a synthetic form of vitamin A caused dozens of APL (*acute promyelocytic leukemia*) sufferers to go into *remission.* A study from Italy involving dozens of patients, revealed that deficiencies in *zinc and thymulin* could throw *acute lymphoblastic leukemia* patients into relapse (551).

*Yourhealthbase.com* reports that researchers in Houston, Texas, have found that *retinoic acid* and *retinal* (forms of vitamin A) could inhibit and fight cancers of the prostate, as well as *acute promyelocyte leukemias* (304).

Dr. Abram Hoffer, M.D., Ph.D., in his book, *Healing Cancer—Complementary Vitamin & Drug Treatment,* says that it is very common for cancer patients to have excessive levels of copper in their body, possibly caused by a lack of zinc (433).

## Vitamin E & Leukemia

According to Ralph Moss, Ph.D., in his book, *Anti-oxidants against Cancer*, vitamin E compounds reduce harmful fats that circulate in the blood, and act as anti-inflammatory agents (507). They help the body fight off leukemias, as well as skin and breast cancers (507). Some researchers believe that the gamma form of vitamin E is superior to the alpha-tocopherol form; others insist that you need both, though the alpha form is more easily used by the body. Try to get the *mixed* tocopherols with tocotrienols, and never use any form of vitamin E that has al- bl- dl- or gl- in the list of ingredients. If you get vitamin E that is made from dl-alpha tocopherol, for example, it is synthetic; if it comes from d-alpha, it is natural. The body often cannot recognize synthetic products and they may do you more harm than good! Be sure your E has tocotrienols. One study that pointed out vitamin E as a culprit in promoting lung cancer noted that it was the SYNTHETIC vitamin E that was at fault. The natural form of vitamin E was not harmful to the body. Many studies have shown that natural vitamin E can help the body fight off cancers. Realize that vitamin E in large doses can thin the blood. Discuss with your physician or Naturopath before supplementing.

Some good **natural sources** of vitamin E are: wheat germ oil, olive oil, sunflower oil (and seeds), dandelion greens, spinach, broccoli, turnip greens, almonds and other nuts, eggs (411) (492) (524), kiwi, mango, fortified cereals, and fresh sprouts (especially wheat berry sprouts).

## Vitamins A, D, E & Selenium

Vitamin A and selenium have been shown to destroy bone cancer cells during in vitro testing. Vitamin E and selenium work together. Vitamin A blood levels can be maintained by juicing fresh fruits and vegetables, such as carrots. Vitamin D helps to normalize the manufacture of bone cells and may help reduce the occurrence of abnormal cells; however, taking synthetic vitamin D as a supplement is not always recommended. It may cause the release of calcium from bones that are already deficient from the cancer (41). Vitamin D is manufactured in the skin when direct sunlight strikes the skin. It takes about 10-20 minutes of full spectrum direct sunlight each day (or at the very least, 3 or 4 times per week) for sufficient vitamin D synthesis in most people, and usually longer if you are dark-skinned. You should consult your physician about sun exposure, especially if you have a history or genetic tendency toward melanoma. Some authorities are recommending sun exposure for 20 minutes a day for at least three days per week for vitamin D production.

Vitamin D not only reduces the risk for colon cancer, but now Harvard scientists and those from the Dana-Farber Cancer Institute, say that it could increase the survival of those fighting the disease (145). While animal studies indicate that vitamin D is critical for slowing the progress of cancer, a **human** study (involving more than 300 people with colon cancer) found that those patients with the *highest* levels of vitamin D had dramatically lower chances of *dying from the disease* (145). It is already known that deficiencies of vitamin D can cause colon cancer.

# IV. Foods & Nutrients That Heal

## AHCC—Mushroom Combo Enhances Immunity

AHCC (*Active hexose correlated compound)* is a substance composed of the mycelia of many mushrooms. In **human** testing, it was found (when given to patients in doses of *3g/day orally for 2-6 months)* to significantly increase the body's natural immunity, thus enabling the immune cells to kill multiple myeloma cells and several other types of cancer cells (206). This compound is found at many natural health food stores and online supplement providers, such as *www.discount-vitamins-herbs.net.* New Chapter® is a company that also makes many important mushroom supplements and other nutritional supplements. Their website is: *http:/ / www.newchapter.com/ product-categories/ lifeshield-mushrooms.*

## Barley Grass Halts Leukemia Cells

As described at *healingcancernaturally.com,* barley grass contains a powerful anti-oxidant which helps the body fight leukemia (as well as prostate cancers and brain cancers). It is also rich in natural chlorophyll, a potent cleanser. Barley grass can be juiced fresh or used in powdered form, which is usually mixed with water. Not only this, but barley grass is very high in calcium content (352) and safer and healthier than cow's milk.

## Beat Leukemia with Beets

A simple garden vegetable may be one of the most powerful detox agents for the human body and blood known to man. It is none other than beets. Beet juice is a very potent and concentrated anti-oxidant (much like wheat grass juice in potency), so much so, that it is always best to combine it with other juices, e.g., carrots, apples, or a green juice like broccoli, celery, or spinach. Never start out drinking several ounces at a time. Begin with two ounces a day, then four, and work up to six or eight ounces at a time, added to small amounts of another juice. (You can also obtain powdered beet root in health food stores that you reconstitute with water.) It is interesting that a vegetable juice that so closely resembles blood (in appearance) is actually GOOD for your blood. Beet juice has proven useful for treating leukemia and other cancers.

Beets can be kept fresh for weeks in the refrigerator. Website *herbs first.com* (now linked with *http:/ / herballegacy.com/ id118.htm*), recommends consuming uncooked beets (a few *pounds…mashed)* daily for *leukemia* and other cancers (250). I prefer to juice beets. Fresh beets are hard as rock. They are difficult enough to slice up for juicing and even harder to mash when raw (unless you are using a food processor to shred them).

## CoQ10 & Leukemia

This is one nutrient you will want to add to your arsenal if you are fighting leukemia or any other type of cancer.

I saw a report, about two years ago, of a little boy who was given Adriamycin for leukemia. He went into remission, but a dangerous side effect of Adriamycin is cardiac muscle damage. This child had such serious damage to his heart from the Adriamycin, that he went into heart failure and was forced to go on the heart transplant-waiting-list. The Oncologist giving him chemo could have prevented the damage to his heart from the Adriamycin by giving him CoQ10. Indeed, it is true that what your physician does not know about natural treatments can be fatal to you or a loved one!

## CoQ10 Deficiencies & Multiple Myelomas

Studies by Dr. Folkers, and his colleagues, revealed that patients with *multiple myeloma* and tumors of the breast often had CoQ10 deficiencies, as compared to their healthier counterparts (507). As a matter-of-fact, evidence over more than three decades revealed that taking CoQ10 increased the lifespan of many cancer patients by years (507).

## Cranberries Halt Progression of Leukemia

The powerful anti-oxidants, also known as *proanthocyanidins* (found in simple cranberries) have been shown, in lab studies, to halt the progression of leukemia. Cranberries also cut the risk for ulcers and bladder infections (22.) Do not use store-bought cranberry juice that is high in sugar. You can get organic cranberry juice and cranberry supplements from health food suppliers, or simply juice your own.

## Flavonoids & Cell Protection

Protecting blood cells from mutation means ensuring that DNA does not mutate. Once cells begin to mutate and the immune system is sick, the end result is often a debilitating cancer, such as leukemia, sarcoma, or multiple myeloma.

The protective ability of phytochemicals (plant chemicals, such as those found in green and black tea) was shown, in a recent report, to have the ability of protecting DNA. Three flavonoids outperformed the rest (351). These three are found in natural foods, e.g., *black currants, celery,* onions, and tea (351). Parsley, silymarin, and ginkgo biloba (high in quercetin) also have ingredients that impede the growth of cancer cells (351). In the fruits that were tested, those with the greatest ability at protecting DNA were found in several fruits and berries, such as blackberries (351). Quercetin, one of the flavonoids, is also found in berries, broccoli, some nuts and seeds, and other foods. Do not take large amounts of quercetin in supplement form. Follow the dosing directions on the label, and always check with your health care provider.

## Folic Acid & Adult Leukemia

Also discussed elsewhere in this chapter, you may want to be sure that you are not deficient in folic acid (vitamin B-9 or folate), first found within leafy green spinach nearly seventy years ago, if you wish to prevent adult leukemia. Because of genetic studies, scientists are convinced that a lack of folic acid in the diet dramatically increases the chance of colorectal cancers, and may also lead to some forms of leukemia, such as *acute lymphocytic leukemia* (507). Can you see how important nutrition is in preventing disease?

Many of today's cases of leukemia are being diagnosed in patients who had prior chemo and radiation for other cancers. Research from one study found that, although taking chemo can increase your leukemia risk, sufficient folic acid in the body may offer some protection for the immune system (551). Some good natural sources of folic acid are leafy greens, sprouts, some fruits (411), and sunflower seeds.

## GLA (Gamma Linolenic Acid) & Leukemia

GLA, already discussed in a previous chapter, is commonly found in borage oil and evening primrose oil. GLA can kill cancer cells and has shown its ability to do so in a variety of cancers. In laboratory tests, when leukemia cells were treated with GLA, nearly half of them died. In the absence of the GLA, only one fifth were killed (351). Apparently, the addition of cortisone increased the effectiveness of GLA, killing a much greater percentage of the unwanted cells (351). Note that the **normal cells were not affected.** More isn't necessarily better, however, in the case of GLA. Larger doses can cause an undesirable immune response with inflammation, which may increase tumors rather than inhibit them. Because of this potential, always follow your health practitioner's recommendation for GLA dosing (351).

Some providers of organic flax oil also add borage oil and/or evening primrose oil as a combination oil supplement in their flax products. Flax itself has been shown to prevent the growth of new cancer cells. See chapter 18 for further information on flax for cancer prevention and treatment, and chapter 14 for the famous Budwig flax oil diet that many people have used to cure their cancers. Flax is a tremendous source of omega-3 oil. (Also, see Moxxor in chapter 34.)

## Grapes (Resveratrol) & Grape Seed Extract Block Leukemia & Myeloma Cells

One of the amazing nutrients in purple grapes, *resveratrol*, was discussed in chapter three, yet it is again coming up as being important in fighting leukemia. Researchers have also noted that this compound inhibits many types of malignant cancers, besides leukemia. Grapes are one of the best sources of resveratrol, which also works to fight the process of cancer by giving cells the ability to differentiate, thereby stopping abnormal cells from growing (131). More than 100 studies have shown the ability of resveratrol at fighting cancer (131). Researchers discovered that resveratrol prevents the formation of an inflammatory agent called *NFkB* that promotes *leukemia viruses* (131). In other words, resveratrol stops the chemicals responsible for the development of leukemia dead in their tracks! Not only that, but scientists have discovered (in lab testing) that this substance works very similar to *Tamoxifen,* a popular chemo drug (131), but without the toxic side effects found in Tamoxifen. This testing has shown that resveratrol may even have the ability to halt the progression of multiple myeloma.

For an excellent 58-page study that was done on resveratrol's role in fighting cancer, including multiple myeloma, lymph and myeloid cancers, see website: *http://www.agrawal.org/PDF/ACR-Resveratrol1.pdf* (346).

The University of Kentucky has just completed a lab study on grapeseed extract. Their findings (published in *Clinical Cancer Research*) showed that grape seed extract could kill more than two thirds of leukemia cells within just 24 hours! It's important when eating grapes, you must eat the seeds too (326a). You can now get resveratrol and grape seed supplements in natural health food stores and on the internet.

## Is it Leukemia—Or is it a Folic Acid, B6 or B12 Deficiency?

If you are diagnosed with leukemia, says Maureen Kennedy Salaman in *Nutrition The Cancer Answer II*, be sure to get more than one opinion. As discussed earlier in this chapter, leukemia could be a misdiagnosis for what is actually a severe deficiency of *folic acid* and/or *vitamin B12—pernicious anemia* (550) [aka *megaloblastic anemia* or *Addison-Biermer* anemia]. A month or two on vitamin therapy and some patient's blood counts were completely normal (550). This may be more common than most people realize.

One such case involved a 43 year-old lady, who presented with nosebleeds, loss of appetite, weight loss, and feeling ill, with a white count over 24,000 (306). After a biopsy, she was told she had leukemia, but she returned to normal after being given 1000 mcg of B12 and 5 mg of folic acid (folate). Her diagnosis was changed to *pernicious anemia* (306). Another 52 year-old who complained of bruising, diarrhea, URI, and other symptoms, was diagnosed with *promyelocytic leukemia;* however, her symptoms all disappeared and her blood tests returned to normal when she was given **folate** (306). She was discovered to have a severe folic acid deficiency. This was 17 years ago and she has had no further symptoms (306).

Have you or a loved one been diagnosed with leukemia? Be sure, first of all, as stated earlier, that you get a second opinion, and next, be sure that what you (or they) have is indeed leukemia and not a lack of B12, folic acid, B6, or even a vitamin C deficiency (550). Vitamin B12 and folic acid are also available in sublingual tablets that you simply place under your tongue and dissolve; however, one of the best ways to be sure you are getting adequate B12, if you are deficient, is with B12 injections from your physician. Check out Dr. Andrew W. Saul's website at: *http://www.doctoryourself.com/nasal.html,* for his recipe on the use of nasal B12. It has also been discovered that many victims of childhood leukemia are critically low in vitamin B6 (pyridoxine). You can also get Vitamin D & CoQ10 in a sublingual tab.

## Kudzu & Boswellia

These herbs help the body's immune system target and fight leukemia cells. As with any herb, never start immediately taking large amounts. Always consult with your physician or Naturopath first.

## LifeMel Honey for Leukemia

Life Mel honey is also discussed in chapter 29 of this book. It is a special honey (developed in Israel) that is used from nectar harvested from 40 herbs, including *Echinacea, Siberian ginseng,* and *Uncaria tomentosa* (with other natural ingredients). Decades of research went into the development of the honey. Two teaspoons per day (one in the morning and one in the evening) are recommended (614). This special honey has been shown, in **human** testing, to prevent the neutropenia (dangerously low white blood count) caused by chemotherapy and to lower the risk of severe platelet drop (thrombocytopenia), often found in chemo patients (614). You can find out more about this amazing honey at website: *http://www.lifemel israel.com* (614). It is often touted to be the most expensive honey in the world. An elderly Canadian man, whose doctor had halted his chemo due to severely depressed immunity, made a rapid recovery after he began taking the honey twice daily (349). Some health food stores do carry LifeMel honey. I have seen it priced (recently) anywhere from thirty to eighty dollars for a 120 gm jar, with some stores giving large discounts for quantity purchases.

## Mangosteen for Leukemia

Mangosteen fruit contains more than two dozen types of anti-oxidants. The ORAC test (*Oxygen Radical Absorbance Capacity*) is a measurement of an anti-oxidant's ability to soak up *free radicals*—and of course—the foods you want to eat are the ones with the highest ORAC rating. Mangosteen is very high on the ORAC list (185). Six different nutrient compounds from this fruit were tested on leukemia cells in the laboratory. All six successfully impeded the cancers. (Note that **mangosteen is not the same** as the mango fruit.)

## Mushroom Extract (Maitake D-Fraction) for Leukemia

Writers Sheri Lieberman, Ph.D., and Ken Babal, C.N., describe Dr. Peter D'Adamo, N.D., as a long term user of maitake mushroom for his cancer patients in their book: *Maitake Mushroom And D-Fraction* (469). In *Eat Right For Your Type,* Dr. D'Adamo recounts the details of a case where he had used *Maitake D-fraction* supplement against terminal leukemia. This particular patient had already taken chemo, but a year later, her spleen was cancerous (469). The tumor was aggressive and grew rapidly. When the patient came to Dr. D'Adamo, she was told to take the Maitake D-Fraction at a *half teaspoon twice a day*. She was eventually found to be cancer-free and, according to Dr. D'Adamo, her case was not at all unusual. He has successfully treated many types of cancer and those with HIV, using a combination of maitake and natural therapies (469). He has also had very good results treating those who came to him after chemo had failed them, including those with *prostate cancer* and cancers *of the liver, breast and colon.* He believes that this mushroom substance enhances the effectiveness of shark cartilage (469). Maitake should never be taken by those with **multiple sclerosis** (184).

Shiitake mushrooms have also been the focus of much research. Oriental populations have used them for thousands of years for treating the immune system. (Fresh shiitake is best if cooked. Always buy organic when possible.) Before consuming any type of mushroom supplement, always check with your physician, especially if you have a chronic illness or are already taking prescriptions medications. Some mushrooms thin the blood, so taking blood-thinners with them can be dangerous. For discounted supplements, see website: *www.swansonvitamins.com.* They also have a great deal of information on current testing of health products at their website, as does *discount-vitamins-herbs.net.* New Chapter® also sells many mushroom supplements and other nutritional products. Their website is: *http://www.newchapter.com/product-categories/lifeshield-mushrooms.*

## Parthenolide for CML & AML Leukemia

Researchers have recently uncovered an ingredient found in the common herb, feverfew (known as *parthenolide)*, which has the capacity (in lab testing) to kill AML and CML leukemia cells more efficiently than the common chemo drug Ara-C (422). An amazing property of this ingredient (also found in magnolia and other natural sources), is that it killed the stem cells that the AML cells originated from, but was harmless to normal cells (422).

## Proteolytic Enzymes for Multiple Myeloma Patients

Proteolytic enzymes are enzymes made by the pancreas. Enzymes such as papain (found in pineapples) and papaya are sometimes referred to as *proteolytic enzymes.* You can find these enzyme supplements in health food stores. They are usually taken 30 minutes before meals.

For information on human trials showing that proteolytic enzymes combined with chemo, could increase the life span (by three years) of dozens of stage II multiple myeloma patients, see details at: *http://www.doctormurray.com/articles/pdfs/ProteolyticsInCancer.pdf* (514).

## Quercetin for Leukemia

Quercetin, discussed earlier, is a very potent flavonoid, protective against cancer. Its effects are increased when combined with ascorbic acid (vitamin C). It may help fight leukemia, and this killing power against leukemia cells appears to be enhanced when combined with *vitamin P* (*rutin*) (551). Good natural sources of quercetin are *cayenne, onions*, and *green tea* (551), as well as berries, broccoli, and some nuts and seeds. Rutin can be found in berries, prunes, paprika, chervil, cherries, grapes, and the skins of citrus fruit, as well as many other foods. Do not take quercetin supplements in excessive amounts for long periods of time. Follow label directions and your doctor's guidelines.

Red and yellow onions are much higher in this nutrient than are white onions (551).

## Rosemary - Ingredient for ALL Leukemia

An ingredient found in the herb, rosemary, known as *carnosol*, had the ability, in laboratory testing, to kill ALL (acute lymphyocytic leukemia) cells (543). Using the herb rosemary in baking wheat bread, for example, slashed the cancer-causing acrylamides by greater than half (361). Even very minute amounts of rosemary, as low as *one per cent of the dough*, was able to cut acrylamides (361).

## Royal Jelly Inhibits Leukemia

According to website *www.cancertutor.com*, in a Canadian study, when mice (pre-disposed to leukemia) were fed royal jelly, they never developed cancer. The mice not receiving the royal jelly died within two weeks, showing the protective effects of royal jelly against leukemia (260).

## Strawberries & Cherries Inhibit Cancer Cells

In a revealing note by Jean Carper, author of *The Food Pharmacy*, researchers placed strawberries at the top of a list of foods that they felt were responsible for decreased fatalities from cancer among more than a thousand geriatric Americans (363). Those eating larger amounts of strawberries decreased their risks for getting cancer three-fold. It was also found that strawberries effectively destroyed viruses, such as herpes, polio, and others (363) (see p. 544). Raspberries, cranberries, cherries, and blueberries have similar cancer-fighting compounds. (Cranberries also cut the risk for ulcers and bladder infections, and they fight leukemia (22.)

An ingredient in cherries, *perillyl alcohol*, was able, in animal testing, to suppress leukemia (370). This ingredient is also described in earlier chapters of this book. (Cherries, especially sour cherries, have long been used as a popular treatment for gout.)

## V. Herbs, Plants & Teas That Inhibit Leukemia

### Abajeru (*Chrysobalanus icaco*) for Leukemia & Other Cancers

Isolated from a tropical plant of the Brazilian Rain Forest (aka as *coco-plum*), abajeru was once used by the locals for fighting arthritic pain and for diabetes (145a). When researchers first conducted lab testing, they found that the bush extract killed not only cancerous *breast-brain-lung-bowel-larynx and pancreas tumors*, but even difficult-to-treat leukemia cells died. In testing **humans**, they were surprised to see that it *worked with 90%* of the people using it (145a). You can find this substance and read more about it on the internet.

### Algae for Leukemia

In recent years, different types of algae are proving to be deadly to cancer cells. According to Dr. R. W. Moss, author of *Cancer Therapy*, it was discovered, in animal testing, that an algae known as *Dunaliella bardawil* could suppress breast tumors (504). This algae and others, like chlorella, are very rich in beta-carotene. Chlorella alga has been the subject of intense study, revealing that it too has impressive tumor-fighting abilities (504). When researchers in Japan fed chlorella to mice, then exposed them to cancer cells, those animals receiving the chlorella outlived the non-treated group. The mice had been given *leukemia* and *breast cancer* cells as well as *Ehrlich's ascites.* It was determined that the chlorella helped the body's natural immunity fight off the abnormal cells (504).

You can purchase chlorella at your local health food store, but be sure to choose an organic brand that is ***broken cell-wall*** chlorella. If the cell wall is not broken, it is not easily absorbed by the body. Also, be sure to purchase algae and seaweed from reputable sources. (Chlorella contains important omega-3, omega-6, ALA fatty acids, B12, and many other vitamins and minerals.)

## Aloe's Anti-Leukemic Factor

Japanese scientists studied the effect of aloe on various kinds of cancer in mice, isolating a chemical by the name of *aloe emodin.* They found that this chemical was responsible for fighting leukemia. They discovered that the compound decreased the proliferation of some tumors in the test animals, and even cured a particular type of malignancy (504). Initial results revealed that it works by stimulating immunity (504). Aloe emodin has also been isolated from the herb, sheep sorrel (270), one of the ingredients that is found in Essiac Tea, discussed in more detail in chapter six of this book. Oriental researchers discovered that aloe-emodin halts a specific type of leukemia cell by preventing its spread.

## Artemisinin & Leukemia

Artemisinin, also known as *wormwood,* has been a popular remedy for centuries for treating parasites, and since it can cross the *blood-brain* barrier, may also be helpful in fighting brain cancers (24). (Poly-MVA, discussed elsewhere in this book, is also capable of crossing into the brain.)

Wormwood has shown promise against intestinal cancers and *leukemia,* with some cancer-fighting activity revealed with kidney and reproductive cancers, as well as those affecting the central nervous system (24). This herb should not be taken on an empty stomach. Be sure to consult with your health care practitioner before taking artemisinin if you are on radiation or have recently been treated with radiation therapy. Note that not all wormwood contains artemisinin (24).

Researchers from the University of Washington recently discovered that they could outfit wormwood (artemisinin) with a *homing device* that sends the substance to cancer cells only, keeping normal cells unharmed (75a). The substance gets inside the cells and acts like a *bomb inside the cell,* as described by Professor Tomikazu Sasaki. It works against the high iron content found in cancer cells (75a).

A word of caution: do not take excessively high doses of this herb. Dosing is usually divided during the day and will depend on individual body weight, so check with your physician first.

## Astragalus & Immunity

This herb is important in restoring depleted immune cells. Check with your physician about using astragalus, especially if you have an infection or are running a temperature (41).

## Autumn Crocus

Autumn Crocus *(Colchicum autumnale)*, long used as a successful remedy for the pain associated with *gout*, has also been used therapeutically for some types of leukemia, and for treating a type of leukemia with ulcers, known as *Behcet's syndrome* (28). Never use this herb without first consulting with your physician; it must be impeccably supervised. Even in low doses, it can be associated with severe adverse effects (28).

## Butcher's Broom

This herb causes the blood vessels in the body to constrict (54). Two plant steroids that were effective at killing leukemia cells were recently isolated from butcher's broom by scientists in Japan (54). Butcher's broom can be found in tea form, as well as supplements.

## Cat's Claw Fights Leukemia

Also known as *Uno de Gato,* this herb has anti-oxidant properties. It can help scavenge and destroy cancer-causing substances (393). Research has shown that the herb can seek out abnormal cells, such as those found in leukemia, and incapacitate them without harming normal cells (393). Cat's claw can be found in supplements, as well as tea bags. See chapter 20 for instances when you should not take this herb.

## Chaparral & Leukemia

Chaparral, an herb that is often consumed in tea form, is believed to have the ability to help the immune system fight tumors and *leukemia* (577). This herb is discussed in greater detail in chapter 32 on teas.

## Essiac Tea for All Cancers

See chapter six for more information on this amazing herbal tea. I would not hesitate to recommend Essiac tea to anyone fighting cancer. Rene Caisse, a Canadian nurse, healed hundreds—possibly thousands—of people of every imaginable cancer using her amazing herbal tea formula. Many people came to her after conventional medicine considered them incurable and hopeless. One of the most amazing books describing the effectiveness of this tea and how it was suppressed by the health industry in Canada is called: *The Essiac Report Canada's Remarkable Unknown Cancer Remedy,* by Richard Thomas. He states that Flor-Essence® Essiac tea is the original (drinkable) formula used by Rene Caisse (580).

Note that there is some competition between the tea produced by Resperin Canada Essiac® and Flor-Essence® Essiac tea. Both companies claim that they have the original Essiac formula (the drinkable formula, not the injectable) that Rene Caisse used in treating her cancer patients. See chapter 16, later in this book, for the story of a young boy who was cured of lymphoma using a natural program that included Resperin Canada's Essiac® tea formula and 714X injections. Both brands of the tea can be found in health food stores and on the internet.

## Garlic Inhibits Promyelocytic Leukemia

Laboratory research studies have recently demonstrated that compounds in garlic can help the immune system fight this type leukemia. Be aware that consuming large amounts of garlic can also thin the blood.

## Goldenseal & Berberine Fight Leukemia

An ingredient isolated in the popular herb, goldenseal (known as *berberine),* was able to **cause leukemia cells to self-destruct** (59). Herbs containing berberine should not be consumed by those with billiary disorders, high blood pressure, glaucoma or heart problems. Do not take them if nursing or pregnant, nor with vitamin B6 or *histidine*, which is an amino acid (178).

## Green Tea Prevents Leukemia & Fights CLL

Certain ingredients in green tea, known as *epigallocatechingallate* (EGCG), have the ability to prevent DNA damage. During testing, this tea was successful at fighting leukemia cells (351). Mixing black and green tea together greatly enhanced their protective power. There is not a great deal of difference between green and black tea. Before black tea ripens, it is referred to as *green tea* (351). It is best to use decaffeinated tea, because caffeine acts as a diuretic, pulling water out of the body, and most cancer patients are already dehydrated. Removing the caffeine does not affect the anti-oxidant potency, however, some believe that tea with caffeine fights arterial plaque better.

Another study reported at *foodnavigator.com* reveals that green tea, in laboratory testing, could interfere with the production of "B-cell chronic lymphocytic leukemia (CLL)," common in people in their sixties, and for which there is no known cure (138). Green tea has also been found (in animal testing by Israeli researchers) to actually regenerate brain cells, something hitherto thought impossible (169). Why are scientists so interested in studying green tea? Countries that consume higher amounts of this herbal drink, have dramatically lower cancer rates.

## Guggul for Leukemia

Guggul is another herb, available in health food stores, that has been used in treating leukemia. It is sometimes combined with Chinese red yeast rice for a natural way of lowering cholesterol. (Check with your Dr. first.)

## Lapacho Used for Leukemia

Lapacho, also commonly known as *pau d'arco* and *taheebo tea*, is described in detail at website *www.rain-tree.com*. It is very popular for treating health disorders, including leukemia and other cancers (509). Be aware that lapacho is actually just an extract from the main tea, *pau d'arco*, but the names get intertwined. When using the herb, you need to be sure that you are using *pau d'arco*—the entire tea. Supporters of this tea say that it is especially helpful in fighting leukemia. They believe that it is unrivaled worldwide for its tumor-fighting properties (173). It is believed that the herb works by activating the body's ability to increase red blood cell production within the marrow cells (173). Lapacho, the main ingredient in this herb, should never be used by itself. When the whole herb was given, it produced clinical anti-cancer effects without the problems that using lapacho alone might cause (173).

It is also important to be aware that when teas, such as this are tested, an extract of one of the tea's main ingredients will sometimes be used in the test, rather than the entire tea. Of course, in using teas such as this, one needs to use the whole tea, not just one or two extracts isolated from the main tea. Not only does lapacho help kill cancer, but it was cleared by the FDA more than twenty-five years ago (173).

Genuine pau d'arco tea should come from the tree's bark, the *inner lining*. It has been used for many years, especially in South America, as an effective way to manage disease, however, getting it from unreliable sources that do not use the tree's inner bark could mean a useless product (98).

## Saffron Destroys Cancer Cells

Some spices appear to be able to destroy cancer cells on contact; saffron is one of them. As noted by Selene Yeager in the *Doctors Book of FOOD REMEDIES*, lab testing showed that ingredients from this common herb could help fight the growth of leukemia cells without harming normal cells (604).

## Scutellaria Fights Leukemia, Myeloma & Lymphoma

A mint herbal remedy used in Chinese medicine, *Scutellaria baicalensis* (sometimes referred to as *skullcap*), in laboratory testing, was found to reduce the spread of acute lymphocytic leukemia. It killed myeloma and lymphoma cells (459).

## Seaweeds, Viva Natural & PTZ Fight Leukemia & Other Cancers

Viva Natural is a nutritional compound taken from seaweed. This extract was effective, in animal studies, against leukemia and lung cancer cells, and was even considered more effective than the drug, *Isoprinosine,* in fighting lung cancer (504).

In his book, *Cancer Therapy,* Dr. Ralph Moss says that, in animal testing, PTZ (a compound taken from narcissus) outperformed the common chemo drug, Methotrexate. The substance halted advanced leukemia. (504).

A kelp known as *Laminaria* may be partly responsible for the fact that the Japanese do not have the high incidence of breast cancers found in the West (504). They consume laminaria and other forms of kelp regularly. Another extract of brown algae, *Sargassum kjellmaniaum,* was effective against sarcomas, and when combined with the compound *sulfated SKCF,* also inhibited leukemia (504). Kelp should only be taken in small amounts, and not by those with thyroid disorders unless cleared with their physician, because it is high in iodine. Other types of seaweed have been discussed elsewhere in this book. (Note that some thyroid disorders are caused by the fact that many people do not get enough iodine in their diets. Others get too much iodine.)

## Turmuric Stops the Spread of Multiple Myeloma

Scientists at the M. D. Anderson Cancer Center, revealed (from laboratory testing in 2003), that *curcumin,* a substance found in turmeric, had the ability to halt the progression of multiple myeloma (203). At the conclusion of the study, they recommended that multiple myeloma sufferers be given this non-toxic remedy (203). For more information, see the website article at: *http://www.discount-vitamins-herbs.net/health-news30.htm #121.* Do you think that physicians treating their cancer patients tell them this? Do you or someone you know have multiple myeloma? If so, has anyone ever told you (or them) that turmeric was shown to halt the spread of this type cancer? This substance is said to be non-toxic and free from the typical side effects found with major pharmaceutical drugs.

Turmeric is safe when used as a spice; however, if you are taking turmeric in supplement form, do not use if you are pregnant, nor if you have gallstones, since it stimulates the gallbladder (571). Like garlic, turmeric can thin the blood, so it should be used in caution by anyone taking blood-thinning medications (571), with blood disorders, ulcers or other gastric disorders, or for anyone recovering from or contemplating surgery. Always check with your physician or Naturopath first.

The cancer hierarchy in India is so impressed with the power of turmeric in cancer prevention, it is highly promoted in that country. In animal testing, it had the ability to cut colon cancers by greater than half, and may inhibit melanoma as well (604). Turmeric has anti-inflammatory properties that assist in wound healing, and may be important in preventing Alzheimer's, as found in animal studies (347). If you are interested in turmeric and other herbal supplements, as well as many vitamins and other nutrients at reasonable prices, see *www.discount-vitamins-herbs.net* and *swansonvitamins.com.* Also, if you want a turmeric capsule that is free of magnesium stearate, see *Nature's Way*® brand. If you want your body to absorb turmeric more easily, eat it with pineapple or supplement with bromelain.

# VI. Other Supplements & Treatments for Leukemia

## Acai Berry Inhibits Leukemia Cells

This little berry from the rain forest is bulging with dozens of anti-oxidants, including many of the same nutrients that are found in the skin of purple grapes and blueberries. *The Journal of Agricultural and Food Chemistry* reports that in vitro studies of acai determined that it can kill leukemia cells (8). Acai berry has become highly popular as a beverage and is also found mixed in many health food drinks.

In laboratory studies at the University of Florida, the acai berry extract caused *86% of the cancer cells* to self-destruct. These were leukemia cells (398).

## Alpha Lipoic Acid Inhibits Leukemia

See other chapters in this book for more information on alpha lipoic acid. It not only protects the liver, but impedes leukemia as well. This is one nutrient you will need to supplement with to get adequate amounts.

## Arsenic & Acute Promyelocytic Leukemia—Perhaps Homeopathy Not As Medieval As Some Have Claimed

Homeopathy, a type of treatment to fight disease that relies on small concentrations, or diluted forms of substances (that in much larger amounts could cause distress or death), has been used for thousands of years by the Chinese. This treatment has often been scorned and ridiculed by the cancer industry. Arsenic, used in very tiny amounts for years to treat a rare form of leukemia known as APL *(acute promyelocytic leukemia)*, is one such example. Once again, however, it appears that many in the modern medical establishment have had to eat their words. Used in China more than a century ago to treat this type of leukemia, it was recently discovered that the Chinese were right all along. Small amounts of arsenic are now being used in—of all places—the USA to treat this rare form of leukemia that attacks adults in their prime years.

Organized medicine claims the ability to cure APL with chemo, but for those who do not respond to chemo, or who relapse, the drug of choice is now *arsenic trioxide* (brand name - *Trisenox*), you guessed it—small amounts of arsenic! It is now being studied for possible use in other leukemias and cancers of the brain, nervous system, and liver, as well as multiple myeloma, and was used in the Dark Ages to fight bubonic plague (231) (533). (You may hear this referred to as *arsenic oxide* and *retinoic acid* therapy.)

## Beta-Sitosterol—Works Against Lymphocytic Leukemia

Beta-sitosterol is a naturally-occurring nutrient that can be found in soy and some brans, but most diets are deficient (33). It helps fight hyperglycemia (type II) and *lymphocytic leukemia.* It is a natural anti-inflammatory, and may also help the body fight ulcers (33). Beta-sitosterol should not be taken during lactation or pregnancy, nor by those with the type of hereditary diseases that interfere with the body's ability to metabolize fats. (See precautions in this book about using whole soy.)

## Burzynski's Antineoplastons: Non-Toxic Help for Hopeless Cancer Cases

Though not discussed at length in this chapter, see chapter 14 and chapter 16 for more information on Dr. Burzynski's antineoplastons and his very successful treatment of **leukemia, lymphomas, bone and breast cancer, as well as inoperable brain cancers,** and many others. The Burzynski Clinic is located in Houston, Texas, the only state in which the FDA had allowed Dr. Burzynski to practice antineoplaston therapy. Their main website is *www.burzynskiclinic.com.* Also, read the remarkable stories of many people who have been cured using non-toxic antineoplastons: *http://burzynskipatientgroup.org/stories.html.* The FDA has finally approved the oral form of antineoplastons (PBs or sodium phenylbutrates) for off-label use, but you will need to ask your physician about prescribing them. Antineoplastons A10 and AS2-1 were recently given orphan drug status by the FDA for use on human brainstem gliomas.

## Burzynski's Treatment - Non-Hodgkin's Lymphoma & Multiple Myeloma Cures

See chapter 16 in this book for the amazing story of Maryjo Siegel, who was completely cured of fatal non-Hodgkin's lymphoma (diagnosed in 1991) after being treated with Burzynski's non-toxic antineoplastons. Also given, is part of her subsequent testimony before the U.S. House of Representatives Government Reform and Oversight Committee on

February 4, 1998 (562). Maryjo, by the way, is still alive and well and completely cancer-free (as of June 2009). You can contact Maryjo at her email address: *maryjo@siegel.net*, and she will be happy to tell you about antineoplastons and her amazing cure. Her full story can also be read at *http://burzynski patientgroup.org/maryjo.htm* (562).

See the following website for additional case testimonials of people who were completely CURED of non-Hodgkins lymphoma at the Burzynski clinic using non-toxic antineoplastons: *http://burzynskipatient group.org/karolr.htm*. Also, see *http:burzynskipatientgroup.org/charlesn.htm*, and a nurse who was cured at: *http://burzynskipatientgroup.org/melodyc.htm*. See *www.burzynskiclinic.com* for their main website.

Website *http://burzynskipatientgroup.org/dagmarb.html*, has the case of a woman cured of multiple myeloma using antineoplastons (after she refused radiation and chemo). She was diagnosed in 1992, and all diagnostics showed her cancer-free in 1995. At last report in 2000, she was still cancer-free and doing well.

## DHEA & Leukemia

DHEA (*Dehydroepiandrosterone*) is a naturally-occurring hormone produced by the adrenals that may play an important role against leukemia (337). Animal testing against viral leukemia with DHEA was hopeful, showing that the compound was effective against free radicals and stimulated the animals' immune systems (337). Before you decide to supplement with DHEA, consult your physician for a blood test to see if you have low blood levels of DHEA and related hormones, especially women who may have other abnormal hormone levels (337). Be sure that you do not indiscriminately begin using the hormone without lab work to determine your current blood levels of DHEA. It is not for people under 30, nor those who have already had some types of cancer, especially those affected by hormones (337). DHEA is a stimulant-type hormone that may be helpful in preventing and fighting muscle loss, obesity, and diabetes (337). This substance has also been used in rejuvenating the skin. You will find it in many skin care products and cosmetics.

## Mullaca - Toxic to Leukemia Cells

Mullaca, also known as *cape goose, wild tomato, winter cherry*, and other common names, is a rain forest herb that fights leukemia cells (200). Website *www.rain-tree.com*, describes the herb in detail and says that the mullaca which is anti-leukemic is actually extracted plant steroids. They help work against several kinds of cancer, such as those of the brain, intestines, skin, and liver (200). In Taiwan, scientists revealed that this herb could help stop the advancement of *acute leukemia*, including *lymphoid (T & B), promyelocytic, myeloid and monocytic* (200). Again, during 2001, Houston scientists discovered a compound in mullaca that was toxic to abnormal cells of the throat and nose and (in animal studies) able to fight leukemia (200). The scientists believe that the herb may function by damaging the DNA of cancer cells so that they are not capable of reproducing (200). Though no drug interactions have been reported, mullaca may lower blood pressure, thin the blood, and produce hypoglycemia. Mullaca is also used as a pain-killer and anti-parasite (200). For more information on mullaca, contact Raintree Nutrition at *www.rain-tree.com*. You may find this supplement sold under the name of *bolsa mullaca*.

## Simarouba, Anamu & Amargo Against Leukemia

- **Simarouba** is an herb used in some cultures for many years, but in vitro testing did not begin until 1976. At that time, it was found to contain anti-leukemia inhibitors, three of which were capable of killing lymphocytic leukemia (272). In spite of this, no testing has been done on humans (272). Excessive doses of this herb may cause side effects, so be sure to discuss with your physician before using the herb for any reason. The herb also has anti-viral properties, and may one day be useful against *West Nile Virus* (272) and other killer viruses.
- **Anamu** kills cancer cells directly and boosts the immune system by triggering the activity of white blood cells. Laboratory research in 1990 showed that substances from this herb could kill leukemia cells and many other types of cancer (16). After three years, the scientists did a follow-up study showing that these same compounds were destroying cancer cells, not just stunting them. The conclusion of the study was that the entire herb (not just isolated extracts of the herb) could kill lymphoma, leukemia, and *breast cancer* (16). Further **lab** studies done in 2001 and 2002 showed anamu to be toxic to cancerous liver and brain cells (16). This herb does contain coumarin, so do not use it without first consulting with your physician, especially if you are already taking blood-thinners. Since extracts of the herb can stimulate the uterus, it should never be used during pregnancy. It can also lower blood sugar (16). Both Anamu and Simarouba are in

Raintree's herbal formula, *N-Tense-2*, available at their website: *http://www.raintree.com/anamu.htm.*

- **Amargo** is another little-known herb found in Raintree Nutrition's *N-Tense-2* that may help the immune system fight leukemia (12).

## Vassourinha's Anti-Leukemic Extracts

Vassourinha is an herb found abundantly not only within the rain forest, but the U.S. as well. Some of the extracts of this herb have been very impressive against leukemia, cancer, and viruses like HIV. It has also demonstrated the ability to work against bone, brain, and skin tumors while being non-toxic to normal cells (302). Be sure to let your physician know if you are taking herbals such as this one, because vassourinha may lower blood pressure (302), and could be incompatible with other herbs or prescriptions.

When Raintree Nutrition found that leukemia was not responding to graviola (in their product *N-Tense)*, they developed *N-Tense-2,* which contains mullaca, cat's claw, and vassourinha, as well as other cancer-fighting herbs specifically for aiding in the fight against leukemia. They are both available at *www.rain-tree.com.* You can also find dosage information there (162). Note that **Raintree Nutrition does not make *curative* claims for their herbs.** They report the results of tests conducted on various herbs, and they suggest that herbs be part of an overall comprehensive health treatment plan. Many of the plants discussed at their website can be purchased bulk-rate by the pound.

# VII. Miscellaneous Herbs & Supplements

## Andrographis Inhibits Leukemia

Andrographis *(Andrographis paniculata)* is an herb found in Asia that has an ancient history of medicinal usage. Research of its use against cancer is very promising, as well as against many pathogens. Studies show that andrographis can help reverse the DNA damage in leukemia cells, causing them to turn back to their normal state, or allowing them to *differentiate* (20). If cells *differentiate* (like they are supposed to), they do not mutate and become cancerous (20). Getting them to revert back to a differentiated state means healthy cells. Extracts taken from andrographis leaves, in some tests, were able to halt abdominal cancers and fight against melanoma, lymphoma (non-Hodgkins), *prostate cancer*, and *breast cancer cells* (20). Andrographis has very low toxicity. In rare cases, it could cause irregular heartbeat, vertigo and/or possible allergic reactions that could be minor or serious (20). Just remember that any hormone, herb, vitamin, prescription, food, or mineral, always has the potential for causing allergic reactions in some individuals.

This herb is available in a brand known as *Androtech,* produced by BioTherapies, in a formula that also contains *Enchinacea and zinc* (20). If you are trying to get pregnant this is not the herb for you, neither should it be used if you are already pregnant or breast feeding.

## Buckthorn Bark Inhibits Lymphocytic Leukemia

Buckthorn bark is one of the ingredients in Harry Hoxsey's tea formula. A research study revealed that some types of buckthorn bark, in animal tests, could halt lymphocytic leukemia (510). See chapter 16 for details on Hoxsey's formula.

## Dyer's Woad Root Extract Cures CML in Humans

Dyers's Woad *(Isatis Indigotica Fortune)* has been part of common medical usage in China for many years. According to *www.nutrition2000.com*, the root of this plant is commonly used in China for treating those with leukemia and tumors (101). One study in particular revealed that a daily dosage of *150-200 mg of purified Dyer's woad* was able to cure CML (chronic myelocytic leukemia) in greater than half of those humans with the disease. (101). These were **humans**, not lab animals! This herb has also been shown to kill various bacteria, parasites, and viruses (101).

## Poly–MVA for Leukemia

See chapter 14 for more information on this amazing nutritional supplement that many cancer survivors have credited to bringing them into total remission, even from leukemia. Their main website can be found at: *www.polymva.net.*

## Shark Liver Oil Inhibits Leukemia

Though shark **cartilage** has been helpful in attacking other cancers, for leukemia, shark liver **oil** (sometimes referred to as *squalene),* is most commonly used. It is often used in cosmetics and facial creams for promoting healthy, wrinkle-free skin.

In one particular case, an elderly woman who had been fighting a form of CLL for more than a decade, experienced a return to normal blood levels within months after her physician prescribed this supplement. She was given a total of eight capsules—each capsule containing *500 mg* of the substance (386). Though no serious problems have been associated with using this supplement in normal dosages, it can cause epigastric discomfort in some people. See your health care practitioner for individual dosing to fit your needs.

## Tian Xian & Multiple Myeloma

*Tian Xian* is a Chinese herb that has been credited with many cancer recoveries, including multiple myelomas. You can read case histories of numerous cancer survivors, some given only two to six months to live, who went into complete remission using Tian Xian at *www.tianxian.com.* Most are still alive today, many years after their ordeal.

## Ukrain Fights Leukemia

Ukrain is given by injection, so it is not exactly gentle or painless; however, it is included here due to its success with several types of cancer, and the fact that it is completely non-toxic. It was discovered in 1978 by Dr. Wassyl J. Nowicky in Austria, who combined two compounds that, when given alone, were toxic. Once merged, however, it was found to be completely non-toxic, except to cancer cells (287)(506). A study that involved 70 cancer patients (all of whom were *terminal),* revealed that Ukrain was toxic to many different types of cancer, including leukemia (506). It can only be found at alternative medicine clinics in the U.S. or in Canada, the Ukraine, or other countries in Europe, where it is commonly used. It is discussed in several other cancer-specific chapters in this book. The main website for Ukrain is at *www.ukrin.com.*

2009 update: because Ukrain is not authorized in Austria, this article (which was described in my first book) is no longer located *at www.ukrin.com.* The website has been changed and is now called *Nowicky Pharma.* You can read detailed information about Ukrain now in the book: *Anti-Cancer Agent Ukrain The Crime Story of an Obstruction,* by Eleonore Thun-Hohenstein. For pictures on how Ukrain works, see website *http://www.ukrain-drug.net/webspeed/index.htm.*

## Xi Shu

Xi Shu *(Camptotheca acuminata)* is an herb that has been used by the Chinese for several millennia. They have used it for treating leukemia, and for this reason, it is often referred to as *the cancer tree* (323).

# VIII. Other Issues Involving Leukemia

## Childhood Leukemia Statistics & Processed Meats

Research involving more than 200 case studies, conducted by the University of Southern California, on the intake of *processed meats* (e.g., lunchmeat, bacon, bologna, hotdogs) and how they affect children, revealed that intake of these foods, which contain nitrates, dramatically increased the risk for leukemia (525). You can read specifics on this study at *http://www.ncbi.nlm.nih.gov/pub med/8167267.*

## Cow's Milk & Leukemia in Cattle

Of great concern is the use of cow's milk, especially in children. It is possible that eliminating cow's milk from your diet may help protect you from getting leukemia, especially since cattle often carry this disease (351). Note that pasteurization does **not** always kill all the viruses in the milk (351). Avoiding cow's milk may also protect your children from juvenile or Type I diabetes.

See chapter 26, later in this book, for more information on why homogenized, pasteurized milk may put you at risk. Unless you are fortunate enough to live near a dairy farm to get raw cow's milk where the farmers are meticulously clean with their cattle and practice organic farming (and have disease-free cattle), it may do you more harm than good.

## Flax Oil & The Budwig Diet

See chapters 14 and 18 of this book for information on the famous Budwig flax oil diet that many have credited to complete cancer cures.

# CHAPTER 9

# GENTLE CURES FOR TOUGH LIVER CANCERS

*"Cast thy burden upon the Lord, and he shall sustain thee:" (Psalm 55:22)*

## I. New Non-Invasive Test for Liver Disease

In the past, most liver disease has been diagnosed by taking a biopsy of the liver, a painful procedure, not without risks to the patient. A new procedure to diagnose "severe liver disease," without needing a biopsy is on the way (218a). It is known as *Transient elastography*, and it *evaluates liver stiffness* in order to *diagnose cirrhosis.* It is also referred to as the *LSM*, *liver stiffness measurement.* This, per a new report from *Clinical Gastroenterology and Hepatology* (218a). See website *www.gastro.org,www.cghjournal.org*, and the full article from website *http://www.eurekalert.org/pubreleases/2008-09/aganta0 82708.php* (218a).

## II. Liver Healers & Protectors

### AHCC—Mushroom Combo that Heals

AHCC (*Active hexose correlated compound*) is a substance that is made up of several different mushroom mycelia. In **human** testing, it was able to strengthen the body's natural immune system and extend the lives of patients recovering from liver cancer surgery (163). You can find this supplement at natural health food stores and online health stores (206).

### Chlorophyll & Chlorophyllin for Liver Cancer Prevention

Scientists have discovered that eating green foods, which are high in natural chlorophyll, could protect from all cancers, but especially those of the colon and liver (76). Many animal studies have shown that natural chlorophyll and chlorophyllin (an extract made from chlorophyll) fight cancer. They discovered that this substance can also protect against the dangerous fungus that often affects nuts and cereals known as *aflatoxin,* a source of liver cancer, especially in nations that do not have adequate safety measures for storing their grains (76). Both chlorophyll and chlorophyllin protect against the DNA damage caused by other cancer-causing substances, especially those found in *grilled meats* and *diesel exhaust.* Dr. George S. Bailey discussed the protective effects of this green substance in the LPI Research Newsletter, "Chlorophylls and Cancer Prevention: passing the First Hurdle," where a **human** study (using chlorophyllin) was done in Eastern China on a group of people who were at risk for liver cancer from *aflatoxin exposure* (76). They were given the chlorophyllin *thrice daily* in 100 mg pills for a total of 300 mg. The participants in the clinical trial experienced a 55% decrease in urinary output of the aflatoxin compounds, which are responsible for *DNA damage* (which leads to liver cancer), indicating that the chlorophyllin was killing the aflatoxin (76).

A new 20 year clinical trial is being done in China for testing chlorophyllin. Eating several servings a day *of green vegetables* would be necessary to obtain the *300 mg per day of chlorophyllin* given in the clinical trial (76). High amounts of chlorophyll in the diet (via green vegetables) could also prevent the type of colon cancer caused by an iron found in red meats (76). There are usually no adverse effects from natural chlorophyll and chlorophyllin.

## Coffee & Liver Cancer

A human study involving over 60,000 people in Finland, revealed that drinking coffee could reduce a person's risk for liver cancer. Those drinking higher amounts of the brew had *68 percent* less risk for liver cancer. Subjects were followed for more than thirty years, and more studies are planned for verification analysis (511). Research also shows that coffee drinking can decrease your risk for type II diabetes (80), but beware, because excess amounts can also raise your risk for developing rheumatoid arthritis (81). Coffee drinking also lowers the risk for developing cirrhosis, a liver disease which often leads to liver cancer.

## CoQ10 & Liver Cancer (Issels Treatment)

Current research conducted by the Leonard M. Miller School of Medicine in Miami (under Niven R. Nerain) revealed that CoQ10 has the ability to kill cancer cells without damage to healthy cells. Not only that, but the National Cancer Institute acknowledged in 2005 that CoQ10 can extend the lives of those with liver cancer and other cancers. Issels Treatment Centers use CoQ10. Their phone #888-447-7357 (290).

For one of America's largest alternative health care centers, the Whitaker Wellness Center, which is in Newport Beach (4321 Birch Street), California, see this link: ***http://whitakerwellness.com/about_us/medical_team.*** Dr. Julian Whitaker, who runs this health care center, has written numerous books on alternative healing. He has an excellent website with a great deal of helpful information. They use many of the alternative health treatments that I have mentioned in my books, including chelation, hyperbaric oxygen, and IV therapies. Dr. Whitaker also writes an excellent newsletter.

## CyberKnife® Therapy for Liver Tumors

See chapter 34 in this book for details on CyberKnife® therapy, which is being used successfully for liver cancers and many other cancers, including hard-to-reach brain tumors. It is a gentle, painless procedure that does not require an incision, surgery, sedation or inpatient stay. It takes very little time, and as soon as the procedure is over, the patient is able to return home. There are very few risks and side effects, though it does involve some radiation (89a), and it can damage nearby healthy cells. Also, see NanoKnife™, chapter 34.

## Cytotron Therapy

See chapter 34 in this book for details on this gentle, painless, non-invasive cancer therapy that many people are also using to restore cartilage in their joints, making joint-replacement surgeries completely unnecessary (90). You may hear this referred to as *QMR* or *Quantum Magnetic Resonance*—they are the same thing.

## ECT—ElectroChemical Therapy for Liver Cancer

Also described as *direct-current* ECT, this therapy originated in China (474). Widespread human testing has not yet been carried out in the U.S. In animals, *platinum electrodes* are placed on the tumor and treated with direct current (474). Animals with *carcinomas* in the colon and rectal areas that had spread to the liver were tested, and it was found that the treatment caused a very dramatic tumor shrinkage (474). More studies are planned in the U.S. on this therapy.

Currently, an ECT machine developed by *Solco Biomedical* (known as the "Solco SET-C21") by Swedish Professor, Nordenstrom, in 1983, is claimed to have minimal side effects, boosts the immunity, and changes the pH of cells via electrochemical reaction. It is available from Korea. The therapy is being used for most cancers, including gastric, breast, lung, skin, and liver (275). It is widely used in Chinese hospitals, Korea, Germany and some cancer treatment centers in the U.S.

## Fungus Cure Also Cures Cancer, Says Oncology Physician

See chapter 34 of this book for the amazing cancer cure that Italian Oncologist, Dr. Simoncini, is using to cure his cancer patients within just days! Cancerous growths are usually WHITE. He says that they are actually a fungus, which can be killed with a non-toxic soda bicarb solution that quickly alkalizes the tumor for destruction (582).

## Holly Mangrove (*Acanthus* or *Harkach Kanta*) for Liver Cancer

Researchers in India discovered that extracts from the leaves of *acanthus* can fight liver cancer in mice (144). This plant is also known as *holly mangrove* and *harkach kanta.* Not only did it prevent liver cancer by protecting DNA from damage, it also extended the lives of the animals. The study was published in the *World Journal of Gastroenterology* 28th Dec. 2007 (144). Though more studies will need to be done to determine use in humans, this test tells us how important herbs and plants are in fighting cancer.

## The Liver Cancer that Vanished

As described by Jean Carper in her book, *Miracle Cures,* when a CAT scan diagnosed a middle-aged man with liver cancer (who had a greater than 20 year history of alcohol use and smoking), a follow-up biopsy was done which confirmed the diagnosis, as well as the fact that the cancer was spreading (364). Doctors sent him home, assuming a rapid death (364). Imagine the surprise of these physicians when their patient showed up alive, well, and much improved within 12 months (364). He told them that he had quit smoking and drinking and that he felt very well and had even gained weight. They were astonished when subsequent diagnostic tests showed no sign of the tumors, and several biopsies done at the prior tumor location were negative (364).

Doctors noted that this was highly unusual, occurring very rarely in the population. So unusual in fact, that very few cases can be found in publicized literature. Though they surmised that giving up cigarettes and alcohol contributed to the patient's healing, they had no real answers to the total regression of the deadly cancer (364). It turns out that the patient himself had the answer. After being given his hopeless diagnosis, the patient began taking an herb, known as *milk thistle,* every day without exception. The dosage he took was *450 mgs* (364). Though the physicians would not admit that it was the milk thistle that cured the liver cancer, they were in favor of using the herb, seeing that there were no toxic side effects. The herb acts as an anti-oxidant, helping the liver repair and renew itself and fend off scavengers (364).

Why were these physicians so reluctant to admit that the only thing that this patient did differently to **cure** his liver cancer was using milk thistle? It does not take a rocket scientist to figure out exactly what cured his inoperable liver cancer. Many people quit smoking and drinking immediately when they are diagnosed with liver cancer (or lung cancer), but that does not cure them. This is simply another case of conventional medicine refusing to admit that something besides a toxic chemo drug cured a deadly cancer. Milk thistle (*silymarin*) can be found at any natural health food store as a supplement and in tea bags. It is also sold in bulk. If you have hemochromatosis, you need to be sure that the milk thistle supplement you purchase does not have iron. Anyone with hemochromatosis should not take large amounts of vitamin C either, since doing so can increase iron in the body. (Also, be aware that if you are diabetic, milk thistle can lower blood sugar.)

## Magnesium for Cancer Prevention

This mineral is critical for the prevention of all types of cancer, including leukemia, and those cancers involving the stomach, prostate, breast, and bones (566). Magnesium taken by mouth can cause diarrhea. See chapter 34 and pages 129 and 400 for information on a new form of magnesium that is absorbed right into the skin, bypassing the stomach.

## Milk Thistle & Other Cancers

Not only has milk thistle proven to protect the liver, but research has shown that the herb could be useful in the fight against cancers of the skin and breast (351).

See chapters five and six of this book for information on how this herb is being used against prostate and colon cancer. Milk thistle has been used for over 2000 years. It is actually the seeds of the plant that are therapeutic, containing the many silymarin flavonoids (571). Milk thistle has many times the anti-oxidant punch that vitamin E has, and it works by helping liver cells to regenerate and throw off toxins (571).

## Milk Thistle, Glutathione, Skin Disorders & Endometriosis

Glutathione is another major anti-oxidant found throughout the human body, and there are few substances you can take that will increase its production. Milk thistle is one of them. Milk thistle also helps raise the body's amount of *superoxide dismutase, (SOD),* another potent anti-oxidant (571). Because the liver can be helped by milk thistle, it may be especially important for people with various types of liver disease (571). It also prompts the regeneration of kidney cells, improves billiary function, and digestion of fats (571). Of course, you will need to check with your doctor before using this herb if you have any type of billiary problems, including stone formation (571), or if you have ulcers.

Though vitamin C aids the body in making more glutathione, milk thistle keeps glutathione reserves from being exhausted in the liver, and it appears to be stronger than either vitamin C or E (337). Other nutrients that increase the body's production of glutathione (besides vitamin C), are natural nutrients that can be found in the sulfur and cruciferous veggies, *avocados*, and some types of nuts such as *walnuts* (337) (338). Milk thistle also acts as an anti-inflammatory for skin disorders, such as *psoriasis.* It may help relieve the painful symptoms of *endometriosis,* since it assists liver cells with estrogen use (288). Scientists have discovered that, in animal testing, if the skin suffers dangerous sun exposure, then they apply silymarin topically, melanoma formation was decreased (288).

No major side effects have been reported from the use of milk thistle. Though it has a reputation for being exceptionally safe, some users of the herb experience diarrhea on initial use for the first 24 to 48 hours (288). It is recommended that the herb be ingested on an empty stomach.

There have been no reports of adverse effects when milk thistle was taken with other routine medications (288). (Of course, as with any herb, there is always the possibility of allergic reactions.)

Do not use this herb if you have allergies to ragweed or daisy-type flowers, dyes, or other allergies (152). Check with your doctor to be certain this herb is appropriate for you. Do not use with alcohol, nor during pregnancy or breast feeding (152), nor as stated earlier, if you have gastric problems, stone formation, or ulcers.

## Milk Thistle & Hepatitis

James A. Duke, Ph.D., author of *The Green Pharmacy Anti-Aging Prescriptions*, recounts the story of a lady with hepatitis A, with severely compromised liver-functioning, who showed an amazing recovery after a vitamin K injection and a three week regimen of milk thistle (388).

When Lloyd Wright contracted hepatitis C from blood transfusions, he healed himself naturally with milk thistle and wrote a book called *Triumph Over Hepatitis C* (603). At his website, *www.hepatitisCfree.com*, he says that he uses only *organic* milk thistle seeds, puts them in water and simmers over heat for *two hours* before consuming the tea mix (603). He also recommends *1000 mg* per day of the herb, even if you are using the tea mix, since silymarin does not dissolve in water (603). Mr. Wright puts the information on his website in hopes that the reports will be seen by physicians who told him it was impossible for any herbal preparation to *regenerate* his liver (603). Mr. Wright has information on new products containing milk thistle and other important liver healing herbs at his website above. He is also a cancer survivor (603).

## Milk Thistle & Toxins

In a research study, when rats were fed poison and silymarin both, the herb prevented liver damage (388). Many chemo drugs are like slow poison. Some chemo drugs are so caustic that the nurses handling the drugs must wear gloves to avoid skin contact.

## Mushroom Poisoning Cure & Super Anti-Oxidant

Is milk thistle the miracle herb many believe? YES! There is no doubt that it helps **protect and *regenerate* the liver.** As noted by Jean Carper in *Miracle Cures*, a German doctor working with milk thistle, found that it had the amazing ability of preventing severe liver damage and deaths normally caused to Europeans who had ingested the lethal *amanita mushroom,* or *death cap* mushroom (364). While amanita kills nearly half of those who ingest it (even with medical treatment), no one given milk thistle experienced a fatality, even though some were not treated for hours (even up to 72 hours), **after** they ate the mushrooms, which is absolutely astounding! The physician believed that the herb competes for poison receptor sites within the liver, thus preventing the toxin from entering (364).

As far as dosing, it is always best to follow your physician's recommendations. Your doctor may start off with a lower dosage (200 mg or less) to see how well you tolerate the herb; however, for those already having liver dysfunction, a higher dosage (e.g., *420 mg* per day taken in 140 mg capsules at the rate of *three* times per day to get a total of 420 mg, or even more per day), may be needed. Once serum levels show an improvement, the amount can be reduced to the lower dosage (364), or as recommended by your physician or Naturopath. (Remember that the liver cancer patient described in the earlier story was ingesting 450 milligrams of silymarin per day for nearly a year.)

James A. Duke, Ph.D., with Michael Castleman, documented a similar study on the power of milk thistle in preventing death from the amanita mushroom in their book, *The Green Pharmacy, Anti-Aging Prescriptions.* Dozens of people received silymarin for mushroom poisoning. There were no fatalities. In another study where more than 150 people were given conventional treatment for amanita ingestion and 16 given silymarin, there were 46 fatalities in those who received conventional care and **no deaths** in those given silymarin (388). Animal studies show that silymarin could help block *acetaminophen* (Tylenol®) from harming the liver (388).

Conventional physicians generally use *activated charcoal* for mushroom and other poisonings, depending on the poison (388). In a nutshell, the patient is given a vile-looking black liquid charcoal to drink. The charcoal is supposed to soak up all the toxins and pull them from the body, preventing damage to vital organs such as the liver; however, it sometimes doesn't work, especially if too much time has passed since the toxin has been ingested. Activated charcoal can also be given through gastric lavage (a tube that goes into the stomach) if the patient is not conscious, for example (e.g., during cases of drug overdose). The charcoal works best if given within a half hour of the time the toxin is ingested. Believe it or not, the U.S. is so far behind Europe in medical technology that silymarin is not even available in emergency rooms for treating mushroom poisoning, yet it is commonly used in European countries. Some U.S. hospitals are finally getting in alpha lipoic acid, but I am sure it is mostly due to the heroic efforts of doctors like Burt Berkson, M.D. (See his book, *The Alpha Lipoic Acid Breakthrough*.)

## Nanotechnology—*Lodamin*—Halting Liver Cancer Spread Without Side Effects

A new drug, Lodamin, which works by halting the blood vessel growth that tumors need to survive, was shown, in animal testing, to be effective against many tumor types, including those of the breast, brain, ovaries, uterus, prostate, neuroblastoma, and glioblastoma (401). It also worked very well in preventing cancer from going into the liver (401). The discovery of the drug, using *nanotechnology* and a derivative from a fungus, was quite accidental. Reports say that it can be taken orally without *side effects* (401). The drug also inhibited melanoma and lung cancer in mice (401). Lodamin is still in the testing phases, and is also being considered for treating macular degeneration and arthritis.

Note that shark cartilage and bindweed, also discussed in this book, work to starve tumors by cutting off blood supply to them, without adverse side effects. (See chapters 7 and 34.)

## Standardized Milk Thistle

Also called *Lady's Thistle* (and many other rural names), be sure to use standardized milk thistle supplements that have *70% and 80% silymarin* (152). This is the strength of milk thistle *used in human studies* (152). If you use a standardized product, you are assured of receiving the potent form of the herb in identical batches (152). Some people confuse milk thistle with blessed thistle; they are two completely different herbs!

As noted earlier, do not use milk thistle if you have allergies to ragweed or daisy-type flowers, dyes, or other allergies (152). Check with your doctor to be certain this herb is safe for you. Do not use during pregnancy or breast-feeding. Do not mix with alcohol (152).

If you purchase the herb in loose bulk format, follow the directions given at the herbal store where it is purchased. Most health food stores where you buy loose herbs should provide you with directions on brewing them. Always consult with your physician or Naturopath for safety precautions, especially if you already have a chronic condition.

## III. Nutrients for Liver Cancer

### Aloe Emodin Effective Against Liver Cancer

Aloe emodin, an ingredient taken from the leafy aloe vera plant, has been researched for its anti-cancer properties in fighting liver cancer, with amazing results. *Life Extension's* website (*www.lef.org*) contains a published report of studies conducted using aloe-emodin to treat cancer. It was useful against liver and lung tumors, in animal studies, and was also able to suppress nerve tissue tumors even though the animal's immune systems were significantly compromised. The substance had no major adverse side effects (7). Other studies reveal that aloe emodin could be an important preventative for liver tumors by causing liver cancer cells to undergo a type of self-destruction. Aloe emodin can also be found in sheep sorrel, one of the herbs used in making Essiac tea (270). Perhaps this is why Essiac tea has a history of being so effective!

Be certain that when you use organic aloe vera jel juice, it must be cold-pressed. The label on the bottle will tell you whether or not it is cold-pressed. Check with your doctor before using, especially if you have a history of chronic illness involving stomach or colon problems.

### Alpha Lipoic Acid Heals Liver Damage, Prevents Cancer, & May Even Eliminate the Need for a Liver Transplant

Alpha lipoic acid is a natural ingredient that our bodies make, but unfortunately, like many other nutrients, we produce less of it as we get older, and we must maintain a high level for good health (344). Dr. Burt Berkson, M.D., Ph.D., author of *The Alpha Lipoic Acid Breakthrough,* lists many of the multiple benefits of this amazing anti-oxidant. It helps the body fight HIV; protects the eyes and other vital organs such as the *kidneys* and liver; wards off diseases like *cancer*, *diabetes,* and *leukemia;* and may even be helpful in preventing the damage caused by a *stroke* or *heart attack* (344).

Dr. Berkson has also successfully treated several of his hepatitis C patients with ALA—patients who were told that they would die without a transplant, yet most returned to jobs or school after treatment, dramatically improved (344). The alpha lipoic acid was part of a structured regimen that included exercise, stress-management, and nutrition. All of the participants received not only ALA, but milk thistle and several vitamins as well. Dr. Berkson believes that, in many cases, patients with liver disorders should try ALA before resorting to a transplant (344).

Have you been diagnosed with liver cancer, hepatitis, or liver failure? Has your physician considered prescribing milk thistle or alpha lipoic acid (ALA) supplements for you? Has he or she explained the importance of lycopene in liver health? Though potatoes, broccoli, brewer's yeast, and spinach are good food sources of alpha lipoic acid, you cannot get sufficient daily amounts without supplementing with this nutrient. Most ALA supplements come in 100 mg capsules.

## Apples for Liver Health

Is it possible that simple ingredients in apples may be powerful enough to prevent cancer and slow its growth? Researchers have discovered, through laboratory testing, that compounds in these fruits can suppress both hepatic and intestinal cancers. Since both the pulp and peelings contain the cancer-fighters, don't peel before eating. Realize though, that all fruits and vegetables (even organic) should be washed thoroughly before consumption.

## Astragalus—Herbal Power for the Liver

Astragalus herb, in capsule or tea form, boosts the immune system, activating immune cells to fight tumors. Check with your physician or Naturopath about using this herb, especially if you have an infection or are running a temperature (178). You can find astragalus tea bags and supplements in natural health food stores.

## Beets for Liver Health

An excellent liver cleansing drink to boost liver health is beet root juice. Hungarian physician, Dr. Alexander Ferenczi, discovered that the juice from this vegetable could fight many types of cancer. He even recommended the powdered form of beet root that is usually reconstituted with water (429). When given to test animals, not only did their tumors disappear, but they had an increased life span over the animals not receiving the juice (429). Truly amazing, isn't it—that something so closely resembling BLOOD, cleanses the blood?

Always start ingesting beet juice slowly to build tolerance. It is very potent, and consuming too much at once can detoxify too rapidly and make you feel worse. Always mix beet juice with another vegetable juice such as carrot, celery, or green juices, rather than drinking it alone. Drinking beet juice without mixing it with other juices can cause choking in some individuals. If you juice beets with some of the pulp and let the juice sit for about an hour, it will thicken and coagulate much like blood does! (Just be aware, especially if you are diabetic, that beets are high in natural sugar.)

## Blueberries Halt Progression of Liver Cancer Cells

An extract from blueberries, *pterostilbene*, was found (in laboratory tests), to halt the progression of liver cancer cells (38). This same ingredient is found in grapes. It also helps lower cholesterol, enhances memory and fights heart disease (37) and colon cancer (38).

## Cherries Prevent Liver Cancer

A compound in cherries (*perillyl alcohol)* can help the body fight off many types of cancer, including those of the abdomen, breast, and liver (604). This was demonstrated, in animal testing, by researcher Charles Elson, Ph.D., who said that the remarkable substance not only helped prevent cancer, but also worked against existing tumors (604).

## Cinnamon for the Liver

Just one teaspoon per day of grated cinnamon can work wonders for your liver because it neutralizes one of the substances (*plasmin*) which causes cancer to spread (178). I purchase cinnamon at a local health food store that sells it by the pound, and use 1 or 2 teaspoons at a time, usually when I make fresh apple juice or even added to homemade grape juice. Cinnamon can help stabilize blood sugar, and may help kill the bacteria responsible for some types of food poisoning. See chapter 31.

## The *390 mg.* Daily Regimen of CoQ10 That Cured Liver, Lung & Breast Cancer in Humans

Research has shown that high dose Coenzyme Q10 given to cancer patients may help them win the fight against several types of cancer. In a 1994 study, two women having breast cancer experienced complete remission during a clinical trial where they were given either *300 mg or 390 mg* of CoQ10 daily (472). In the patient receiving 390 milligrams, the tumor completely vanished within a 60-day period (472). A year later, another human study was conducted, and a middle-aged patient experienced total remission of a liver cancer previously marked by multiple tumors. Every single tumor vanished. Another patient on CoQ10 enjoyed complete remission of lung cancer after a period of several months. An elderly patient with breast cancer experienced no further cancer after she had lump removal and was on the CoQ10 treatment (473). CoQ10 supplements are available in health food stores, pharmacies, popular grocery chains, and many internet sites.

Most nutritionists will recommend that you start off with a low dose of CoQ10, such as 50 mg per day, then progress to higher doses as needed. For example, start with 50 mg/day; after two weeks, take the 50 mg twice a day; two weeks later, take it three times a day. Depending on your situation, you may want 100 mg/day, 200 mg/day or more. If you are fighting cancer, you will probably want to work up to 300—400 mg daily. Always check with your physician or Naturopath. If you have a conventional doctor, I would advise getting an opinion from an alternative medicine physician, because many conventional physicians are totally in the dark about CoQ10 (see below).

## Essiac Tea & Other Herbs

See chapter six of this book for information on Rene Caisse and the many patients she cured of various cancers with Essiac tea, including her own mother. There are preparations on the market that contain the herbs already pre-mixed. One example is known as *Flor-Essence*®, which not only has the Essiac herbs, but kelp, blessed thistle, and red clover for boosting the immune system. *Flor-Essence*® comes already made into a tea, or in a dry mix that you can brew to make the tea yourself. It is available at many health food stores.

Rene Caisse, a Canadian nurse, healed hundreds (probably thousands) of people of every imaginable cancer using her amazing herbal tea, many of whom came to her after conventional medicine considered them *incurable* and *hopeless.* One of the most amazing books describing the effectiveness of this tea and how it was suppressed by the health industry in Canada is called *The Essiac Report Canada's Remarkable Unknown Cancer Remedy.* Author is Richard Thomas, who states that Flor-Essence® is the original (drinkable) formula used by Rene Caisse (580).

Note that there is some competition between the tea produced by Resperin Canada Essiac® and Flor-Essence® Essiac tea. Both companies claim that they have the original Essiac formula (the drinkable formula, not the injectable) that Rene Caisse used in treating her cancer patients.

See chapter 16 (later in my book) for the story of a young boy who was cured of lymphoma using a natural program that included Essiac® Resperin tea formula and 714X injections. (A website that has Essiac® Resperin is given in that chapter, as well as information on where to obtain 714X.) Also, see Appendix II at the back of this book for some important resource websites.

Chapter 16 also has the amazing story of Maryjo Siegel (diagnosed in 1991 with a fatal non-Hodgkin's lymphoma), who was cured of her cancer with Burzynski's non-toxic antineoplastons (562). As of an email from her in June 2009, she is alive and well, living a healthy, normal lifestyle and has never had a reoccurrence of her cancer!

Marie Nadine Antol, author of *Healing Teas,* recommends many nutrients and herbs for their benefit in promoting liver health. Some of these *are dandelion…milk thistle, pau d'arco, and propolis* (333). (Note that some herbs have blood-thinning effects, may increase bile secretion or gastric acids, or elevate your blood pressure. Do not use them without first consulting with your health practitioner.)

## Graviola - Help From The Rain Forest

Refer to chapters five and six for more information on how this herb has been successfully used by cancer patients to cure their cancer.

## Goldenseal Inhibits Liver Cancer Cells

As described at *www.herbs2000.com,* goldenseal contains *berberine*, which impedes the formation and growth of abnormal cells in the liver (178). This herb (and its components) should not be used in women who may be pregnant, nor those who are nursing, or have billiary problems; it should not be combined with vitamin B6, *histidine,* hormones or *insulin;* it should not be used by those with blood pressure problems, *glaucoma,* or heart-lung problems (178).

## Grapes (Resveratrol) Fight Liver Cancer

Research credits resveratrol (a super anti-oxidant) to the prevention of liver cancer. It works by preventing malignant cells from invading the body, and halts the formation of a compound identified with malignant breast cells as well. See chapter three of this book for more information on the amazing curative powers of this nutrient, which is found in common table grapes, pomegranates, and other foods. One grape that you may want to consider is the **muscadine grape**, so high in anti-oxidants that many health articles have been written on them. Resveratrol is also being touted as a way to fight obesity, as well as high cholesterol levels since it keeps the body from storing fat. You can purchase resveratrol in supplements online and at most local health food stores, as well as some chain grocers and pharmacies.

## Green Foods & Liver Health

Chlorella is an algae harvested from rivers and ponds that is even richer in chlorophyll than wheat grass, alfalfa, and all other green foods, including other alga. It has higher levels of chlorophyll than any other plant, including spirulina. C. M. Hawken, author of *Green Foods "Phyto Foods" for Super Health,* says that chlorella stimulates the immune system by producing extra white blood cells and increasing levels of interferon. It has been shown to inhibit some cancers and even cause the cells to revert to normal (426). Chlorella has magnesium, beta-carotene, calcium, zinc, protein, many other vitamins and minerals, and several carotenoids, which are heart-protective and cancer-preventative (426). Be sure, in purchasing chlorella, that you obtain a brand that has *broken-cell-wall.* Without the cell wall of this one-celled organism being broken, you cannot absorb it.

If you are wondering about chlorella dosages for those with cancer, Dr. Joseph Mercola of *www.mercola.com,* says that people fighting cancer have taken chlorella at the rate of *30 grams* in one day. He also described the case of a patient (with bone cancer), who had amazing benefits after only six months of taking this nutrient at the rate of *20 grams* a day (485).

In Ann Wigmore's, *The Wheat grass Book*, chlorophyll is described as being so similar in structure to hemoglobin that physicians have actually used it for anemic patients (600). It can help carry oxygen to all the cells of the body, including the brain (600). Wheat grass (though not as high in chlorophyll as chlorella) is another green food that greatly enhances the immune system. Ms. Wigmore believed that there are three important compounds in wheat grass that benefit the liver: *choline* which fights fat build-up; *magnesium* which helps extract fats; and *potassium* which rejuvenates (600). Remember too, that when you keep your body highly oxygenated and alkaline, cancer cells cannot survive. Greens alkalize!

## Green Tea for Liver Health

Green tea is rich in bioflavonoids which fight destructive free radicals. As noted in the book: *Dr. Earl Mindell's What You Should Know About The Super Antioxidant Miracle,* tea bioflavonoids have been known to eliminate dangerous lipids in the blood, lower *blood pressure*, inhibit processes that trigger cancer, stop the growth of pathogens, help the body assimilate food, and protect against dangerous blood clots and *strokes* (492). These compounds also keep the liver and brain healthy, and fight bacteria and gum disease (492). Green tea is much higher in catechins (the bioflavonoids) than black tea. As discussed earlier, for some cancers, combining both teas is more effective. Green tea catechins are available at health food stores in supplement form if you do not wish to drink the tea. Note that cancer patients should stick to caffeine-free tea, as caffeine is very dehydrating; however, it is possible that the caffeine-free tea does not remove plaque in blood vessels as well.

Many studies have shown impressive abilities of green tea to inhibit all types of cancer. In animal studies, green tea cut lung cancer nearly in half. It has also reduced *stomach…liver* [and] *skin cancer* rates dramatically, not only preventing them, but stopping the active spread (492). Green tea has also been found (in animal testing by Israeli researchers) to regenerate brain cells, something hitherto thought impossible (169). This is something to consider if you have loved ones battling dementia, alzheimers, or brain damage.

## Hormones & Liver Cancer

Recent studies have shown that using birth control pills increase a woman's risk of liver cancer three times over those who do not use them. See chapter 22 in this book for more information on how pharmaceutical companies knowingly promoted their potentially toxic synthetic estrogen and progesterone prescriptions to the public, when they knew full well that natural estrogen and natural progesterone (found in nature) were already available, and without toxic side effects. Synthetic hormone replacement therapy (HRT) has been proven to increase the risks of blood clots, breast cancer, and uterine cancer. Many women who are placed on HRT, then develop breast cancer (sometimes years later in life), are then placed on Tamoxifen. One of the side effects of Tamoxifen is uterine cancer, as well as visual problems. After going through breast cancer, then taking Tamoxifen, many of these same women THEN develop uterine cancer. (Taking a drug that causes cancer, then taking another drug (that causes cancer) for the cancer caused by the second drug—is this not total insanity?)

## IP-6 for Cancer Prevention

IP-6 can be found in health food stores. It is a natural, non-toxic and inexpensive anti-oxidant found in many plants, and is said to boost the body's immunity. Some naturopaths routinely recommend IP-6 to their patients fighting cancer.

## Limonene Halts the Growth of Tumor Cells

Laboratory research shows that an ingredient in citrus fruit, known as *limonene,* has anti-cancer properties (604). University of Wisconsin's Michael Gould, Ph.D, said that limonene could help kill cancer cells (604). This is detailed by Selene Yeager, author of *Doctors Book of Food Remedies.* In animal studies, she says that limonene shrank tumors by *70 percent* (604). These studies involved mostly lung and breast cancers. When scientists fed laboratory animals a derivative of orange juice, their liver lesions were reduced by nearly half. They had first removed the *vitamin C* from the juice (604).

## Liver Cancer & Alkalinity – A Cure?

One of the most important ways to keep the liver healthy is by alkalizing the body. Dr. Simoncini was mentioned earlier in this chapter for his emphasis on treating cancer with soda bicarb to destroy the tumor by alkalizing it. See chapter 34 for more information on his exciting results in curing many of his patients within just days by simply destroying the fungus (cancerous tumor) with a simple alkaline solution!

## Lycopene Power & Liver Health

If you are interested in a drink that will rapidly improve the health of your liver, try tomato juice. For low blood sugar, mononucleosis, *chronic fatigue,* and *yeast* problems, John Heinerman in *Heinerman's Encyclopedia of Healing Juices*, recommends this lycopene-rich drink, which will rejuvenate the adrenals and liver (429). He also recommends adding a very small amount of seasoning (cayenne and hot sauce) if tolerated (429). Research on **humans** demonstrated that lycopene can cut the risk for cancer of the liver in half. Other good food sources of lycopene, besides cooked tomatoes are: watermelon, guavas, dried tomatoes, and red peppers.

It is best to consume a fat with lycopene for better absorption (337).

## Mushrooms That Prevent Liver Cancer & Metastasis

Animal studies proved that liver cancers could be reduced in mice receiving maitake powder and *Maitake D-fraction*, derived from maitake mushrooms. Of the group receiving no mushroom at all, every single one of them developed liver tumors (469). It was also found, in these same tests, that maitake prevented the spread of cancer (469).

Maitake should not be taken by those with *multiple sclerosis.* It can increase a substance that destroys nerve tissue in people with MS (184).

Lentinan injections, from the shiitake mushroom, help stop the progression of cancerous liver cells (178); however, since they are not considered conventional medicine, you will have to seek an alternative practitioner for this treatment.

Reishi mushroom extract may also help fight liver cancer (178). It is available in supplement form.

Another mushroom that helps in the fight against liver cancer is the agaricus mushroom *(Agaricus Blazei Murill).* It has a polysaccharide that helps fight rectal, liver, breast, lung, and ovarian cancers (10). These mushrooms can be ordered at *www.agaricus.net*, and other websites (10). They can also be found in supplements in some natural health food stores. New Chapter® has many mushroom supplements. You can find their brand in most health food stores and on the internet.

The School of Medicine at Ehime University in Japan found (through studies in mice) that agaricus blazei murill extract is a potent cancer preventative (447). Not only did the mushroom prevent the growth of tumors, but it slowed their spread as well. The mushroom also enhanced and increased immune cells (447). The substance that was extracted from the agaricus mushroom was *sodium pyroglutamate* (447).

There are many websites that provide agaricus or ABM mushroom, some in dried form and some fresh. (See chapter 25 of this book for more information about the amazing healing and curative powers of mushrooms and their extracts.) Other mushrooms important in fighting cancer are the mesima, chaga, tinder polypore, and split-gill mushroom (15). Some of these mushrooms have multiple names.

## Oleander Soup for Liver & Lung Cancer

Used by an attorney in Texas, who cured his mother of *lung and liver cancer* (as well as a sister who was fighting *Hepatitis C*), you can read more about this cancer remedy at *http://www.buzzle.com/articles//father-of-the-oleander-soup-cancer-remedy.html* (437). It has also been said to cure rheumatoid arthritis in a patient using it, and helping in cases of psoriasis and HIV (437). A physician from Turkey (Dr. H. Z. Ozel) developed the remedy, which was being considered by the FDA; however, after successfully going through a Phase I trial, it sank into relative obscurity due to funding problems (437). You will find this treatment under the name Anvirzel™ (437). There are many precautions in regards to making your own oleander soup. The leaves are considered poisonous.

## Onions Prevent Liver Cancer

Researchers at Cornell University believe that it is very possible that an *onion a day* in your diet can make a dramatic difference in your overall health (471). Details on this study can be found at *www.news.cornell.edu/releases/Oct04/onions.cancer.ssl.html*. It also appears that the variety of onion you eat makes a big difference. In the article, scientist Rui Hai Liu, M.D., Ph.D., says that the best varieties for their anti-oxidant potency are *shallots, Western Yellow, pungent yellow and Northern Red*. According to him, onions also kill viruses, inhibit allergies, and fight inflammation. Apparently, the stronger-smelling onions are best for anti-cancer potency. The *Western Yellow* onions far surpassed *Western White* onions for flavonoid content (471). Choose red, purple, or yellow onions, rather than the white onions.

## Other Liver Nutrients

Animal testing shows that deficiencies in the nutrients lecithin and/or choline may promote liver cancer (551). You can find both supplements at health food stores; however, if you take lecithin, your body can produce choline (551).

A substance known as *borage oil* can keep toxins from harming your liver. Borage oil is sometimes used for dangerous cases of *mushroom poisoning* (551). Two other substances used for this purpose are milk thistle and alpha lipoic acid, as discussed earlier in this chapter.

Many other nutrients help fortify the liver. Even patients fighting hepatitis have been helped by drinking beet root juice, but only if they consume at least four or more cups of the juice every day, regardless of the type of hepatitis (551). Do not suddenly start drinking large amounts of beet juice. It detoxifies the body so rapidly, initially, it may make you worse! Start by drinking small amounts (two ounces at a time) and always mix it with a few ounces of another vegetable juice, such as carrot or celery. Drinking it alone may cause choking in some individuals.

From what I have researched on garlic, I believe that next to eating fresh organic garlic, the best garlic extract is Kyolic®. They received an award from the National Nutrition Foods Association, and use a stringent manufacturing and aging process. When cooking, it is best to use fresh, organic garlic. Chicory, a close relative of milk thistle, also has liver-protective abilities.

## Probiotics Cut Liver Cancer Risk

In a controlled **human** study of the probiotics, *Lactobacillus* and *Propionibacterium,* individuals who received two capsules daily had lower levels of a common liver cancer-causing toxin in their body. Those conducting the research summarized that the probiotics decreased levels of the toxin. Those receiving a placebo did not achieve these results (240).

## Phyllanthus for the Liver

This herb, *Phyllanthus niruri*, also known as the *kidney stone tree*, can help fend off cancerous liver cells, and is the source of a vaccination that was developed against *hepatitis-B* (233). It should not be used without your physician's advice, since it may lower blood pressure. It may also lower blood sugars and strip fluids from the body, resulting in dehydration (233).

## Red Clover for Liver & Prostate Health

Red clover, with its wealth of isoflavones, has a beneficial amount of naturally-occurring plant estrogen (497). Red clover can enhance the body's natural immunity, helping it fight cancer, inflammation, and chronic disorders (497). These natural plant estrogens lock onto estrogen receptors in the body, blocking the more harmful synthetic estrogens from entering the cells.

You can find red clover supplements in capsules, tablet form, teas, and other preparations at natural health food stores (497). This herb can thin the blood.

## Sea-Based Oceanic Help for Curing Liver Cancer

Shark cartilage is discussed in chapter seven in more detail for its treatment of cervical, ovarian, and uterine cancers, however, it has also been effective against other cancers. Dr. Ernesto Contreras, Jr., of Panama, used this supplement for 60 days to cure eight of his cancer patients, all of whom had been considered terminal (550). All of them had tumor shrinkage from *30-100* percent, and one experienced a total cure from terminal **liver cancer** within two months of starting the supplements (550). Shark cartilage is not for use with children, nor during pregnancy, or if you have recently had a heart attack, transplant, surgery, chemo, or radiation. It is not for those with seafood allergies, liver disease (though it was used successfully in the case above for liver cancer), high blood pressure, pheochromocytoma (adrenal tumor which can cause excessively high blood pressure), ulcers or circulatory diseases. See chapter seven for more information on dosing. You should always consult with your chosen health practitioner for dosing to fit your individual needs before taking this supplement.

See chapter 34 of this book for information on an herb, known as *bindweed*, that is said to have *100 times* the ability at blocking blood vessel formation as that found in shark cartilage (150) (301a), also without toxic side effects. See chapter 12 in this book for the case of a woman with pancreatic and liver cancer who had positive results using this compound. Do not use bindweed in its wild state. It must be processed to be toxin-free.

## Selenium Prevents Liver Cancer

Selenium is vitally important for liver cancer prevention. Testing of 100,000 humans in China revealed that this mineral could reduce liver cancer deaths by more than one-third! The study lasted eight years. This mineral is particularly important for anyone fighting *hepatitis-B* (178). Though too much selenium can be toxic, most people don't get enough of this mineral on a daily basis.

Hard as you may try, you cannot get enough of this mineral in the normal daily diet without, for example, eating about 30 bushels of parsley or two acres worth (337), or unless you eat a a few handfuls of Brazil nuts (grown in selenium-rich soil) every day. Most nutritionists will recommend 100-200 ***micrograms*** of selenium per day, though much higher doses have been used by some individuals, without problems. Too much can be toxic.

Good natural sources, as listed in Dr. H. Winter Griffith's *Vitamins Herbs, Minerals & Supplements,* are *whole-grain* foods, *cabbage,* and *onions* (411). Brazil nuts (507), leafy greens, and kelp are also rich in selenium.

## Soy Lecithin, Arginine & Jerusalem Artichokes - Nutrition to Help Prevent the Progression of Liver Cancer

Soy lecithin works against free radicals to fight against cancer. Arginine is a protein building-block found in many foods, e.g., *sunflower seeds* and *chocolate* (178). It helps suppress abnormal liver cells, but does so in such a way that the body does not suffer protein-starvation. Jerusalem artichokes have an ingredient (known as *inulin*), which was discovered, in lab studies, to suppress the growth of abnormal liver cells (178). (This is INULIN, **not insulin.**) Do not use arginine if you have genital herpes or the herpes virus that causes fever blisters and shingles.

Be sure to get organic artichokes, because most artichokes are heavily sprayed. Also, realize that there is a wide controversy about what types of soy to use. Many soybeans are now being genetically modified (referred to as *GMO foods*), and their long-term health effects on human beings is questionable. If you would like more information on this health controversy, just go on the internet and google the words "the world according to Monsanto," and you will be shocked. Use only fermented soy. Avoid all other soy products.

## TheraSphere Therapy for Liver Cancer

TheraSphere is a new type of concentrated radiation that uses millions of tiny glass particles with attached radiation to treat liver cancer, cholangiocarcinomas, or cancers that have gone into the liver. Though certainly not a natural treatment, it is being mentioned here because it is considered gentle, free of serious side effects, and the patient can go home the same day as treatment. It is considered conventional therapy without the side effects that would normally be found if undergoing chemo. See website *herald-review.com/articles/008/01/16/lifefeatures/1029341.txt* for an article on this treatment (407). Also, see this website: *cancercompass.com/message-board/message/all,19011,0.htm.*

## Tian Xian for Liver Cancer

Tian Xian, a Chinese herb, is said to be effective in fighting several forms of cancer, including liver cancer. As reported at *www.tianxian.com*, in November of 1992, 83 year-old Mr. N. Zentaro of Japan, was diagnosed with liver cancer as well as stomach cancer. His physician felt that due to his age and the fact that the cancer was in two sites, surgery would not be feasible. Not only that, but even if he had opted for surgery, he was given only months to live (611). His daughter told him about Tian Xian, which he began taking. Not only was he cured, but six years later, alive and well, he reported in a testimonial that he is still taking the herb with completely normal health checkups (611). This supplement is available at some health food stores and on several websites including *www.tianxian.com,* where you can find many testimonials from cancer survivors.

## Vitamin K for Cancer Prevention

A human study, published in *JAMA,* revealed that participants supplementing with vitamin K could dramatically lower their liver cancer occurrence (408). The study was done from 1996 to 1998 and involved more than three dozen participants, all having viral cirrhosis and hepatitis C (408). The participants were given vitamin K2 at the rate of *45 mg*/day. Researchers discovered that the group receiving vitamin K decreased their chances of liver cancer by *90 percent* (408).

Note that leafy greens (e.g, spinach, kale, chard, and broccoli) are rich in vitamin K. In eating fresh produce, you must use scrupulous handling and cleaning to prevent bacterial contamination. There are many recent cases of food poisoning from e-coli and salmonella (and other bacteria) from raw fruits and vegetables. Also, use products like cinnamon, garlic, turmeric, cayenne, wild oil of oregano, pumpkin seeds, grapefruit seed extract, grape juice, wine, and cloves to kill bacteria. Use alpha lipoic acid, borage oil, amla fruit (see below), lycopene, and milk thistle to protect the liver.

## IV. Miscellaneous Liver Protectors

- **Actinidia** is a root popular in China for medicinal uses. When test animals were given injections of this herb, liver tumors were dramatically suppressed (504). Note that **Kiwi fruit** is a type of actinidia.

- ***Amla fruit*** **(aka the *Indian gooseberry, tamalaki and katuki rhizome),*** was found, in laboratory testing, to dramatically protect the liver by preventing toxic chemicals from causing cancer (14). Testing also shows that the juices from this fruit could lower cholesterol. This was revealed in animal and **human** testing (14).

- **Bitter orange** has potent anti-oxidants, known as *monoterpenes*, which help suppress mutant liver cells (178).

- **Bupleurum** has something in common with an herb that **is used to fight liver cancer**—milk thistle! Bupleurum rejuvenates a sluggish liver. It has a reputation as an anti-inflammatory and is used in Japan to successfully treat liver diseases, such as hepatitis (50). It has also been used for bone cancer (50). Be aware that excessive dosing of this herb can cause epigastric problems and swelling. It should not be taken if you are running a temperature or taking other medications. If bupleurum causes epigastric problems, your herbalist or health practitioner may need to lower the amount that you are taking (41).

- **Chinese peony** (different species) demonstrated the ability, in animal studies, to prevent liver damage caused by chemicals (388). It is recommended by the World Health Organization for liver health. Medical practitioners in China generally give a daily dosage of this root of *3—20* grams (388). Do not use this herb if you have endometrial cancer (10). Never take this supplement without consulting your physician or Naturopath. It can be dangerous if use is not closely monitored.

- **Dandelion** has been used for hundreds of years in rural areas for treating jaundice (388). This herb is a powerhouse of anti-oxidants that help the liver (388). Although it is non-toxic and has many medicinal uses (235), be aware that dandelion can increase hydrocholoric acid and bile secretion, something to consider if you have ulcers, gallstones, billiary disease, or other G.I. tract disorders.

- **Indian Almond** *(Terminalia catappa)* extract can protect the liver against chemical damage, as found in animal testing. This herb grows wild in some states (388).

- **Kudzu** *(Pueraria Montana)* is another herb containing liver protective anti-oxidants (388).

- **Macela** *(Achyrocline satureoides)* is a potent herb from the rain forest of the Amazon. Laboratory research has shown that a compound taken from these flowers can suppress abnormal cells (183). Lab studies from Argentina reported that the herb causes death to cancerous liver cells, and was also effective against the AIDS virus and *Pseudorabies* (183). Animal studies have shown no reports of toxicity with the herb. It is used in Brazil as a tea, and has been used in herbal medicine for years—sometimes the floral parts of the plant—and sometimes the plant in its entirety (183). Macela has a blood sugar-lowering effect as well (183). For more information on this herb, see Raintree Nutrition at *www.rain-tree.com.*

- **Picrorrhiza** *(Picrorrhiza kurroa)* is an herb from which the extract *picroliv* comes. This extract is currently undergoing human testing in India, where it is popular for treating hepatitis (388).

- **Schisandra** has over two dozen compounds in its seeds that protect the liver (388). It is yet another popular Chinese herb for use against liver disorders, such as hepatitis, given in dosages of *1 to 7 teaspoons* per day (388). Schisandra berries have been used in treating many ailments, including diabetes and tumors of the liver (264). When human studies were done in China on patients with liver disease, substances in schisandra increased levels of an important anti-oxidant known as *glutathione,* and were said to be helpful to patients suffering from cancerous livers and liver inflammation, whether caused by chemicals or by viruses (264). Most health food stores have schisandra in capsule supplements and tea bags.

- **Scutellaria and licorice**—While scutellaria can help destroy abnormal cells in the liver, it can also be used in tea form with licorice for those who have hepatitis and wish to keep from developing cancer of the liver (178). Licorice should not be taken by anyone with hypertension, eye problems (such as *glaucoma*), or for those with *estrogen*-related *disorders* (178).* If you decide to use this herbal combo, only use it for *six weeks* at a time, then go off the herbal tea for a *two-week* period (178). Take the tea with foods that are potassium-rich and do not take the scutellaria if you have or should develop diarrhea (178). (*One way to prevent the problems associated with licorice use is to obtain DGL or *de-glycyrrhizinated* licorice, available in health food stores.) Chewing a few tablets of DGL before meals can help heal GERD, indigestion, and prevent ulcers.

- **Tamarind juice and bottle gourd** protect the liver from damage. Dr. James Duke, author of *The Green Pharmacy Anti-aging Prescriptions,* said that one of the highest sources for choline is the *bottle gourd,* which is normally served like squash (388). You can find liver-protective tamarind juice in Latin America and in the U.S. in some hispanic grocery stores (388).

- **Turmeric** is a popular cooking spice. It contains curcumin, a protective ingredient for liver cells, and a great anti-inflammatory agent. It has performed impressively in studies inhibiting cancer growths and has been discussed in several other chapters in this book. See chapter 20 for instances when you should not use curcumin (turmeric). If you want your body to absorb turmeric more easily, eat it with pineapple or supplement with bromelain.

## Keeping the Liver Healthy

It is important to realize that prevention of liver damage in the first place is your priority for liver health. The liver is important for the metabolism of amino acids, carbohydrates, and fats. It is so important in detoxifying harmful chemicals, that we cannot survive long without it. Chemicals, including prescription drugs and excessive use of over-the-counter medicines, such as Acetaminophen (Tylenol®), are toxic to liver cells. The liver must work overtime to flush what it considers to be poisons from the system, as well as harmful food additives that the body does not recognize. Also, be aware that certain vitamins, such as vitamin A and D are not water soluble and are stored in the liver. Excess amounts of these vitamins can be harmful. This is why your best source of vitamin D is sunshine, and your best source of vitamin A is NATURAL beta-carotene, not the synthetic form found in pills. The body turns natural beta-carotene into vitamin A. Drink carrot juice and eat orange and yellow vegetables (e.g., squash, yams, and pumpkin) for natural beta-carotene.

Many patients are on the transplant-waiting-list because of adverse drug reactions to medications they have taken. Some are there because they thought it was safe to consume RAW seafood which contained viruses capable of destroying liver cells. Stay away from raw seafood and any type of undercooked meat. Other substances (e.g., hormones, pesticides, and herbicides) used recklessly in commercial farming, are harmful to the liver. Bacterial contamination of foods with e-coli, salmonella, and other pathogens can also damage the liver. Alcohol consumption is very damaging to the liver. The thousands of people who succumb to cirrhosis and other diseases caused by excess alcohol consumption, are a sad testimony to this fact every single day.

Note that you should always check with your physician before beginning any herbal regimen, including relatively safe herbs such as milk thistle. If you have already received a transplant, there are certain herbs, vitamins, hormones, or minerals that may interfere with the anti-rejection medications that you must take. If your liver damage was caused by excess iron (a genetic disorder known as *hemochromatosis*) for example, you must be sure that if taking milk thistle, you use a standardized preparation that is **not** high in iron, or it could do you more harm than good. Anyone with hemochromatosis should not take large amounts of vitamin C either, since doing so can increase iron in the body. This is another reason you should discuss supplements with your physician before ingestion.

There are many herbs that, if consumed in large amounts, or taken over long periods of time, can cause liver damage. A few of these are *comfrey, germander…and pennyroyal*, and of course, be sure to purchase your mushrooms in your local grocery store or natural health food store (preferably organic). Don't take chances gathering them in the wild if you are not familiar with varieties that can be deadly (388). You may want to keep a bottle of milk thistle (silymarin) in your first-aid kit for emergencies. Also, see the information in this chapter about the benefits of alpha lipoic acid for liver health.

## V. Other Treatments for Liver Cancer

Though some of these treatments are not exactly what I would consider *painless, gentle, or natural,* they do not involve the use of toxic chemo-therapy and are being included here for informational purposes for that reason.

- **Bland Embolization, Ablation & Radiofrequency Thermal Ablation for Liver Cancers, & SIR-Spheres®**

***Bland embolization*** and ***ablation*** are both procedures that researchers believe may prolong the lives of some liver cancer patients. In ***radio-frequency ablation,*** heat is used in an attempt to destroy malignant cells, an alternative to riskier surgery (247a). The procedure uses ultrasound to guide the surgeon to the area needing treatment. It is used for primary liver cancer or liver tumors that have spread and is considered a safe treatment that patients seem to tolerate quite well. Some patients treated with this type therapy experience a cure with no later reoccurrence of their tumors. It is generally used for those who are not surgical candidates. ***Radiofrequency ablation*** treatment is gaining popularity, especially among those with liver cancer and those having primary lung growths, as well as those that have spread from other sites (247a). A probe is placed as close as possible to the tumor, then radio waves are sent through the probe to destroy the cancer cells (247a). A recent clinical trial, known as *the RAPTURE study*, was conducted on more than a hundred lung cancer patients treated with this therapy. Within two years of the treatment, the majority of the patients were still alive, and none had died from the treatment. There is little damage to healthy cells during the ablation (247a).

Though I discussed radiofrequency ablation for liver tumors in my first book, *Painless Cancer Cures*, I recently saw a website article describing this very same procedure being used successfully in hundreds of **human** trials for those with inoperable liver tumors. Apparently, it is gaining more and more popularity and extending lives. It is used for liver cancers (e.g., hepatocellular carcinoma) and spreading colon cancers. Some Oncologists are using this procedure on other cancers, not just those of the liver and colon.

In ***Embolization*** (aka *radioembolization*), a procedure is done that cuts off blood supplies to the tumor, thus starving the tumor to death. These procedures are likewise being used for other forms of cancer, besides those of the liver. You may also hear them referred to as ***embolization particle therapy,*** or ***radioembolization spheres***. (Shark cartilage and bindweed also work by cutting off blood supply to tumors.)

***SIRT, or Selective Internal Radiation Therapy***, sends "Millions of microscopic, radioactive spheres called SIR-Spheres®" right to the site of the tumor to "deliver 40 times more radiation to the liver tumors," than can possibly be done using conventional radiotherapy. This kills the cancer cells and usually leaves most of the healthy cells unharmed (265a). Though it isn't considered a "cure," often the tumors are shrunk so much that they can then be surgically removed, "resulting in a long-time cure" for the patient (265a). Since this is a form of radiation, there is always the potential for adverse effects, but it is being mentioned here because conventional doctors may offer it as a last resort for those with inoperable liver cancer, or inoperable liver cancer that has spread from the colorectal area (265a). For information on this procedure, as well as potential side effects and who is eligible (or may not be eligible) for the procedure, see article at website *http://www.umgcc.org/sir-spheres/about_ sirt.htm* (265a). (You may hear these referred to as *chemoembolization.*)

- **LITT—Laser-Induced Thermotherapy**

There is a great deal of information on the internet and in medical journals on a laser procedure that is apparently increasing survival time (over surgery) for some patients with primary tumors that have spread to other organs, such as the liver or bone. It is called *LITT* or *laser-induced thermotherapy*, and it is also used for some cancers which are considered inoperable. The treatment uses a laser to eradicate cancerous growths. Thousands of patients have already been treated successfully with this procedure. Most have a primary cancer that has spread into other organs.

## Light Infusion Therapy (Litx™) for Hepatocellular Carcinoma

This is a new light therapy that does not cause the serious side effects commonly found with conventional radiation treatments, and it not only kills the tumor cells, but it destroys the blood vessel networking that they need for survival (176a). It is undergoing clinical trials (now in Phase III trials in humans) for hepatocellular carcinoma, a difficult-to-treat liver cancer. It uses a light-activated drug that kills cancerous cells without killing massive amounts of healthy cells (as standard radiation tends to do). It is not considered a non-invasive treatment, however, the entire procedure takes less than three hours, after which time the patient returns home. You can see a video on exactly how the therapy works, and read more about this remarkable new technology at Light Sciences website: *http://www.lsoncology.com/litx_therapy* (176a).

## Liver Flush

Refer to chapter 36 for a nutritious liver flush recipe.

## Poly–MVA for Liver Cancer

See chapter 14 in this book for more information on an amazing nutritional supplement known as Poly-MVA, a palladium lipoic complex that contains several vitamins, alpha lipoic acid, and amino acids that many cancer survivors are crediting to bringing them into total remission. For testimonials of people who used this substance to cure their cancers, see website *http://www.polymvasurvivors.com/testimonials.html.* Many of these testimonials are given ten or more years ago, yet all survivors are still here as of March 2007.

## Rexin-G™ for All Solid Tumor Cancers

Rexin-G™ has been undergoing clinical trials at Mayo Clinic, M.D. Anderson, and a few other facilities. It is a drug for cancers that have spread, and those types of cancer that conventional medicine says do not respond to chemo (256). **Human** clinical studies, thus far, have had good results. In the very first human trial, 83% of the patients experienced tumor shrinkage. The patients all had spreading pancreatic cancer (256).

Good responses were also achieved in **human** studies involving several other types of metastatic cancer. Due to the reports, this drug is now used for treating all forms of *solid tumors* in the Philippines that are resistant to conventional therapy (256). The U.S. FDA has given the drug its *orphan drug status* for use with pancreatic cancers in the US, as well as other types of cancer metastases, which means that trials will continue (256). It is given intravenously, so isn't exactly natural or painless, but could be considered gentler than older chemo drugs because it is said to be a non-chemo drug, showing itself in **human** clinical trials, not to have the adverse side effects normally associated with chemo drugs (256). You can get more information on this drug at *epeiusbiotech.com/rexin_g-factsheet.asp.* Epeius Biotechnologies are the producers of Rexin-G™ (257).

## Ukrain for All Cancers, Including Cisplatin-Resistant

Nearly every chapter in this book describes Ukrain and its various clinical trials against cancer. Ukrain is non-toxic and has been shown to stimulate the body's natural immunity.

Cisplatin is a commonly known chemo drug used for various types of cancer. Many people who choose this conventional treatment go on to develop cancers that are resistant to this drug. Laboratory testing has shown that Ukrain, which is non-toxic, acts very much like the drug cisplatin—and for those who have chosen chemo and now have Cisplatin-resistant cancers—it is believed that Ukrain may be helpful in overcoming this problem (458). For more information on this study, see PubMed NCBI website, PMID 10190087 (458). You will not find Ukrain therapy at most conventional medicine facilities. It can be found at natural treatment centers and alternative centers in some areas of the U.S. and other countries, such as Europe, where it is very popular.

# VI. New Treatment for Bile Duct Cancers

This is a rare type of cancer that involves the bile duct, rather than the liver. Prognosis is good if it is caught before it has spread to other areas (442a). Problem is, this type cancer isn't usually detected until it has spread, so removing the cancer surgically isn't always possible. A new study that was published in *Clinical Gastroenterology and Hepatology,* revealed that combining *photodynamic therapy (PDT)* and *endoscopic retrograde cholangiopancreatiography (ERCP)* could increase survival in these patients

(442a). During ERCP, a *stent* is placed into the clogged bile ducts for a return to *normal function*. The stent opens up the duct. On the other hand, photodynamic therapy (with CT assist) uses light to *burn the tumor*. These procedures have been done on dozens of humans, some having very good results (442a). For details, see: *http://patient.Cancerconsultants.com/CancerNews_Liver_Cancer.aspx?Document Id=41944* (442a).

## VII. ALA, Silymarin & Selenium Enable Patients to Cancel Liver Transplants

When three men with hepatitis C were involved in a study where they were treated with ALA (alpha lipoic acid), silymarin (milk thistle), and selenium, they had such dramatic improvements, that they were able to go off the liver transplant-waiting-list. For details on this study, see the National Library of Medicine's website article: "A Conservative Triple Antioxidant Approach to the Treatment of Hepatitis C. Combination of Alpha Lipoic Acid (thioctic acid), Silymarin and Selenium: Three Case Histories by Berkson, B.M." See PubMed website *http://www.ncbi.nlb.gov/pubmed /10554539?dopt=abstract* (344a). Remember too, that hepatitis can progress into liver cancer.

## VIII. Iodine Removes Harmful Toxins & Protects the Liver

See Dr. Mark Sircus' book, *Iodine Bringing Back the Universal Medicine*, for reasons why most people are deficient in iodine, which causes a build-up in the body of parasites, yeasts, viruses, mercury, bromide and other heavy metals, all of which cause cancer and other diseases. He also discusses how certain diseases, like malaria, have been killed simply by taking iodine (566a). It was by ingesting iodine that victims of the Chernobyl disaster in Russia were saved from thyroid cancer (566a). See website *www.magnascent.com* and *www.magneticclay.com* for sources of a superior form of natural, food-grade, gentle iodine (Magnascent or Nascent iodine) that is rapidly absorbed into the body and used by all cells.

# CHAPTER 10

# GENTLE CURES FOR TOUGH LUNG CANCERS & MESOTHELIOMA

*"I shall not die, but live, and declare the works of the Lord." (Psalm 118:17)*

## Cancer of the Lungs - Types & Diagnostics

Lung cancer and the type of diagnosis given is sometimes *non-small cell* or *small cell lung cancer,* depending on the cell's appearance under magnification, and as noted at NCI's (National Cancer Institute) website, there are several forms of "non-small cell lung cancer…Squamous cell carcinoma…also called epidermoid carcinoma…Large cell carcinoma… Adenocarcinoma…" and rarer forms, such as: "pleomorphic, carcinoid tumor, salivary gland carcinoma, and unclassified carcinoma" (219).

Your physician will want to do a lung biopsy if cancer is suspected. In the past, this is usually done by an invasive procedure, which goes through the chest to obtain a small piece of the suspected area. There are now less invasive ways to check for lung cancer. Some physicians are getting lung biopsies via an endoscopy, which passes through the mouth and into the throat.

## AHCC - Mushroom Combo Enhances Immunity

AHCC (*Active hexose correlated compound)* is actually a compound from the mycelia of many mushrooms. In **human** testing, it was found (when given to patients in doses of *3g/day* by mouth over 2-6 months) to significantly increase the body's natural immunity at killing lung cancer cells and several other types of cancerous cells (206). This compound is found at many natural health food stores and online supplement providers (e.g., *www.discount-vitamins-herbs.net).*

## Cranberries Halt Lung Tumors

The powerful anti-oxidants (also known as *proanthocyanidins)* found in simple cranberries, have been shown, in research studies, to halt the progression and formation of lung growths. Cranberries also help fight leukemia, and they cut the risk for ulcers and bladder infections (22).

## CyberKnife® Therapy for Lung Tumors

See chapter 34 in this book for details on CyberKnife® therapy, which is being used successfully for lung cancers and many other cancers, including hard-to-reach brain tumors. It is a gentle, painless procedure that does not require an incision, surgery, sedation or inpatient stay. It takes very little time, and as soon as the procedure is over, the patient is able to walk out and return home. There are very few risks and side effects, though it does involve some radiation (89a), and it can damage nearby healthy cells. Also, see under NanoKnife™, chapter 34, for a non-toxic, gentle new therapy.

## Cytotron Therapy

A new cancer (and arthritis) treatment developed and available in India that you will not yet be able to get in the U.S., is being successfully used on humans and is known as *Cytotron Therapy*. It is gentle, completely painless, and non-toxic. See chapter 34 in this book for more details on what is also called *QMR* or *Quantum Magnetic Resonance* (90).

## ECT—ElectroChemical Therapy for Lung Cancer

Also described as *direct-current* ECT, this therapy originated in China (474). Widespread human testing has not yet been carried out in the U.S. In animals, *platinum electrodes* are placed on the tumor and treated with direct current (474). Animals with *colorectal carcinomas* that have spread to the liver were tested, and it was found that the treatment caused dramatic tumor shrinkage (474). More studies on this therapy are planned in the U.S.

Currently, an ECT machine developed by *Solco Biomedical* (known as the "Solco SET-C21") by Swedish Professor, Nordenstrom, is claimed to have minimal side effects, boosts the immunity, and changes the pH of cells via electrochemical reaction. It is available from Korea. The therapy is being used for most cancers, including gastric, breast, lung, skin, and liver (275). It is widely used in Chinese hospitals, Korea, Germany and some cancer treatment centers in the U.S.

## Flavenols (Fruits & Vegetables) Prevent Lung Cancer

New studies involving nearly 1400 people, show that ingesting three or more servings per day of *fruits and vegetables*, along with *green or black* tea consumption can help protect those who smoke from getting lung cancer (120). The UCLA researchers credit the protection to *plant-pigments* (flavenols) found in the substances. These flavenols are found in many fruits, vegetables, greens and teas, and the protection may extend to other cancers that are *smoking-related*, including those of the *bladder, head and neck, and kidney*...(121). Research on humans in China proved that people consuming the most vegetables in their diet had 60% fewer lung cancer rates, and those eating large amounts of fruit could cut their incidence for lung cancer one quarter. Even smokers benefited from increasing flavenols in their diets.

## Fungus Cure Also Cures Cancer, Says Oncology Physician

See chapter 34 of this book for the amazing cancer cure that Italian Oncologist, Dr. Simoncini, is using to cure his cancer patients within just days! Cancerous growths are usually WHITE. He says that they are actually a fungus, which can be killed with a non-toxic soda bicarb solution that quickly alkalizes the tumor for destruction (582).

## Intensity Modulated Radiotherapy (IMRT) for Lung Cancer

This radiation treatment is currently under testing in Europe and is being used in the U.S as well. It uses targeted radiotherapy to help minimize damage to nearby normal cells. It is used for lung tumors, thyroid and breast cancers, as well as prostate, esophageal, nasal, head cancers, liver, brain, ovarian, cervical cancers, and uterine growths. You may also see this treatment referred to as ***TOMO Therapy*** or *TOMO Treatment*—they are the same thing.

IMRT was first used at Memorial Sloan-Kettering Hospital for treating cancer of the prostate (163a). Rather than using one large radiation beam to target the tumor, this type radiation uses many beams to target cancer tumors more precisely, thus (hopefully) preventing excess damage to nearby normal cells (163a), though it is still considered radiation and will have some of the same side effects as any radiation would cause.

IMRT has been popular at treating tumors located around or near critical, vital organs (163a).

## Magnesium for Cancer Prevention

This mineral is extremely vital for the prevention of all types of cancer, including leukemia and those involving the stomach, prostate, breast, and bones (566). Some researchers believe that 90% of the population in the U.S. could be magnesium deficient due to magnesium-poor soils, leading to a vast array of chronic illnesses. See chapter 34 for more details on using magnesium and soda bicarb against cancer.

## Megadose Vitamin C Cures A "Terminal" Lung Cancer

When 59 year-old, Arlindo O., was told that his advanced lung cancer had gone into his brain, physicians sent him home to die (149a), yet today he is *cancer-free* (149a), and he credits his survival to vitamin C. Recent studies *from the National Institutes of Health* showed that vitamin C given *intravenously* could halt the growth of "aggressive brain, ovarian and pancreatic tumors…" in mice (149a). The treatment is non-toxic to healthy cells, having none of the adverse, damaging side effects associated with standard *chemotherapy and radiation.* According to Dr. Scott Greenberg, who treated Arlindo with high intravenous doses of vitamin C, "it is a valuable option for those who don't respond to other treatments," and "can be used along with traditional chemo and radiation" (149a). He said that the vitamin C creates "hydrogen peroxide," which kills the cancer cells much "like chemotherapy does," (149a) except that vitamin C is non-toxic to healthy cells. He even talked about a woman he treated with massive intravenous vitamin C, who had "a large breast mass protruding out of her chest" (149a). Within just "a few months of treatment," the mass disappeared. It has been five years and her cancer has not returned (149a).

Mega-dosing vitamin C by intravenous therapy is discussed in several other chapters of this book. New research continues to prove that Abram Hoffer, Irwin Stone, Linus Pauling, Bernard Rimland, Dr. Robert Cathcart, Dr. Thomas Levy, and many others were correct in their assessment of the anti-oxidant effects of this wonder-vitamin.

## Proteolytic Enzymes for Lung Cancer

Proteolytic enzymes are enzymes made by the pancreas. They also include papain (found in pineapples) and enzymes found in papaya. You can find these enzyme supplements in health food stores. They should be taken 30 minutes before meals for digestive help.

Human trials have shown that combining proteolytic enzyme therapy with chemo could extend the lifespan of those with inoperable lung cancers, as well as diminish adverse chemo effects (514).

## Rexin-G™ for Metastatic Cancers

Rexin-G™ has been undergoing clinical trials at Mayo Clinic, M.D. Anderson, and a few other facilities. It is a drug for cancers that have spread, and those types of cancer that conventional medicine says do not respond to chemo drugs (256). Human clinical studies, thus far, have had good results. In the very first human trial, 83% of the patients experienced tumor shrinkage. The patients all had spreading pancreatic cancer (256). Good responses were also achieved in human studies involving several other types of metastatic cancer. Due to the reports, this drug is now used for treating all forms of *solid tumors* in the Philippines that are resistant to conventional therapy (256). The U.S. FDA has given the drug its *orphan drug status* for use with pancreatic cancers in the US, as well as other types of cancer metastases, which means that trials will continue (256). It is given intravenously, so isn't exactly natural or painless, but could be considered gentler than older chemo drugs because it is said to be a non-chemo drug, showing itself in **human** clinical trials, not to have the adverse side effects normally associated with chemo drugs (256). You can get more information on this drug at *epeiusbiotech.com/rexin_g-factsheet.asp.* Epeius Biotechnologies are the producers of Rexin-G™ (257).

## Stereotactic Body Radiotherapy for Lung Cancer

Stereotactic Body Radiotherapy has recently been introduced at Northwest Indiana's Methodist Hospital for destroying lung tumors. An *Elekta Stereotactic Body Frame* is used in the procedure, which gives very precisely-controlled *radiation beams* for lung tumor destruction. Many people diagnosed with lung tumors are not physically able to undergo surgery, and this is another option available to those with lung cancer, especially stage I. Considered painless with few complications, and requiring less than an hour (and only three treatments), it is done on an outpatient basis. See website *insideindianabusiness.com/newsitem.asp?ID=27347* for more details (220). Though it is considered radiation, it is more precisely-controlled than standard radiation, supposedly having milder side effects. Realize that this type radiation treatment, like any other, may depress the immune system, albeit not as severely.

## I. Nutrients To Prevent & Halt Lung Cancer

## Apples Cut Lung Cancer Risk by 50%

Eating apples appears to cut in half the risk for lung cancer (180). Juicing organic fresh apple juice and adding cinnamon is doubly nutritious, and liver healthy; however, remember not to discard the vitamin-rich peelings, and use scrupulous cleaning to prevent food-borne illnesses.

## The Lung Cancer That Disappeared

- **<u>Case #1:</u> Beets & Broccoli for Lung Cancer**

A physician in Budapest, who treated a lung tumor patient with beets [raw], discovered after six weeks that there was absolutely no trace of the tumor left, and within one month of treatment, the patient had gained over twenty pounds (429). Vegetables containing sulfuric compounds, (e.g., from the cabbage family [and] *onion*, are effective at not only inhibiting tumors, but useful for fighting those already formed) (430).

According to Dr. Ralph W. Moss, author of *Cancer Therapy,* a sulfur extract taken from broccoli, known as *sulphoraphane*, was believed by a prominent medical college to be possibly the greatest cancer-fighting substance ever discovered (504). This cancer-fighting compound is not just in broccoli. It is also found in all the cruciferous vegetables and sulfur-containing vegetables. Apparently, *steaming* or *microwaving* does not reduce its potency (504). Human studies show that eating raw vegetables with sulphoraphane can also help fight lung cancer in those who smoke. There are compounds in raw broccoli that also prevent and fight ulcers and heart disease. (These vegetables (raw) also alkalize the body.)

## <u>Case #2</u>: Phytoplankton for Lung Cancer

When T. Harper was told that he had terminal lung cancer and he began ingesting small quantities of marine phytoplankton from his own facility that grows the substance, not only did his cancer totally disappear, but he was able to achieve a healthy weight and go off the insulin that he had used for 17 years. His story, and others, can be found at *http://www.shirleys-wellness-café.com/cancer.htm* (187). Phytoplankton supplements can be found at most natural health food stores and internet health food sites.

## Beta-Carotene

Beta-Carotene is effective at lung cancer prevention; however, studies show that natural beta-carotene (rather than the synthetic supplemental form) is much more effective. When a popular **human** study was conducted on the effects of beta-carotene on smokers, it was reported that taking the vitamin could increase their incidence for cancers of the lung (68); however, there is one very big fact that was left out of the media reports on this study. They neglected to report that the beta-carotene used in the study was SYNTHETIC beta-carotene, NOT **natural** beta-carotene (68). The media also failed to report that this increased tendency to develop lung cancer rose only for those who consumed alcohol and more than *a pack of cigarettes a day* (68). As further described at *jrussellshealth.com*, the study did not include men who had no deficiencies of vitamin E or beta-carotene. It was flawed, because the study used only human subjects who were already at *high risk* for lung cancer *(poor diets and heavy smoking)*, and the government disbanded the research when the participants taking SYNTHETIC forms of beta-carotene had increased risks for cancer development (68).

Studies point to the need for natural forms of beta-carotene and vitamin A for health, rather than the synthetic forms. Research from China proves that synthetic beta-carotene may damage cellular DNA, while the natural beta-carotene fights tumor formation (507). When scientists from Israel emphasized that one should be closely aware of what type of beta-carotene was being used (natural as opposed to synthetic), **they were ignored** (507). An excellent source of beta-carotene (and B12) is chlorella. Just be sure to get the broken cell-wall chlorella. Chlorella also has the highest concentration of chlorophyll of any green food!

Is it possible that the body does not distinguish synthetic beta-carotene and vitamin A as it does when the natural forms are provided by nature, as given to us by our great Creator, God? As a matter-of-fact, a scientific study revealed that malignant changes in stomach cells could be returned to normal with the use of *natural beta-carotene* (507). Is it any wonder that something synthetic is far inferior to what God intended for us in nature?

Another study involving more than 20,000 doctors, found beta-carotene supplementation to be non-toxic (305). The study can be found at *http://ods.od.nih.gov*. It was further noted that using synthetic beta-carotene was only bad for participants who consumed alcohol at the rate *of one drink per day* (305). Those conducting the study determined that eating foods rich in natural beta-carotene could help cut as many as *15,000-20,000* lung cancer fatalities a year, and it wouldn't take much—just ONE carrot (305). Have you had YOUR carrot today?

Once people quit smoking, they are at increased risk for throat cancer until the larynx heals. Adequate amounts of natural beta-carotene are vital in the healing process to prevent this type of cancer (305). Even in those who are non-smokers, consuming carrots is probably their best cancer insurance, as revealed by a study from Sweden (180). Beta-carotene can be taken in large doses, as long as it is the NATURAL form [e.g., from foods like carrot juice and yams], because once the body stores enough vitamin A, excess amounts are excreted. Even though consuming high levels of *carotenoids* may color the skin a slight yellowish-orange, this is temporary and not harmful (316). Though carrots, cantaloupe, and yams are high in beta-carotene, one of the best sources of this nutrient is the blue-green alga, spirulina. Spirulina is anti-viral, having the ability to boost the immunity in fighting the HIV-1 virus (426).

## Cherries Inhibit Lung Cancer

An anti-oxidant found in cherries, called *perillyl alcohol,* in animal tests, was shown to prevent many types of cancer, including those of the lung (604), more evidence for the health-promoting benefits of fresh fruit. Cherries and their juices are also popular natural remedies for treating gout. Tart cherries are especially effective.

## CoQ10 - The Super Anti-oxidant

CoQ10 (also known as *ubiquinone*) is one of the greatest anti-oxidants of the new millennium, and the human body cannot function without it. It is a naturally-occurring ingredient in all cells, much like a vitamin, though it is not classified as one. Some amounts are produced by our body, but levels decrease as we age (507). Low blood levels of this nutrient have been linked to many diseases and disorders. A complete lack of CoQ10 in your body results in death. The amount of food that has CoQ10 that would have to be eaten in order to give you adequate daily amounts would be impossible for most people to consume (507). CoQ10 has proven so critical that there are actually individuals who have been able to get off the heart transplant-waiting-list after taking CoQ10 supplements. There are no toxic side effects with this nutrient, however, it may take considerably large doses for some people to get the desired effect (87).

In humans, research has demonstrated that using this vital nutrient in doses of 390 mg/day has enabled some stage IV breast cancer patients to go into total remission (564). This, according to Dr. Stephen T. Sinatra, cardiologist, author of the book *The Coenzyme Q10 Phenomenon*. Dr. Karl Folkers, a pioneer in studying this nutrient, believed that insufficient levels of CoQ10 is why pancreatic cancer kills so many people (564). Dr. Sinatra considers this nutrient a *miracle*. He tells of one case study in particular when a man asked him to take over the care of his elderly mother, who was suffering with heart failure and pneumonia. His mom had been ventilator-dependent for nearly a month and was not expected to live, yet when her son asked her physicians to put her on CoQ10, they refused because it was not on the hospital *formulary*, besides being unconventional (564).

The patient, already semi-comatose, was transferred to another hospital and Dr. Sinatra took over her care. He immediately began giving her CoQ10 through a nasogastric tube (*450 mg/day*). She was also given 1000 mg/day of magnesium, along with a balanced mineral and vitamin regimen that Dr. Sinatra had developed (564). He noted that the CCU doctors and nurses were all skeptical of his alternative therapy; however, within three days after starting the CoQ10, the patient began to rouse from her comatose state. Ten days later, she came off the vent. In another four days she was out of bed, sitting up, requiring merely minimal *oxygen* and was released from the hospital. Since that time, Dr Sinatra said that he has seen the patient in his office several times. He said that she stays on *360 mg* of CoQ10 every day, and when last contacted, she was active and working (564).

Dr. Sinatra has used CoQ10 to treat many of his cardiac patients, only to discover that it has also helped fight gum disorders, auto-immune problems, arthritic disease, *neurodegenerative disorders*, and cancer (564). He believes that the indifference of modern medicine toward this nutrient is costing lives, and he cannot understand the reluctance of the medical profession to use it (564).

Research has shown that Parkinson's disease, periodontal disease, and accelerated aging may all be linked to deficiencies in CoQ10, and that this supplement may prevent dementia, *stroke,* and *cancer* due to its tremendous ability at fighting free radicals (337).

Current research conducted by the Leonard M. Miller School of Medicine in Miami (under Niven R. Nerain), shows that CoQ10 is deadly to cancer cells, but causes no damage to healthy cells. Not only that, but the NCI acknowledged in 2005 that CoQ10 can extend the lives of those with lung cancer and other cancers. Issels Treatment Centers use CoQ10. Their phone #888-447-7357 (290).

A cardiologist by the name of Dr. Peter Langsjoen (from the University of Texas) agreed with Dr. Folkers to use CoQ10 on his severely ill patients. Six of them had congestive heart failure (four of those six had lung cancer). They all went into remission after using 500 mg a day of CoQ10 (435). Another patient that Dr. Folkers treated had lung cancer (*small cell),* which had spread. He had been given a few months to live. He improved using only CoQ10 as his therapy. After a year, there was no sign of the spreading cancer. Fifteen years later, he was still free of cancer (435).

Are you struggling with cancer, such as pancreatic cancer or breast cancer, an auto-immune disorder, heart disease, or a lung disorder? Does your physician have you on CoQ10? If not, ask them, **WHY?** If you have a chronic disorder or disease, small doses of CoQ10 will not be effective; however, you should begin with a small dose, such as 30 mg to 50 mg, then gradually increase the dosage until you are taking 300 mg to 400 mg daily in divided dosages. Check with your physician as he or she can instruct you on gradually progressing your dosage of this nutrient, depending on your condition. Your physician may prefer that you take one large dosage daily, rather than dividing the doses. Just be sure to get the opinion of a natural health physician, because many conventional doctors know very little about CoQ10. Most are trained in handing out prescription medications, not natural substances. There is so much overwhelming evidence in favor of using CoQ10, it is difficult to understand why any physician would be reluctant in recommending this very valuable, non-toxic supplement to their patients.

For one of America's largest alternative health care centers, check out the Whitaker Wellness Center, which is in Newport Beach (4321 Birch Street), California. See this link: ***http://whitakerwellness.com/ about_***

***us/medical_team.*** Dr. Julian Whitaker, who runs this health care center, has written numerous books on alternative healing. He has an excellent website with a great deal of helpful information. They use many of the alternative health treatments that I have mentioned in my books, including chelation, hyperbaric oxygen, and IV therapies.

## Cranberries & Lung Cancer

Recent animal tests by the University of Massachusetts at Dartmouth, showed that a cranberry compound could halt lung tumors. Earlier studies found that the fruit may help the brain to heal itself after stroke damage. Cranberries also cut the risk for ulcers and bladder infections, and they help fight leukemia (22).

## Ellagic Acid

Nuts and berries contain an anti-oxidant known as *ellagic acid*, an important cancer-fighter. When two researchers in Ohio fed test animals a diet rich in this nutrient, then injected them with cancer 14 days later, the group of animals receiving the ellagic acid had a reduction in cancerous tumors by greater than half (504). One of the richest sources of ellagic acid is raspberries. Other sources are cherries, strawberries, pomegranates, grapes, cranberries, walnuts, and pecans.

## Glucomannan (Konjac-Mannan) & Lung Cancer

Konjac-mannan (*Amorphophallus konjac*) is a complex sugar (made up of mannose and glucose), which you may also hear referred to as konjac fiber, devil's tongue, voodoo plant or voodoo lily, konjaka, elephant foot, konnyaku, konnyaka, konjac fiber, or similar names. When ingested, this plant forms a gel in the stomach which fights toxins and acts like a slow laxative. Since it has a filling effect, it has been used in weight loss supplements. It helps good bacteria flourish in the intestines, but it also may prevent the absorption of the fat soluble vitamins, so should not be taken when you are taking vitamins A, D or E. The supplement can cause gas, diarrhea, nausea and/or vomiting in some individuals.

In an animal study on dozens of mice, konjac-mannan inhibited lung cancer. It was noted that there were fewer cancers and a longer lifespan in the treated animals (17).

## Grape Seed Extract - Pycnogenol®

*Pycnogenol®* is a product extracted from the bark of pines, and is rich in bioflavonoids. These *bioflavonoids* are also found in the seeds of grapes and are popular supplements. They are super anti-oxidants, important in preventing disease and boosting the immune system (507). They are many times more powerful than vitamin E and vitamin C, and according to one researcher, the only thing better at zapping free radicals is *green tea extract* (507). If you are fighting cancer, grape seed extract and CoQ10 should be in your nutritional arsenal for healing your immune system. Do not take grape seed extract at the same time that you take other nutrients, such as Vitamin C. Research suggests that taking them at the same time may raise blood pressure in some individuals.

## Green Tea Fights Lung Cancer, Breast & Prostate Cancer & May Even Help Regenerate Brain Cells

Green tea is said to boost the body's metabolism. Green tea may be important in helping the body prevent cancer of the prostate, breast, gastric cancer, and its spread (135). Green tea has also been found, in animal testing by Israeli researchers, to actually regenerate brain cells, something hitherto thought impossible (169). Oolong tea is often called the quickest fat-burner among all tea types (135).

## IP6 - Inositol Hexaphosphate & Lung Cancer

Cancer cells use a lot of iron and must have iron to survive. Drugs that remove iron from the body, thus fighting cancer cells, have adverse side effects; however, IP6 effectively robs cancer cells of iron without depleting the body's natural stores of iron. It is said to be a gentle, safe ingredient, relatively inexpensive, and without the high toxicity of chemo drugs. Extensive human trials have yet to be done on IP6. (554). This nutrient, derived from rice bran, is also discussed elsewhere in this book.

## Lentinan - A Mushroom Extract for Lung Cancer

Lentinan, which boosts the natural immunity of the body, comes from **shiitake mushroom** *(lentinus edodes).* In animal testing, it reduced malignancies and increased lifespan by nearly 50%. In one particular study, test animals with early cancers of the lung, receiving lentinan, experienced a cure rate of *25 to 75 percent* (504). You can find shiitake mushroom in tea form by Alvita®. (Some alternative health care providers give lentinan injections.)

## LifeMel Honey for Cancer Patients

This amazing honey, developed in Israel, is also discussed later in chapter 29. It is a special honey made from the nectar of 40 herbs, including *Echinacea, Siberian ginseng,* and *Uncaria tomentosa*, with other natural ingredients. Two teaspoons per day (one in the morning and one in the evening) are recommended (614). This special honey was able, in **human** testing, to prevent the neutropenia (dangerously low white blood count) caused by chemotherapy and to lower the risk of severe platelet drop (thrombocytopenia), often found in chemo patients (614). You can find out more about this remarkable honey at website *http://www.lifemel israel.com.* (614).

## Limonene Prevents Lung Cancer

Lemon (citrus limon) has a potent anti-oxidant protection in its peeling, fruit, and juice in the form of *limonene,* a proven cancer preventative. Dr. James Duke and Michael Castleman, authors of *The Green Pharmacy Anti-Aging Prescriptions*, explain that test animals with lung cancer (treated with limonene) had decreased tumors over those not given the limonene (388). If you think your best source of limonene is lemons, guess again. Says Dr. Duke, it is *caraway seed* (388). (Rye bread is helpful in some individuals for lowering blood pressure, and if you bake your own, be sure to add plenty of caraway seeds.)

## Lycopene

Lycopene is a potent anti-oxidant found in fruits and vegetables like tomatoes and guavas. It has a ten-fold greater strength at fighting tumors than beta-carotene and has *four times* the power of alpha-carotene (507). Lycopene should always be taken with a fat source for best absorption (337). A good example would be tomatoes and olive oil, tomatoes with flax seed oil, tomato sauce mixed with olive oil, or fresh avocados mixed with tomatoes or salsa.

## Niacin, Vitamin C, & Lung Cancer

Dr. Abram Hoffer, M.D., Ph.D., has been a pioneer in Orthomolecular Medicine (using megadose vitamins and minerals to heal the body). When a patient with lung cancer and psychiatric problems was referred to him, he prescribed high dose vitamin therapy, which included *1000 mg* of *niacin* and *1000 mg* of *vitamin C* after meals. The patient fully recovered, not only physically, but mentally (432). [Note that niacin also lowers cholesterol, but it works best if you get the niacin that causes the body to flush. The *flush-free* niacin (usually niacinamide) that many stores sell, will not cause the veins to dilate and will not lower cholesterol as well. Never use the *timed-release* form of niacin.] According to Dr. Hoffer, in rare instances some persons using this vitamin could experience a type of jaundice. Discontinuing the niacin reverses the problem (432). Taking a baby aspirin or two about 20 minutes before you take niacin will reduce the flushing sensation; however, it is believed that the flushing is beneficial! Niacin removes histamine from the body. If you take 300 mg of niacin and get a warm flush, then an hour later, take the same amount and there is no flush, it is because your histamine levels are still low. (For this reason, niacin could be helpful in preventing allergic responses.)

At one time, niacin was given to people who worked in arctic climates to keep them warm. Humans have tolerated thousands of milligrams daily of this B-vitamin for lowering their cholesterol without toxicity. Niacin, in lab testing, was shown to fight Alzheimers. It has already been widely used in humans for depression, bi-polar disorders, and migraines. Always check with your physician or Naturopath first.

## Omega-3 Shrinks Lung Tumor by 90%

When a 78 year-old was given only months to live in 2000 (after being diagnosed with lung cancer), he began a drastic dietary change with the help of his neighbor, a professor of biochemistry. That has been several years ago. He slashed all corn from his diet, including anything remotely related to corn products. This is because of their high omega-6 content, which he believed contributed to the cancer. He began increasing his intake of omega-3 fatty acids by taking *golden algae oil* and *fish oil* on a daily basis (181). He began taking *EPA and DHA* every day. He also discontinued the use of any type of vegetable oil, other than very limited use of *olive oil and canola oil* (181). See website *http://www.discount-vitamns-*

*herbs.net/n-119-lung-cancer_omega-3.htm,* for details on the supplements that he used. Another great source for omega-3 is found in ground flax seed and flax seed oil. Another extremely healthy source is Krill oil.

## Pomegranate Extract Halts Lung Cancer Cells

Animal studies have shown that pomegranate extract can halt the progression of lung cancer cells. Although it did not overtly kill the cells themselves, it prevented further growth (238).

## Resveratrol for Fighting Lung Cancer

Resveratrol, an ingredient in **grapes,** has proven so potent against cancer cells, that an entire chapter in this book has been devoted to it. Please see chapter three for more information on resveratrol. Researchers have discovered, in **human** studies, that this compound and others in grapes, may impede lung cancer and keep it from spreading. Animal studies also bear this out. They attributed this fact to its ability to prevent *angiogenesis* (blood vessel growth) and to prevent the formation of DNA within the abnormal cells (446). Resveratrol is also being touted as a way to fight obesity, as well as high cholesterol levels, since it keeps the body from storing fat. Shark cartilage and bindweed (discussed elsewhere in this book) also block the formation of blood vessels in tumors, without toxic side effects.

## Sushi Fights A Rare Lung Cancer

A rare type of lung cancer (*adenocarcinoma*) may be prevented by ingesting sushi. This, according to researchers from Japan, who studied the diets of thousands of individuals. They concluded that those who ingested this fish cut their risk for cancer by 50% (281). Just realize that if you consume raw fish, seafood, or meat, you may be gambling with your health in other ways.

## II. Minerals, Vitamins & Nutrients for Lung Cancer Prevention

### Alpha Lipoic Acid

Alpha lipoic acid is an important nutrient, considered by some to be the *universal anti-oxidant.* There is a great deal of documentation supporting its ability to prevent cancer. It can also help remove poisonous metals from the body (337). ALA can be purchased in supplement form. As we grow older, our bodies produce less and less of this vital nutrient, making it next to impossible to get the amount we need from diet alone. For example, to get what you need in dietary amounts, get ready to ingest about 50-70% of your weight in spinach every day (344)! Other food sources of this nutrient (besides spinach) are potatoes and brewer's yeast.

If you are looking for a place to find herbs, vitamins and supplements that are reasonably priced, check internet site: *www.discount-vitamins-herbs.net.* Not only do they provide a tremendous variety of supplements, but they also have a wealth of information from scientific studies on nutrients. They provide timed-released supplements, such as alpha lipoic acid, which are not always easy to find. (Never take niacin in the timed-release form.) You may have a need for niacin without realizing it. An ailment known as **Meniere's Syndrome** can often be reversed simply by supplementing with niacin, zinc and vitamins B12 and B6.

### Glutathione Prevents Lung & Other Cancers

Glutathione is another amino acid important in cancer prevention that the body is able to produce, if we are not nutritionally-deprived (337). This nutrient helps fight obesity, food addictions, cataracts, and several forms of cancer, including those of the urinary system and the lungs (337).

It may not be wise to take glutathione in supplement form (orally) because of poor absorption. Taking Vitamin C keeps levels elevated, but does not produce more (337). Glutathione helps the body maintain constant supplies of vitamins C and E by *recycling* these vitamins once the body has *oxidized* them (337). (Cooking destroys much of the glutathione in foods.) Some excellent sources of this nutrient include: avocados, uncooked spinach, apples, carrots, and tomatoes. According to Steven Petrosino, Ph.D., at website *www.nutritionadvisor.com,* you can also increase your body's glutathione levels *with undenatured whey protein isolate,* as well as with "the herb milk thistle...[and] curcumin...alpha lipoic acid...vitamin B6, riboflavin…selenium...asparagus, avocados, squash, okra, cauliflower, broccoli, potatoes, spinach, walnuts, garlic, and raw tomatoes…." (85)

You can find *undenatured whey protein isolate* at their website (above) in a brand known as *Immunocal,* as well as more information on the scientific studies performed on this supplement. It is the only whey protein isolate listed in the *Physician's Desk Reference* (PDR), but you do not need a prescription to obtain it.

## Melatonin—Anti-oxidant

Melatonin is described at *healthyroads.com* as a *miracle hormone.* This is another hormone that the body produces naturally, but as we get older, we make less and less (192). Long popularized as a remedy for *insomnia,* especially for shift workers, this anti-oxidant fights aging, cancer, heart disease, and boosts the body's immunity (192).

In a **human study,** melatonin had anti-cancer properties, stimulated the body's natural immunity, and fought advancing cancer with doses of 10 mg/day, without significant side effects (191). Melatonin crosses into the brain, something many other anti-oxidants, such as vitamin E, are not capable of doing (191). Melatonin is useful in the prevention of *cachexia,* a type of *wasting* away experienced by many sufferers of terminal cancer, however, there are some restrictions to the use of the hormone. It is not recommended that patients with *leukemia, lymphoma and myeloma* take melatonin. There is a possibility that melatonin may accelerate the advancement of these type cancers (507). In addition to this precaution for melatonin, the supplement could cause depression and worsening of allergies in some individuals, and should not be taken by those on cortisone, nor those who are pregnant (192). It is also possible that the hormone "may cause constriction of blood vessels," problems with libido and infertility, temperature drops, and "retinal damage" (192). Significant amounts of natural melatonin can be found simply in eating tart cherries (61). Recent studies have shown that insufficient levels of melatonin in the body increase the risk for breast cancer.

Note that glutamine, an amino acid, can also help prevent the wasting syndrome *(cachexia)* that haunts many cancer patients (507).

## Selenium Prevents Lung Cancer

During 1973 in a scientific study known as *The Willett Study*, blood was drawn from over four thousand healthy men, after which they were followed for *5 years*. Cancer was later found in more than a hundred of the participants (507). Blood comparisons were made to the men who were still healthy. It was found that those men who developed cancer had very low amounts of selenium. Those having the lowest levels of selenium were twice as likely to have cancer as the men with higher amounts. Their greatest risk was for gastric and prostate cancer (507). The *Willett study* generated so much interest that the National Cancer Institute sponsored yet another study on selenium that lasted for eight years, whose primary intention was to test the mineral's effects on skin cancer. They wanted to see if selenium could help prevent melanoma. They were in for a surprise, however, because the mineral did not influence the incidence of melanoma, but the participants given selenium experienced half as many deaths from deadly *lung, colon, rectum, and prostate* cancers as those not receiving the selenium (507).

Some good natural food sources of selenium are: cruciferous vegetables, whole-grains and *garlic* (411). Brazil nuts are also very rich in selenium (507). Realize however, that this is only true if the foods are grown in soils that are not stripped of selenium.

In taking selenium supplements, it is always good to do so in combination with *vitamin E* (180). See the last chapter in this book for a look at some of the most recent vitamin E and selenium studies (for prostate cancer). A physician by the name of Emanuel Revici developed a cancer therapy with *selenium* at its heart. For 40 years he was very successful in treating cancer patients at his New York clinic; however, as is commonly found in those promoting natural cures, he was eventually harassed to the point of being forced out of practice by the AMA (106). Selenium is one of the few minerals that will remove dangerous mercury from the body (566b).

## Vitamin C

Vitamin C appears to protect cells, and apparently it does not take much to do the job. Research revealed that participants ingesting less than 200 milligrams per day (or the equivalent of eating just *two oranges*), were able to cut their risk of lung cancer in half (148). Recent studies have also shown that two servings of orange juice per day can dramatically reduce your risk for heart attack.

Dr. Gladys Block, affiliated with the National Cancer Institute, confirmed that Vitamin C plays an important role in the prevention of cancer (367).

See chapters eight and sixteen in this book for the story of a biochemist who cured his teenage daughter of Hodgkins disease using high dose vitamin C therapy, also known as *Ortho-molecular* Medicine. (Also, see the new studies just out on vitamin C, E, and selenium in relation to lung cancer and prostate cancer in chapter 34.)

## Vitamin E & Lung Cancer Growths

There is a proven link between vitamin E deficiencies and several cancer types. Research studies have linked high levels of vitamin E to a decrease in the risk for getting either stomach or lung cancer. In one particular animal study, when test animals were subjected to a known cancer-causing agent, none of the animals on vitamin E developed cancer. Every single one of those not receiving the vitamin developed cancer (492). It appears that the anti-oxidant effect of vitamin E is most effective when you combine it with vitamin C.

Be sure in buying vitamin E to purchase the natural form (***d**-alpha-tocopherol)* and other *mixed tocopherols*. You should not purchase the man-made form (***dl**-alpha tocopheryl acetate)* which is more difficult for the body to absorb. If you purchase the dry form of natural vitamin E, it is more easily absorbed by the body. Some researchers believe that the gamma form of vitamin E is superior to the alpha form in fighting cancer, though the alpha form is more easily used by the body. Much of the supplemental vitamin E you see on the market comes from soybeans. Always use organic natural products whenever possible. There are 4 tocopherols and 4 tocotrienols in vitamin E, and you need all of them.

Some good **natural sources** of vitamin E are: wheat germ oil, olive oil, sunflower oil (and seeds), dandelion greens, spinach, broccoli, turnip greens, almonds and other nuts, eggs (411) (492) (524), kiwi and mangoes, fortified cereals and fresh sprouts, especially wheat berry sprouts.

Many of our crops are now being genetically manipulated. They are referred to as GMO foods, and there is a great deal of concern about the long-term safety of these foods. If you want to read and hear some frightening facts about the effects of GMO foods, and how those who are engineering them are attempting to control the world's food supply, just go to the internet and google the words: *the world according to Monsanto.*

## III. Herbs Effective Against Lung Cancer

### Abajeru (*Chrysobalanus icaco*) for Lung Cancer & Other Cancers

Isolated from a tropical plant of the Brazilian Rain forest (aka as *coco-plum*), abajeru was once used by the locals for fighting arthritic pain and diabetes (145a). When researchers first conducted lab testing, they found that the bush extract killed not only cancerous *breast-brain-lung-bowel-larynx and pancreas tumors*, but even difficult-to-treat leukemia cells died. In testing humans, they were surprised to see that it *worked with 90% of the patients.* You can find this substance at many internet sites and in health food stores (145a).

### Aloe Vera Juice for Smokers

Aloe vera juice may be important in preventing the progression of cancer in smokers. It halts the conversion of toxic compounds (found *in tobacco smoke*) into cancer-causing chemicals. If you have diarrhea, stomach cancer, or any type of chronic disease, discuss aloe with your physician or Naturopath before ingesting large amounts (180). Be certain that when you use aloe vera jel juice (the type that you drink) it must be cold-pressed. Check the label. Use organic only.

### Aspilia & Lung Cancer

Aspilia *(Aspilia mossambicenisis),* also known as *Wild Sunflower*, not only kills parasites, but acts much like an antibiotic. *Herbs2000.com* reports that the herb may help in the destruction of breast and lung cancer cells (27).

### Astragalus for the Immunity

Astragalus has a healing effect on the lungs, and is reported to enhance the body's natural immunity (504). When researchers took an alkaloid from a variety of this herb *(oxyphysus),* they found, in animal testing, that it stopped melanoma, and it took only one day for it to halt more than *80 percent* of the cancerous lung cells (504). Check with your physician or Naturopath about using this herb, especially if you have an infection or are running a temperature (180).

## Cat's Claw

Cat's Claw, also known as *Uno de' Gato*, is a known immune stimulant. This herb has been able, in some cases, to bring about remission in lung cancer. See chapter 20 for instances when you should not take cat's claw.

## Cayenne Powder

Cayenne pepper powder may be useful for smokers, as it appears to be able to prevent one of the chemicals in tobacco smoke from becoming harmful (180). Realize though, that there are thousands of other chemicals released in tobacco smoke that are highly toxic.

## Espinheira Santa

This herb *(Limaosinho maytenus)* is widely used in South America for medicinal purposes. It has been popular in ulcer healing since it appears to balance the body's hydrochloric acid output, and lab studies have confirmed that it may work just as well as the drug *Cimetidine (Tagamet)* (109). Also, researchers believe that compounds extracted *from the trunk bark* are toxic to some types of lung cancer, ovarian cancer cells, and other cancers as well (109).

## Essiac Tea for All Cancers

See chapter six for more information on this amazing herbal tea. Rene Caisse, a Canadian nurse, healed hundreds (possibly thousands) of people of every imaginable cancer using her herbal tea formula, many of whom came to her after conventional medicine considered them hopeless.

One of Rene's patients was a man with terminal lung cancer. He came to the Brusch Clinic for seven weeks. Afterwards, his pain and breathing problems disappeared and he resumed his favorite sport—swimming (580). Note that there is some competition between the tea produced by Resperin Canada Essiac® and Flor-Essence® Essiac tea. Both companies claim that they have the original Essiac formula (the drinkable formula, not the injectable) that Rene Caisse used in treating her cancer patients. See chapter 16 in this book for the story of a young boy who was cured of lymphoma using Essiac® Resperin Canada's tea formula and 714X injections. A website that has Essiac® Resperin

Canada is also given in that chapter. You can find both tea brands (and others) in health food stores as well.

## Graviola & Cancer

See chapters five and six for information on the ability of the herb, graviola, from the Amazon Rain forest, to bring about some cancer cures without toxic side effects.

## Green Tea Inhibits Lung Cancer

One of the main ingredients in green tea is *epigallocatechin gallate (EGCG*). Green tea not only prevents skin and gastrointestinal tumors, but laboratory animals receiving EGCG grew far fewer cancers of the lung than those not fed the tea (504). It was also found to drastically reduce the occurrence of lung and gastric cancers in animals given only green tea as their drink. Nearly all the test animals not receiving the tea came down with cancer (504). Studies show that drinking black tea can also reduce lung cancer risk (180).

## Milk Thistle for Lung Cancer

This herb, in animals studies, halted lung cancer. Pure silibinin was used, rather than milk thistle supplements that you would find in health food stores. Authors of the study contend that the human-sized dose for someone weighing in at 150 lbs would be *2 to 20 grams per day*. The herb is non-toxic (196).

## Oleander Soup - for Lung Cancer & Liver Cancer

Used by an attorney in Texas to cure his mother of *lung and liver cancer (*as well as a sister who was fighting *Hepatitis C),* you can read more about this cancer remedy at *http://www.buzzle.com/articles//father-of-the-oleander-soup-cancer-remedy.html* (437). It has also been said to cure a woman's rheumatoid arthritis, and help cases of psoriasis and HIV (437). A physician from Turkey, Dr. H. Z. Ozel, developed the remedy, which was being considered by the FDA; however, after successfully going through a Phase I trial, it sank into relative obscurity due to funding problems (437). You will find this treatment under the name Anvirzel™ (437). There are many precautions in regards to making your own oleander soup. The leaves themselves are considered poisonous.

## Parsley Inhibits Lung Tumors

Parsley is an overall cleanser. The seeds have an anti-inflammatory effect. The herb is often dried and used in teas. It contains a compound known as *myristicin*, which inhibits the development of cancerous growths in the lung (180). Do not use parsley if you are pregnant; it can cause premature labor. It should not be used during an infectious process, especially involving the kidneys. Parsley oil can cause skin irritations and is highly toxic (228). Fresh, organically grown parsley (in small amounts) is best. If you buy it in herb form, be aware that if the tea comes from the root, it is much more potent than tea made from the leaf.

## Psoralea Seed Inhibits Lung Cancer

Psoralea seed is popular in traditional Japanese and Chinese herbal medicine for many different ailments. It is used for lung cancer because it contains compounds which fight *osteosarcoma and lung cancer cells* (245). Since this herb can increase your sensitivity to sunlight, limit sun exposure, or avoid the sun altogether during and immediately after use (245).

## Rhodiola Rosea for Carcinoma

Rhodiola Rosea is a native herb from Siberia. According to *planetherbs.com,* it is not unusual for those who regularly drink the tea made from this herb to live over a century (259). It is very popular in middle Asia and was named *rosea* because it smells like roses. It has been able to increase the life span of *lung carcinoma* patients, as well as those having other types of cancer (259). See the website above for more information. The tea can be found in some health food stores and many internet sites.

## Seaweed

Many sea vegetables (seaweed) are healing and curative. An extract taken from seaweed, known as *Viva Natural,* has anti-cancer activity. It proved effective against lung cancer and leukemia, in animal testing, and was even more effective than the common chemo drug, *Isoprinosine* (504). Viva-Natural is made from drying out *wakame* seaweed (363). In one animal study, it cured some of the lung cancers. Scientists participating in the study were amazed that this seaweed nutrient was so potent at boosting the immunity (363). **Laminaria** is another species of seaweed important in cancer prevention. Scientists in Japan discovered several species of the weed were effective at preventing and suppressing cancerous colon cells (363). It is important to note that many seaweeds, like kelp, are very high in iodine and should be ingested taking this into consideration. Those with thyroid disorders (and other health problems) should consult their physician before consuming herbs and seaweed. Sometimes an underactive thyroid is caused by a lack of iodine in the diet. Your physician can run tests to determine your thyroid functioning.

## Tian Xian - Herbal Treatment for Lung Cancer

Tian Xian (*pronounced Dianne Sean*) is an herbal supplement from China promoted for its ability to control, inhibit, and destroy cancer cells (293). There are many testimonials at their website of cancer patients from all over the world who have experienced complete cancer cures using this herb, several of them with lung cancer (293).

## Turmeric (Curcumin)

This herbal spice has been able to differentiate between normal and abnormal cells and has the ability to protect against radiation (89) and in human studies, to halt the spread of multiple myeloma (203). It is available as a spice that you can get at your local grocers, or in more concentrated forms at natural health food stores as a supplement. There is a gene known as the *p53* gene that has the ability to prevent cancer cells from replicating. Turmeric appears to have the ability to activate this gene against *small lung-cell cancer* (180). Turmeric may also be beneficial for those fighting COPD and asthma, due to its anti-inflammatory properties. You will find more curcumin in turmeric than you will in curry powder. Use organic turmeric rather than curry! If you want a turmeric capsule that is free of magnesium stearate additive, see *Nature's Way*® brand. See chapter 20 for instances of when you should not use turmeric (curcumin). If you want your body to absorb turmeric more easily, eat it with pineapple or supplement with bromelain.

## IV. Other Supplements & Treatments for Lung Cancer

### Beta-Glucan & Lung Cancer

Beta-glucan is an extract of *baker's yeast* and is available in supplement form at most health food stores. It is also extracted from mushrooms (e.g., *shiitake...and maitake*). Human research, described in the *Journal of the National Cancer Institute,* showed that injecting this nutrient into tumors made them shrink in less than a week. The nine human participants in the study had either *skin, breast, or lung cancer.* The beta-glucan caused the body's *immune cells* to concentrate at the site of the cancer, thus destroying it (354).

Lentinan, discussed earlier, is a beta-glucan extracted from *shiitake* mushrooms. It is used in Japan to treat late stages of cancer, and when given intravenously, it has often extended the lives of cancer patients by several years (354).

One website in particular, *http://www.cancer-treatments.net/cancer.html,* promotes the use of *oat beta-glucan*, which they claim is superior to the yeast form most popular in health food stores. However, the website says that there is now available an even more *potent whole cell beta-glucan from baker's yeast* (221). If interested, you can contact them at: *http://www.cancer-prevention.net.*

### Burzynski's Antineoplastons—Non-Toxic Cancer Cures

Antineoplastons are non-toxic cancer treatments provided by Dr. Stanislaw Burzynski at his clinic in Houston, Texas, which have cured many cancer patients. They are mentioned in several other cancer-specific chapters of this book and in great detail in chapter 14 due to their remarkable success with terminal brain cancer patients, including young children. They are also used for lung cancer patients and nearly every other cancer imaginable, including mesothelioma cancers, discussed below. See their main website at: *www.burzynskiclinic.com,* and read some of the many testimonials of patients who have successfully used antineoplastons to cure their cancers at *http://burzynskipatientgroup.org/stories.html.* The FDA has finally approved the oral form of anti-neoplastons (PBs or sodium phenylbutrates) for off-label use, but you will need to ask your physician about prescribing them. Note that antineoplastons A10 and AS2-1 were recently given orphan drug status by the FDA for use on human brainstem gliomas. Some individuals can have side effects from antineoplastons, but they are quickly reversible, unlike toxic chemo drugs that often cause fatal adverse reactions.

## Calcium D-Glucarate™

D-Glucarate™ is a *naturally-occurring* ingredient found in whole foods, such as leafy greens, apples, and sprouts (394). It is described in detail by Rita Elkins, M.H. in her book: *D-Glucarate™, Powerful Protector Against Breast and Prostate Cancers.* D-Glucarate™ was isolated and patented in 1986. It decreases levels of harmful estrogen (estradiol) and testosterone in the body, and it assists the body in ridding itself of harmful toxins (394). This nutrient is organ-protective, and it reduces serum cholesterol levels. It works by binding itself with toxic compounds and neutralizing them. Ms. Elkins also notes that the substance is so efficient, researchers discovered that when they gave an antibiotic, *Kanamycin* (which was known to have toxic effects) to rats, along with the D-Glucarate™, it protected them from the kidney impairment that this antibiotic usually causes (394). A report, published in *Anti-Cancer Research,* revealed (in the test animals that received it) that the nutrient could slash the risk for cancer in half (394).

Calcium D-Glucarate™ is an important supplement for *ex-smokers* because it effectively blocks carcinogens. Also, this compound was helpful, in *animal testing*, at halting and even reversing some cases of breast cancer (394). There has been no evidence of toxicity in using D-Glucarate™, however, you should still discuss it with your physician or Naturopath before supplementing (394).

## Noni Juice & Lung Cancer

According to research studies, noni juice (*Morinda citriolia)* can inhibit malignancies of the lung (Lewis lung carcinoma). It is believed that it works by stimulating immune cells. The juice may also help fight infections. Noni can kill e-coli, *salmonella…shigella…and staphylococcus aureus germs* (396). You can find noni juice in most health food stores.

## Poly–MVA for Lung Cancer & All Other Cancers

See chapter 14 for more information on Poly-MVA, a potent nutrient compound that many cancer patients are crediting with curing them. Also, read the many testimonials of cancer survivors who describe using Poly-MVA to help cure their lung cancer, as well as Stage IV adenocarcinoma;

*hopeless* brain cancers; ovarian, uterine, endometrial and breast cancers; anaplastic carcinoma; bladder and prostate cancers; ALL leukemia; Hodgkins and non-Hodgkins lymphomas; multiple myelomas; osteosarcoma and pancreatic cancers, at website *http://www.S94567060.onlinehome.us/survivors/testimonials.html.* The main Poly-MVA website is located at *www.polymva.net.* Many of these patients refused chemo and radiation and opted only for alternative therapies, such as Poly-MVA. Some began with chemo and radiation, but their cancers returned much more aggressively. Others successfully used Poly-MVA against cancers CAUSED by the radiation and chemo that they received. Some used Poly-MVA in conjunction with other alternative or conventional treatments. Be sure you get the genuine supplement. Go to *polymva.net.*

Poly MVA contains a proprietary blend of palladium and alpha lipoic acid, molybdenum, some important B vitamins, rhodium, ruthenium, formylmethionine, and acetyl cysteine. Also, see testimonials at website *http://www.polymvasurvivors.com/testimonials.html.* Many of these testimonials were given ten or more years ago, yet all survivors are still here as of March 2007. Poly MVA alkalizes the body.

## Transfer Factor™ for Lung Cancer

See website *http://www.shirleys-wellness-cafe.com/tf/s/cancer-testimonials.htm,* for testimonials of people who have used this compound to heal their cancers or fortify their immune system, including a woman who had lung cancer that invaded her lymphatic system, and a woman with lung cancer that had gone into her bones and spine (592).

## Ukrain - An Effective Non-Toxic Cancer Treatment

Ukrain, as discussed earlier, combines two common ingredients which are both toxic when given alone; however, once combined they were found to be only toxic to cancer cells (287). See other cancer-specific chapters in this book for more detailed information on this amazing, non-toxic cancer treatment.

2009 update: note that because Ukrain is not authorized in Austria, this article (as discussed in my first book, *Painless Cancer Cures)* is no longer located *at www.ukrin.com.* The website has been changed and is now called *Nowicky Pharma.* You can read this information about Ukrain now in the book: *Anti-Cancer Agent Ukrain — The Crime Story of an Obstruction* by

Eleonore Thun-Hohenstein. For pictures of how Ukrain works, see website *http://www.ukrain-drug.net/webspeed/index.htm.*

## V. Flax Oil, GLA & Miscellaneous Items

See chapter 18 for more information on the curative, healing properties of flax oil. Gamma-linolenic acid (GLA) is found in *borage seed oil* and *evening primrose oil* and helps promote normal cell growth. It can help the immune system in suppressing abnormal cells in the lung. Do not use GLAs without consulting your physician or Naturopath, especially if you are taking chemo (180).

## Water, Hydration & Cancer Patients

The importance of adequate fluid intake cannot be over-emphasized for cancer patients and for prevention of all illnesses. Be sure to consult with your physician about salt and fluid intake, especially if you are on a low salt, fluid-restricted diet or any other type of special diet. Do not use water with chlorine and fluoride. If you do not have a filtration system at home, you may want to resort to steam-distilled water for drinking and cooking purposes, or a reputable purified water from your local health food store. See chapter 23 in this book for more information on the importance of water drinking in cancer prevention and treatment.

## A Word About Smoking & Lung Cancer

Smoking is actually the culprit most responsible for lung cancer. One simple reason is because the smoke that comes out of a cigarette actually creates toxic free radicals that have the capacity to change the DNA in your cells. Once this genetic material in your cells begins to change or mutate, the new defective cells begin multiplying rapidly, especially when *exposed* to additional carcinogens. You may not even be a smoker, but when you inhale secondhand smoke, the same toxic free radicals are entering your cells as those of the person who lit the cigarette! Inhaling secondhand smoke can increase your risk for many cancers, including bladder cancer. Every time a person smokes just one cigarette, thousands of toxins are released into the air and into their lungs (371).

Being sure that you have sufficient amounts of beta-carotene may be one of your best health measures in keeping your lungs healthy and cancer-free (550). Breathing in toxic air pollutants causes the body to use up excessive amounts of all nutrients and anti-oxidants, including *vitamin A*, prompting the liver to change beta-carotene into more vitamin A. Selenium and vitamin E are other crucial anti-oxidants needed to combat free radicals. It is always important to remember, especially for smokers—or ex-smokers—that you should be taking beta-carotene in its NATURAL form, rather than synthetic forms of the vitamin. For example, when you drink carrot juice, or eat sweet potatoes, you are taking in a natural form of beta-carotene. The body takes the natural beta-carotene that you ingest and converts it into natural vitamin A, which is a great deal healthier than synthetic vitamin A or synthetic beta-carotene. The body always recognizes natural substances, but often has no idea what to do with synthetic compounds. The same is true of SYNTHETIC vitamin E! Do not take vitamin A supplements. Use food sources.

## Zeolites (Megamin)

See chapter 34 for more information on zeolites.

# VI. Mesothelioma Helps

Note that there are many other items in this book that may help with mesothelioma, such as Essiac Tea and Poly-MVA. Those given below may prove especially helpful and they are NON-toxic:

## • Burzynski's Antineoplastons

Mesothelioma is a very rare cancer caused by asbestos exposure. It usually affects the thoracic cavity where the heart and lungs are located, but can affect other areas of the body. Non-toxic antineoplastons (discussed above) have been used at Burzynski's Clinic in Houston, Texas, for treating this disease. See their website at: *www.burzynskiclinic.com.* The FDA has finally approved the oral form of antineoplastons (PBs) for off-label use, but you will need to ask your physician about prescribing them. Note that antineoplastons A10 and AS2-1 were recently given orphan drug status by the FDA for use on human brainstem gliomas.

## • Cholesterol Drug for Mesothelioma

For detailed information on a new cancer-treatment regimen that includes combining "low-dose interferon with lovastatin," so far used in melanoma (but also being considered for other cancers like mesothelioma—doctors saw tumors start to regress—often in a matter of *a few weeks*) (76a), see website *www.neoplas.org,* and chapter 34 in this book. The treatment has no toxic side effects as found in chemo and *radiation* (76a). Just be aware that statin drugs strip CoQ10 out of the body. If you agree to this treatment, you will need to supplement with CoQ10.

## • Onconase for Mesothelioma

This drug (aka *Ranpirnase*) is a new pharmaceutical drug developed for treating mesothelioma, and is claimed not to have the adverse effects that are normally seen in common chemo drugs (222). It is said to work on other cancers, such as those of the lungs. It was developed by a company known as *Alfacell* (222). The drug is also supposed to make it possible to give lower dosages of standard chemo drugs with the same cancer-killing effects. It is said to fight *solid tumor cancers,* such as *carcinomas*, as well as those of the *kidney, breast, lung, and prostate* (222). Just be aware that even though this new drug is said to be relatively free of toxic side effects, drugs such as this one are sometimes combined with conventional chemo drugs that **do** have potentially toxic side effects.

# VII. Iodine For Lung Cancers

In his book, *Iodine Bringing Back the Universal Medicine*, Mark Sircus, Ac., OMD, discusses the rampant iodine-deficiency in U.S. diets, mostly due to decreasing levels in the soil, destruction of iodine by chlorine in our water supply, and its drastic effects on the health of millions (566a). The Japanese enjoy the best health statistics of any other nation, yet they consume 12 or more **milligrams** of iodine every day (mostly in the form of seaweed), while the U.S. recommends a paltry 300 **micrograms** of iodine for its citizens (566a). Is it any wonder that cancer statistics and chronic diseases are so high in this nation? See page 129 and 400 for a superior form of iodine that is taken by mouth, and more information in chapter 34 on soda bicarb, iodine, and magnesium for fighting cancer.

# CHAPTER 11

# GENTLE CURES FOR TOUGH MOUTH, NOSE, THROAT & THYROID CANCERS

*"Deal bountifully with thy servant, that I may live, and keep thy word." (Psalm 119:17)*
*"Let My Mouth be Filled with Thy Praise and With Thy Honor all the day." (Ps 71:8)*

## I. Mouth, Throat & Nose Cancers

## Abajeru (*Chrysobalanus icaco*) for Cancer of the Larynx & Other Cancers

Isolated from a tropical plant of the Brazilian Rain Forest (aka as *coco-plum*), abajeru was once used by the locals for fighting arthritic pain and diabetes (145a). When researchers first conducted lab testing, they found that the bush extract killed not only cancerous *breast-brain-lung-bowel-larynx and pancreas tumors*, but even difficult-to-treat leukemia cells died. In testing **humans,** they were surprised to see that it *worked with 90% of the patients.* You can find this substance in health food stores and on the internet at many websites (145a).

## Beta-Carotene & the Mouth Cancer that Disappeared

Once again, beta-carotene has shown evidence of curing yet another type of cancer—cancer of the mouth. As described by Jack Challem in his book: *All About Carotenoids Beta-Carotene, Lutein & Lycopene,* multiple studies on humans at the University of Arizona in Tucson (*and others*) have shown that this nutrient can cause leukoplakia (a precancerous type of oral lesion) to revert back to normal. If leukoplakia is not treated, it will eventually progress to cancer (366). This condition, which has been linked to alcohol and tobacco consumption, has also been reversed with *vitamin A and vitamin E* (366). (Mr. Challem has a new book out: *Stop Prediabetes Now,* with co-author Ron Hunninghake, M.D. Also see his new book: *The Food-Mood Solution.)*

Halting mouth cancer does not necessarily even require natural vitamin A. When Steve Otto of Washington, D.C., developed cancer of the mouth, he underwent several months of chemo and radiation, which did absolutely nothing to stop the progression of his tumor. He jumped at the chance for something new when he was offered a synthetic vitamin A known as *retinoic acid.* He only took *eight pills per day* for a few months before the tumor began to shrink and totally vanished (507). This was not laboratory or animal testing. This was a case of vitamin A CURING MOUTH CANCER in a human, yet how much publicity did it receive from the medical community? How much media attention was given to it? Most of mainstream America never heard of it.

It is worth noting that even though a synthetic form of vitamin A cured this patient's oral cancer, *natural beta-carotene* has been shown to revert malignant gastric cells back to normal—something the *synthetic* pill was unable to do. Taking the synthetic beta-carotene caused blood levels of lycopene to drop, another reason why natural beta-carotene is best (507). Fresh carrot juice is beta-carotene-rich, as are most of the green juices and seaweed. Increased consumption of veggies and fruit is linked to lower rates for mouth, throat, and head cancers, as well as reduced occurrence of *second primary tumors* (507).

## Black Raspberries for Throat Cancer Prevention

Scientists from Ohio State University found that rodents ingesting black raspberries had *60 percent* fewer esophageal tumors and *80 percent* fewer colon tumors. Gary D. Stoner, Ph.D., leader of the study group, says that clinical trials on humans are currently underway (213). Multiple **human** studies have been done to show that eating more veggies and fruit reduces the risk for many types of cancer, including those of the mouth and throat.

## Brazilian Peppertree Inhibits Throat Cancers

Brazilian peppertree is not only *antimicrobial,* but Health Sciences Institute at *www.hsibaltimore.com,* says that, in laboratory testing, it helps in the fight against cancers of *the throat, esophagus, and other areas* (162). This herb may cause uterine stimulation and a drop in blood pressure. It is not for long term use (45). For more information on the herb, contact *www.rain-tree.com.*

## Burzynski's Antineoplastons for Head & Neck Cancers

Antineoplastons are non-toxic cancer treatments developed by Dr. Stanislaw Burzynski at his clinic in Houston, Texas, which have cured many cancer patients. They are used for cancers of the head-and-neck, as well as nearly all other cancers, and are discussed later in this chapter in more detail under the section on *thyroid cancer.* They are also discussed in great detail in chapter 14 of this book. Dr. Burzynski's webpage is at *www.burzynskiclinic.com.* The FDA has finally approved the oral form of antineoplastons (sodium phenylbutrates or PBs) for off-label use. Note that antineoplastons A10 and AS2-1 were recently given orphan drug status for use on human brainstem gliomas.

## Chlorella, Folic Acid, Resveratrol, Limonene & Cherries

Other nutrients that fight the ravages of head-and-neck cancers include: wheat grass, algae (such as chlorella and spirulina), limonene, cherries, and grape juice (resveratrol). These nutrients and herbs are discussed in several other chapters of this book. For an excellent 58-page study that was done on resveratrol's role in fighting cancer, including *head-and-neck squamous cell carcinoma*, see website *http://www.agrawal.org/PDF/ACR-Resveratrol1.pdf.* The study was conducted by M.D. Anderson Cancer Center and the UCLA Center for Human Nutrition (346).

## Cryospray Ablation—Non-Toxic, Gentle Treatment for Barrett's Esophagus & Throat Cancer

A new type of gentle, non-toxic treatment for throat cancer, which uses liquid nitrogen to freeze the cells, is being used at Loyola Medical Center in Chicago (480). This procedure is also being used for the abnormal *esophageal* cells known as *Barrett's esophagus,* which is usually caused by GERD or *acid reflux* disease (480). Barrett's esophagus often deteriorates into cancer. Cryospray ablation may be used to treat other cancers, such as those of the *colon,* in the not-so-distant-future. Though the treatment may need to be repeated, reports say that usually the first treatment takes out *70 to 90 percent* of the unwanted cells. Physicians were amazed that the response was so rapid. The treatment typically requires only *15 minutes to a couple of hours,* with patients going home the same day and resuming normal activities. Before now, the use of liquid nitrogen has been limited to *warts and skin cancer* (480). (Note that orange peel extract may also help with GERD, as well as DGL tablets, available at health food stores. See page 262.)

## CyberKnife® Therapy for Mouth, Nose & Throat Tumors

See chapter 34 in this book for details on CyberKnife® therapy, which is being used successfully for many cancers, including hard-to-reach brain tumors. It is a gentle, painless procedure that does not require an incision, surgery, sedation or inpatient stay. It takes very little time, and as soon as the procedure is over, the patient is able to walk out and return home. There are very few risks and side effects, though it does involve some radiation (89a) and can damage nearby healthy cells. Also, see info under NanoKnife™, chapter 34.

## Cytotron Therapy for Cancer & Arthritis

A new cancer (and arthritis) treatment developed and available in India that you will not yet be able to get in the U.S., is being successfully used on humans and is known as *Cytotron Therapy.* It is gentle, completely painless, and non-toxic. See chapter 34 in this book for more details on what is also called *QMR* or *Quantum Magnetic Resonance* (90).

## Ellagic Acid Prevents Esophageal Cancer

Commonly found in nuts, cherries, berries, grapes, tea and apples, ellagic acid inhibits esophageal cancers. Scientists in Ohio tested the nutrient's proficiency in stopping cancer of the throat in animals. Test results showed a *21 to 55 percent* drop in tumor formation in the test animals. *Precancerous growths* were also inhibited (504). One of the richest sources of ellagic acid is raspberries. When test animals were given the berries as part of their daily diet, there was a dramatic decrease in malignancies of the throat—in some cases—greater than 50%, and strangely enough, in this particular instance, more wasn't necessarily better. Smaller amounts worked best. When researchers doubled the amount of berries, results were not as remarkable. Berries used in the study were black raspberries. This nutrient has also shown effectiveness at halting prostate cancer cells and inhibiting cervical cancer. Other good food sources of ellagic acid are cranberries, cherries, strawberries, pecans, walnuts, and pomegranates. (Cranberries also help fight leukemia, and they cut the risk for ulcers and bladder infections) (22.)

## Essiac Tea for Lip, Throat, Mouth & Gastric Cancer

See chapter six for more information on this amazing, healing herbal tea. Rene Caisse, a Canadian nurse, healed hundreds (possibly thousands) of people of every imaginable cancer throughout Canada and the United States using her amazing herbal tea, many of whom came to her after conventional medicine considered them hopeless. One of the most amazing books describing the effectiveness of this tea and how it was suppressed by the health industry in Canada, is called: *The Essiac Report Canada's Remarkable Unknown Cancer Remedy,* by Richard Thomas, who claims (per Dr. Charles Brusch) that Flor-Essence® is the original (drinkable) formula that Rene Caisse used (580).

Note that there is some competition between the tea produced by Resperin Canada Essiac® and Flor-Essence® Essiac tea. Both companies claim that they have the original Essiac formula (the drinkable formula, not the injectable) that Rene Caisse used in treating her cancer patients.

See chapter 16 in this book for the story of a young boy who was cured of lymphoma using a natural program that included Essiac® Resperin Canada's tea formula and 714X injections. A website that has Essiac® Resperin Canada is also given in that chapter.

In Richard Thomas' book, he has a copy of a letter written to the manufacturer of Flor-Essence® Essiac tea from patient W. Gaspard describing his mother's battle with gastric and throat cancer. She had been given a few months to live at most. She began drinking Flor-Essence® tea. Within five months, her physician told her son that his mom's cancer had nearly disappeared, almost a year after she had been given three months to live (580). Mr. Thomas also discusses a case of lip cancer that Rene Caisse treated with her Essiac formula. When the patient first came to Rene, she commented that the cancer had horribly *disfigured* him. Within six months of starting on the tea formula, he went back to his job and lived cancer-free for another 40 years (580). Another patient, with *basal cell carcinoma* in his *right cheek* (which had been biopsied), was completely cured within five weeks. He had received only *four Essiac treatments* (580). When questionnaires were mailed out to survivors of Rene's Caisse's formula, many of them responded. Richard Thomas discussed eleven of them in his book. The shortest interval since treatment was 11 years for one patient. The longest interval since treatment (in the replies received) was 31 years (580).

## Fungus Cure Also Cures Cancer, Says Oncology Physician

See chapter 34 of this book for the amazing cancer cure that Italian Oncologist, Dr. Simoncini, is using to cure his cancer patients within just days. Cancerous growths are usually WHITE. He says that they are a fungus, which can be killed with a non-toxic soda bicarb solution that quickly alkalizes and kills them (582). This chapter will also tell you about Dr. Mark Sircus' oral soda bicarb for treating cancer rapidly and inexpensively, without having to resort to intravenous use. Both believe in treating cancer with soda bicarb for quickly alkalizing the cells.

## Garlic Inhibits Cancer of the Esophagus

Physicians from M.D. Anderson were shocked to discover that mice treated with a compound found in garlic (*diallyl sulfide*) were two-thirds less likely to develop malignant cells, even when given a toxin that caused colon cancer. When they tried the same test against esophageal cancer, the results were even more dramatic (337). According to Dr. Michael Wargovich, the animals receiving garlic, though pre-disposed to cancer, did not develop the disease (337). He believes that the garlic somehow activated processes in the liver that reduced the toxicity of the cancer-causing agents (337). Garlic not only prevents cancer, but it can help normalize blood pressure; kill bacteria, viruses and *parasites*; reduce harmful lipids and high *blood sugar, and* fight *yeast infections* (337).

## Gene Therapy (Advexin) Trial Less Toxic for Some Head & Neck Cancer Patients

The p53 gene is normally the cancer-fighting gene, but it can mutate and cause cancer (121a). As described at *consultantlive.com* website, researchers led by John Nemunaitis, M.D, Medical Director at the Mary Crowley Medical Research Center in Dallas, conducted a scientific study involving 123 participants, all of whom had *end-stage* "recurrent squamous cell carcinoma of the head and neck" (121a). The new gene therapy, known as ***Advexin***, revealed milder side effects over those receiving the chemo drug, *methotrexate* (121a). Though this certainly is not a painless, gentle or natural treatment, it is being included here for those people who are end-stage, and do choose the conventional medicine route, simply because this particular therapy may be less toxic than other chemo drugs (121a).

## Grapefruit Flavonoids Reduce Risk for Oral Cancers

Flavonoids from grapefruit were recently tested at Texas A & M University on animals with mouth cancers, and the results were eye-opening. Two flavonoids from grapefruit, known as *naringin* and *naringenin,* decreased both number and size of growths in the animals tested (491). Their conclusion was that the compounds (especially those in grapefruit) could help ward off cancer (491). Just be sure if eating grapefruit, you are not taking medications that can be incompatible with grapefruit juice.

## Graviola for Cancer

Refer to chapters five and six in this book for information on this herb (from the Amazonian Rain Forest) that has cancer-fighting properties.

## Green Tea Protects Against Esophageal & Stomach Cancer

*Life Extension's* webpage at *www.lef.org,* discusses the important anti-cancer properties of green tea. Stomach cancer rates decreased dramatically in humans ingesting *seven or more cups* of this tea every *day* (59). A Chinese study found that stomach cancer risk could be cut in half in those who were long time consumers of green tea. Apparently, green tea helps reduce nitrite injury against stomach cells better than vitamin C does (59). Research from 1994, on human subjects, revealed that this tea can decrease the chances of esophageal cancer by 60% (137). The polyphenols in the tea are powerful anti-oxidants. They are being put into many skin care products for their ability at fighting skin cancers (137). Green tea has also been found, in animal testing by Israeli researchers, to actually regenerate brain cells, something hitherto thought impossible (169).

Research has shown that simply rinsing your mouth out with green tea cannot only kill abnormal cells in the mouth, but help prevent new ones from forming (512). While not touted as a *cure,* it is certainly worth practicing. Just realize that if you drink a lot of caffeinated tea every day, it can act like a diuretic and remove valuable minerals from your body. De-caffeinated tea will not do so, but also does not fight plaque as well. Always use organic teas.

## Intensity Modulated Radiotherapy (IMRT) for Head & Neck Cancers

This radiation treatment is currently under testing in Europe and is being used in the U.S as well. It uses targeted radiotherapy to help minimize damage to nearby normal cells. It is used for lung tumors, thyroid and breast cancers, as well as prostate, esophageal, nasal and head cancers, liver, brain, ovarian, cervical cancers, and uterine growths. You may also see this treatment referred to as ***TOMO Therapy*** or *TOMO Treatment*—they are the same thing.

IMRT was first used at Memorial Sloan-Kettering Hospital for treating cancer of the prostate (163a). Rather than using one large radiation beam to target the tumor, this type radiation uses many beams to target cancer tumors more precisely, thus preventing excess damage to nearby normal cells (163a). It is still considered radiation, and will have some of the same side effects as any radiation would cause. IMRT has been popular at treating tumors located around or near critical, vital organs (163a).

## LifeMel Honey for Cancer Patients

This amazing honey is also discussed in chapter 29 in this book. It is a special honey (developed in Israel) that is taken from the nectar of 40 herbs, including *Echinacea, Siberian ginseng,* and *Uncaria tomentosa,* with other natural ingredients. Two teaspoons per day (one in the morning and one in the evening) are recommended (614). This special honey has been shown, in **human** testing, to prevent the neutropenia (dangerous white blood cell drop) caused by chemotherapy and to lower the risk of severe platelet drop (thrombocytopenia), often found in chemo patients (614). You can find out more at website *http://www.lifemelisrael.com.* (614).

## Lycopene Decreases Risk for Mouth & Throat Cancers

Lycopene intake, mentioned at length in earlier chapters, is also associated with decreased risk for cancers of the mouth, throat and pharynx, by more than one third (507). Good natural sources of lycopene are: red tomatoes, guavas, watermelon, carrots, and red peppers, as well as many other vegetables and fruits. Lycopene should be taken with a fat source for best absorption (337), e.g., tomatoes and olive oil, or tomatoes, peppers and avocado slices.

## Magnesium for Cancer Prevention

This mineral is critical for the prevention of all types of cancer, including leukemia, and those involving the stomach, prostate, breast, and bones (566). See page 129.b

## Molybdenum Prevents Esophageal Cancer

Lack of molybdenum, a common *trace mineral*, may be responsible for the occurrence of some cancers (504). Part of the problem may be linked to its lack in the soil. When this mineral (along with *vitamin C)* is added to the soil and *food*, cases of esophageal cancer are reduced; apparently it does not take much. When added to the water supply at minute amounts, both stomach and throat cancers were dramatically reduced (504).

## Mullaca Effective Against Gliomas & Nasopharynx (Nose & Throat) Cancers

Mullaca is a rain forest herb that is toxic to gliomas. [Gliomas are a type of brain tumor.] Clinical research is ongoing with this fascinating herb, and preliminary laboratory and animal studies have shown that it reinforces the immune system, is deadly to many cancers (including leukemia), and it kills some bacteria and parasites (200). In laboratory testing, says Raintree Nutrition *(rain-tree.com)*, extracts of mullaca, known as *physalins,* have shown impressive anti-cancer effects toward multiple forms of cancers, including intestinal, head-and-neck, lung, and liver (200). Because Mullaca may intensify or lessen the effects of some prescription medications, be sure to consult with your physician or Naturopath before supplementing (200). You may find this substance sold under the name of *bolsa mullaca.* Also, see chapter 14 for more information on gliomas and other brain tumors.

## Niacinamide & Esophageal Cancers

Several **human** studies have shown that patients with head-and-neck cancers have an 80% *response rate* when given large doses of this B vitamin in combination with radiation. Without the niacinamide, the response rate was only 10% (592). Though I do not advocate radiation therapy, you may find this information helpful should you choose this treatment.

## Onions Inhibit Oral Cancer

Harvard animal studies revealed that a substance (used for treating mouth cancer) taken from onions, greatly reduced some of the abnormal cells in the test subjects, and even destroyed other cancer cells (363). Onions can also help lower blood sugar levels (363).

## Photodynamic Therapy for Oral Cancers

See chapter 12 and chapter 34 for more information on the use of photodynamic therapy (PDT), also called *Cytoluminescent Therapy*®. Though it is discussed in chapter 12 in conjunction with pancreatic cancer, this procedure has also successfully treated other forms of cancer, including mouth and throat cancers. I have read some negative comments about it. Patients using the infrared lights had deteriorating health, with complaints of pain, malaise, overall weakness, and weight loss. Now, when given, it is recommended that it is only done by professionals in an outpatient setting, rather than having the patients activate the treatment at home.

## Poly–MVA (Palladium Lipoic Complex)

See chapter 14 for more information on this amazing nutritional supplement that many cancer survivors credit with bringing them into complete remission. The main website for Poly-MVA is: *www.polymva.net.*

## Resveratrol & Thyroid Cancers

See chapter three in this book for more information on this potent substance that can be found in common table grapes and pomegranates. Resveratrol is also being touted as a way to fight obesity, as well as high cholesterol levels, since it keeps the body from storing fat.

## Rexin-G™ for All Solid Tumors & Metastatic Cancers

Rexin-G™ has been undergoing clinical trials at Mayo Clinic, M.D. Anderson, and a few other facilities. It is a drug for cancers that have spread, and those types of cancer that conventional medicine says do not respond to chemo (256). **Human** clinical studies, thus far, have had good results. In the very first human trial, 83% of the patients experienced tumor shrinkage. The patients all had spreading pancreatic cancer (256). Good responses were also achieved in **human** studies involving several other types of metastatic cancer. Due to the reports, this drug is now used for treating all forms of *solid tumors* in the Philippines that are resistant to conventional therapy (256). The U.S. FDA has given the drug its *orphan drug status* for use with pancreatic cancers in the US, as well as other types of cancer metastases, which means that trials will continue (256). It is given intravenously, so isn't exactly natural or painless, but could be considered gentler than older chemo drugs because it is said to be a non-chemo drug, showing itself in **human** clinical trials, not to have the adverse side effects normally associated with chemo drugs (256). You can get more information on this drug at *epeiusbiotech.com/rexin_g-factsheet.asp.* Epeius Biotechnologies are the producers of Rexin-G™ (257).

## Riboflavin (B-2), Chinese Herbs, Vitamin A, Selenium & Zinc Help Prevent Mouth & Esophageal Cancer

Experiments done in China to see if vitamins could stop the high rate of esophageal cancers, rampant in some parts of the country, had remarkable results. In his book, *Cancer Therapy*, Dr. Ralph Moss says that in one area, out of thousands of people, more than half already had signs of cancer of the esophagus with significant abnormal cell growth (504). Over two thousand had precancerous cells. Patients were given either *riboflavin or a placebo*, or a specially prepared herbal mix called *anti-tumor B*, or vitamin A (retinamide), depending on how extensive the dysplasia was. When the participants were checked 36 months later, the group receiving the herbal formula had more than fifty-percent **fewer cancers** than the placebo group. Those receiving vitamin A and riboflavin had *33.7 and 19 percent* fewer esophageal cancers (504). (The ingredients in the herbal mix, *anti-tumor B*, were not listed in the reference.)

The combined nutrients, *zinc, vitamin A...riboflavin, and selenium*, can reduce the incidence of oral cancer (507). In 1995, researchers from India discovered that using a combo of these 4 nutraceuticals decreased the incidence of damaged DNA by *72 to 95 percent* in a group of volunteers receiving it (507). Out of hundreds of *heavy smokers* that were tested, Dr. Moss says that 150 were given the vitamin-mineral combo and the other half, a placebo. Of those participants given the nutritional regimen, more than half experienced a total remission from their oral cancer; however, in those not receiving the vitamins and minerals, *only 8 percent* went into remission (507). Research has proven that oral doses of zinc, taken by those with increased susceptibility to cancer, can decrease their incidence of mouth and throat cancer. In lab studies, scientists were able to reverse abnormal cell growth (potentially cancerous) in animals by merely feeding them zinc.

## Simarouba Inhibits Cancer of the Pharynx

Simarouba is another rain forest herb that helps impede throat carcinomas (272). Excessive dosages (triple what is normal) may result in stomach upset, sweating, and excess urinary output (272). As with any herbal remedy, be sure to consult with your physician first. Do not give herbal preparations to children without first consulting their physician.

## Spirulina Inhibits Oral Cancers

*Spirulina-Dunaliella* is a type of blue-green algae, high in beta-carotene and other anti-oxidants. Animal studies have shown that this alga is important in helping to prevent the formation and spread of mouth cancers (558). In a human study involving mouth cancer, half the patients given spirulina improved. They were given one gram daily (571).

## Transfer Factor™ Heals An Aggressive Esophageal Cancer

See website *http://www.shirleys-wellness-café.com/tf/s/cancer-testimonials.htm,* for a testimonial from Dr Robertson, M.D., whose patient's aggressive esophageal cancer was healed by taking Transfer Factor™ alone (without radiation, chemo or surgery). The patient used "Transfer Factor, 3 capsules, 3 times a day [and] Transfer Factor Plus, 3 capsules, 3 times a day" (592).

The initial development of this substance can be credited to Dr. H. Sherwood Lawrence in 1949. He was researching T.B. and discovered that he could take the immunity found in white blood cells and transfer it from a donor to a recipient. This factor (that contained the immunity), he referred to as *transfer factor* (295). Since that time, thousands of papers have been written on this nutrient and billions spent on research (295). This immune enhancer has recently become available to the public in supplement form (295). As described at *realsuccess4life.com,* a report from a study by [the] Institute of Longevity Medicine was done in 1999 on Transfer Factor™, comparing it to nearly 200 *of the world's most popular nutrients* (3). The testing (according to Jeunesse, Inc.) claims that "Transfer Factor™ is 500% more powerful than any other nutrient or substance found in any nutritional or medical literature" (3). They say that it outperformed "Noni... Aloe Vera... Cordyceps Formula, Shiitake Mushroom, Echinacea...[and] IP6," and it works by increasing natural killer cell activity within the immune system (3). Transfer factor™ is available at websites *http://www.4lifeweb.com/pb* and *http://www.4tf.com/home.htm,* as well as other internet sites.

A research company has recently developed a patented high anti-oxidant liquid blend containing not only Transfer Factor E-XF™, but juice from the popular Brazilian Rain Forest berry—the acai berry—as well as pomegranate, purple grapes, elderberries, blueberries, and other anti-oxidants in a drink known as *RioVida.* You can read more about *RioVida* at *www.RioVida.com.* The anti-oxidant power of the acai berry is claimed to be ten times more potent than grapes and twice as potent as blueberries. For those interested in this product, *RioVida* can be ordered from several internet sites.

## Transfer Factor™ & Papillary Thyroid Cancer

See website *http://www.shirleys-wellness-cafe.com/tf/s/cancer-testimonials.htm* for the testimonial of a woman who had surgery for papillary thyroid cancer and also used Transfer Factor™ to rid herself of cancer.

## Ukrain Effective Against Esophageal Cancer, Without Toxic Side Effects

The plant, *greater celandine,* is very toxic to humans, and so is the drug *Thiotepa*, however, one physician discovered that when the two are combined, a new drug (they named *Ukrain)* was birthed that was only toxic to **cancer cells** (287)(589). Ukrain has been effective against cancer in clinical trials involving hundreds of people, yet it is non-toxic to normal cells in humans (589). My first book, *Painless Cancer Cures,* has details on squamous cell cancers of the throat that were successfully treated with Ukrain after standard conventional treatment (chemo and radiation) failed completely. Ukrain is only available through alternative health clinics in the U.S., Canada, and Europe.

2009 update: note that because Ukrain is not authorized in Austria, this article is no longer located *at www.ukrin.com.* The website has been changed and is now called *Nowicky Pharma,* however, you can read this information about Ukrain now in the book, *Anti-Cancer Agent Ukrain—The Crime Story of an Obstruction,* by Eleonore Thun-Hohenstein. See *www.ukrin.com,* for more information. Ukrain is considered alternative therapy, so you will have to seek an alternative health care physician in the United States for Ukrain therapy, or travel to Canada or Europe, where Ukrain is widely used. For pictures on how Ukrain works, see website *http://www.ukrain-drug.net/webspeed/index.htm.*

A case study on a human, who was diagnosed with esophageal cancer (considered inoperable) after having many months of swallowing difficulty, is described at *http://www.ncbi.nlm.nih.gov/pubmed/8899345?Ordinalpos=3&itool=EntrezSystem2.PEntrez.Pubmed.Pubmed_resultsPanel.Pubmed_RVDDocSum,* or go to the U.S. National Library of Medicine website at NCBI PubMed and enter the PMID 8899345 (589). Having already undergone conventional treatment without success, the patient was given Ukrain (*46 ampoules*), and went into total remission, and—as of last report—was still cancer-free after four years (589).

## II. Thyroid Cancers

There are four types of thyroid cancer, depending on the location and cellular origin: papillary, medullary, follicular, and anaplastic. This cancer is usually treated by surgical removal, which may involve a partial or total thyroidectomy, depending on the extent of the cancer. Afterwards, of course, thyroid hormone replacement therapy is prescribed. Other treatments involve the use of radioactive iodine therapy, CAAT or Controlled Amino Acid Therapy (an alternative therapy), as well as the usual chemo and radiation that orthodox medicine advocates.

One of the best ways to protect the thyroid is a highly nutritious diet, including the use of natural sea salt containing iodine; however, you need to use any type of iodine supplement under medical supervision, especially if you already have a thyroid disorder. (Also, see p. 129.)

Some of the other alternative therapies mentioned in this book have been successful with thyroid cancers. For example: hydrazine sulfate, developed by Dr. Joseph Gold, details of which can be read in chapter 16 of this book. Dr. Gold's clinic does not take calls from patients, but you can have your health practitioner call them at #315-472-6616. They are located at Syracuse Cancer Research Institute, Inc., Presidential Plaza, 600 East Genesee St., Syracuse N.Y. 13202.

## Conventional Treatments

Just a note to advise that if your Oncologist tells you that they are going to put you on Nexavar® (Sorafenib) for your thyroid cancer, this chemo drug has many potential side effects—some mild, some very severe—as with any other standard chemo drug. Some patients have very good response to it, others do not. This book will give you a great deal of information that will help you make a choice on the type treatment you are interested in pursuing. Always write your questions down and present them to your physician at your next visit, and be sure you know all the side effects of treatments before agreeing to them!

## Alternative Non-Toxic Treatments - Burzynski's Antineoplastons & Thyroid Cancers

Antineoplastons are non-toxic cancer treatments, developed and provided by Dr. Stanislaw Burzynski at his clinic in Houston, Texas, which have cured many cancer patients. They are mentioned in several other cancer-specific chapters of this book, and in great detail in chapter 14 due to their remarkable success with brain cancer patients. They are also used for thyroid cancer patients and nearly every other cancer imaginable. See their main website at: *www.burzynskiclinic.com*, and read some of the many testimonials of patients who have successfully used antineoplastons to cure their cancer at: *http://burzynskipatientgroup.org/stor ies.html*. (Many of those cured with antineoplastons at the above website have left their email addresses or phone numbers where they can be contacted if you wish to discuss their experience at the Burzynski Clinic with them.)

Antineoplastons are not always *gentle* or *painless* because they are given intravenously, however, they are developed from natural substances and are non-toxic, and they are sometimes given in capsule form, known as PBs or sodium phenylbutrates (which **is** gentle and painless). If patients do have side effects from them (e.g. electrolyte problems), they are easily reversible!) The FDA has finally approved the oral form of antineoplastons (PBs) for off-label use, but you will need to ask your physician about prescribing them. Note that antineoplastons A10 and AS2-1 were recently given orphan drug status for use on human brainstem gliomas.

## Intensity Modulated Radiotherapy (IMRT) & Thyroid Cancers

This radiation treatment is currently under testing in Europe and is being used in the U.S as well. It uses targeted radiotherapy to help minimize damage to nearby normal cells. It is used for lung tumors, thyroid, and breast cancers, as well as prostate, esophageal, nasal, head cancers, liver, brain, ovarian, cervical cancers, and uterine growths. You may also see this treatment referred to as ***TOMO Therapy*** or *TOMO Treatment*—they are the same thing.

IMRT was first used at Memorial Sloan-Kettering Hospital for treating cancer of the prostate (163a). Rather than using one large radiation beam to target the tumor, this type radiation uses many beams to target cancer tumors more precisely, thus preventing excess damage to nearby normal cells (163a). Keep in mind that it is still considered radiation, and will have some of the same side effects as any radiation would cause. IMRT has been popular at treating tumors located around or near critical, vital organs (163a).

## Radiofrequency Ablation Treatment (RFA) & Thyroid Cancers

Discussed in other areas of this book, RFA is also being used for thyroid carcinomas, along with the use of an *ethanol* injection. It is used as an alternative for those who are not good surgical candidates, or who do not wish to undergo surgery, and is especially useful for liver tumors. Anesthesia and surgical incision are not needed for the procedure. A needle electrode is carefully manipulated into the growth, and the tumor is destroyed by heat generated from electrical currents given off by the electrode. In a human study of those experiencing *recurrent local and distant well-differentiated thyroid carcinoma,* there were no serious complications from the procedure, and some of the patients had total remission from their cancer. For more information, see the study described in detail at PubMed's website PMID 16858194 (502).

# CHAPTER 12

# GENTLE CURES FOR TOUGH PANCREATIC CANCERS

*"Let my soul live, and it shall praise thee; and let thy judgments help me." (Psalm 119:175)*

## Cytotron Therapy

See chapter 34 in this book for more details on this gentle, painless, non-invasive cancer therapy that many people are also using to restore cartilage in their joints, making joint-replacement surgeries completely unnecessary (90). You may hear this referred to as *QMR* or *Quantum Magnetic Resonance*—they are the same thing.

## The Pancreatic Cancer That Disappeared

## Case #1—Gerson Therapy

*The Complete Encyclopedia of Natural Healing* by Gary Null, Ph.D., details the story of a patient with pancreatic cancer, who followed Gerson Therapy for a year and experienced a total cure. He had no chemo, no surgery, and no radiation. This was more than *14 years ago* (519).

Max Gerson, a graduate from the University of Freiburg Medical School, moved to New York and practiced medicine there for many years until his death. Afflicted with migraine headaches that nearly disabled him, he ended up finding a cure for them using a restricted sodium, raw veggie-fruit diet. He believed that cancer could be prevented and controlled by dietary means, much to the fury of the AMA, which was completely against him and what they considered his absurd ideas of preventing and halting cancer with dietary methods (504). In no uncertain terms, they told him that dietary intake had absolutely nothing whatsoever to do with controlling cancer (504)!

Even though we now understand how important nutrition is in cancer prevention, the cancer establishment really hasn't changed much. They have only recently admitted that certain foods may decrease your risk of cancer, but they still believe the main answer to treating this dread disease is in toxic chemicals and radiation, rather than helping the body get well with the right nutrients, as provided by our Creator God, to heal and restore an immune system gone awry.

One of Gerson's patients was none other than the famous Albert Schweitzer, M.D., who spoke very highly of Gerson and praised his work, calling him a *medical genius* (504). It is interesting that one of the components of Gerson Therapy included over a dozen glasses a day of freshly-squeezed fruit and vegetable juices, mainly carrot juice. Ann Wigmore and Eydie Mae Hunsberger also used several glasses of fresh juices daily for optimal health. Realize that there is an element of *New Age* Philosophy in Gerson Therapy, something that I do not promote. I believe that those cancer patients who have done well on Gerson Therapy, have done so primarily because of the **13 glasses a day** of healthy fruit and vegetable juices the diet promotes. This sort of diet is very detoxifying and puts the body in a balanced state of alkalinity, enabling the immune system to heal diseases in some individuals.

At one time, Gerson was so popular that he was published in *JAMA*, but the same magazine later ridiculed him, calling him a *quack* (519). Gerson worked on ways to help *lupus* and *tuberculosis* patients. At that time, very little had been done in the medical field for either disease; however, he successfully reversed these diseases in some of his patients by recommending a natural juicing diet of green grasses and raw vegetables. He was extremely popular *in Europe until the 1930s* (519). His work still prospers today, kept alive (in Mexico) by Charlotte Strauss, Gerson's daughter (519). You can contact them for more information at their website: *www.gerson.org*. At one time, Gerson was even commended by Senator Claude Pepper of Florida in a U.S. committee.

## Case #2—Vitamin C Therapy

Dr. Abram Hoffer, a long time advocate of Orthomolecular and Complementary Medicine, says that conventional medicine considers pancreatic cancer not only untreatable, but usually gives little hope of surviving beyond five years, once the diagnosis is made (433); however, he goes on to describe a middle-aged patient who came to see him with *terminal* pancreatic cancer. She was seeking advice about a high dose vitamin C regimen, and had been told that she only had a few months to live. Dr. Hoffer not only started her on vitamin C megadoses of 40 grams per day intravenously, but also prescribed other nutrients, including vitamins and minerals (zinc, niacin, selenium) (432). Before she came to see him, she had been taking daily divided doses of *10,000 mg* of vitamin

C. Within six months of seeking Dr. Hoffer's treatment, diagnostics could find no tumor! Her physician was so disbelieving that he ordered the tests a second time. The results were the same—the tumor was gone. She survived her ordeal, going on to live a normal life for more than twenty years (432).

There has been much controversy about megadosing with vitamin C for cancer, but most researchers agree that giving vitamin C directly into the bloodstream (intravenously) gets best results. Linus Pauling, Dr. Abram Hoffer, Dr. Irwin Stone, Dr. Robert Cathcart, and many other chemists and researchers have believed and taught this for years. It seems that the modern medical community may finally be taking them seriously.

Recently, the National Institute of Diabetes and Digestive and Kidney Diseases in Bethesda, Maryland, discovered that giving large amounts of this vitamin intravenously to mice with ovarian cancers, glioblastoma, and cancers of the pancreas, halted the tumors by more than half (329a). The study was headed up by Mark Levine, who said that the vitamin C worked by forming *hydrogen peroxide,* which destroyed the *cancer cells* (329a). Cancer Treatment Centers of America *(CTCA)* in Zion, Illinois, is also testing intravenous Vitamin C on patients with advanced cancer (329a). (Also, see page 544 of this book for a new form of C.)

## Abajeru (*Chrysobalanus icaco*) for Pancreatic & Other Cancers

Isolated from a tropical plant of the Brazilian Rain Forest (aka as *coco-plum*), abajeru was once used by the locals for fighting arthritic pain and diabetes (145a). When researchers first conducted lab testing, they found that the bush extract killed not only cancerous *breast-brain-lung-bowel-larynx and pancreas tumors*, but even difficult-to-treat leukemia cells died. In testing **humans**, they were surprised to see that it *worked with 90% of the patients.* You can find this substance in health food stores and on the internet at many websites (145a).

## Bindweed Herb (*Convolvulus arvensis*) Fights Pancreatic Cancer

A common field weed, that you may find sold as *VascuStatin/Angioblock*, or under the name *PGM* or *MPGC,* is being described as a cancer-fighter (150) (301a). It is being used successfully by health practitioners for fighting many forms of cancer, including ovarian and pancreatic cancers, and it is said to be non-toxic and "100 times stronger than shark cartilage" at preventing the growth of new blood vessels, a property known as anti-angiogenesis (150) (301a). For details see website *http://organicpharmacy.org/products/VascuStatin,* and this website *springboard4health.com/notebook/health_bindweed.html.* Also, see page two at *http://organic pharmacy.org/products/VascuStatin,* for warnings about when this substance should not be used.

Many physicians are giving this herb to their cancer patients. Also, see the Nov. 24, 2000 letter from a pancreatic cancer patient at website *springboard4health.com/notebook/health_bindweed.html,* who used bindweed extracts WPGC (*Muramyl polysaccharide-glycan complex*) and then PGM, *2 oz. daily*, along with other nutritional supplements to fight stage IV pancreatic cancer that had gone into the liver (150). She was diagnosed (via *biopsy*) with "invasive adenocarcinoma of the pancreas – Stage IV." She had already refused chemo and radiation. Her best results did not begin until AFTER September 29th, when she began taking the PGM. By November 19th, her *liver* had "returned to its normal size" (150).

## Burzynski's Antineoplastons—Non-Toxic Cancer Cures

Antineoplastons are non-toxic cancer treatments discovered and provided by Dr. Stanislaw Burzynski at his clinic in Houston, Texas, which have cured many cancer patients. They are mentioned in several other cancer-specific chapters of this book, and in great detail in chapter 14 due to their remarkable success with terminal brain cancer patients. They are also used for pancreatic cancer patients and nearly every other cancer imaginable. See their main website at: *www.burzynskiclinic.com,* and read some of the many testimonials of patients who have successfully used antineoplastons: *http://burzynskipatientgroup.org/storieshtml,* to cure their cancers. The FDA has finally approved the oral form of antineoplastons (PBs or sodium phenylbutrates) for off-label use, but you will need to ask your health care practitioner about prescribing them. Note that antineoplastons A10 and AS2-1 were recently given orphan drug status for use on human brainstem gliomas.

## Cherries & Limonene Shrink Pancreatic Tumors

*Perillyl alcohol*, a powerful ingredient found in cherries, limes, and lemons helps kill cancer cells, but is harmless to normal cells. It helps to prevent breast, liver, and skin cancers (97). This substance caused a 50% reduction in tumors of the pancreas (in animal testing) and a total regression of the cancers in 16% of them. Those not given the perillyl alcohol had no such results. The substance is also said to help in preventing cancers of the intestines, lungs, and prostate (97). A Swedish study found that the most important way to prevent pancreatic cancer was by plenty of *citrus fruits (and carrots)*...in the diet (363). These foods also decrease the incidence of gastric cancers. In animal studies, Japanese scientists found that an extract injection (from the rind of grapefruit) could stop cancers and even cause remission in those already having cancer (363).

## Cholesterol Drug for Pancreatic Cancer - No Toxic Side Effects

For detailed information on a new cancer-treatment regimen that includes combining "low-dose interferon with lovastatin," so far used in melanoma, but also being considered for other cancers like pancreatic cancer (76a), see website *www.neoplas.org* [and chapter 34 in this book]. Doctors saw their patient's tumors start to regress—often within *a few weeks!* The treatment has no toxic side effects as found in chemo and *radiation* (76a). Just be aware that statin drugs strip CoQ10 out of your body. If your physician recommends this treatment, let him or her know about this so that they can advise you on CoQ10 supplementation. Some physicians are not aware of this side effect of statin drugs.

## CoQ10—Low Levels Linked to Pancreatic Cancer

This nutrient, also called *ubiquinone*, has been the subject of many scientific double-blind **human studies**, and is so important in fighting cancer, it is mentioned in several other cancer-specific chapters in this book. It is found in all of our cells and in some foods, but amounts decrease as we age. Some natural food sources of this nutrient are: nuts, leafy greens, and salmon (564). The late Dr. Karl Folkers was a prominent scientist, greatly interested in the effects of ubiquinone on cancer. In his studies, he found that cancer patients had drastically low levels of CoQ10, and patients with pancreatic cancers had the lowest levels of CoQ10 than with any other cancers studied. He believed that insufficient amounts of this nutrient accounts for the high death rate in cancer of the pancreas (550). The same low blood levels of CoQ10 were discovered in children with *leukemia* (550).

Current research conducted by the Leonard M. Miller School of Medicine in Miami (under Niven R. Nerain), revealed that CoQ10 has the ability to kill cancer cells without damage to healthy cells. Not only that, but the National Cancer Institute (NCI) acknowledged in 2005 that CoQ10 can extend the lives of those with pancreatic cancer and other cancers. CoQ10 therapy is used at the Issels Treatment Centers. Their website is: *http:/www.issels.com.* Their phone #888-447-7357 (290).

For one of America's largest alternative health care centers, see the Whitaker Wellness Center, which is in Newport Beach (4321 Birch Street), California. Refer to this link: ***http://whitakerwellness.com/about_us/medical_team.*** Dr. Julian Whitaker, who runs this health care center, has written numerous books on alternative healing. He has an excellent website with a great deal of helpful information. They use many of the alternative health treatments that I have mentioned in my books, including chelation, hyperbaric oxygen, and IV therapies.

## CyberKnife® Therapy for PancreaticTumors

See chapter 34 in this book for details on CyberKnife® therapy, which is being used successfully for pancreatic cancers and many other cancers, including hard-to-reach brain tumors. It is a gentle, painless procedure that does not require an incision, surgery, sedation or inpatient stay. It takes very little time, and as soon as the procedure is over, the patient is able to return home. There are very few risks and side effects, though it does involve some radiation (89a), and can damage nearby healthy cells. Also, see NanoKnife™, chapter 34.

## Essiac Tea for All Cancers

See chapter six for more information on this amazing herbal tea. Rene Caisse, a Canadian nurse, healed hundreds (probably thousands) of people of every imaginable cancer using her amazing herbal tea, many of whom came to her after conventional medicine considered them hopeless. One of the most amazing books describing the effectiveness of this tea and how it was suppressed by the health industry in Canada is called: *The Essiac Report Canada's Remarkable Unknown Cancer Remedy,* by Richard Thomas, who claims that Flor-Essence® Essiac is the original (drinkable) formula that Rene Caisse used (580).

Note that there is some competition between the tea produced by Resperin Canada Essiac® and Flor-Essence® Essiac tea. Both companies claim that they have the original Essiac formula (the drinkable formula, not the injectable) that Rene Caisse used in treating her cancer patients. See chapter 16 in this book for the story of a young boy who was cured of lymphoma using a natural program that included Essiac® Resperin Canada's tea formula and 714X injections. A website that has Essiac® Resperin Canada is also given in that chapter. You can find both formulas at health food stores and on the internet, as well as other brands. I have tried Flor-Essence®; it tastes like a tea blend.

## Figs That Fight Cancer

An anti-cancer chemical isolated from figs, known as *benzaldehyde,* can shrink tumors by more than one-third in mice injected with the compound. Japanese scientists gave this extract by mouth to **human** participants, with good results; however, when they used injectables containing the extract, results were much more remarkable. More than 50% of participants having late stage cancer got better. Many of them experienced total *remission,* some had *partial remission.* The fig nutrient extended their life span, and it worked much better in **human** growths than in mice studies (363). Juice from figs also had the ability to destroy parasites and bacteria (363). There is a story in the Bible concerning Israeli leader, Hezekiah, who was healed of boils using a fig poultice.

## Fungus Cure Also Cures Cancer, Says Oncology Physician

See chapter 34 of this book for the amazing cancer cure that Italian Oncologist, Dr. Simoncini, is using to cure his cancer patients within just days! Cancerous growths are usually WHITE. He says that they are actually a fungus, which can be killed with a non-toxic soda bicarb solution that quickly alkalizes the tumor for destruction (582).

## Geraniol Effective Against Pancreatic Cancer

Geraniol is a fruit phytochemical that is capable of inhibiting tumor growth, as demonstrated by laboratory testing. Extensive testing on humans has not yet been done. It is also found in certain spices (e.g., ginger and rosemary).

## GLA Increases Survival Rates in Pancreatic Cancer

A human study in Canada showed that gamma-linolenic acid (GLA) could dramatically increase the lifespan of more than two dozen people with terminal pancreatic cancer (551). The nutrient also worked on some humans with intestinal and breast cancers, without adverse problems (551). The best source of GLA is *borage* oil (also called *starflower oil).* Other good sources are *black currant, hemp* and *evening primrose* oil (43).

## Graviola & Resveratrol

See chapter three for an amazing ingredient in common table grapes (and pomegranates) credited to preventing and curing cancer, and chapter five and six for information on *graviola,* an herb from the rain forest. Both of these chapters describe case histories of people that credit their total cure from cancer to natural substances. (Some patients have used graviola to help cure their pancreatic cancer.)

For an excellent 58-page study that was done on resveratrol's role in fighting cancer (including pancreatic cancer), see website *http://www.agrawal.org/PDF/ACR-Resveratrol1.pdf.* The study was conducted by M.D. Anderson Cancer Center, and the UCLA Center for Human Nutrition (346). Just be sure to check with your health care provider before taking graviola, or any other herb or supplement, especially if you already have a health condition.

A recent study from the journal: *Advances in Experimental Medicine and Biology,* revealed that resveratrol in grapes and red wine kills pancreatic cancer cells by attacking the center of the cell's *mitochondria,* where all the cellular energy is produced (252) (255).

## LifeMel Honey

This amazing honey is also discussed in chapter 29 of this book. It is a special honey, developed in Israel, that is taken from the nectar of 40 herbs, including *Echinacea, Siberian ginseng,* and *Uncaria tomentosa,* with other natural ingredients. Two teaspoons per day (one in the morning and one in the evening) are recommended (614). This special honey has been shown, in human testing, to prevent the neutropenia (serious white blood cell drop) caused by chemotherapy and to lower the risk of severe platelet drop (thrombocytopenia), so often found in chemo patients (614). You can find out more about this remarkable honey at website *http://www.lifemelisrael.com*. (614). I have seen LifeMel honey in health food stores.

## Lycopene & Beta-Carotene Cut Pancreatic Cancer Risk

Already mentioned earlier, lycopene is an important nutrient in preventing pancreatic cancer. More than 28,000 people in the U.S. died from pancreatic cancer during the year 2000 (351). Though this deadly disease kills nine out of ten people diagnosed, there is more than enough evidence to substantiate that its cause could be dietary (351). A human research study revealed that those people who exclude vegetables from their diets are four times as likely to develop this deadly cancer. Consuming several servings (*of vegetables*) per day was found to be protective (351). The type of vegetables eaten mattered as well—most importantly—the consumption of lycopene-rich and beta-carotene-rich foods (351), e.g., tomatoes, carrots, guavas, squash, papaya, and watermelon.

If you are still not convinced, as some in the scientific community, that food and the dietary choices we make greatly influence the chances of having pancreatic cancer, consider the research done by George Comstock in Hagerstown, Maryland (551). After studying more than *25,000* people, he discovered a definite link between lycopene deficiency and this type of cancer. Some good natural sources of lycopene are watermelon, guavas, pink grapefruit, papaya, and tomatoes, as mentioned earlier.

## Magnesium & Iodine for Cancer Prevention

These minerals are critical for the prevention of all types of cancer, including leukemia, and those involving the stomach, prostate, breast, and bones (566). Also, see p. 129.

## Nigella Sativa Seed Oil Extract (Thymoquinone) Fights Pancreatic Cancer

In a study from Thomas Jefferson University in Philadelphia, researchers have discovered, in laboratory testing, that an extract taken from the Middle Eastern (and Indian) herb, *nigella sativa,* can kill pancreatic cancer cells (331) This herb is also known as *black cumin.* More studies on the extract are planned (331) .

## Onions & Berries Dramatically Decrease Pancreatic Cancer Risk

In a **human** study, involving more than 183,000 participants in California (over an eight-year period), flavonols found in berries and onions were discovered to reduce pancreatic cancer risk by *25 percent* (in non-smokers) and by greater than *59 percent* in smokers (418). The flavonol that produced the greatest protection for non-smokers was *kaempferol (in spinach and some cabbages).* The flavenols consumed by the participants, besides the kaempferol, included *quercetin (from onion and apples*), and *myricetin (from berries and red onions)* (418).

## Poly–MVA for Pancreatic Cancer

See chapter 14 for more information on this nutrient-rich formula, which may be helpful in reversing pancreatic cancers (as well as brain cancers).

## Photodynamic Therapy for Pancreatic Cancer

Though I do not look at this treatment as particularly *gentle* or *painless,* since it is an invasive procedure done in an operating room, it is being included in this section for informational purposes, and because it has been a successful alternative to toxic chemo drugs and radiation for many people.

This therapy, in **human** testing, extended the lives of *many of the 16 pancreatic patients* who used it during the trial. They are first given a drug that causes the cancer cells to be more sensitive to light. When they are then exposed to a *fibre-optic* light source, the cancer cells die (177). The procedure aims at cancer cells rather than healthy cells, though it is possible to harm healthy cells if the light is not aimed *precisely* enough, and because the sensitizing drug can also sensitize healthy cells. This study was conducted with terminal, inoperable cancer patients (177). After the procedure, because of the increased light sensitivity, patients are told that they have to avoid the sun and any type of bright lighting. Even after the treatment, they are ushered into darkened rooms (177). Other professionals are trying to develop substances that will make cells even more light-sensitive, yet be able to discern better between healthy and abnormal cells (177), in order that healthy cells are not destroyed in the process. This procedure appears to be gaining popularity. It has also been successfully used for those with mouth and esophageal cancers. (Also, see Cytoluminescent Therapy® in chapter 34.)

I have read some negative comments about this treatment. Patients using the infrared lights had deteriorating health with complaints of pain, malaise, overall weakness, and weight loss. Now, when given, it is recommended that it is only done by professionals in an outpatient setting, rather than having the patients activate the treatment themselves at home.

## Proteolytic Enzymes

These are enzymes produced by the pancreas. Substances in papaya and pineapple are also considered proteolytic enzymes. (See below info under pancreatic enzymes.) They are given in enteric-coated supplements so that they do not digest until they reach the intestines. **Human** studies have been done showing that these enzymes can prolong the lives of those with pancreatic cancer. They should always be enteric-coated and are usually taken 30 minutes before meals. Also, for several **human** trials on those with colon, lung, stomach cancers, and multiple myeloma, using proteolytic enzymes in combo with chemotherapy, see website *http://www.doctormurray.com/articles/pdfs/ProteolyticsInCancer.pdf* (514).

Pancreatic enzymes have been used to treat not only pancreatic cancer, but chronic diseases as well, including those involving the immune system. The enzyme therapy appears to work by halting the spread of the disease (551). Physicians in Germany have been able to completely wipe out tumors with these enzyme injections, given together with *vitamin A* (551). Many foods contain vitamin A, including most of the leafy green vegetables and several types of fruits and other vegetables. Most of the time, raw is best (551). The best way to heal your pancreas, is to help it out by letting it take an occasional break by fasting, or by ingesting *digestive enzymes* (551). Maureen Kennedy Salaman has two enzyme supplements, *Multi-Enzyme* and *Enzyme Ease*® at her website: *www.mksalaman.com*. Just go to the product section at her website for the *Maximum Living Quality Supplements* for ordering either formula. (And of course, don't forget that ounce-for-ounce, chlorella and spirulina are highest of all in natural beta-carotene.) Chlorella is highest in chlorlophyll of any green plant. Just be sure to use the broken cell-wall chlorella.

You can also find proteolytic enzyme supplements at natural health food stores, as well as nattokinase (used to dissolve life-threatening blood clots) and wobenzyme. Nattokinase is derived from fermented soy beans.

Do not take nattokinase or vitamin K-2 without consulting with your doctor, especially if you are taking blood-thinners or you have had a heart attack, stroke, or blood clot in the past. You will usually take enzymes about 30 minutes before you eat.

## R.N. Cures Her Own Pancreatic Cancer with Diet

See chapter 24 for the story of an R.N., who cured her pancreatic tumor with dietary changes and **topical** applications of hydrogen peroxide gel.

## Rexin-G™ for Pancreatic Cancer & Metastatic Cancers

Rexin-G™ has been undergoing clinical trials at Mayo Clinic, M.D. Anderson, and a few other facilities. It is a drug for cancers that have spread, and those types of cancer that conventional medicine says do not respond to chemo (256). **Human** clinical studies, thus far, have had good results. In the very first human trial, 83% of the patients experienced tumor shrinkage. The patients all had spreading pancreatic cancer (256). Good responses were also achieved in **human** studies involving several other types of spreading cancers. Due to the reports, this drug is now used for treating all forms of *solid tumors* in the Philippines that are resistant to conventional therapy (256). The U.S. FDA has given the drug its *orphan drug status** for use with pancreatic cancers in the US, as well as other types of cancer metastases, which means that trials will continue (256). It is given intravenously, so isn't exactly natural or painless, but could be considered gentler than older chemo drugs, because it is said to be a non-chemo drug, showing itself in **human** clinical trials, not to have the adverse side effects normally associated with chemo drugs (256). You can get more information on this drug at *epeiusbiotech.com/rexin_g-factsheet.asp*. Epeius Biotechnologies are the producers of Rexin-G™ (257). (**Orphan* drugs are approved for rare diseases.)

## Saw Palmetto Inhibits Pancreatic Cancer

The herb, saw palmetto, popular in Europe for prostate health, was shown, in a study from Purdue University, to have the ability to fight malignant pancreatic and kidney cells (547). Physicians conducting the study used extracts from saw palmetto known as *mono-laurin* and *mono-myristin*, which were responsible for the above results (547).

## Tian Xian for Pancreatic Cancer

Tian Xian is a Chinese herb that has been promoted for its usefulness in controlling, halting, and killing cancer cells. When Maribel C. Lim (Philippines) was put through a battery of testing and diagnosed with pancreatic cancer, she was told that even if she opted for surgery, she would not survive longer than 6-12 months. Her physician insisted she have surgery, but she refused, opting instead on an herbal regimen of Tian Xian. She also changed her diet, eliminating *sugar, salt, fat, oil [and] white flour.* Two years later, she was still alive, still taking the herb and doing very well (227). Tian Xian has been credited with many cancer recoveries, including pancreatic cancers. You can read case histories of multiple cancer survivors, some given only months to live, who went into total remission using Tian Xian, described at *www.tianxian.com.* Many are still alive today and cancer-free, years after their ordeal. Realize that I am not against surgery for pancreatic cancer. Some pancreatic cancer surgeries are very successful. This is a decision and choice that you will have to discuss with your health care practitioner.

## Turmeric Inhibits Pancreatic Cancer

Curcumin, the ingredient in turmeric that gives it that golden glow, has been discussed in other chapters in this book for its cancer-fighting properties. Research revealed recently that scientists testing varying strengths of curcumin on (human) cancerous cells of the pancreas, discovered that the curcumin restricted the tumors. It may also offer some protection against Alzheimers. See chapter 20 for instances of when you should not use turmeric (curcumin). If you want your body to absorb turmeric more easily, eat it with pineapple or supplement with bromelain.

## Ukrain Retards Growth of Pancreatic Cancer Cells

In a controlled study involving 42 people with pancreatic cancer in Kiev, Ukraine, patients had longer survival times who were treated with Ukrain therapy *(10 mg every second day, repeated 10 times)* (609). In another study that involved 126 people, none of those treated with chemo lasted more than 19 months, however, many of those treated with Ukrain survived longer than four years (609). For details of this study, see the U.S. National Library of Medicine website NCBI PubMed, PMID 11345025 (609).

Ukrain is popular in Europe, Canada, and many other countries outside the U.S.

Ukrain was developed by combining two ingredients that when given individually are very toxic, but once combined, they are **no longer toxic**, except to **cancer cells** (287). Note: since this compound is generally given by injection, I wouldn't exactly classify it as *painless*, but it is being included in this section because it is completely non-toxic, **gentle** on the body, and because of its success against pancreatic cancer.

Ukrain has very powerful anti-tumor effects. Many cancer patients, who have been treated outpatient with Ukrain, have gone into complete remission lasting *19 years* beyond treatment (287). The National Cancer Institute conducted lab studies showing that Ukrain was deadly to all of the solid cancer cells that were studied, including intestinal cancer cells that had stubbornly resisted all other forms of treatment, yet without having any toxic side effects (287). It was also effective against cancerous pancreatic cells that had hitherto not responded to *Cisplatin*, a common chemo drug given, though healthy cells were not harmed (287). The dosage of Ukrain effective at killing cancer cells would have to be multiplied **100 times** before it would ever harm normal cells (287). Or, in other words, it would be difficult to overdose a cancer patient with this non-toxic substance.

The most amazing thing about the study results to me was the lack of further testing and publicity the results were given. How many people are aware of the non-toxic effects of Ukrain at killing cancer cells? Most cancer patients are never told about Ukrain or antineoplastons. Since it is considered alternative therapy, if you desire to use Ukrain, you will have to seek an alternative health physician in the United States, Canada, or Europe for Ukrain therapy. It is a sad fact that since it **isn't toxic to healthy cells**, it is not widely promoted in the U.S.

2009 update: note that because Ukrain is not authorized in Austria, this article is no longer located at *www.ukrin.com*. The website has been changed and is now called *Nowicky Pharma*. You can read this information about Ukrain now in the book: *Anti-Cancer Agent Ukrain—The Crime Story of an Obstruction*, by Eleonore Thun-Hohenstein. Also, see website: *http://www.ukrain-drug.net/papers/153.htm*, for information regarding Ukrain and pancreatic cancer. For pictures showing how Ukrain works, see website: *http://www.ukrain-drug.net/webspeed/index.htm*.

## Vitamin B6 Halts Pancreatic Cancer & Folate (B9 or Folic Acid) Cuts Risk for This Type Cancer

Laboratory tests indicate that vitamin B6 is important in halting the progression of pancreatic cancer. Extensive testing in humans has not yet been done (307). A human study, as reported in the *Journal of the National Cancer Institute* (Mar. 2006), involved "81,922 men and women from Sweden, for an average of 6.8 years," to see if there is a link between folate intake and the risk for pancreatic cancer (601b). Scientists discovered that the participants who ingested "more than 350 micrograms of folate from food per day," were "75% less likely to develop pancreatic cancer" in comparison to those who took "less than 200 micrograms per day" (601b). They found that the best protection came not from folate *supplements*, but from natural foods containing *folate* (601b), showing once again, that we cannot improve upon what our Great Creator God has given us! Some natural food sources of folic acid include: citrus, leafy greens (e.g., *spinach, lettuce, kale, and turnip greens*), *eggs*, *peanuts*, *corn*, fortified cereals (601b), and steel cut oats.

## Vitamin C Lowers Risk for Pancreatic Cancer

When researchers in Europe studied nearly 200 human cases and compared pancreatic cancer rates, they discovered lower rates of this type cancer among people consuming vitamin C-rich foods, and those limiting unhealthy fats in their diet (551). There are also impressive success stories of people healing their pancreatic cancer with mega-doses of vitamin C (given intravenously).

An email friend of mine was diagnosed with pancreatic cancer in December 2004. She immediately started taking megadose vitamin C (intravenously through an alternative health care practitioner). She is currently cancer-free. She started with "50 gm three days a week; went to four days a week, then 5 days a week." In her words, she said that she "felt wonderful the whole time and kept working without any side effects except the first few days when" she was "detoxing." She reports that "I continue to feel great and go once a week." (This is also known as Orthomolecular Medicine.) When last tested at the end of April 2005, her doctor claimed that he must have "made a mistake" (in the original diagnosis). All her tests are negative; she is cancer-free.

## Vitamin D Reduces Risk of Pancreatic Cancer 43%

A human study, described in the September 2006 issue of *Cancer Epidemiology Biomarkers & Prevention,* found that taking as little as *400 IU*/day of this vitamin could cut the risk for pancreatic cancer by 43%. Those taking under *150 IU*/day cut their risk by 22%. Individuals taking more than the *400 IU*/day did not seem to have an advantage. This study reaffirms other research, which shows that populations getting adequate sunshine (which triggers the natural production of vitamin D in the skin) have much lower incidence for not only pancreatic cancers, but also breast and colon cancers (308). Most people need about ten to twenty minutes a day (at least three times weekly) of natural sunshine (without sunscreen) for vitamin D synthesis. Current research is also showing that sufficient vitamin D can extend the lives of colon cancer patients. Always check with your physician or Naturopath about individualized sun exposure.

## Zapping Pancreatic Cancer Cells with Two Simple & Safe Treatments – ALA & Naltrexone

A **human** study carried out by B.M. Berkson, D.M. Rubin and A.C. Berkson proved that even a deadly pancreatic cancer (that had already spread to the liver) could be stopped and reversed! This was done by using intravenous ALA (alpha lipoic acid) and **low dose** Naltrexone. For details, see the full article at National Library of Medicine PubMed website. PMID 16484716 (344b).

## ZoonCan for Pancreatic Cancers

ZoonCan, also known by its Chinese name of *Zhongjiefeng Pian,* is an herbal remedy which contains *Herba sarcandrae* or *Sarcandra glaber (Thunb) Nakai,* and may be important in helping the body fight cancers, especially those of the pancreas, colon and rectal area. It has also been used in human studies for several other cancers. For more details, see website: *4uherb.com/cancer/colorectal/treat.htm* (63a).

# CHAPTER 13

# GENTLE CURES FOR TOUGH BLADDER & KIDNEY CANCERS

*"He sent his word, and healed them, and delivered them from their destructions." (Psalm 107:20)*

## Newer, Gentler Diagnostics for Bladder Cancer

The best way (in the past) for your physician to diagnose bladder cancer was usually by doing a painful cystoscopy in order to get a biopsy sample of the tissue lining the bladder (553a). There are newer, less invasive diagnostic tests coming available (some already are) that merely require a urine sample to check for bladder cancer, though your physician may still decide to confirm diagnosis with a cystoscopy, if these tests show positive (553a). Some of these tests include: "BTA STAT, NMP22, fibrin-fibrinogen degradation products (FDP), and telomerase," as well as "chemluminescent hemoglobin, and hemoglobin dipstick…" (553a). Reports, thus far, indicate that the "Urinary telomerase" has "outperformed" other urine screening tests (553a); however, be aware that newer products are coming on the market and being approved by the FDA on a regular basis.

It is expected that within the next 12-24 months, *UroSens*, a simple blood test that can help find bladder cancer, and may also help in diagnosing other cancers, such as oral cancers, intestinal, prostate, and cervical cancers, will be on the market (284a).

## Astragalus Inhibits the Spread of Kidney Cancer

Astragalus is an herb that enhances the body's immunity. It may be important in preventing kidney cancer (172) because it activates a gene which prevents abnormal cells from spreading. Check with your physician or Naturopath about using this herb, especially if you have an infection or are running a temperature (36).

## Berberine for Bladder Cancer

Herbs that contain this substance fight inflammation in the body and may help the immune system fight cancer of the bladder (58). *Herbs2000.com* recommends that you do **not** take goldenseal, other herbs that have berberine, or similar herbs longer than *two weeks*, nor should it be used for those who have bile disorders or may be pregnant. It is also advised not to use this herb in combo with *vitamin B6* or with *histidine*, nor for those with *glaucoma* or heart problems, lung problems, or blood pressure disorders (83).

## Broccoli Sprouts Fight Bladder Cancer

Scientists found that they could slash the risk of *bladder cancer* in *half* simply by feeding test animals a substance from *broccoli sprouts* that had been *freeze dried* (making it more concentrated); further proof that cruciferous vegetables could save your life (49). The substance responsible is known as *ITC* or *isothyiocyanates,* powerful plant chemicals found in these vegetables that seem to target bladder cells. They found that *broccoli sprouts* "have approximately 30 times more" ITCs than broccoli that is fully-grown (49). The *freeze dried extract* that the researchers used in their study had *600 times as much* ITC as the sprouts (49). Cooking your broccoli and other cruciferous veggies destroys the ITC.

Here is something to be greatly concerned about: the FDA is now undertaking a plan to irradiate ALL fruits and vegetables! Irradiating food destroys all the vitamins and enzymes! You might as well shoot it, because it will certainly be dead! This is one reason why many nutritionists are against microwaving food. They say that microwaving also destroys some of the nutritional benefits in food.

## BCG—*Bacillus Calmette-Guerin* for Inoperable Upper Urinary Tract Cancers

For a report on the successful use of BCG (Bacillus Calmette-Guerin) for *upper urinary tract urothelial tumors* in humans, see the U.S. Library of Medicine NCBI, PubMed study at PMID #12352398. The results, involving 37 patients, revealed that "BCG perfusion therapy of the upper urinary tract for papillary tumors or carcinoma in situ," for those who could not undergo *radical surgery,* could extend their lives, though the only ones that experienced a cure were those with *carcinoma in situ* (578).

Though this treatment has some potentially adverse effects, it is being mentioned in this book because—for some patients who are inoperable—it might help prevent them from needing to resort to dialysis and may even "cure those with carcinoma in situ of the upper urinary tract" (578). BCG is used in many countries to vaccinate against TB.

## Burzynski's Non-Toxic Antineoplastons for Curing Bladder Cancers

Stanislaw R. Burzynski, M.D., Ph.D., working with peptides and amino acids, developed *peptide fractions* that he believed would treat cancer effectively. These came to be known as *antineoplastons*. He manufactured the non-toxic substances in his own lab and eagerly shared his findings with other scientists (505). When he gave more than a dozen patients with cancer of the bladder his antineoplastons, the results were amazing. They were all treated, then studied over the next decade. At the study's completion, the following results were reported: out of the original 19 participants, *thirteen* were in complete "remission…two [in] partial remission…one [had] stable disease [and] three" were advancing in the disease. Antineoplastons have been found to be safe and non-toxic, even in large doses (505). Note that they are **not** the same as antineoplastics.

Dr. Burzynski's story is an interesting one. He has had a great deal of success in treating cancer patients, and many of them diagnosed as *terminal*, he has completely cured, but he has spent a good portion of his life fighting constant harassment by the modern medical establishment in much the same way that Rene Caisse did. Apparently, their success rate against cancer made those who were promoting toxic treatments uncomfortable. After much struggle, the FDA has finally approved the oral form of antineoplastons (PBs or sodium phenylbutrates) for off-label use. Note that both antineoplastons A10 and AS2-1 were recently given orphan drug status for use on human brainstem gliomas.

## Cat's Claw Fights Bladder Cancer

Cat's claw herb enhances the body's natural immunity against cancer cells. See other chapters in this book for when you should not use this herb.

## Chlorine Causes Bladder Cancer

You can greatly add to your health risks by drinking water containing chlorine or fluoride. Some excellent filters are available that keep unwanted chemicals out of your drinking water, as well as the option of using spring water or distilled water. See chapter 23 of this book for more information on the importance of adequate water consumption. Recent reports have admitted that common tap water has become contaminated with residues of prescription drugs!

## Cholesterol Drug for Kidney Cancer - No Toxic Side Effects

For detailed information on a new cancer-treatment regimen that includes combining "low-dose interferon with lovastatin," so far used in melanoma, but also being considered for other cancers like kidney cancer (76a), see website: *www.neoplas.org*, and chapter 34 in this book. Doctors saw tumors start to regress—often in *a few weeks*. The treatment has no toxic side effects, as found in chemo and *radiation* (76a). Be aware that statin drugs can strip CoQ10 out of your body. If your doctor chooses this treatment, let them know this so that they can advise you on CoQ10 supplementation. Some physicians are not aware of this statin side effect.

## CyberKnife® Therapy for Bladder & Kidney Tumors

See chapter 34 in this book for details on CyberKnife® therapy, which is being used successfully for kidney cancers and many other cancers, including hard-to-reach brain tumors. It is a gentle, painless procedure that does not require an incision, surgery, sedation or inpatient stay. It takes very little time, and as soon as the procedure is over, the patient is able to return home. There are very few risks and side effects, though it does involve some radiation (89a), and it can damage nearby healthy cells. Also, see NanoKnife™, chapter 34.

## Cytotron Therapy

A new cancer (and arthritis) treatment developed and available in India that you will not yet be able to get in the U.S., is being successfully used on humans and is known as *Cytotron Therapy*. It is gentle, completely painless, and non-toxic. See chapter 34 in this book for more details on Cytotron, also known as *QMR* or *Quantum Magnetic Resonance* (90).

## EFAs (Essential Fatty Acids) & Bladder Cancer

When a group of urologists from Aberdeen Royal Infirmary compared blood from nearly 100 people (with cancer of the bladder) to the general population, they found that those with bladder cancer were lacking efficient levels of fatty acids, thus showing that lower amounts of these EFAs may greatly contribute to the incidence of bladder cancer in humans (504). According to Siegfried Gursche in his book, *Good Fats and Oils,* some natural sources of essential fatty acids are: "unrefined pumpkinseed oil," unrefined "walnut oil…[and] flax seed oil," to name a few. These oils (pumpkinseed, flax and walnut) should never be heated (416). Always choose organic. A few other essential fatty acid sources include fish oils, borage oil, perilla oil, evening primrose oil, krill oil, and avocados. The best fish are Atlantic mackerel, wild salmon, tilapia, and sardines. Avoid *farm raised* salmon, tile fish, swordfish, king mackerel, wild striped bass and blue fish. If you eat tuna, it is best to get the organic chunk light, not the white or albacore. (One of the healthiest and richest sources of omega-3 is krill oil.)

## Essiac Tea for All Cancers

See chapter six for more information on this healing, herbal tea. I would not hesitate to recommend this tea remedy to anyone fighting cancer. Rene Caisse, a Canadian nurse, healed hundreds (possibly thousands) of people of every imaginable cancer over several decades, using her remarkable herbal tea formula, many of whom came to her after conventional medicine considered them hopeless.

One of the most amazing books describing the effectiveness of this tea and how it was suppressed by the health industry in Canada is called: *The Essiac Report Canada's Remarkable Unknown Cancer Remedy,* by Richard Thomas, who claims that Flor-Essence® is the original (drinkable) formula that Rene Caisse used (580).

Note that there is some competition between the tea produced by Resperin Canada Essiac® and Flor-Essence® Essiac tea. Both companies claim that they have the original Essiac formula (the drinkable formula, not the injectable) that Rene Caisse used in treating her cancer patients.

See chapter 16 in this book for the story of a young boy who was cured of lymphoma using a natural program that included Essiac® Resperin Canada's tea formula and 714X injections. A website that has Resperin Canada Essiac® is also given in that chapter. You can find both brands (and others) at health food stores and internet sites.

## Fungus Cure Also Cures Cancer, Says Oncology Physician

See chapter 34 of this book for the amazing cancer cure that Italian Oncologist, Dr. Simoncini, is using to cure his cancer patients within just days! Cancerous growths are usually WHITE. He says that they are actually a fungus, which can be killed with a non-toxic soda bicarb solution that quickly alkalizes the tumor for destruction (582).

## High Fruit & Vegetable Intake Dramatically Decreases Risk for Bladder Cancer

An *analysis* that involved *38 research studies* on the effects of food and bladder health, according to the *American Journal of Epidemiology* (April 2000), discovered that deficient amounts of *fruit and vegetables* and *high fat* in the diet were the main risk factors (601a) for bladder disease. How risky are we speaking? *Low* levels of *fruit* in your diet, for example, will increase your risk for bladder cancer by *40%*. Too much unhealthy *fat*, and your risk goes up by *37%*. Too little veggies increase the risk by *16%* (601a).

## Garlic Fights Bladder Cancer

Aged garlic extract was found, in U.S. testing on animals, to be better at fighting cancer of the bladder than the cancer vaccine "BCG" *(Bacillus Calmette-Guerin)* (363). Multiple animal tests have proven that not only can garlic boost the immunity for fighting cancer, but it can also *reverse* the abnormal cells that have already formed (363). Japanese researchers were able to cure breast cancers in mice with *fresh garlic*, and they were further amazed to find that garlic out-performed vitamin E's ability at reversing trauma to the liver. Garlic is so potent that doctors in China have even used it to cure a normally fatal form of *cryptococcal meningitis* (363). Also, scientists studying the spice found that, when taken by mouth, garlic can suppress a highly destructive type of malignant bladder growth.

## Grapes (Resveratrol) & Bladder Cancer

Chicago researchers noted, in the journal *Science*, that resveratrol can halt the development of cancer during any of its three stages of formation (130). Resveratrol is found naturally in grape juice and pomegranates and is also available in supplemental tablet form (130). See chapter three (in this book) for more information on resveratrol and how Johanna Brandt cured her own abdominal cancer without chemo, surgery, or radiation by using common table grapes and a raw food diet. Reservatrol supplements are now available in most health food stores and internet sites. Do not consume raw meat or fish. Those who consume a steady diet of cooked meats and processed meats increase their risk for nearly all cancers, including liver, colorectal, esophageal, and lung cancer.

## Graviola

See chapters five and six for this and other herbs that have been used effectively in fighting cancer.

## Green Tea Fights Bladder Cancer

Impressive animal studies have shown that injections of EGCG (an extract found in green tea) destroyed 64% of their bladder tumors. All of the animals not receiving the green tea extract experienced rapidly growing tumors. The report was published in *The Journal of Urology* September 2003 (134). More recently, research shows that green tea can help regenerate brain cells, something scientists hitherto thought impossible (169). Also, recent **human** studies verify that drinking green tea can slash the risk for bladder cancers.

## Indoles - Vegetables That Can Save Your Life

Cruciferous vegetables, those containing indoles, such as cabbage, cauliflower and kohlrabi, are important for keeping bladder cancer patients in remission (36). Recent studies, involving nearly 48,000 male participants, revealed that having several servings of these cruciferous veggies every week can significantly reduce the incidence of this type of cancer (36). (These were **human**, not animal studies.)

## Intravesical Immunotherapy for Superficial Bladder Cancer

In this procedure, the bladder is treated with medication (most commonly BCG, *Bacille Calmette-Guerin*), which is inserted via a tube into the bladder itself. Side effects may include blood in the urine, irritation and fever, which are usually temporary. A very small percentage (1%) of people may develop TB from the procedure (164). (Also, see info on BCG earlier in this chapter.)

## IP6 - Inositol Hexaphosphate & Bladder Cancer

Cancer cells use a lot of iron and must have iron to survive. Drugs that remove iron from the body, thus fighting cancer cells, also have adverse side effects; however, IP6 effectively robs cancer cells of iron without depleting the body's natural stores of iron. It is a safe ingredient, without the high toxicity of chemo drugs, and relatively inexpensive. Extensive human trials have yet to be done on IP6 (554), though many people are using the substance. This natural nutrient, derived from rice bran, is also discussed in other chapters of this book.

## LifeMel Honey for Cancer Patients

This amazing honey is also discussed in chapter 29. It is a special honey (developed in Israel) produced from the nectar of 40 herbs, including *Echinacea, Siberian ginseng,* and *Uncaria tomentosa,* with other natural ingredients. Two teaspoons per day (one in the am and one in the pm) are recommended (614). This special honey has shown the ability, in **human** testing, to prevent the neutropenia (serious drop in white blood cells) caused by chemotherapy and to lower the risk of severe platelet drop (thrombocytopenia), often found in chemo patients (614). You can find out more about this protective honey at website: *http://www.lifemel israel.com* (614). You will see LifeMel in specialty health food stores and internet sites.

## Magnesium & Iodine for Cancer Prevention

These minerals are critical for the prevention of all types of cancer, including leukemia, and those involving the stomach, prostate, breast, and bones (566). Also, see page 129.

## Mushrooms That Fight Cancer

**Shiitake** mushrooms have been the focus of much research and are popular in Japan for abdominal cancers. One of their extracts, lentinan, discussed elsewhere in this book, revealed significant anti-cancer properties, in test animals. Lentinan is usually given as an injection by alternative health care providers, so it isn't exactly what I would consider *gentle* or *painless,* however, it is a natural substance, and is being included here for its non-toxic benefits to the immune system. Its ability to fight viruses was demonstrated, in one particular case, when an AIDS patient went into complete remission after receiving lentinan injections. **Maitake** mushroom may help reduce the incidence of bladder cancer return after surgery (36). Maitake should not be taken by those with *multiple sclerosis.* It can increase a substance that destroys nerve tissue in people with MS (184). Also, see below for info on the polyporus mushroom. Note that oyster mushrooms have been found to fight colon and breast cancers.

## Onconase—New Non-Toxic Drug for Kidney Cancer

Onconase (aka *Ranpirnase*) is a new pharmaceutical drug developed for treating mesothelioma, and is claimed not to have the adverse effects that are normally seen in common chemo drugs (222). It is said to work on other cancers, such as those of the kidneys. It was developed by a company known as *Alfacell* (222). The drug is also supposed to make it possible to give lower dosages of standard chemo drugs with the same cancer-killing effects. It is said to fight *solid tumor cancers,* such as *carcinomas*, as well as those of the *kidney, breast, lung, and prostate* (222). Just be aware that even though this new drug is said to be relatively free of toxic side effects, drugs such as this are sometimes combined with conventional chemo drugs that **do** have toxic side effects. Human trials are currently underway on Ranpirnase.

## PH & Bladder Cancer

See chapter 30 of this book for the story of a cancer patient who was completely cured of Stage III bladder cancer, simply by changing his body's high acidity level to an alkaline pH. Just remember that cooking food increases its acidity, and the acid effect on the body. Raw foods are much more alkaline and have an alkaline effect on the body. Constant stress will also reduce the body's alkalinity. It will do little good to consume a raw diet for alkalinity if you are overwhelmed with stress, which has an acidic effect on the body.

## Poly–MVA for Bladder Cancers

See chapter 14 for more information on this palladium lipoic acid complex that contains vitamins, alpha lipoic acid, and amino acids that many cancer survivors are crediting to bringing about total remission from their cancers; some even sent home to die, who recovered completely using this nutritional drink. Their main website is: *www.polymva.net.*

## Polyporus Umbellatus Mushroom for Recurring Bladder Cancer

This immune-boosting mushroom is one of ten mushrooms found in *Garden of Life's RM-10* product developed by Jordan Rubin (317). His 80 year-old grandmother used the product to heal her advanced ovarian cancer. See chapter six and website: *http://www.crohns.net/Miva/education/testimonial_rosemenlowe.shtml* (30). It has also been helpful for those with urinary tract infections, and may help the immune system in stopping the spread of leukemia (317). For information and resources where you can obtain RM-10, see website: *http://www.crohns.net/Miva/productinfo/whatsinRM10.shtml* (317). This mushroom has also been helpful in cutting in half the reoccurrence of **bladder cancer** in a test involving 146 **human** participants (317).

## Rexin-G™ for Pancreatic Cancer & Metastatic Cancers

Rexin-G™ has been undergoing clinical trials at Mayo Clinic, M.D. Anderson, and a few other facilities. It is a drug for cancers that have spread, and those types of cancer that conventional medicine says do not respond to chemo (256). Human clinical studies, thus far, have had good results. In the very first **human** trial, 83% of the patients experienced tumor shrinkage. The patients all had spreading pancreatic cancer (256). Good responses were also achieved in **human** studies involving several other types of metastatic cancer. Due to the reports, this drug is now used for treating all forms of *solid tumors* in the Philippines that are resistant to conventional therapy (256). The U.S. FDA has given the drug its *orphan drug status* (meaning it is okay to use for rare diseases) for use with pancreatic cancers in the US, as well as other types of cancer metastases, which also means that trials will continue (256). It is given intravenously, so isn't exactly natural or painless, but could be considered gentler than older chemo drugs because it is said to be a non-chemo drug, showing itself in **human** clinical trials, not to have the adverse side effects normally associated with chemo drugs (256). You can get more information on this drug at *epeiusbiotech.com/rexin_g-factsheet.asp*. Epeius Biotechnologies are the producers of Rexin-G™ (257).

## Rhodiola Rosea—A Simple Herb for Bladder Cancer

Rhodiola Rosea is an herb from Siberia with an odor much like that of *roses*, says *planetherbs.com*, hence its name. It is very popular in Asia for treating many ailments, including stress-related issues and high cholesterol. It is also used for performance improvement in athletes, hearing improvement, blood sugar regulation, liver protection and cancer prevention (259). Rhodiola is a very powerful anti-oxidant. Researchers in Russia discovered that oral ingestion could prevent the formation of tumors, as well as their spread (in animal testing). In **humans**, the herb not only boosted the immunity of patients with tumors of the bladder, but it also extended the lives of those with lung and breast cancer (259). You can find rhodiola in many health food stores and internet sites.

## Saw Palmetto Fights Kidney Cancer

Saw Palmetto, long popular for fighting prostate problems, was shown in a 1997 study, to help fight pancreatic and kidney growths (547).

## Selenium & Bladder Cancer

Though cigarette smoking greatly increases the risk for bladder cancer, **human** studies show that including selenium in the diet can decrease the risk for this type cancer.

## Shark Cartilage

See other chapters in this book, including chapters seven and fourteen, for further information on how shark cartilage has been used to fight various cancers and their spread. Also, see chapter 34 of this book for information on an herb (known as *bindweed)* that is said to have *100 times* the ability at blocking blood vessel formation, which starves tumors, as that found in shark cartilage (150).

## Skullcap Extract—Baicalein Against Bladder Cancer & Prostate Cancer

An extract from the Chinese herb skullcap (baicalein), in laboratory and animal testing, inhibited bladder cancer cells (488). The extract was also used in **human** studies to help stabilize and extend the lives of prostate cancer patients (488).

## Ukrain Effective Against Bladder Cancer

Ukrain, discussed in many other cancer-specific chapters of this book, is a cancer treatment composed of two ingredients, both of which are toxic individually, but once combined, they are toxic only to cancer cells (287). A **human** research study was conducted using Ukrain on 28 patients having bladder cancer (588). They were split into three groups of 9, 10, and 9. The first group was given *100 mg of Ukrain*; the second group, *200 mg;* and the third group *300 mg* (all received the Ukrain *I.V.* at *10 mg per day*). The final result was that more than half of all patients experienced *complete or partial regression of tumors.* Details of the study can be seen at the U.S. National Library of Medicine website under PMID 10190079, or go to this website: *http://www.ncbi.nlm.nih.gov/pubmed/10190079?ordinalpos=1&itool=EntrezSystem2.PEntrez.PubMed.PubMedResultsPanel.Pubmed_RVAbstractPlus* (588).

It is noteworthy that with most drugs, the dosage between what is therapeutic and what becomes toxic is a slim margin. This is not the case with Ukrain. Unlike toxic chemotherapy, **human testing has revealed no adverse side effects from Ukrain** (287). This treatment is only available at alternative therapy clinics in the U.S. and Europe.

2009 update: note that because Ukrain is not authorized in Austria, their website has changed and is now called *Nowicky Pharma.* You can read this info about Ukrain now in the book: *Anti-Cancer Agent Ukrain—The Crime Story of an Obstruction,* by Eleonore Thun-Hohenstein. See *www.ukrin.com* for more information. Also, for pictures of how Ukrain works, see website: *http://www.ukrain-drug.net/webspeed/index.htm.*

## Ukrain Heals Renal Cancer in Human Study

A human case study of a man with renal cancer, who received chemo and underwent surgery, can be found at the U.S. National Library of Medicine, Institute of Health PubMed website PMID 11345035. The chemo didn't work. His cancer progressed into his liver and *vena cava inferior.* He was then given Ukrain therapy and experienced a total remission, which at last report, was more than three years ago (529).

## Ukrain for Successful Treatment of Urethral Cancer

A **human** study, involving the use of Ukrain for urethral cancer, can also be found at *www.pubmed.gov.* The case report describes a patient who underwent surgery for urethral cancer. Two months later, the cancer returned. Rather than choosing another surgery, the patient was given only Ukrain therapy. Within four months, there was no trace of cancer, nor three years later. The case ID is 8899346 (441).

## Vitamin C Megadosing for Advanced Bladder Cancer

In a report from Irwin Stone, presented to his colleagues 14 February, 1976, as described in the website article from Dr. Stone, "The Genetics of Scurvy and the Cancer Problem," he tells of a bladder cancer patient, an adult male, whose cancer had spread "to the spine at the level of the 10th thoracic vertebra" (571a). After having the tumor removed, the "patient [was] completely paraplegic" (571a):

> The report says that 'He was put on 50,000 mg of ascorbate and to quote the doctor, 'he is now coming along beautifully.' There has been a return of bladder and bowel function and the patient is now able to walk with braces. The cancers are under control and dormant. During the day, the patient takes the powdered ascorbic acid and sodium ascorbate, and at bedtime takes eight of the time-release ascorbic acid tablets' (571a).

## Vitamin C for Bladder Cancer Prevention

Bladder cancer occurs more commonly in smokers than in nonsmokers. At the end of the sixties, researchers from Tulane University discovered that large doses of vitamin C can help eliminate the carcinogens that promote cancer of the bladder in people who smoke (549). For purposes of the study, the vitamin was given in split dosages of 500 mg (3 x per day or 1500 mg total). The results of the study prompted Dr. Schlegel to suggest such a regimen for those susceptible to bladder cancer, e.g., cigarette-smokers (549). Natural vitamin C can be found in leafy green vegetables, rose hips, currants, fresh sprouts, cruciferous vegetables, chlorella, spirulina, berries, citrus fruits, pomegranate, and some types of lettuce, as well as many other fruits and vegetables.

When choosing your vitamin C, if you use supplements (rather than natural food sources), it is best to choose natural derivatives from acerola or rose hips (ascorbic acid) rather than the sodium ascorbate form of vitamin C. The sodium ascorbate may aggravate *symptoms* (36). The ascorbic acid form of vitamin C (as opposed to the sodium ascorbate form) also keeps the urine acidic and will help prevent bladder infections, however, some people cannot tolerate the acidity of ascorbic acid. Either take it with food or use the less acidic *Ester-C*®. Even taken with food, large amounts of ascorbic acid can cause diarrhea. This diarrhea effect will diminish as the body grows more tolerant to larger levels. When given intravenously, most people have no uncomfortable side effects in massive doses, e.g., some as large as 130 grams per day. Try to get your vitamin C without additives like magnesium stearate and titanium dioxide, and it is best to use the entire form of vitamin C, not just the ascorbic acid.

Many elderly people in nursing homes (with catheters) could be greatly helped by giving them 1000 mg/day of vitamin C and plenty of water to help prevent bladder and kidney infections. I have a friend in an assisted-living center who nearly died from a kidney infection. She had been on every antibiotic imaginable and none of them were helping. When I asked her doctor to try her on 1000 mg./day of ascorbic acid, and he did so, she improved rapidly. Her infection cleared and she has never had another kidney infection. This was several years ago. She continues to take the same dosage of vitamin C daily and drinks plenty of fresh water. (Dr. Irwin Stone, a pioneer in studying scurvy and vitamin C, believed that most humans need much larger amounts of vitamin C a day than this.) Be sure, in taking vitamin C, that you are also getting plenty of B vitamins and magnesium. See chapter 34 for more details on vitamin C and most importantly, see page 544 on the amazing new *liposome-encapsulated vitamin C*, which a physician used to heal dengue fever.

## Vitamin D & Sunlight Inhibit Cancer Spread

There are so many warnings about sunlight causing skin cancer that many people are going overboard and avoiding any sun exposure whatsoever, forgetting that the sun is our most natural, important source of **vitamin D.** When sunlight hits the skin, a natural process occurs that creates vitamin D in our bodies. We need about 10—20 minutes of sunlight (without sunscreen) every single day for vitamin D synthesis, because it also boosts the immune system and helps normalize blood pressure. This is why it is so easy to fall asleep when you are lying on a beach sunbathing. Sunshine lowers blood pressure, stimulates the immune system, and it relaxes you.

Vitamin D may be important in preventing renal cancer from spreading, as well as preventing tumor formation in the kidneys (172). Some parents are becoming so over-anxious about bundling up their children against the sun, there is an alarming increase in this country of ricketts—a bone growth disorder caused by a lack of vitamin D in the diet—especially critical for children with their fast-growing bones. Check with your physician or Naturopath as well, especially if there is a genetic tendency in your family (or history) for skin cancer.

## Vitamin E Protects Against Bladder & Prostate Cancer

New research shows that vitamin E can help fight several types of cancer, including those of the bladder and prostate (524). A controlled study showed that increasing dietary amounts of *alpha-tocopherol* (vitamin E) could cut bladder cancer in half. Researchers also concluded that the gamma and alpha-forms of tocopherols cut prostate cancers by *53 percent and 39 percent* (524). Note that some research has shown that the gamma-tocopherol form of vitamin E is more powerful at cancer prevention than the alpha-tocopherol, however, the alpha form is most easily used by the body. If the alpha-tocopherol is the only kind you are able to find, at least be sure you use the d-alpha tocopherol and not the dl-alpha tocopherol which is synthetic, and more difficult for the cells to absorb. It is best to get the mixed tocopherols in natural foods or supplements, rather than synthetic, along with the tocotrienols. Good food sources of vitamin E are wheat germ oil, olive oil, sunflower oil (and seeds); dandelion greens, spinach, broccoli, turnip greens; almonds and other nuts; eggs (411) (492), kiwi, and mangoes; fortified cereals and fresh sprouts; especially wheat berry sprouts.

## Vitamin Combo Therapy for Bladder Cancer

When researchers gave patients with this type cancer 40,000 IU of vitamin A every day (as well as *B6 (100 mg), C (2000 mg), and E (400 IU)*, they experienced a dramatic decrease in tumors *(40%)* over those not taking the supplements, plus their life span doubled! This study was reported in *Earl Mindell's What You Should Know About The Super Antioxidant Miracle.* It was concluded that the vitamin therapy probably lowered the incidence of recurrence often found in these type cancers (492). It is important to note in this study (and the one discussed below), that we are talking about clinical trials involving **humans,** not lab mice.

In another controlled study to determine the efficacy of using mega-dose vitamins for 65 bladder cancer patients (conducted at the West Virginia School of Medicine), participants were treated with a common cancer vaccine known as BCG (507). (BCG is a weakened strain of the microbe that is administered in TB vaccinations.) They gave 30 of the patients the recommended daily allowances of anti-oxidants, and the rest were given megadoses, which were not particularly large amounts, e.g., two grams of vitamin C (507). Although the recurrence for bladder cancer is usually very high, less than a year later, the recurrence of bladder cancer in those receiving the megadoses were dropping. Five years later, those taking high dose vitamins experienced less than half as many reoccurrences as those given the lower dosages. By the completion of the study, eighty percent of those not receiving the mega-doses relapsed, and forty percent of the rest developed reoccurrence of tumors (507). This was startling evidence, in a **human trial,** that giving bladder cancer patients mega vitamin/mineral doses, slashed their cancer recurrence rate by nearly half (507). **(Yet, how many bladder cancer patients do you think are being placed on a mega-dose, anti-oxidant therapy**

**program like the one described above to keep their cancer from recurring?)**

It is important to realize that if you take high doses of synthetic vitamins (e.g., vitamin A and D), you should be monitored by a physician. These are *fat-soluble vitamins* and they can be stored in body tissues and organs and cause toxicity if excessive amounts are taken (507). One way that you can avoid this problem (e.g., in the case of vitamin A), is to take natural sources of beta-carotene, such as fresh carrot juice or chlorella, which the body then converts into NATURAL vitamin A. In the case of vitamin D, get natural sunshine.

Many alternative physicians are providing vitamin mega-dosing for their cancer patients, otherwise known as *Orthomolecular Medicine.* It is also good news that there are some conventional physicians now using complementary medicine, and after many years of public outcry, a few pharmaceutical companies are working at producing less toxic drugs for cancer.

Also, see page 544 of this book for the amazing breakthrough promoted by Dr. Thomas Levy on an oral form of vitamin C, known as *liposome-encapsulated vitamin C* (466b). That page will also tell you where you can find this new form of vitamin C (*Lypo-Spherion*™). Dr. Levy has used only 10-12 packets of this new vitamin C to cure a woman of hemorrhagic dengue fever! He says that 5-6 grams of this oral vitamin C is more potent than *50 grams* given intravenously due to its excellent total absorption by the body at the cellular level (466b). If you know someone who is desperately ill and cannot get to a physician for intravenous vitamin C therapy, this new oral *liposome-encapsulated Vitamin C*, may be exactly what they need!

## Water Prevents Bladder Cancer

So important to our survival, research has shown that drinking adequate water can decrease your overall risk for developing cancer. Though recent media reports said that you only need to drink water when you feel thirsty, others believe that the signal for thirst means your body is already dehydrated! Studies have shown that men who drink 88 ounces or more of water per day can cut their chance for *bladder cancer* by 50% (36). Dehydration is common in cancer patients. Years of chronic dehydration have been linked to the cause of asthma, lupus, arthritis, degenerative disc disease, and all auto-immune disorders. Be sure that the water you are drinking does not contain chlorine and fluoride. If you do not have access to a good filtration system, you may want to try a reputable spring water from your local health food store, or more inexpensive steam-distilled water. (See Chapter 23 in this book for more details on the importance of water for optimal health and disease recovery.)

# CHAPTER 14

# GENTLE CURES FOR TOUGH BRAIN CANCERS, ASTROCYTOMAS & NEUROBLASTOMAS

*"Bless the Lord, O my soul, and forget not all his benefits: Who forgiveth all thine iniquities, who healeth all thy diseases; who redeemeth thy life from destruction; who crowneth thee with loving kindness and tender mercies."* (Psalm 103:2-4)

## I. Antineoplastons - Miracle Non-Toxic Cures Used for Inoperable, "Terminal" Brain Tumors

Have you or a loved one been told that you (or they) have an inoperable brain tumor, or that you (or they) are terminal, and the type tumor that you (or they) have cannot be cured? Do not let someone convince you of that—because there are many people who have been cured of *terminal* brain cancer without chemo and without radiation. This chapter will tell you about case histories of several of them, but they are not unique or isolated cases. They are routine cures for an alternative, non-toxic cancer therapy that most cancer patients are never told about. This is a blatant *cover-up*, and make no mistake about it, it is very intentional. There is one website, in particular, where you can read about the individual case histories of more than two dozen people who were told that their brain cancer was incurable, many of them children; people who are in complete remission today, living normal, healthy lives without brain tumors.

Some of the patients initially received chemo and/or radiation, but the tumors returned. See website: *http://burzynskipatientgroup.org/stories.html.* Many of the people you will read about at this website have included their email addresses, or home addresses where you can feel free to write to them. Some of those cases are described briefly in this chapter. Antineoplastons are not always painless, since they are often given intravenously, however, they are also given in capsules in a painless, oral form known as sodium phenylbutrates or PBs. The FDA has finally approved the oral form of antineoplastons for off-label use, but you will need to ask your physician about prescribing them. Note that antineoplastons A10 and AS2-1 were recently given orphan drug status by the FDA for use on human brainstem gliomas. Some individuals can have mild side effects from antineoplastons, but they are quickly reversible, unlike toxic chemo drugs that often cause fatal adverse reactions.

## • Astrocytoma Treated Successfully with Antineoplastons

Besides treating many other types of cancer with antineoplastons and PBs, Dr. Burzynski has successfully treated pilocytic astrocytoma. See website: *http://burzynskipatientgroup.org/jonathanc.html*, for the case of a woman given two years to live (1997), who used antineoplastons to shrink a pilocytic astrocytoma. Seven years since being given a *terminal* diagnosis, she has been planning a college degree and a real estate major. Antineoplastons are sometimes first given in I.V. form and in oral form (known as sodium phenylbutrates or PBs). The oral form has been approved for off label use by the FDA. Note that antineoplastons A10 and AS2-1 were recently given orphan drug status for use on human brainstem gliomas.

## • Antineoplastons Cure Deadly Medulloblastoma in Children

**Case #1:** When a three-year-old little boy, Dustin K., was diagnosed with medulloblastoma, his parents were given little hope. This is a rare and deadly form of cancer (52). He initially had surgery, however, doctors were not able to remove all of the tumor. They wanted to follow-up with chemo and radiation, to which the parents objected. Instead, they sought treatment at the Burzynski Clinic in Houston, Texas. Dustin was treated with antineoplastons and within months, his tumor had disappeared. When it returned a short while later, he was treated again with antineoplastons, and the tumor again disappeared and has not recurred (52). He is now totally cancer-free at 13-years-of-age and living a normal, healthy life. His uncle is a practicing physician, who had advised his parents not to treat with Burzynski, initially; however, in reading the case history of this child, it is his uncle who had a change of heart, and tells part of the story. You can read the details for yourself at *http://burzynskipatientgroup.org/dustink.htm* (52). What's more, this is NOT an isolated case!

**Case #2:** Roy H. was only fifteen-months-old when he was diagnosed with this deadly brain cancer. After having a huge tumor surgically taken from his brain, his parents decided to treat the remaining two tumors (that had spread to the other side of his brain) with Dr. Burzynski's antineoplastons, rather than the chemo and radiation which Roy's pediatrician had recommended. The antineoplastons totally cured the little boy. He is now eight-years-old, enjoying school, and has had no reoccurrence of the cancer. For details on his case, see website: *http://www.burzynskipatientgroup.org/royh.htm* (53a).

- ## Atypical Teratoid/Rhabdoid Tumors of the Central Nervous System in Children

For a study using antineoplastons on this type of rare tumor, see the Burzynski Research Institute article at *http://www.burzynskiclinic.com/ph/media-corner-publications.html*, and greater details at: *http://www.burzynskiclinic.com/assets/documents/Pub_SRB_2004_Phase_II_studies_ofANP_A10_and_AS2_1_in_children_with_a_typical.pdf*, or go to the site and do a search.

- ## Malignant Rhabdoid Brain Tumor

This same website describes the story of a four-year-old little girl who was diagnosed with a rhabdoid brain tumor, Crystin S. (51), whose parents were advised that the tumor was incurable, and all they could hope for was to possibly extend her life briefly by giving both chemo and radiation at the same time, which they agreed to. The tumor initially shrank, then returned. Her parents took her to Burzynski's Clinic in Houston, Texas, for antineoplaston treatment, which ultimately resulted in a complete cure. For several months, the little girl seemed fine; however, her parents were later to find out that something dreadful had happened to her (51). The Oncologist, certain that Crystin was going to die anyway, had given her double the radiation dosage that she should have received. After being completely cured of brain cancer on Burzynski's antineoplastons, the little girl died several months later. Upon autopsy, her parents were told that her death was caused by the massive doses of chemo and radiotherapy she had been given, which had resulted in irreversible injury to her brain (51). Had the child never received chemo and radiation to begin with, she would probably still be alive today!

## • Inoperable Brain Stem Tumor Cured With Antineoplastons

Jason M. was only thirteen-years-old when he was first diagnosed with a benign inoperable brain stem tumor in 1994. Because of hydrocephalus, a shunt was inserted and he did fine until July of 2001, when the tumor had transformed into a high-grade brain stem glioma (487). When his parents were offered BBBD (a form of "intra-arterial platinum therapy," a therapy that most patients don't even live through), they opted instead to go to the Burzynski clinic in August of that year (487).

As described by Jason's mother, Patty:

> We sought opinions from several major cancer centers. John Hopkins, Brigham and Women's, Henry Ford Brain Tumor Center, University of Michigan and MD Anderson. The consensus was the same from all the doctors. Jason's condition was terminal. Radiation and chemotherapy were the recommended forms of treatment, both of which are non-curative. Success, by these doctors standards, with radiation and chemo is determined if the patient lives 3 months after the treatment. The side effects of radiation in the brain stem are devastating, plus there is the risk of radiation necrosis. Chemotherapy does not penetrate the blood brain barrier. It is accepted, but not effective in brain tumors. None of the doctors could give us a success story. Jason's local neurosurgeon told us if he were in our position, he would not radiate or do chemo because of the devastating side effects they create in terms of quality and length of life. Just "let him die" (487) [they were told].

Though none of their physicians supported the decision, they forged ahead with non-toxic antineoplastons at Dr. Burzynski's Texas clinic (487). Jason was able to live a normal lifestyle while on the antineoplastons, even having the ability to go on a safari, as told by his mom:

> In July 2002, Jason, his dad and I were sent to South Africa for a hunting safari. Jason was able to go hunting, and shot a warthog, an impala, a kudu and a zebra. He also darted a white rhino and implanted microchips in its horns to guard against poachers. All of this was done while he was on the

antineoplastins. We transported the medicine to Africa with us and continued on with the daily routine. This was a dream come true. God brought some very gracious and generous people into our lives because of this tragedy (487).

Patty describes the difficult months that lay ahead of them:

> For four months the tumor continued to grow. We spent a lot of time in prayer. There were people all around the country praying for Jason and our family. Jason was beginning to have some neurological problems because of the size of the tumor. He couldn't hear very well, his eyes were only partly open and he had a very difficult time staying awake. The FDA wanted to pull Jason out of the trial, but the doctors at the Burzynski Clinic convinced them to give Jason a little more time. Finally in December 2001, the tumor quit growing. For three months there was no change. In February the tumor started to respond. It was 20% smaller. Jason's hearing came back, his eyes opened and he was able to stay awake all day. The tumor continued to shrink. Not rapidly, but nonetheless it was getting smaller. The side effects of the antineoplastons are minimal. Watching sodium intake, drinking lots of water and taking supplements to keep the electrolytes in balance became part of the daily routine. Once the tumor began to shrink, Jason was able to resume a fairly normal life style…December 4, 2002 the MRI showed no tumor. Jason had a PET Scan in January which showed no active cancer cells. Jason continued on the infusion treatment and the next three MRI's showed no cancer. On April 21, 2003 we returned to the Burzynski Clinic. Jason is in remission (487).

By December of 2002, Jason's brain tumor had completely disappeared. He had also made several dietary changes, including the elimination of all "sugars, white flour, rice, simple carbs, dairy…" and ate "vegetables and meat." He also incorporated routine exercise into his schedule (487).

As of the most recent communication I have received from Jason and his mom (in the Summer of 2008), his cancer has never returned, he has graduated from college and has a full-time job. I have seen Jason's chart. I have seen the diagnostic tests that were done on him before and AFTER he was treated with antineoplastons. He truly is a miracle case, and fortunately for him and his parents, he was not forced against his will by the FDA and AMA to accept toxic drugs and chemo for his cancer!

- **Stage III Inoperable Anaplastic Astrocytoma Cured Without Chemo or Radiation**

See the amazing story of Jodi. G., who was completely cured of an inoperable, stage III Anaplastic Astrocytoma (brain tumor), using only Burzynski's antineoplastons (53). Jodi refused chemo and radiation because doctors never talked *cure*, to her. All they discussed was possibly extending her life. Details of her story are posted at website: *http://burzynskipatientgroup.org/jodig.htm.* Four years have passed since Jodi was diagnosed. She remains cancer-free (53).

- **Myxopapillary Ependymoma Treated Successfully With Antineoplastons**

For details on a little boy who was diagnosed with myxopapillary ependymoma and successfully treated with antineoplastons, see website: *http://burzynskipatientgroup.org/kylel.htm.*

- **More Inoperable Brain Tumors That Disappeared**

Antineoplaston treatment was devised by Stanislaw Burzynski, M.D., Ph.D., and is still being used at his Houston, Texas, clinic. It is the only place in the country that the FDA allows his treatment, apart from the fact that they have finally approved the oral form of antineoplastons (PBs or sodium phenylbutrates) for off-label use.

Dr. Burzynski found that, secondary to the body's *immune system*, there is another defense system in the body (chemically) that is programmed to protect us from abnormal cells (21). He developed a group of peptides he called *antineoplastons,* that were found to be effective against a variety of cancer cells in lab studies, yet they **were non-toxic to normal cells** (21). It is believed that antineoplastons work by causing cancer cells to revert or re-program back into normal cells. The compounds do occur naturally in humans, but for some unknown reason, at very **low levels in cancer patients**. Extensive **human** testing has been done with antineoplastons, so do not let your physician tell you that they are "experimental" or "untested"! (Also, they are not the same thing as antineoplastics.) Antineoplastics are toxic; antineoplastons are not!

Dr. Burzynski's discovery has been used successfully against "breast cancer, lymphoma, leukemia, and bone cancer," and many other cancers, and have been especially effective against malignant brain cancer cells (21). In 1988, he "treated twenty patients" diagnosed with a rapidly-advancing form of cancer growth known as *astrocytoma*. They were all in an advanced stage of the disease (21). (This is a malignant-type of brain tumor with a dismal chance of survival. Very few patients live longer than two years, once they are diagnosed.) All the patients, several of them very young children, received the antineoplastons administered (outpatient intravenously) over a seven-hour-period during the night as they slept. As a result of the treatment, most of the patients had dramatic improvements (21). Within *six weeks*, all the children and most of the adults were able to return to school or *part-time work*. There was a positive response in *80 percent* of those tested. A checkup **four years later on all of them** revealed that many were still in total remission carrying out their *normal activities* (21).

This is remarkable when you consider that every one of these people had advanced, inoperable brain cancer, yet four years later, they are all still very much alive!

Dr. Burzynski presented diagnostic MRIs to the World Research Foundation Congress (1990) of a woman with a very *fast-growing astrocytoma*. Within 60 days of antineoplaston treatment, there was obvious *shrinkage* of the tumor, and six months later, no trace of the tumor (21). Not only that, but Dr. Burzynski revealed that the space where the tumor had once been—was **completely healed over with normal brain tissue**—there were no gaping holes or shadows showing scar tissue. Five years later, the patient still has no traces of cancer and is alive and well (21).

## Antineoplastons for Glioblastoma

Glioblastoma is another very deadly and difficult-to-treat type of brain tumor. Most people survive less than a year from the time they are diagnosed. When Dr. Burzynski realized that this type of cancer was not responding to his overnight *IV drip*, he created *a small pump* device that the patient could attach to their clothes, thus, the antineoplastons could be given in continuous infusion over a 24-hour period, rather than just at night (21). One of his first patients to try the pump was a child with "a brain stem glioblastoma…" an inoperable location. He underwent radiation first and the tumor shrank initially, but then began **growing again a short time later** (21). Dr. Burzynski started the child on the pump he developed. **The brain tumor disappeared completely within**

**4 weeks, replaced by *normal, brain tissue.*** Dr. Burzynski revealed diagnostic pictures of this case in 1990 from the child's MRI results. A follow-up (three years later) showed that the child was still cancer-free. The new pump delivery system has had "favorable results in approximately 60 percent of the patients who have been treated with it" (21). This is particularly remarkable when you realize that most of the patients receiving this treatment are **terminal cases of inoperable brain cancer.** (Note that antineoplastons A10 and AS2-1 were recently given orphan drug status for use on human brainstem gliomas.)

## Antineoplastons Cure Child's Pineoblastoma

When Sophia G. was ten-and-a-half months old, she was diagnosed with pineoblastoma. Surgery removed the tumor, but it returned—and her parents were told that the only treatment available was chemo and radiation—that there was nothing else available for her. The parents knew that most children treated for brain tumors with chemo and radiation suffer irreversible brain damage, and many never recover. When they asked the Oncologist if their little girl would ever get on a bus for school, the response was "no," and when they refused the chemo and radiation, they took their little girl home, contacted Hospice, and expected to watch her die. Instead, relatives who were researching for them, discovered antineoplastons. Sophia was treated by Dr. Burzynski with antineoplastons and cured. Today she is cancer-free, normal, healthy, happy and in the first grade at school! For details on her case history, see website: *http://burzynskipatientgroup.org/sophiag.htm* (53b).

## Antineoplastons & the FDA

It is noteworthy that Dr. Burzynski has had great success at curing some of the most aggressive, deadly cancers, especially terminal patients having malignant brain cancers. I wonder how many patients in the U.S. (and other countries) diagnosed with *hopeless,* inoperable brain tumors are ever told about antineoplastons by the physicians treating them? Do YOU know someone recently diagnosed with an inoperable brain tumor? Has their physician mentioned this non-toxic, alternative treatment?

Some insurance companies are **finally** getting around to covering antineoplastons. Be prepared, however, to butt heads with the FDA if you try to pursue antineoplastons. Only those with lymphomas or malignant brain tumors can use them. Any other type of cancer and the FDA will usually tell you that you must first use chemotherapy or radiation before trying I.V. antineoplastons, even though chemo and radiation are toxic treatments, and **antineoplastons are NON-TOXIC.** Some individuals can have mild side effects from antineoplastons, but they are quickly reversible, unlike toxic chemo drugs that often cause fatal adverse reactions.

As noted earlier, the FDA has finally approved the oral form of antineoplastons (sodium phenylbutrates or PBs) for off-label use. Antineoplastons A10 and AS2-1 were recently given orphan drug status for use on human brainstem gliomas.

The FDA has vigorously attacked Burzynski from day one of his discovery. They charged that one of his patients died of blood-poisoning (from an intravenous infusion), yet the report never gave any specifics, and not at any time did Dr. Burzynski ever receive documentation of a patient of his having fatal septicemia. All studies ever done on these compounds have shown them to be safe. They are *natural products*, accepted into the cells, "even in high doses, without any of the serious side effects" found in chemotherapy agents (51). The trumped-up attack by the FDA was just one more attempt to try to find something negative, in a desperate attempt to discredit this very successful alternative cancer therapy. Their tactics over the years haven't changed in the least. They will abruptly remove an herb from every shelf in America if three people have an allergic reaction to it, yet leave a deadly drug (like Vioxx®) on the market for years even AFTER it kills thousands of people! Their hypocrisy is totally amazing!

Dr. Burzynski's story has been mainly a *fight to survive* since he has had to spend a great deal of his time and finances fighting legal and political battles "brought against him by the FDA, the American Cancer Society, National Cancer Institute, large insurance companies [and], the medical board and health department of Texas…" However, during this same period of time, he has gained global fame for his work. Clinical trials are still being conducted around the world with his discovery (21).

During the time that Maryjo Siegel testified before the U.S. House of Representatives Government Reform and Oversight Committee (February 4, 1998), in defense of Dr. Burzynski, this is what was reported to the committee by another physician, Dr. Nicolas Patronas, when he was asked about Dr. Burzynski's non-toxic antineoplastons:

> **Dr. Nicolas Patronas, Chief of Neuroradiology at the National Cancer Institute, testified under oath that antineoplastons are the most effective treatment for brain tumors he has ever seen**

> [emphasis added]. Top oncologists have lauded Dr. Burzynski's work, including those at the University of Washington and Georgetown University. Doctors and scientists around the world eagerly await the approval of antineoplastons. [In 1991] Dr. Michael Friedman [past] commissioner of the FDA, wrote that "Antineoplastons deserve a closer look…the human brain tumor responses are real." So why is the FDA so determined to impede the progress of a drug with such promising results (562)?

Antineoplastons are given intravenously and PBs are taken orally. PBs are converted by the liver into antineoplastons. See Burzynski's Clinic website at: *www.burzynskiclinic.com.* Additional information can also be found at: *www.curezone.com.* At Burzynski Patient Group website: *http://burzynskipatientgroup.org/stories.html,* you can also read the case histories of more than 38 people with brain tumors, glioblastomas, astrocytoma, astrocytoma III, anaplastic astrocytoma, brain stem gliomas, ependymoma, pineoblastoma, and neuroblastoma, brought into remission with antineoplastons and PBs. There are also case histories of remarkable remissions in many other cancers at this website, including: multiple myeloma, lymphocytic lymphoma, non-Hodgkins lymphoma, prostate cancer, breast cancer, ovarian cancer, and esophageal cancer. There is even a case history of a patient who has had good results using antineoplastons with a rare type of lymphocytic lymphoma known as *Waldenstrom's* macroglobulinemia (see website *http://burzynskipatientgroup.org/margaretl.htm*), and a patient whose lupus was brought into remission (see website: *http://burzynskipatientgroup.org/darlenen.html).* Dr. Burzynski has treated more than **8000** cancer patients.

Dr. Burzynski also treats other auto-immune disorders. What I find most disturbing about so many of these cases, including those involving young children, is that when (the parents) were given a poor prognosis and asked their Oncologist if there was anything available that could offer hope, apart from devastating chemo and radiation, they were told ***no.*** In one case in particular, a doctor knew the history of a patient who had been cured of an aggressive brain tumor at the Burzynski Clinic, and still never revealed this information to the parents of his brain cancer patient, pushing them instead to put their child through chemo and radiation!

In many cases, cancer patients were also told that the only thing chemo or radiation could do was *possibly* gain them a few more months of life at the most, yet they were not told about antineoplastons! The Burzynski Clinic also treats many other cancers and disorders including: CLL and CML (leukemias), fibrous histiocytoma, mesothelioma, neuro-endocrine tumors, Wilm's tumor, mantle zone lymphoma, Hodgkins &

non-Hodgkins lymphoma, mycosis-fungoides-sezary syndrome, choroid plexus neoplasm, craniopharyngioma, mixed olioma, high-grade gliomas, visual pathway gliomas, and many others, too numerous to mention here. The main webpage for the Burzynski Clinic is: *www.burzynskiclinic.com.* See the section in this chapter under *Mullaca Inhibits Brain Cancer (Gliomas),* for more information on several types of brain tumors, including some very rare brain tumors.

## • Burzynski Therapy for Neuroblastoma & Optic Pathway Gliomas

Also see website *http://burzynskipatientgroup.org/tavism.htm,* for the case of a little boy cured of neuroblastoma using Dr. Burzynski's antineoplaston (ANP) therapy. He first received surgery, radiation and chemo—all of which failed.

Note that neuroblastoma cancers usually form in the *nerve tissues* found in the *adrenal gland, neck, chest, or spinal cord,* and are more common in children (336a). It is believed that if the cancer is due to faulty DNA (specifically the *Unb11qLOH and 1p36 LOH* chromosomes), their survival chances are less likely than victims who do not have these genetic defects. Their treatment choices may be more aggressive than those not having the chromosomal abnormality (336a).

For Burzynski Research Institute studies on optic pathway gliomas and treatment with antineoplastons, see the article at this website: *http://www.tradingmarkets.com/print.site/news/Stock%20News/2038966,* and information at the Burzynski Research Institute website: *http://www.burzynskiclinic.com,* as well as clinical trial reports at website: *http://www.burzynskiclinic.com/ph/media-corner-publications.html.*

# How to Prevent Neuroblastoma, Brain Tumor & Leukemia in Your Children Before They Are Born

Seven studies by researchers at the University of Toronto from 1960-2005, looking at how a mother's vitamin intake could affect her child's later development of cancer, had some surprising results (407a). As noted by *CancerConsultants.com* website, all vitamins were studied, including *folic acid.* Mothers who took vitamin supplements (that included folic acid) had children with *36%* fewer cases of *pediatric leukemia; 18% reduction in pediatric brain tumors*, and *47% reduction in neuroblastoma* in their children. Authors of the study theorized that folic acid might have been the most important of the vitamins (407a), and it is already a well-known fact that women who take folic-acid can help prevent neural-tube birth defects in their babies.

This study is described in the Journal *Clinical Pharmacology and Therapeutics* (retrieved from website article: "Vitamins During Pregnancy Decrease Childhood Cancer Risk" from *http://patient.cancerconsultants.com/CancerNews_Neuroblastoma.aspx?DocumentId=39373* (407a); more proof that nutrition plays a critical role in disease prevention, even in the womb!

## Non-Toxic Alternative Treatment for Curing Glioblastoma Multiforme

BEFORE you choose conventional treatment for glioblastoma multiforme, please see the case of Susan H. at Dr. Burzynski's patient group website: *http://www.burzynskipatientgroup.org/susanhale.htm* (280a). Susan's brain tumor returned after radiation (Gamma Knife®). She then went to the Burzynski Clinic and received antineoplaston therapy. She was completely cured of glioblastoma multiforme using Dr. Burzynski's antineoplastons (280a). You can call the Burzynski Clinic and ask for her dad (his name is at the end of the article), and he will give you more details about his daughter's amazing recovery.

## Non-Toxic Conventional Vaccine for Glioblastoma Multiforme & Using Drugs With Minimal Damage

Though I have mentioned the fact that Dr. Burzynski has had great success curing brain cancers, I will also mention here, a conventional treatment that is said to have no major adverse effects, though it is still in the *investigative* phase (220a), and you may wish to ask your physician about this treatment as one of your options. It is known as **CDX-110**, an *investigative vaccine*, which might help improve survival for those with glioblastoma multiforme, a cancer that affects *10,000* people every year in the *United States* (220a.) Realize, however, that this vaccine is often combined with chemo drugs that DO have very toxic side effects. Conventional physicians usually give *surgery, radiation and chemo,* but even with treatment, average survival…is *one year*, once *newly diagnosed.* What's worse, the past four decades have seen little change in these dismal statistics. For more information on getting into one of the trials on CDX-110, contact *www.cancer.gov* and *eCancerTrials.*

Another tactic, recently developed, is giving a monoclonal antibody, such as the drug *Neuradiab*, during surgery on the tumor, right into the tumor cavity to destroy any remaining cells. This drug uses radioactive iodine to kill the cancer cells. It is also used for lymphoma cancers.

## Non-Toxic Immunotherapy, Including Individualized Vaccines

More and more health care researchers are studying the effectiveness of using immunotherapy for fighting cancer. This is taking on many new forms, such as removing white blood cells from patients and mixing them (in the laboratory) with the cancer cells. Once the white blood cells form antibodies against the cancer, the new individualized vaccine that has been developed is re-injected into the patient. Since the patient's own cells are used, there is no danger of rejection. Sometimes, as described elsewhere in this book, the cancer-fighting substances are taken from a close relative, allowed to multiply in the laboratory, then injected into the patient. A great deal of research is being done on customized-vaccines.

## Vitamin C & Glioblastoma

There has been much controversy about megadosing with vitamin C for cancer, but most researchers agree that giving vitamin C directly into the bloodstream (intravenously), gets best results. Linus Pauling, Dr. Abram Hoffer, Dr. Irwin Stone, Dr. Robert Cathcart, and many other physicians and researchers have believed and taught this for years. It seems that the modern medical community may finally be taking them seriously.

The National Institute of Diabetes and Digestive and Kidney Diseases in Bethesda, Maryland, discovered recently, that giving large amounts of this vitamin intravenously to mice with ovarian cancers, glioblastoma, and cancers of the pancreas, restricted the *growth by up to 53%* (329a). The study was headed up by Mark Levine, who said that the vitamin C worked by forming *hydrogen peroxide,* which destroyed the *cancer cells* (329a). Cancer Treatment Centers of America *(CTCA)* in Zion, Illinois, is also testing intravenous Vitamin C on patients with advanced cancer (329a). Also, see page 544 of this book for an exciting new form of vitamin C taken orally. It is called *liposome-encapsulated vitamin C* (466b). Dr. Thomas Levy has actually used this new oral form of vitamin C to cure a woman who had hemorrhagic dengue fever. (466b). He believes that 5-6 grams of this new C by mouth is more effective than 50 grams of intravenous vitamin C. Page 544 will also tell you where you can find it.

## II. Other Brain Cancer Therapies

### Abajeru (*Chrysobalanus icaco*) for Brain & Other Cancers

Isolated from a tropical plant of the Brazilian Rain Forest (aka as *coco-plum*), abajeru was once used by the locals for fighting arthritic pain and diabetes (145a). When researchers first conducted lab testing, they found that the bush extract killed *breast-brain-lung-bowel-larynx and pancreas tumors*, and even difficult-to-treat leukemia cells died. In testing **humans**, they were surprised to see that it *worked with 90% of the patients* (145a).

### Artemisinin & Brain Cancer

Artemisinin, also called *wormwood,* has been popular in killing parasites, however, in scientific studies, it was also successful in fighting many types of cancer, most remarkably those of the colon and blood (*leukemia)* (322). Artemisinin has the ability of crossing over into the brain, something very few drugs can do (322). Excessive doses of artemisinin can be harmful. The safety of using artemisinin for extended periods is unknown (322). Do not take this herb without consulting your physician, especially if you are already taking radiation therapy or have recently had radiation therapy. Do not take it on an empty stomach. Also, see Poly-MVA, later in this chapter, which has the ability of crossing over into the brain.

### Cartilage Supplements & Dietary Changes Cure A Child's Neuroblastoma

Neuroblastoma is a very aggressive cancer that affects mostly newborns through fourteen-year-olds. This type cancer is described in detail at website: *www.chemtox.com/neuroblastoma/default.htm* (528). Neuroblastoma tumors are usually found in the body cavity (rather than the limbs), and outcome is not good. If the tumor has not spread, it is usually removed by surgery. Once it has gone into the bones, it is considered likely to be fatal (528). A link between this disease and a common pesticide (known as *chlordane)* has been found. Supposedly, it was no longer used after 1988, but it was so widely used before that, that people living in 75% of the homes that were built before 1988 will still find it in the air (528). You may want to check out that next home you buy for chlordane levels (if it was built before 1988), especially if you have small children toddling around.

When eleven-year-old Kyle S. awoke one morning with unbearable pain, he had no idea what was happening to him. Less than a day later, he was unable to walk, and a short time later, he was diagnosed with *stage IV neuroblastoma.* Trusting in the modern medical establishment, Kyle's parents promptly took him to St. Judes' Hospital "for whole body radiation and Autologous Bone Marrow Transplant (ABMT)" (73). As noted by a writer at website: *www.karlloren.com,* his father describes what happened next as a horror story. Though his young son endured a year "of chemotherapy using different drugs and transfusions for neutropenia, and…weeks of solitary isolation, there was no change in Kyle's tumor." His parents were told that the tumor was *chemo-resistant,* and that nothing further could be done for the child (73), however, Kyle's parents were not about to give up. (Note that when chemo or radiation fails, parents are often given the excuse that their child's cancer is *chemo-resistant.*)

During the next few months, Kyle was given "oxygen therapy, chelation therapy," and dietary and nutritional changes, including supplements. His parents also got in touch with John Prudden, MD, "Harvard graduate and former professor of medicine at Columbia College of Physicians and Surgeons. Prudden prescribed Bovine Cartilage (VitaCart®) at 9 grams per day as a non-toxic means of killing tumor cells" (73).

Kyle's family also set up an appointment with Dr. Jack Taylor at the Taylor Wellness Center for his *Metabolic Assessment Program.* (See their website below.) This nutritional program helped Kyle to detoxify. (Note that the VitaCarte® I have seen on the internet is spelled with an "e.") Not only was Kyle taking VitaCarte® and other supplements, as noted above, but his family was involved in a prayer support group, and were determined to help their son undo the harmful effects that the chemo had inflicted upon his young body (73).

The type of cartilage Dr. Prudden used, *VitaCarte®*, is made *by Phoenix Biologics, Inc.*, and can be ordered by contacting #800-947-VITA. Their website is *www.vitacarte.com.* Dr. Jack Taylor's Wellness Center website is located at *www.biotor.com.* Dr. Taylor's program is not promoted as a cancer program—it is a metabolic nutritional wellness program. (Note that recent lab studies show that the carotenoid, astaxanthin, can help fight neuroblastoma cells. Natural sources include krill, salmon, and shrimp.)

## Cayenne - A Spice Cures An Inoperable Brain Cancer

Cayenne pepper has been used to promote heart health for years. Dr. Christopher, *often called Dr. Cayenne*, has given his patients this natural remedy for nearly every chronic ailment imaginable (69). For gastric ulcers, he prescribes *one teaspoon of cayenne pepper in a glass of water three times a day.* If you opt to take capsules, always take them with food. For heart attacks, he says that you cannot take the capsules (69), and recommends using cayenne pepper in hot water, as a tea mixture, or even using a few drops on the tongue in an emergency (69). (Check with your Dr. first!)

Dr. Richard Shulze described an account of a gentleman cured of inoperable brain tumor by consuming cayenne pepper tea. The patient was given a very slim chance (5%) of living if he chose chemo. He refused the chemo (69). Instead, he went home and began drinking a tea made from cayenne at the rate of *ten cups per day.* His tumor was gone within 90 days (69). Dr. Shulze explained that the high level of phytochemicals and other nutrients in the tea cleared the blood and boosted the immune system in the patient. Countries that consume spicy foods have a much lower incidence for cardiac disease and cancer than those who do not (69). (Do not use cayenne with bleeding ulcers!)

Note that many people have used not only cayenne pepper, but **hibiscus tea and rye bread** for lowering their blood pressure and cholesterol levels, as well as celery juice and the vitamin, niacin. Niacin lowers cholesterol, but only if you get the niacin that causes the body to flush. The *flush-free* niacin that many stores sell (niacinamide) will not cause the veins to dilate as well and will not lower cholesterol as well. Do not ever take niacin in the *timed-release* form. It may harm the liver. Niacin may also be important in helping the body build collateral blood vessels around the heart, thus preventing heart attacks or repeat heart attacks.

Policosanol can be just as effective at lowering harmful cholesterol as common pharmaceutical drugs, but without any toxic side effects. You can get policosanol in health food stores. Chinese red yeast rice with guggul also lowers harmful cholesterol. RESVERATROL (in grapes and pomegranate) has cholesterol-lowering and blood-pressure-lowering effects. Check with your physician before switching to herbal formulas. Chinese red yeast rice has the same ingredient as one of the cholesterol-lowering drugs on the market, which means that it too could cause liver problems in some individuals.

## Chaparral & Brain Cancer

Chaparral tea is derived from an evergreen shrub called *greasewood or creosote bush*. The active ingredient of the creosote bush is NDGA (*nordihydroguaiaretic acid*) (504). When cancerous cells from a brain *glioma* were exposed to NDGA, the cells were killed within hours. It is very important if using chaparral tea, to purchase from a reliable supplier (504). Trying to concoct home remedies of chapparal from unreliable sources is unsafe, since NDGA ingested in large amounts or combined with certain drugs can be harmful.

## Curcumin & Resveratrol for Neuroblastoma & Gliomas

Discussed in great detail in chapter three of this book, resveratrol is a substance found in common table grapes and pomegranates. Animal studies show that this substance helps destroy neuroblastoma cells. Laboratory testing showed that curcumin also had this capacity (546). Curcumin is a powerful antioxidant discussed in many other cancer-specific chapters of this book. Get your curcumin from turmeric, rather than curry, and always use organic turmeric. See chapter 20 for instances of when you should not use turmeric (curcumin). If you want your body to absorb turmeric more easily, eat it with pineapple or supplement with bromelain.

A study described at *Clinical Cancer Research* stated that resveratrol was lethal (in animal testing) to glioma cells, not only working against tumor formation, but preventing the spread of blood vessels necessary to sustain tumor growth (560a).

## Cytotron Therapy for Cancer & Arthritis

See chapter 34 in this book for more details on this gentle, painless, non-invasive cancer therapy that many people are also using to restore cartilage in their joints, making joint-replacement surgeries completely unnecessary (90). You may hear this referred to as *QMR* or *Quantum Magnetic Resonance*—they are the same thing.

## Essiac Tea & Central Nervous System Cancers in Children

See chapter six of this book for more detailed information on the nurse who cured hundreds, perhaps thousands, of cancer patients in Canada using a formula from four herbs that she called *Essiac tea.* (Her last name spelled backwards.)

Richard Thomas wrote a detailed book on the Essiac formula, known as Flor-Essence®. In his book: *The Essiac Report Canada's Remarkable Unknown Cancer Remedy,* he has a copy of a letter from Dr. E. Bruce Hendrick, M.D. F.R.C.S. who was, at the time (Oct. 1983), Chief of the Division of Neurosurgery at The Hospital For Sick Children in Toronto, Canada (580). In the letter, Dr. Hendrick wrote to The Minister of Health & Welfare (House of Commons, Parliament Building in Ottawa, Ontario), describing the excellent results that eight of his ten patients had when they began ingesting Essiac tea. All the children had central nervous system tumors and none had undergone chemo or radiation. Eight of the ten improved neurologically. He was especially impressed with the fact that Essiac had no adverse *side effects* (580).

Dr. Charles A. Brusch, who worked with Rene Caisse and who was also personal physician to John F. Kennedy, stated that: "The results we obtained with thousands of patients of various races, sexes and ages with all types of cancer definitely proves Essiac to be a cure for cancer" (580). Dr. Brusch also wrote a letter explaining that he and Rene Caisse had even used the tea for healing burns that patients had experienced as a result of radiation therapy (580). Dr. Brusch said that Rene gave him the Essiac formula (oral formula), which was later developed into the Flor-Essence® tea (580). You can obtain Flor-Essence® Essiac tea at most health food stores. There is some competition between this tea and Resperin Canada Essiac® brand. Both claim that they have the original (drinkable) formula given to Dr. Brusch from Rene Caisse. You can find both brands (and others) in health food stores and on the internet.

## Flavenols in Citrus Fight Brain Cancer

Studies have shown that certain types of flavenols help clear toxins from the liver, and the flavenols found in tangerine skins help in the destruction of brain cancer cells, as well as helping in prevention of their further spread (55). The best way to use the peelings is shredding or grating them in dishes or steeping them in hot tea or water (55).

## Flax Oil Used To Cure Inoperable Brain Cancer

Many testimonials have been given of patients brought back from terminal illness to amazing health by the Johanna Budwig flax oil diet. Dr. Johanna Budwig, a nobel prize nominee (seven times) and German biochemical expert, found that the blood of cancer patients is lacking essential fatty acids. Her diet revolves around very specific ingredients, including flax oil and cottage cheese (601). These two ingredients, as described at *www.healingcancernaturally.com*, are combined as follows:

> For each tablespoon of flaxseed oil, add 2 tablespoons of low-fat cottage cheese (or quark) or 6 tablespoons of yoghurt. The flaxoil/cottage cheese or flaxoil/yoghurt mixture should be fully blended until no traces of oil remain visible, proving that the highly unsaturated fatty acids have become water soluble (a hand-held mixer or a blender works well) (99). [Quark is a pasty type of white cheese.]

As you can see, the ingredients are very simple. It works because the flax oil reacts with the sulfuric contents of the cottage cheese, and dramatically increases oxygenation at the cellular level. This combination binds the fats to protein, thus making them readily available at the cellular level. The body is also supplied with natural essential fatty acids that prevent cancer cells from running rampant in the body (601). Note that this is not all of the famous Budwig diet. There are other facets included as well. For example: the diet forbids the ingestion of margarine, any type of animal fats (e.g., including butter, and fats found in other animal products), and no sugar whatsoever, though raw juicing from vegetables is encouraged, as is *apple juice*. Herbal teas are also recommended at least three times a day (601). It is important to realize that the Budwig diet is a complete protocol. It is a "lacto-vegetarian diet except that fish is allowed, flax seeds, fruit juices, vegetable juices, sauerkraut, sunshine, emotional and spiritual peace and stress control," as well as the ingredients above (170). More than "50% of Dr. Budwig's patients were doctors or relatives of doctors…" (99). See *www.healingcancernaturally.com,* for more specifics on the Budwig diet, as well as chapter 18 of this book. Dr. Budwig described her work in the following way:

> And what do I actually do? I give cancer patients simple, natural foods. That is all. I take sick people out of the hospital, when it is said that they do not have more than an hour or two left to

> live, that the scientifically attested diagnosis is at hand and that the patient is completely moribund. In most cases I can help even these patients quickly and conclusively (99).

There are many amazing cancer cures attributed to Dr. Budwig's flax oil diet. One example is that of Sandy A., who was diagnosed with an *inoperable brain tumor* (601). When the tumor began to bleed, he was told that there was nothing more to offer him. He started on Dr. Budwig's formula and improved so that he could partially resume normal activities. He is still being considered a medical marvel ten years later (601).

Ms. Budwig admitted that for those patients in the most severe stages (who had been told that surgery was useless), "even in these cases health can be restored, usually within a few months, I would say in 90% of cases" (99). The Budwig diet uses a natural formula that inhibits the formation of cancer. It is known throughout the world. Many people have followed this regimen, people who were said to be *terminal.* They were cured on the Budwig diet, and are now going about their usual everyday activities without restriction (601). The substances in the Budwig diet heal the immune system, giving the body the ability to heal itself.

See Chapter 18 for more information on the amazing healing and curative properties of flax oil. Further details of the Budwig diet are also discussed in that chapter. Dr. Johanna Budwig authored several books, including *The Oil Protein Diet Cookbook*, which contains many recipes using the Budwig protocol. Her books are available in major bookstores. Website: *www.healingcancernaturally.com*, contains a great deal of information on the Budwig diet, as does *http://www.barleans.com/budwig.html.* Be sure that you **never heat flax oil**, and that you always keep it refrigerated. Also, if you choose the Budwig diet, be sure to use only certified organic dairy products—raw—if you can get them.

If you are fighting terminal cancer, I would certainly recommend the Budwig diet. If you go with dairy, just be sure you use organic and get raw dairy (the cottage cheese or yogurt) from a dairy farmer near you that has healthy, disease-free herds and practices scrupulously clean farming (you don't need parasites). The very last thing you need in your diet is the addition of hormones, herbicides, and pesticides that are often found in non-organic dairy. These are the substances that may have caused your cancer in the first place. Read chapter 26 of this book.

## Fungus Cure Also Cures Cancer, Says Oncology Physician

See chapter 34 of this book for the amazing cancer cure that Italian Oncologist, Dr. Simoncini, is using to cure his cancer patients within just days. Cancerous growths are usually WHITE. He says that they are actually a fungus, which can be killed with a non-toxic soda bicarb solution that quickly alkalizes the tumor for destruction (582).

## Garlic & Glioblastoma

An ingredient in garlic, *diallyl trisulfide,* helps kill glioblastoma cells.

## Ginkgo Slows Brain Cancer Growth

Animal studies at Georgetown University Medical Center showed that this herb (taken from ginkgo leaves), stopped cancerous cells by 80%. Not only was the extract used on breast cancer cells, but it worked (albeit not as well) on cancers of the brain (125).

## GLA & Brain Cancer Treatment

GLA, *Gamma linolenic acid* (found in *evening primrose oil and borage oil)* has potent cancer-fighting abilities. In one study on brain tumors, giving the GLA into the tumor by hypodermic shrank the growths (351). Not only does GLA destroy many types of cancerous cells, but it does not affect healthy cells. It is best not to take over two grams per day (351).

## Gliadel® Wafer for Gliomas & Glioblastomas

This is a type of chemo in the form of a wafer that is placed into the brain when a tumor is removed. It dissolves slowly as it delivers the chemo drug, BCNU. It is said not to have the severe toxic side effects that may be experienced when this chemo drug is given intravenously.

## GMO Foods - Genetically Modified Foods Nightmare

We are now being bombarded with the problem of GMO (genetically-modified organisms) foods, without evidence of how they will affect our health in the years to come. Many soybeans (and corn) in this country (and overseas) are now coming from genetically-modified seeds.

## Goldenseal Fights Brain Tumors

This herb, which contains an ingredient known as *berberine* (and others like it), helps the body fight inflammation and cancers, such as those of the brain, bladder, skin, and intestines, as well as leukemia (58). In animal testing, goldenseal (berberine) had double the cancer-destruction rate for cancer cells as that of BCNU, a chemotherapy drug (58). If purchasing berberine, be sure to use a *standardized* form (58). Berberine has been shown to prevent cancer cells in the liver from multiplying. For times when you should not use goldenseal, see chapter 6, and ask your doctor.

## Grapes (Resveratrol) & Grape Seed Extract

In 1989, Johanna Brandt's *Grape Cure* book was published under the title: *How to Conquer Cancer, Naturally*, by Tree of Life Publications, Joshua Tree, California. This edition included several pages of testimonials, including a brain cancer patient who had been sent home to die (cured on the grape diet), and a woman who was given up as terminal when it was discovered that she had an aggressive abdominal cancer. The physician taking care of her testified to her astounding and complete recovery while using only *The Grape Cure* diet (356).

Remember too, that grape seed extract is a super anti-oxidant that has the ability to cross the blood-brain barrier. Compounds that can cross the blood-brain barrier are important in the treatment of brain tumors as well as other disorders, such as Alzheimers. Resveratrol is found in red wine, purple and red grapes, pomegranates, and other fruits.

## Graviola & Brain Cancer

For information on using graviola for cancer, see chapters five and six. See this website as well: *http://clem.mscd.edu/~boettner/CancerTutor/Cancer/Graviola.html.*

## LifeMel Honey for Cancer Patients

This amazing honey is also discussed in chapter 29 of this book. It is a special honey (developed in Israel) produced from bees that gather nectar from 40 herbs, including *Echinacea, Siberian ginseng,* and *Uncaria tomentosa,* with other natural ingredients. Two teaspoons per day (one in the morning and one in the evening) are recommended (614). This special honey has been shown, in **human** testing, to prevent the neutropenia (serious drop in white blood cells) caused by chemotherapy and to lower the risk of severe platelet drop (thrombocytopenia), often found in chemo patients (614). You can find out more about this remarkable honey at website: *http://www.lifemelisrael.com* (614).

## Macrobiotics Cure A Brain Cancer

When Mona S. of Columbus, Ohio, lost consciousness playing tennis, she was told that she had a grapefruit-sized tumor in her brain and given a few months to live (391). Her story can be found in J. L. Eftekhar's book, *Heal Yourself*, from *Globe Digests*™. She gave up on traditional medicine (after only three chemo doses) and started on a macrobiotic diet. She also developed a positive attitude, telling herself that the growth was shrinking (391). Four months after starting the diet, Eftekhar says that diagnostics showed no traces of the growth. She was completely healed and has had no reoccurrences. She credits her healing to prayer, her spiritual faith in God, sticking with the macrobiotic diet, and her *positive* approach to life and healing. She also used tapes and videos to reinforce her determination to get well (391).

Macrobiotics, developed by *Michio Kushi,* relies on a diet of mostly whole grains, as well as certain percentages of fresh vegetables, soup, *beans and seaweed.* Seafood and fish are allowed on the diet, as well as fresh fruits (504).

Though there are many health benefits to some of the ingredients in the macrobiotic diet, it is being included here for informational purposes only. I do not agree with all of it, especially the emphasis that it places on Eastern philosophies, some of which I feel are in direct conflict with Christianity. For informational purposes, macrobiotics are discussed in greater detail in chapter 27 of this book.

## Magnesium & Iodine for Cancer Prevention

These minerals are critical for the prevention of all types of cancer, including leukemia, and cancer of the stomach, prostate, breast, and bones (566). Also, see page 129.

## Marijuana - Medical Usage

When scientists from Madrid revealed that *medical marijuana* (*Tetrahydro-cannabinol)* could destroy inoperable brain growths in animals (when it was injected into the tumors), not a single newspaper in the United States reported the findings, and the story only ran one time on mainstream media wires (285). This was not *new* information. As far back as 1974, researchers announced that medical marijuana could inhibit leukemia (viral) in mice, as well as breast and lung cancer (285). This information was all documented in a book written by Jack Herer, *The Emperor Wears No Clothes,* however, the government silenced the report (285). *Cancertutor.com* website reports that in 1976, the Executive Office outlawed all research studies on this drug and handed over all rights to the drug industry for the manufacture of a synthetic marijuana that worked identically to the natural form, but they failed (285).

Use of marijuana, especially over long periods of time has shown to be detrimental to overall brain health, however, I find it interesting that research studies proving that injections can cure animals with inoperable *brain tumors,* was aggressively silenced by the government. Though I would never advocate any sort of illicit drug use, I am not against the use of medicinal marijuana for pain relief in cancer patients, as long as use is closely monitored, and the recipients are not out driving the highways while relieving their pain! Of course, people who drink alcohol aren't supposed to be out on the highways either, yet they are, and they are killing thousands every year! Today, more than 30 years after former President Gerald Ford ended cannabis research, there is still much controversy over the use of medicinal marijuana for pain control in cancer patients, though some states have legalized it for this purpose only. It is said to kill pain better than narcotics.

## Melatonin

When studies involving dozens of patients, who were given melatonin over a *one year* period were completed, it was found that those who received the melatonin had longer survival time, no tumor growth, and fewer adverse effects and *complications*, as compared to those given *supportive care* only (507). It is not recommended that patients with *leukemia, lymphoma and myeloma* take melatonin. There is a possibility that melatonin may accelerate these type cancers (507). In addition to this precaution for melatonin, the supplement could cause depression and worsening of allergies in some individuals, and should not be taken by those on cortisone, nor those who are pregnant (192). It is also possible that the hormone can reduce blood flow and libido and lower body temperature. It may also cause *retinal damage* (192). Significant amounts of natural melatonin can be found simply in eating tart cherries (61).

## Mullaca Inhibits Brain Cancer (Gliomas)

Mullaca is another rain forest herb that is toxic to brain tumors. Clinical research is still going on with this fascinating herb, and preliminary laboratory and animal studies have shown that it can boost the immune system, is deadly to many different forms of cancer cells, and kills microbes (200). You may find this supplement sold as *bolsa mullaca.*

Typical brain stem gliomas are usually found in children and are often considered inoperable. This is because they invade once healthy brain tissue that could end up causing paralysis and death if surgery is done. Most children with this diagnosis do not survive more than a year, however, see the earlier information in this chapter on antineoplastons! Atypical gliomas, on the other hand, may carry a longer survival rate. A very ominous symptom children may first develop, indicating the presence of this type tumor, is double-vision. As described at *www.braintumor.org*, other symptoms may include: neuro changes (frequent falling, loss of balance, speech problems), abdominal upset, and choking when swallowing (44). Other types of gliomas described at the website above include: "ependymoma, ganglioneuroma, juvenile pilocytic, mixed glioma, oligodendrogliomas [and] optic nerve glioma" (44). Some non-glioma types of brain tumors include: "chordoma, craniopharyngioma, medullo-blastoma, meningioma, pineal tumors, pituitary tumors, pituitary adenoma, primitive neuroectodermal tumors (PNETs), Schwannoma [and] vascular tumors" (297). Other types of cancerous brain conditions include: "CNS [central nervous system] lymphoma, meningeal carcinomatosis, pseudo-tumor cerebri [and] tuberous sclerosis" (298).

Substances that are taken from mullaca that inhibit cancer cells are plant steroids that have shown impressive abilities during lab and animal studies in fighting many types of cancer, including those of the brain, intestines, skin, liver, throat, cervix, and nasal passages (200). Mullaca should not be taken by those on blood thinners, blood pressure medications, diabetic medications, or heart medications without the supervision of their physician. It can affect blood pressure, clotting time, and blood sugar levels (200).

For details on painless treatment of many of these tumors (above), such as meningiomas, pituitary tumors, schwannomas, arterial venous malformations, oligodendrogliomas, hemangioblastomas, craniopharyni-giomas, orbital tumors, spinal tumors, etc., see chapter 34 under the heading of **CyberKnife®** therapy. Also, see NanoKnife™, same chapter.

## Mushroom Extract Cures A Brain Cancer

Though a popular mushroom, maitake, is presented here because of its ability to fight **brain cancer.** Its healing properties are discussed in other chapters of this book. One of the extracts from maitake, known as *Maitake D-Fraction,* has become popular as an immune booster and cancer-fighter. Maitake should not be taken by those with *multiple sclerosis* (184).

In the book by Shari Lieberman, Ph.D., and Ken Babal, C.N., *Maitake Mushroom And D-Fraction,* the amazing curative power of this mushroom is documented in a middle-aged man who was totally cured of an enormous brain tumor after using the substance for only *four months* (469). You can find this supplement in some health food stores as well as several internet sites, including *www.iherb.com.*

## Myrrh

In laboratory testing, compounds from this biblical herb not only killed breast, brain, and prostate cancer cells, it killed the drug-resistant cells, without harming nearby healthy cells. Large scale human testing has not yet been done on this herb.

## Nanotechnology—*Lodamin*—Curing Glioblastoma & Neuroblastoma Without Side Effects

A new drug, Lodamin, which works by halting the blood vessel growth that tumors need to survive, was shown in animal testing, to be effective against many tumor types, including those of the breast, brain, ovaries, uterus, prostate, neuroblastoma, and glioblastoma (401). It also worked very well in preventing cancer from going into the liver (401). The discovery of the drug, using *nanotechnology* and a derivative from a fungus, was quite accidental. Reports say that it can be taken orally without *side effects* (401). Lodamin is still in the testing phases, and is also being considered for treating macular degeneration and arthritis.

Note that shark cartilage and bindweed (chapter 34) also work to starve tumors by cutting off the blood supply to them, without adverse side effects.

## Poly–MVA for Brain Tumors

Poly-MVA is a highly nutritious drink and proprietary blend of palladium and alpha lipoic acid, molybdenum, some important B vitamins, rhodium, ruthenium, formylmethionine, and acetyl cysteine.

This is one cancer treatment that can cross into the brain—good news for those fighting brain tumors—and it may be helpful in *reversing* other cancers, such as *multiple myeloma* and *pancreatic cancer* (235). Poly-MVA can be ordered at their main website: *http://www.polymva.net.* Be aware that there are bogus forms of this formula floating around. The website above has the original formula. For testimonials of people who used this substance to cure their brain cancer (and many other types of cancer), see website: *http://www.polymvasurvivors.com/testimonials.html.*

## Rexin-G™ for Metastatic Cancers

Rexin-G™ has been undergoing clinical trials at Mayo Clinic, M.D. Anderson, and a few other facilities. It is a drug for cancers that have spread, and those types of cancer that conventional medicine says do not respond to chemo drugs (256). Human clinical studies thus far, have had good results. In the very first human trial, 83% of the patients had tumor shrinkage. The patients all had spreading pancreatic cancer (256). Good responses were also achieved in human studies involving several other types of spreading cancers. Due to the reports, this drug is now used for treating all forms of *solid tumors* in the Philippines that are resistant to conventional therapy (256). The U.S. FDA has given the drug its *orphan drug status* for use with pancreatic cancers in the US, as well as other types of cancer metastases, which means that trials will continue (256). It is given intravenously, so isn't exactly natural or painless, but could be considered gentler than older chemo drugs because it is said to be a non-chemo drug, showing itself in **human** clinical trials, not to have the adverse side effects normally found with chemo drugs (256). You can get more information on this drug at *epeiusbiotech.com/rexin_g-factsheet.asp.* Epeius Biotechnologies are the producers of Rexin-G™ (257).

## Scorpion Venom from Israel for Gliomas

University of Alabama researchers are studying the effects of scorpion venom on glioma (brain) cancers (449). Physicians are looking at a giant Israeli scorpion which kills cockroaches with its venom, but does not harm humans. When they isolated a drug made from the venom and directly injected it into glioma cells, they discovered that only the cancer cells died—the surrounding cells were left untouched. They are still testing the substance (449). One of the drugs being tested from the venom is TM-601. See chapter 34 for more information on scorpion venom and gliomas.

## Taheebo Tea for Cancer

Lapacho, also commonly known as *pau d'arco* and *taheebo tea*, is very popular for treating health disorders, including leukemia and other cancers (509). Be aware that lapacho is actually just an extract from the main tea, *pau d'arco*, but the names get intertwined. When using the herb, you need to be sure that you are using *pau d'arco*—the entire tea. Supporters of this tea say that it is especially helpful in fighting leukemia. Not only that, but they believe it is unrivaled worldwide for its tumor-fighting properties (229). The herb is said to work by activating the body's ability to increase red blood cell production within the marrow cells (229). Lapacho is the main ingredient in this herb, and should never be used alone. When the whole herb was given, it produced clinical anti-cancer effects without the problems that isolating the lapacho and using it alone can cause (229).

It is important to be aware that sometimes when teas such as this are tested, an extract of one of the tea's main ingredients will be used in the test, rather than the entire tea. Of course, in using teas such as this, one needs to use the whole tea, not one or two extracts isolated from the main tea. Not only does the herb kill cancer, but it was cleared by the FDA more than 25 years ago (229).

Genuine pau d'arco tea should come from the tree's bark (the *inner lining*.) It has been used for many years, especially in South America, as an effective way to manage disease, however, getting it from unreliable sources that do not use the tree's inner bark could mean a useless product (98). Since lapacho has blood-thinning properties, you need to discuss the tea with your physician before consumption, especially if you are already taking blood-thinning medications or supplements.

## Ukrain Effective Against Brain Cancer Without Toxic Side Effects

Ukrain is a product that was combined from two common ingredients in 1978 by Dr. Wassyl J. Nowicky in Austria. Given individually, they are toxic, but when combined, they are toxic only to cancer cells (287). Dozens of articles have been written on this compound. It was tested and shown (in vitro) to have the ability to kill nearly *100%* of the many types of cancer cells it was used against (506). Though it is an injection, thus not exactly gentle, natural or painless, it is discussed in several cancer-specific chapters of this book, because it is completely non-toxic and has been effective with so many different forms of cancer, including many of those considered *hopeless* and *terminal.* Apparently, Ukrain aggressively congregates at the tumor cells once administered. It boosts the immune system and keeps tumors from forming a blood supply network (287). Ukrain has been successful against many cancers, including rectal, colorectal, breast, pancreatic, bladder, prostate, bronchial, brain, testicular and neuroblastoma (287). When hundreds of terminal patients, who had failed conventional treatment were tested with this non-toxic substance (over a 5.5 year period), more than half of those with astrocytomas (brain tumor) and neuroblastomas went into remission (287).

This compound has repeatedly outperformed conventional medicine, and these are **humans** we are talking about, not lab mice! The late Dr. Atkins regarded Ukrain as the single best anti-cancer agent he had ever used. He said of Ukrain: "Like chemotherapy, it kills cancer cells…" However, "it spares normal…healthy tissue. If the medical community were willing to give it a try, Ukrain could replace chemotherapy in treating almost all cancers" (287). Ukrain is only available through alternative health clinics in the U.S., Canada, and Europe.

2009 update: note that because Ukrain is not authorized in Austria, this info is no longer located *at www.ukrin.com.* The website has been changed and is now called *Nowicky Pharma;* however, you can read this information about Ukrain in the book*: Anti-Cancer Agent Ukrain—The Crime Story of an Obstruction* by Eleonore Thun-Hohenstein. Also, for pictures of how Ukrain works, see website: *http://www.ukrain-drug.net/webspeed/index.htm.*

## Ukrain for Astrocytoma & Neuroblastoma

Another human case study, involving a *frontal anaplastic grade III astrocytoma* which was greatly reduced with Ukrain, can be found at *http://www.ncbi.nlm.nih.gov/sites/entrez*. The identification number for this case is #8899347 (570). For a study involving a young child with neuroblastoma, see the National Institutes of Health and U.S. National Library of Medicine (case PMID 10190082) (336). The child involved in this study had stage IV neuroblastoma. After having the tumor extracted and kidney removal, he was treated with Ukrain (336). Within two months, he had extensive spread through many areas of his body. He was again given Ukrain. The tumors stopped growing, shrank and some of them disappeared completely. The cancer was stopped (336).

## Vassourinha & Anamu

These are two rain forest herbs that have anti-tumor properties. **Vassourinha** *(Scoparia dulcis)* contains the plant compound *betulinic acid*, which has undergone much recent testing for its ability to fight tumors, viruses (HIV), and even leukemia (302). Raintree Nutrition, at website *www.rain-tree.com*, reports that the herb has been toxic to malignant growths in the skin, bone, and brain, yet is not toxic to normal cells (302). This herb should not be used by pregnant women; it may cause uterine contractions. It can also lower blood sugar in some individuals, and it increases the effects of barbiturates and antidepressants, so be sure to consult with your physician or Naturopath before using this or any other herbal products, especially if you are already on prescription medications, or have a chronic illness (302).

**Anamu** *(Petiveria alliacea)* is sometimes referred to as *garlic weed*, because of its *odor*. This herb can help the body fight tumors and leukemia. Extracts from anamu were found, during in vitro studies, to kill cancers of the brain, lymphatic system, liver, and blood (leukemia) (16). One animal study showed that anamu boosted the natural killer cells of the immune system by 100%. This herb should not be used by pregnant women (may start contractions). Raintree Nutrition also reports that Anamu can lower blood sugar, and it may interfere with blood coagulation (16).

Note that Raintree Nutrition does not make *curative* claims for their herbs. They report the results of tests conducted on various herbs, and they suggest that herbs be part of an overall comprehensive health treatment plan. Many of the plants discussed at their website can be purchased by the pound.

## Zeaxanthin for Neuroblastoma

Zeaxanthin is an antioxidant carotenoid that, in laboratory testing, effectively killed *neuroblastoma cells* (546), an excellent reason for eating leafy greens (e.g., kale, spinach, collards, and mustard greens).

# III. Popular Non-Natural Brain Cancer Treatments

## Gamma Knife® & CyberKnife® for Inoperable Lesions & Tumors

See chapter 34 for details on Gamma Knife® and CyberKnife® surgery, neither of which actually involves using a knife or incision. One is painful and is only used for brain tumors, the other is painless (CyberKnife®) and used for brain and other areas of the body. (Also, see chapter 34 for information on the new non-toxic, painless NanoKnife™ therapy for solid tumors elsewhere in the body.)

## IMRT (Intensity Modulated Radiation Therapy) for Medulloblastoma & Neuroblastoma

This radiation treatment is currently under testing in Europe and is being used in the U.S as well. It uses targeted radiotherapy to help minimize damage to nearby normal cells. It is used for lung tumors, thyroid, and breast cancers, as well as prostate, esophageal, nasal, head cancers, liver, brain, ovarian, cervical cancers, and uterine growths. You may also see this treatment referred to as ***TOMO Therapy*** or *TOMO Treatment*—they are the same thing.

Rather than using one large radiation beam to target the tumor, this type radiation uses many beams to target cancer tumors more precisely, thus (hopefully) preventing excess damage to nearby normal cells (163a); however, it is still considered radiation and will have some of the same side effects as any radiation would cause.

IMRT has been popular at treating tumors located around or near critical, vital organs (163a). It has been successfully used in treating children with many types of cancers, including those with rhabdomyosarcomas, who otherwise had little hope of survival (163a). One side effect of treating children with medulloblastomas (with standard radiation) has been not only severe radiation side effects, but possible hearing loss as well. With IMRT, medulloblastoma has been treated without the hearing loss, due to the ability to more precisely direct the beams (163a). For more information on pediatric treatment of tumors using IMRT, see website: *http://www.mskcc.org/mskcc/html/8442.cfm* (163a). Also, see the information (earlier in this chapter) on the successful treatment of children's brain tumors with non-toxic antineoplastons before you make a choice on this or any other therapy.

## 3F8 Monoclonal Antibody Treatment for Neuroblastoma

Neuroblastoma, a cancer that most commonly is diagnosed in young children, varies greatly in the way it acts in the human body. Some are successfully treated with surgery, yet some do not need any treatment at all before disappearing, however, 50% of the cases are lethal and quickly spreading (205). The disease is sometimes treated (if high-risk) with 3F8, a monoclonal antibody, which is not at all *painless*, *gentle*, or *natural,* but is being mentioned here because it has been effective in bringing about some remissions of neuroblastoma. The drug is in fact, a painful treatment, simply due to the way that it works.

Memorial Sloan-Kettering Cancer Center uses this therapy for those with *high-risk neuroblastoma.* Those with *low risk* neuroblastoma are not usually given radiation or chemo at Memorial Sloan-Kettering. For more information about this treatment for neuroblastoma, see website *http://www.mskcc.org/mskcc/html/62107.cfm* (205).

When your child's immune system functions normally, it makes antibodies that destroy invading bacteria, viruses, and mutant cells, however, their immune cells won't fight neuroblastoma, because this cancer growth disguises itself as a tissue that their immune cells "see" as normal, not as cancerous. Scientists developed 3F8 from the immune system cells of mice. The drug contains substances that lock onto markers on the cancer cells so that your child's own immune system can "see" them as cancer and not as normal cells, thus attacking and destroying them. This treatment has been used (and improved) over a period of 20 years. It is given intravenously over a 30 minute period. You may hear your physician refer to *HAMA* or *"human anti-mouse antibodies"* (2). Since the drug is made from mouse immune cells, it is possible for your child's own body to develop immune cells against the 3F8 (a situation called *HAMA)*, so further treatment is stopped until tests show that their body is no longer fighting the 3F8; then treatments resume. See *http://www.mskcc.org/mskcc/html/3215.cfm* (2), for more information on monoclonal antibody 3F8.

## IV. Pituitary Tumors

These type tumors, though rare, are found growing in a tiny gland near the heart of the brain known as the *pituitary* (234). As described at website: *http://www.ninds.nih.gov,* the pituitary manufactures "hormones that affect growth and the functions of other glands in the body. These type tumors are usually benign, which means they are non-cancerous, grow slowly and do not spread to other parts of the body" (234). They can, however, cause the body to manufacture excessive levels of other hormones, which can have drastic effects on the health (234). There are many "symptoms of pituitary tumors," including: "headaches, vision problems, nausea and vomiting, or any of the problems caused by the production of too many hormones, such as infertility or loss of menstrual periods in women, abnormal growth, high blood pressure, heat or cold intolerance, and other skin and body changes" (234).

Tumors of the pituitary gland, though rarely cancerous, respond best with early diagnosis and treatment. Current orthodox treatment includes "surgical removal of the tumor; radiation therapy, using drugs or radiation to kill the abnormal cells," or "using certain medications to block the pituitary gland from producing too many hormones. The most common treatment is surgery" (234). This type growth is generally considered *curable*, depending on what kind of tumor, "patient's age and general state of health" (234). If the tumor is *producing* excess amounts of *prolactin,* it may be treated with *medication,* like *cabergolide* (233a). There are many alternative treatments for brain tumors given in this chapter, though surgery for pituitary tumors is usually very successful. See more detailed information in chapter 34 of this book on the CyberKnife® and Gamma Knife®, which are often used successfully on pituitary tumors, since their location makes them difficult to reach. The CyberKnife® is painless, the Gamma Knife® is not.

The CyberKnife® is a newer procedure and is said to have few risks and side effects (89a), though it can damage nearby healthy cells. (Also, see chapter 34 for NanoKnife™ therapy.)

An "endonasal endoscopic approach," *EEA*, which involves going up through the nose to remove the tumor, may only require an inpatient stay of two days or less (233a). The University of Pittsburgh uses this approach for removing pituitary tumors. It is also referred to as: "endoscopic transnasal brain surgery," and can even remove growths "as large as baseballs, all through the nose…requiring no incisions" (233a). Their phone is: #1-800-533-8762. You may also hear this referred to as *MINC* or "Minimally Invasive EndoSurgery Center" (233a).

## V. Cell Phones, Brain & Mouth Cancers & How to Protect Yourself

There is much new research coming forth about our exposure to electromagnetic radiation via cell phones, which are placed against the head and ear. Multiple human studies indicate that cell phone use can lead to not only brain cancer, but mouth tumors (e.g., salivary gland tumors). To limit your exposure to this type radiation, and the dangers associated with it, use the popular hands-free cell phone appliances or stick to the non-cellular phones. The department of public health, in some countries, is advising against the use of cell phones, especially in teens and young children. Some people think that using headsets is protecting them. This may not be the case. When using cell phones, do not carry on lengthy conversations. Keep your conversations short. Think—*a few MINUTES* a few times a day—not hours!

For your peace of mind, if you are spending hours a day on a cell phone, headsets may not be giving you the protection you think they are (251a). Check out the use of *Ferrite Beads*, which may protect you by helping block out radio frequencies that otherwise would be impacting your brain (251a). You can read more about this safety measure at Dr. Mercola's website: *http://www.mercola.com/forms/ferrite_beads.htm,* where the product is also available for purchase (251a). If you don't choose this for yourself, you may wish to do it for your children, especially if they are spending long hours on cell phones every day talking and texting.

# CHAPTER 15

# GENTLE CURES FOR TOUGH SKIN CANCERS (MELANOMA)

*"Come, and let us return unto the Lord: for he hath torn, and he will heal us; he hath smitten, and he will bind us up." (Hosea 6:1)*

## Skin Cancer Types

Melanomas arise from the skin cells found at the deepest levels *of the epidermis.* If you are diagnosed with *basal cell* or *squamous cell* cancers, these are normally found on areas of your body (e.g., legs, arms, face, scalp, ears) where you are most likely to get sunlight while outdoors (or inside a car) (48). These type cancers are considered *curable* if diagnosed early. Melanomas are likely to be discovered in the form of *moles* that may have already *spread* to other areas of the body (as well as other skin areas), and because of their ability to do so, are much more deadly (48). Many times they are not diagnosed until they have already spread, and melanoma does not respond well to chemo and radiation.

## Grapes - Prevention for Skin Cancer & Prostate Cancer

According to a CNN interactive article from their *Health Story Page* entitled "Study: Grapes inhibit cancer growth" (from the journal *Science*), resveratrol may be a potent protection against prostate cancer, and animal research has shown that it can help fight skin cancers as well (132).

## Gene Immunotherapy Cures Man Dying From Stage IV Melanoma

In a history-making case, Seattle scientists at the Fred Hutchinson Cancer Research Center and Memorial Sloan-Kettering Cancer Center, were able to bring about a total cure of a terminal melanoma patient, by injecting the patient with his own treated cells to fight his cancer (269). The article was published in *the New England Journal of Medicine.* White blood cells (called *T-cells*) had been *cloned* and grown in a lab setting until there were *5 billion* of them (269). They were then re-injected into the patient's body.

Eight weeks later, the cancer had completely vanished (269). It has been over two years and the patient continues to be doing well and cancer-free. This type therapy is also known as *immunotherapy* (269). This is more proof that the body's own immune cells, if given in massive doses, can overwhelm and destroy cancer cells. Continued human testing is underway on this procedure. Since the patient receives their own cells, there is no problem with rejection.

## Organ Transplant Increases Risk for Melanoma

Unfortunately, after going through the trauma of an *organ transplant*, studies show that these patients have an *increased risk* for several kinds of *cance*r, *including skin cancers,* which may go undetected at first (361a). As described in an article at website: *CancerConsultants.com,* the information "was presented at the 2008 annual meeting of the American Academy of Dermatology" (361a). It is believed [of course] that this increased risk for skin cancer (and other cancers) is due from immunosuppressives often given in the transplant process. These patients are cautioned against sun exposure (361a). *Immunosuppressives* are things like cortisone, chemo and radiation, and anything else that depresses the immune system.

## Vitamin A, C & E for Skin Health & Cancer Prevention

Anti-oxidants protect the skin against UV damage. If your skin is well-fortified with the nutrition that it needs, skin cells will not usually change under normal sun exposure. According to author Maureen Kennedy Salaman, in her book: *All Your Health Questions Answered Naturally,* scientists discovered that by spreading *vitamin C* on the surface of the skin of *live pigs*, the animals could be protected from harmful UV rays up to *five times* as much as would normally burn their skin (551). Not only did it protect their skin from being burned, but it prevented damage at the cellular level. The topical C lasted for days and its effects could not be removed, not *even* when the skin was thoroughly washed (551). Other skin protectors are vitamin A and E (551). Applying tocopherol vitamin E to the skin (as well as taking it in the form of supplements at *100 U*/day can reduce cancer by *70 percent.* If taking vitamin A daily, you would need greater than *5,000 IUs* in order to cut the risk of skin cancer by *90 percent*...(551) Other skin protectors are discussed later in this chapter. If you are juicing beta-carotene-rich foods (e.g., carrot juice), the body converts beta-carotene into natural vitamin A.

## Andiroba & Berberine Inhibit Skin Tumors

See other chapters in this book for more information on the herb andiroba, used against sarcomas and skin cancers, and the herb goldenseal (berberine), which fights the formation of melanoma and many other cancers. (Also, see indications for when this herb should **not** be used.)

## Azelaic Acid

In laboratory testing, azelaic acid [topical] kills melanoma cells, but leaves normal cells unharmed. According to researchers, this compound caused regression in malignant skin cancers by not merely killing them, but inhibiting their growth (504). It has also been effective in treating acne and various skin problems due to its bactericidal properties. Azalaic acid was researched (in over two dozen various laboratory tests) with the cells of human melanoma (504). It effectively restricted further growth of melanoma in every single culture. Adding *B vitamin, carnitine,* to this ingredient, enhanced its effect (504).

## Basal Cell Carcinoma & Topical Vitamin C

I received an email 11/09/2007 from Dr. Andrew Saul's website (see *www.doctoryourself.com)* explaining that using vitamin C in topical form can help stop *Basal Cell Carcinoma.* He says that using a high concentration of vitamin C on top of the skin to kill this type cancer was known in 1971. Frederick R. Klenner, MD, described the use of vitamin C in an ointment form (30% vitamin C) to kill cancerous basal cell growths.

## Basal Cell Carcinoma & GDC-0449 - New Drug with Mild Side Effects

In the conventional arena of drug development for cancer, a new drug, still being tested, but said to be without major side effects, is **GDC-0449** (588b). As described by *CancerConsultants.com* website, the findings were "presented at the 2008 Annual Meeting of the American Association for Cancer Research" (588b). A trial was done with *nine* participants, all of whom had "advanced basal cell carcinoma." They were given oral dosages of the new drug. In "eight of the nine patients," there was "shrinkage or stabilization of the cancer" [and] it was said that "Side effects were reported as mild with GDC-0449" (588b). Those wishing to participate in such clinical trials can contact the National Cancer Institute at *www.cancer .gov* (588b). Note that this drug is still in Phase I trials. It has a long way to go, but the fact that it appears to have few side effects, thus far, is certainly a plus.

## Beta-Glucan Fights Skin Cancer

Beta-glucan is an extract from yeast and mushrooms (e.g., *shiitake...and maitake*). It is available in supplement form at most health food stores (354). A study involving nine people *having skin, breast, or lung cancer*, showed definite tumor shrinkage within just a few days after injection of this substance into the growths (354). Lentinan is a shiitake beta-glucan extract used widely in Japan to treat late stages of cancer. When given intravenously, survival times can often be prolonged by several years (354). For more information, see web pages at: *www.cancer-prevention.net* (221) and *www.cancer-treatments.net/cancer.html.*

## Burzynski's Antineoplastons Cure Stage IV Melanoma in Child

Jessica K. was only three-years-old when she was diagnosed with stage IV melanoma. It started on her foot in 1984, and it was removed, but returned in 1985, and had spread as a large malignant tumor in her groin and into nearby lymph nodes. Not wishing to subject their daughter to chemo and radiation, her parents took her to Dr. Burzynski in Houston, Texas (444a). She was put on antineoplastons and completely cured. As of 2004 (her most recent update—nearly twenty years after being diagnosed), she is still cancer-free and leading a normal life. See her complete report at website: *http://burzynskipatientgroup.org/jessicak.htm* (444a). Also, see chapter 14 of this book for more amazing cases of cancer patients completely cured of what they were told were terminal cancers, people who were basically sent home to die, then chose non-toxic antineoplastons from the Burzynski Clinic in Houston, Texas *(www.burzynskiclinic.com)*. Also, see many of the patient's own stories about their success in fighting cancer with antineoplastons at website: *http://burzynskipatientgroup.org/stories.html.* Many were hopeless, very aggressive brain tumors, but several other forms of cancer are also treated successfully with antineoplastons. They are either given I.V., or in an oral form known as *sodium phenylbutrates* or *PBs*. The FDA has finally approved the oral form of antineoplastons

(PBs) for off-label use, and antineoplastons A10 and AS2-1 were recently given orphan drug status for use on human brainstem gliomas.

## Chaparral Tea & Melanoma

Chaparral *(Larrea tridentata or Larrea divericata),* also called the *creosote bush*, has been around for years, popular as a medicinal tea for anything from common colds to cancer (72). NDGA (*nordihydroguairetic acid),* a highly potent substance, was extracted from chaparral in the early forties. Studies show that this extract can kill some viruses, pathogens, and cancer cells without the toxic adverse reactions found in chemo drugs (72). Scientists also discovered that NDGA works by preventing cancer cells from using glucose, and cancer cells thrive on sugar. If you destroy their capacity to use glucose, they will die (72). *Curezone.com* describes an article by Drs. Dean Burk and Mark Woods...*NDGA The Penicillin of Quinones*, which reports on the tumor inhibiting ability and basic non-toxicity of chaparral. They determined that although NDGA has such *low toxicity*, in laboratory testing it proved to be one of the most formidable cancer-*fighting anti-metabolic agents.* Unlike healthy cells in the body, cancer cells function without oxygen, however, they rely on huge amounts of sugar for their existence (72).

One very impressive case study demonstrated the effects of chaparral tea on melanoma in an elderly man, who also had a neck mass. He had endured several surgeries (72). According to *Curezone.com,* the patient brewed his own chaparral tea by using *7 to 8 grams* of the "leaves to a quart of hot water" and consuming "2 to 3 cups per day" (72). After several months, the melanoma on his face was dramatically reduced, and he no longer had the neck tumor (72).

Many people simply gather chaparral leaves and brew their own tea, but this can be dangerous if you consume too much. Chaparral grows abundantly in many western states. It has been reported that chaparral can cause liver damage if taken in excessively large amounts. It can also cause severe cramping and abdominal discomfort. It was recently removed from the marketplace by the FDA, based on reports of four people, who developed *liver toxicity* from the herb. *Curezone.com* says that the specifics from those four occurrences are not yet available (72).

Did you note those **FOUR cases of liver toxicity** above? This is an HERB we are discussing, NOT a pharmaceutical drug. Did you notice how quickly the FDA acted to remove this herb from shelves in America? If you have seen the reports on Vioxx®, Rezulin, Baycol, and other drugs, and read other chapters in this book, you already know that it is possible for a pharmaceutical drug to harm or kill thousands of people before the FDA forces if off the market. When more than two dozen cases of brain hemorrhage were reported to the FDA with the use of the drug PPA, it was **NOT** removed from the market. Dr. Strand, in his book *Death By Prescription*, explains that the drug was believed responsible for more than two dozen strokes (572). When reports of deaths began pouring in from the use of the drug Baycol, it was not removed from the market, but was prescribed to more than **half-a-million** patients (572). It was also believed to be the cause of more than a thousand reports of rhabdomyolysis (572), a devastating disease that destroys muscles.

More than 300 people died before the drug Propulsid was finally taken off the market, many of whom were children (385). The drug, Vioxx®, may have caused thousands of deaths before it was finally removed from the market (just recently), and now there are accusations that MERCK may have been involved in covering up data showing that the drug could cause fatal heart attacks. What is wrong with this picture? All DRUGS mentioned above were controlled by huge pharmaceutical conglomerates! The drug companies were making millions off the concoctions, and they fought to keep them in the marketplace, regardless of the death reports. The FDA had no interest in chaparral and there were no drug companies fighting to keep it on the shelves. And why the big secrecy about not revealing the details of the **four cases** of liver toxicity reported?

The FDA would love to control every mineral, vitamin, and herb on the market to keep them from the public, and make it impossible for consumers to obtain them, so you will be left in a state of total dependency on pharmaceutical drugs for staying alive. That is their ultimate goal. Their main concern is not the drugs manufactured by the pharmaceutical companies. They wait with bated breath for any minuscule report of an herb or vitamin preparation that gave somebody a sour stomach, headache or *buzz*, or isolated allergic reaction, so that they can find an excuse to take away YOUR right to purchase herbs, vitamins, and alternative therapies. Above is just one small sample of the blatant hypocrisy of the FDA. If you think that your safety is their ultimate concern, you are sadly mistaken. They are not concerned with keeping you safe, they are concerned with taking away your freedom, and keeping you and your loved ones locked into a future of total dependency on multiple chemicals concocted by the pharmaceutical industry!

## Chili Peppers

One of the main ingredients in these spicy little veggies, *capsaicin,* in lab tests, destroyed cancer cells. It is believed that capsaicin heats the cells from within, choking off the oxygen supply to the cells. Problem is, researchers won't be sure if capsaicin can be used topically for skin cancers until more testing is done to determine the full effects on healthy cells. There are, however, some capsaicin-containing skin creams on the market already for other uses, such as back and joint pain. It seems to me that if capsaicin is harmful to healthy cells, these other topical skin creams would have been discontinued years ago (593). This cream is even being used to ease the pain from shingles!

## Cholesterol Drug Kills Melanoma in Human Studies

As described by NeoPlas Innovation Director of Research, Dr. Stephen Cantrell, when they gave melanoma patients a "regimen of low-dose interferon with lovastatin," a common cholesterol-lowering drug, they saw tumors start to regress, often *in a few weeks* (76a). Not only that, but the most complained-about side effect was *fatigue* (76a). Most participants did not have the adverse effects usually found with chemo drugs and *radiation* (76a). Amazingly enough, they are also considering this new treatment for other lethal cancers, such as "pancreatic cancer, colon cancer, renal (kidney) cancer, mesothelioma, and a group of sarcomas, including osteosarcoma, chondrosarcoma and malignant fibrous histiocytoma" (76a). For more information on this exciting new development, see the NeoPlas website *www.neoplas.org* (76a). This treatment has "arrested or eradicated tumors in more than 80% of initial patients" (76a). They first used the treatment in 2000 on a man with "stage 4 melanoma, he remains disease-free today" (76a).

## CoQ10 - Low Levels Could Indicate Danger of Melanoma

A human study found very low CoQ10 levels in those with melanoma, and even lower levels in those who had melanomas that had spread to other areas of the body. This indicates that insufficient levels of this nutrient may increase a person's risk for melanoma and its spread (190).

## Cryo Treatment for Cancer

Usually guided by doppler imagery, cryo treatment involves freezing cancerous growths with a controlled method that seeks to leave healthy tissue undamaged. It has been used effectively in many types of cancer. It usually causes less damage to the body than radiation or chemo and is less invasive. It can't be considered entirely *painless* or *gentle*, but is being mentioned here, simply because it may be a more favorable choice than chemo or radiation, depending on the type cancer. Cryotherapy has been successfully used for abnormal cells of the cervix, retinoblastoma, skin cancers (before they become malignant), prostate cancer, liver growths, and others. It is sometimes used in combination with other therapies.

## Curaderm BEC5 - An Eggplant Extract (Topical) for Curing Non-Invasive Skin Cancers

Curaderm BEC5 is a topical cream, derived from eggplant, for treating superficial, non-invasive, non-melanoma skin cancers (basal cell and squamous cell cancers) and *actinic keratoses* (357). There is a lot of information on this cream on the internet. One such site is: *http://www.cura-care.com*. Also, see website: *http://www.bellaonline.com/articles/art56016.asp*. It is intended only for external use, and not for those who are allergic to aspirin or eggplant.

## CyberKnife® Therapy for Tumors

See chapter 34 in this book for details on CyberKnife® therapy, which is being used successfully for many cancers, including hard-to-reach brain tumors and other difficult-to-reach tumors. It is a gentle, painless procedure that does not require an incision, surgery, sedation or inpatient stay. It is quick, and as soon as the procedure is over, the patient is able to return home. There are very few risks and side effects, though it does involve some radiation (89a), and it can damage nearby healthy cells. Also, see NanoKnife™ therapy, chapter 34.

## Cytotron Therapy

See chapter 34 for more details on this gentle, non-invasive cancer therapy that many people are also using to restore cartilage in their joints, making joint-replacement surgeries completely unnecessary (90). You may hear this referred to as *QMR* or *Quantum Magnetic Resonance*—they are the same thing.

## ECT - ElectroChemical Therapy for Skin Cancer

Also described as *direct-current* ECT, this therapy originated in China (474). Widespread human testing has not yet been carried out in the U.S. In animals, *platinum electrodes* are placed on the tumor and treated with direct current (474). Animals with *colorectal carcinomas* that have spread to the liver were tested, and it was found that the treatment caused *significant* tumor shrinkage (474). More studies are planned in the U.S. on ECT.

Currently, an ECT machine developed by *Solco Biomedical* (known as the *Solco SET-C21*) by Swedish Professor, Nordenstrom, is claimed to have minimal side effects, boosts the immunity, and changes the pH of cells via electrochemical reactions (275). It is available from Korea. The therapy is being used for most cancers including: gastric, breast, lung, skin, and liver (275). It is widely used in Chinese hospitals, Korea, Germany, and surprisingly, some cancer treatment centers in the U.S.

## Espinheira Santa for Skin Cancers

Espinheira Santa (*Maytenus* species) is an evergreen holly from South America, where parts of the plant (*bark or leaf*) are popular for relieving *pain* (109). Researchers have identified extracts from this plant for skin cancer treatment. It is believed that the cancer-fighting qualities can be linked to the substances found in the bark of this evergreen. The herb is available in *tincture* form, or sold in bulk leaf tea format (109).

## Essiac Tea

See chapter six for more information on this healing herbal tea. You can find Essiac at many natural health food stores in an already prepared drinkable form, or a dry form that you brew yourself. Rene Caisse, a Canadian nurse, healed hundreds (possibly thousands) of people of every imaginable cancer using her amazing herbal tea, many of whom came to her after conventional medicine considered them hopeless. One of the most amazing books describing the effectiveness of this tea and how it was suppressed by the health industry in Canada, is called *The Essiac Report Canada's Remarkable Unknown Cancer Remedy,* by Richard Thomas, who claims that Flor-Essence® is the original (drinkable) formula that Rene Caisse used (580).

Note that there is some competition between the tea produced by Resperin Canada Essiac® and Flor-Essence® Essiac tea. Both companies claim that they have the original Essiac formula (the drinkable formula, not the injectable) that Rene Caisse used in treating her cancer patients. See chapter 16 in this book for the story of a young boy who was cured of lymphoma using a natural program that included Essiac® Resperin Canada's tea formula and 714X injections. A website that has Essiac® Resperin Canada tea is also given in that chapter. 714X isn't painless, gentle, or natural, but is being included since it was successfully used in combination with Essiac.

## Fungus Cure Also Cures Cancer, Says Oncology Physician

See chapter 34 of this book for the amazing cancer cure that Italian Oncologist, Dr. Simoncini, is using to cure his cancer patients within days. Cancerous growths are usually white. He says that they are a fungus, which can be killed with a non-toxic soda bicarb solution that alkalizes and kills the tumor. He uses topical 7% iodine for skin cancers (582).

## Garlic & Skin Cancer Prevention

Scientists in Japan have found that garlic inhibits skin cancer. If you are looking for the best type of garlic to use, use fresh organically-grown garlic or the garlic that has been aged (liquid form), which does not contain undesirable chemicals (551). Other important protectants against skin cancer, as well as aged garlic, are topical vitamin C and E, and vitamin A taken orally, discussed earlier in this chapter (551). Researchers believe it is possible that caffeine may also provide some skin protection.
I believe that Kyolic® brand is superior garlic. Kyolic® received an award from the National Nutrition Foods Association, and uses a stringent manufacturing and aging process. Whenever possible, it is best to use fresh, organic garlic.

## Ginseng & Skin Cancer

Recently, scientists found that a ginseng isolate could help reverse *melanoma* (504). Note that more than 5 to 10 grams of panax ginseng a day can cause nervousness and over-stimulation, as well as problems with hypertension and *headaches* (494). Women who have already gone through menopause may find, after using panax ginseng, that they have developed *vaginal bleeding,* but this side effect is highly unusual. Do not take Vitamin C at the same time you take ginseng. Space them apart by at least two hours for best usage (494).

## Grape Seed Extract for Skin Cancer

Scientists from the University of Alabama found (in animal testing) that *proanthocyanidins* in grapeskin resulted in up to *65 percent* less tumors and *78 percent smaller* tumors in those with skin cancer that had been caused by sunlight exposure (214).

## Green Tea Protects Against Skin Cancer

The anti-oxidant protection in green tea is so formidable that using it topically on the skin of mice (previously exposed to carcinogens), gave the animals close to perfect cancer immunity (551).

## Green Tea, Quercetin & Silibinin Protect Against Epidermoid Cancers

Another study showed that a substance found in green tea, known as EGCG or *epigallocatechin 3—gallate*, along with the nutrients quercetin and silibinin, offer significant protection against skin cancer (348). Green tea, silibinin and quercetin are also discussed in other chapters of this book.

Silibinin is found in milk thistle, and quercetin can be found in many foods including: red onions and apples (440), *teas…beans* (378), nuts, seeds, broccoli, and in the herb, ginkgo biloba.

## Hoxsey Formula & Skin Cancers

Though Harry Hoxsey was most famous for his tea recipe, he also developed a topical salve for skin cancer made primarily of *zinc chloride, antimony trisulfide and blood root* that is now used in a *related orthodox version* against skin cancer (504). A type of skin cancer treatment that has a nearly perfect *cure rate,* when used in treating *primary basal cell carcinomas,* is known as *Moh's surgery* (504). This surgery for skin cancer involves shaving off the cancerous growth layer by layer, until it is completely removed. The layers are reviewed microscopically.

## Krill Oil, Powerful Cancer-Fighter

Krill are tiny shrimp-like creatures that are found by the billions in Antarctic waters. Animal studies have shown that *Neptune Krill Oil* ™ may help prevent skin cancer. This oil is high in EPA and DHA essential oils and many other nutrients. Not only were the mice in the study given krill oil by mouth, but it was also applied topically to their skin. Melanomas were cut by nearly half in all animals receiving the krill oil (whether orally or topically), and those receiving both oral and topical application of krill oil, had their **risk** for melanoma cut by over 66%. The dose given to the mice was comparable to "2 g of Krill Oil per day for a 150-pound man or a 130-pound woman" (174). Website *http://www.discount-vitamins-herbs.net* has this supplement, as well as information on the research.

## LifeMel Honey for Cancer Patients

This amazing honey is also discussed in chapter 29 of this book. It is a special honey (developed in Israel) produced from the nectar of 40 herbs, including *Echinacea, Siberian ginseng,* and *Uncaria tomentosa,* with other natural ingredients. Two teaspoons per day (one in the am and one in the pm) are recommended (614). This special honey has been shown, in human testing, to prevent the neutropenia (serious drop in white blood cells) caused by chemotherapy and to lower the risk of severe platelet drop (thrombocytopenia), often found in chemo patients (614). You can find out more about this remarkable honey at website: *http://www.lifemel israel.com.* (614).

## Marine Phytoplankton & Skin Cancer Prevention

Another amazing sea nutrient may be helpful in the prevention of skin cancer. This, according to the findings of the PNAS - Proceedings of the National Academy of Sciences. See the full story at *http://www.shirleys-wellness-café.com/cancer.htm* (187) on marine phytoplankton.

## Milk Thistle Protects Against Skin Cancer

Milk thistle, discussed earlier in this book because of its importance in protecting the liver, can also help decrease problems with *psoriasis*. It may even be important in treating endometriosis. It enables estrogen to be processed by the liver, helps bile output from the body, and may one day be considered an important anti-cancer herb for fighting melanoma (288). As noted in *The Healing Power of Vitamins, Minerals, and Herbs*, from the Reader's Digest Association, Cleveland scientists discovered that topical applications of *the active ingredient, silymarin* (on the *skin of mice*), resulted in 2/3 less *skin tumors* after the animals were dosed with UV rays (288).

## Nanotechnology—*Lodamin*—Curing Cancer Without Side Effects

A new drug, Lodamin, which works by halting the blood vessel growth that tumors need to survive, was shown, in animal testing, to be effective against many tumor types, including those of the breast, brain, ovaries, uterus, prostate, neuroblastoma, and glioblastoma (401). It also worked very well in preventing cancer from going into the liver (401). The discovery of the drug, using *nanotechnology* and a derivative from a fungus, was quite accidental. Reports say that it can be taken orally without *side effects* (401). The drug also inhibited melanoma and lung cancer in mice (401). Lodamin is still in the testing phases, and is also being considered for treating macular degeneration and arthritis.

Note that shark cartilage and bindweed, also discussed in this book, work to starve tumors by cutting off blood supply to them, without adverse side effects. Bindweed should not be taken in its wild state.

## Poly–MVA (Palladium Lipoic Complex)

See chapter 14 for more information on this non-toxic nutritional formula that many cancer survivors are crediting to their complete recovery. Their main website is *www.polymva.net*. Many patients were sent home to die using only Poly-MVA for alternative therapy, yet they recovered fully and are alive years later. Their testimonials can be read at *http://www.S94567060.onlinehome.us/survivors/testimonials.html*, as well as their other website: *http://www.polymvasurvivors.com/testimonials.html*.

## Pomegranate Fruit Extract for Skin Tumors

This juice (*extract PFE*) can fight the development of cancerous skin growths (in animal testing) (237). Though these are animal studies only, it may not be long before you are able to purchase a sunscreen with natural pomegranate extract as a protectant against skin cancer. (See chapter five of this book for **a human study** showing that drinking pomegranate juice can help in the prevention of recurring prostate cancer.)

## Resveratrol Analog for Melanoma

If you go to the U.S. National Library of Medicine (which is also a service of the National Institutes of Health) on the internet, you can type in *resveratrol* and immediately find more than 2000 scientific studies conducted on resveratrol. Resveratrol is found in wine and grapes. See chapter three of this book for all the health benefits of resveratrol. A very similar plant phenolic acid known as *piceatannol*, also found in dark wines and grapeskin, is a popular component of many historical folk remedies, and has been found (in laboratory tests) to inhibit colorectal cancer cells. Details of the laboratory study on piceatannol and **melanoma** can be found at *http://www.springerlink.com/content/patxrdbrgml9yacg* (403).

An excellent study on the ability of resveratrol's cancer-fighting properties (including fighting melanoma), can be found in a detailed 58-page article at: *http://www.agrawal.org/PDF/ACR-Resveratrol1.pdf*, from the M.D. Anderson Cancer Center and the UCLA Center for Human Nutrition (346). Since excess use of fermented wines can cause liver damage, your best source is natural products such as grapeskin, cranberries, blueberries, pomegranates, and other food sources. Resveratrol is also available as a supplement in health food stores and internet sites.

## Rexin-G™ for Solid Tumors & Spreading Cancers

Rexin-G™ has been undergoing clinical trials at Mayo Clinic, M.D. Anderson, and a few other facilities. It is a drug for cancers that have spread, and those types of cancer that conventional medicine says do not respond to chemo (256). Human clinical studies, thus far, have had good results. In the very first human trial, 83% of the patients experienced tumor shrinkage. The patients had spreading pancreatic cancers (256). Good responses were also achieved in human studies involving several other types of metastatic cancer. Due to the reports, this drug is now used for treating all forms of *solid tumors* in the Philippines that are resistant to conventional therapy (256). The U.S. FDA has given the drug its *orphan drug status* for use with pancreatic cancers in the US, as well as other types of cancer spread (256). It is given intravenously, so isn't exactly natural or painless, but could be considered gentler than older chemo drugs because it is said to be a non-chemo drug, showing itself in **human** clinical trials, not to have the adverse side effects normally associated with chemo drugs (256). You can get more detailed information on this drug from website: *epeiusbiotech.com/rexin_g-factsheet.asp*. Epeius Biotechnologies are the producers of Rexin-G™ (257).

## Selenium Prevents Skin Cancer

Hairless mice were given selenium, then treated with harmful doses of *ultraviolet rays*. Those mice receiving the largest doses of the selenium in their diet experienced the fewest malignancies (551). Further testing revealed that this anti-cancer ability is probably because selenium increases glutathione levels (551). When researchers studied the effects of this important mineral on skin cancers, they found that insufficient amounts of selenium increased the participant's risk for *skin cancer*…5.8 *times* (507). It has also been discovered, in **human** research, that sufficient levels of selenium can dramatically reduce your risk for asthma.

## Shark Cartilage Kills Human Melanoma Cells

Shark cartilage, discussed in several other chapters, was able to reduce melanoma cells, in animal testing. When mice treated with skin cancer cells were also given shark cartilage supplementation on a daily basis, within 21 days, mice receiving the shark cartilage had a reduction in the size of their tumors, while tumors in the control group grew twice as large without the shark cartilage (550). Shark cartilage is not for use with children, nor during pregnancy, or if you have recently had a heart attack, transplant, surgery, chemo or radiation. It is not for those with high blood pressure, pheochromocytoma (adrenal tumor which can cause excessively high blood pressure), liver diseases (though it has been used successfully to treat liver cancer), allergies to seafood, ulcers or circulatory diseases. More information on dosing is given in chapter seven.

See chapter 34 of this book for information on an herb known as *bindweed* that is said to have *100 times* the ability at blocking blood vessel formation as that found in shark cartilage (150) (301a). Note that you should be consulting with a naturopathic health physician about your own individual dosing needs for this supplement.

## Skin Problems & Psoriasis

For psoriasis, be sure you are getting essential fatty acid omega-3's in your diet, and juice at least 3-4 glasses a day of fresh carrot juice. You need the vitamin A that you will be getting from the beta-carotene. Also, be sure that you are taking at least 3 glasses a day of barley green (powdered drink) juice, or another green powdered drink, such as Dee Simmon's *Green Miracle,* available at her website: *http://ultimateliving.com.* Be certain that you are juicing greens (e.g., fresh kale, spinach, broccoli, cabbage, and *celery) on a daily basis and getting plenty of water, if you are not on a water-restricted diet. You should also include a good complete vitamin supplement daily, as well as a mineral supplement, such as Maureen Kennedy Salaman's *Mineral Rich*®. (*Celery also fights colon cancer, high cholesterol and high blood pressure.) You may also want to try **low sodium** V8® Juice.

Others have had great success using shark cartilage supplements for psoriasis, as well as aloe and milk thistle. If you are a woman, you may want to get on a NATURAL progesterone cream supplement for psoriasis help, such as *ProgestiMax*®. You can order *ProgestiMax*® (and *Mineral Rich*®) at Maureen K. Salaman's website: *www.mksalaman.com.* See chapter 22 of this book on hormone replacement therapy for more information about when you should (and shouldn't) take natural progesterone.

Also, see pp 591-594 for information on the Italian Oncologist who has determined that cancer is a fungus, curable by alkalizing the tumor. He also believes that psoriasis is caused by a fungus.

## Soy (Fermented) Heals A Precancerous Skin Lesion

Haelan is nothing more than a soy drink that has undergone a fermentation process, yet it has shown impressive abilities, in some individuals, for treating different forms of cancer. An article from *Well Being Journal (www.wellbeingjournal.com)* by Donna Sage, M.S.S.A., tells the story of an eight-year-old who used Haelan to heal a *precancerous skin condition.* The boy's family history was positive for melanoma. Drinking an ounce of Haelan per day caused the lesion to completely heal (541). There are several websites that market Haelan, including *http://www.haelan partners.com.*

For information on Haelan, see the company's website at *www.haelan951.com.* Information on Haelan's Research Foundation's website was accumulated from clinical studies performed on fermented soy beverages manufactured by Haelan Products, Inc. of Woodinville, Washington. The Haelan fermented soy beverages are sold in the United States, without medical claims, and are available directly from the company or one of their distributors (143). If you are going to use soy products, fermented soy is best. Avoid the rest.

## *Trienelle®* Cream

This is a new cream that is applied topically to the skin for preventing skin cancer. It is rich in vitamin E, mushrooms, and many anti-oxidants, which also help stop the aging process. For information on this cream, see their website at: *http://www.trienelle.com.*

## Ukrain for Treating Melanoma

A human case study, involving the use of Ukrain only, a non-toxic therapy that is popular in Europe, resulted in a cure for malignant melanoma. For the last 12 years, there has been no reoccurrence of the disease in the patient who was treated. Ukrain has been proven, in **human** testing, to be totally safe, without toxic side effects (424).

## Vassourinha - Betulinic Acid

Vassourinha is an herb found abundantly within the rain forest and in the U.S. as well. Betulinic acid is one of the compounds taken from this herb. This extract has been very impressive against leukemia, cancer, and viruses such as HIV, and it has also demonstrated the ability to work against bone, brain, and skin tumors, while being non-toxic to normal cells (302). Vassourinha may lower blood pressure (302). Studies demonstrate that betulinic acid helps to seek out and destroy human malignant skin cells without harming normal cells, something chemo drugs fail miserably at, and it was also able to inhibit HIV I. The herb's affinity for skin cancer cells is remarkable, especially when the data was put alongside that of several toxic chemo drugs (302).

## Soda Bicarb, Iodine & Magnesium for Cancer

For an amazing study on the importance of alkalizing the body with a rapid, powerful ingredient as simple as soda bicarb, see the book: *Sodium Bicarbonate Rich Man's Poor Man's Cancer Treatment* by Dr. Mark Sircus, Ac., OMD. Although Dr. Simoncini (see chapter 34) uses topical iodine for skin cancer, Dr. Sircus says taking soda bicarb orally can accomplish much the same thing. He discusses a detailed step-by-step program that a man with prostate cancer (that had spread into his bones) used to alkalize his body with oral soda bicarb, curing his cancer within 11 days (566c). You can get *Arm & Hammer*® soda bicarb at your local grocers for about a dollar–a-pound. They do not advertise the product for cancer use, but it is used for alkalizing a "sour stomach." There has been some controversy about aluminum in baking soda, but *Arm & Hammer*® says that their product contains no aluminum. For a company that sells a soda bicarb that they guarantee to be aluminum-free, see Bob's Red Mill products at: *http://www.bobsredmill.com* (566c). Simply use pH testing strips that you can get at your local health food store to check your urine or saliva pH.

Dr. Sircus also has much to say about the pervasive lack of magnesium and iodine in the average diet, and why these deficiencies are causing heart disease, cancer, and many other diseases. These minerals are required in every single metabolic process of the body without which we cannot survive. See his amazing books, *Magnesium The Ultimate Heart Medicine* and *Magnesium Medicine The Lamp of Life,* available at: *http://www.magnesiumforlife.com* (566b). He also discusses a new transdermal form of magnesium that you simply spray onto your skin (or use as flakes in your bath or in a footbath), which can be found at website: *http://www. ancient-minerals.com* or *www.magneticclay.com.*(566b).

Also, see Dr. Sircus' book, *Iodine Bringing Back the Universal Medicine,* on the importance of iodine in fighting yeast (and killing cancer in the process), bacteria, malaria, flu, and many other ailments caused by a deficiency in this critical mineral (566a). You can find a food-grade, gentle form of superior iodine called *Magnascent* (or *Nascent* iodine) at *http://www.magnascent.com* and *http://www.magneticclay.com.* Also, see Appendix II.

## Yucca Root Extract (Topical)

An extract from the yucca plant root is used topically, not only for skin disorders, but many believe it can help fight skin cancer.

# CHAPTER 16

# GENTLE CURES FOR TOUGH LYMPHOMAS & SARCOMAS

*"Have mercy upon me, O Lord; For I am weak: O Lord, heal me; for my bones are vexed." (Psalm 6:2) "Be not wise in thine own eyes: fear the Lord, and depart from evil. It shall be health to thy navel, and marrow to thy bones." (Proverbs 3:7-8)*

## Sarcomas

Sarcomas usually begin as a bone mass, but can be found in nearly every part of the body, including fat and muscle. Types of sarcomas (see website: *www.cancer-healing.com* and *www.life-enthusiast.com/usa*) are:

- Osteosarcoma or osteogenic sarcoma (bone)
- Chondrosarcoma (cartilage)
- Leiomyosarcoma (smooth muscle) involuntary muscle
- Rhabdomyosarcoma (skeletal muscle) voluntary striated muscle
- Mesothelial sarcoma or mesothelioma (membranous lining of body cavities)
- Fibrosarcoma (fibrous tissue)
- Angiosarcoma or hemangioendothelioma (blood vessels)
- Liposarcoma (adipose tissue)
- Glioma or astrocytoma (neurogenic connective tissue found in the brain)
- Myxosarcoma (primitive embryonic connective tissue)
- Mesenchymous or mixed mesodermal tumor (mixed connective tissue types) (263).

## AHCC—Mushroom Combo Enhances Immunity in Human Study With Rhabdomyosarcoma

AHCC *(Active hexose correlated compound)* is a complex compound composed of the mycelia of many mushrooms. In **human** testing, it was found (when given in doses of "3g/day orally for 2-6 months") to significantly increase the body's natural immunity at killing *rhabdomyosarcoma* cells and several other types of cancerous cells (206). This compound is found at many natural health food stores and online supplement providers (e.g., *www.discount-vitamins-herbs.net).*

## Hodgkin's Versus Non-Hodgkin's Lymphoma

Lymphomas are cancers that arise from the body's lymphatic system, the system in your body that works like a filter, straining out pathogens and abnormalities. There are two main forms of lymphoma: *Hodgkin's Disease,* or *Hodgkin's lymphoma* and *non-Hodgkin's lymphoma* (218). Lymphomas (except for Hodgkins) are known as *non-Hodgkin's lymphoma* (155). The only way to tell them apart is to look at the cells under a microscope (usually done after a biopsy), as discussed at website: *www.oncology channel.com/nonhodgkins.* You will find a cell known as *Reed-Sternberg cells* in Hodgkin's lymphoma. They do not occur in non-Hodgkin's lymphoma (155).

Lymphomas are also staged according to their progression or severity, with Stage I being the least severe, meaning that the cancer is in at least one lymph node. Once the cancer has spread beyond the lymph system to other areas of the body, it is considered Stage IV. There are more than a dozen different types of non-Hodgkins lymphoma, and its severity depends on its type, location, whether or not it has spread, and how fast it is growing. Some cancers are aggressive, growing and spreading very rapidly; others grow very slowly.

## CDA-II & Non-Hodgkin's Lymphoma

CDA-II is a type of nutritional therapy combined with a urine therapy that was studied extensively in Taiwan by Dr. Ming C. Liau, who also spent 14 years working with Dr. Burzynski in Houston, Texas. Clinical trials were done at Anhui Medical University showing that this treatment was safe and effective. The only adverse effect was vein irritation and rarely, a potential for venous thrombosis. It is sometimes combined with B17 and vitamin C with very good results (468).

## Chemo Pill for Advanced Lymphoma & Leukemia

A new chemo pill that developers claim does not have the adverse side effects normally seen with usual chemo drugs, is being touted as a way to fight several types of lymphoma and leukemia. It is known as *fostamatinib disodium* and thus far, in **human** trials, is showing great promise for aggressive lymphomas and leukemia. For details, see website: *http://insciences.org/article.php?article_id=570*, and study information per the University of Rochester Medical Center (72a).

## CyberKnife® Therapy for Spinal Cord Tumors, Sarcomas & Other Tumors

See chapter 34 in this book for details on CyberKnife® therapy, which is being used successfully for many cancers, including hard-to-reach brain tumors, sarcomas, and spinal cord tumors. It is a gentle, painless procedure that does not require an incision, surgery, sedation or inpatient stay. It is very quick, and as soon as the procedure is over, the patient is able to return home. There are very few risks and side effects, though it does involve some radiation (89a), and it can damage nearby healthy cells. Also, see NanoKnife™, chapter 34.

## Cytotron Therapy

See chapter 34 in this book for more details on this gentle, non-invasive cancer therapy that many people are also using to restore cartilage in their joints, making joint-replacement surgeries completely unnecessary (90). You may hear this referred to as *QMR* or *Quantum Magnetic Resonance.*

## Extracorporeal Photopheresis with Autologous Dendritic Cell Vaccine for T-cell Lymphoma (UV Light Therapy)

Another treatment that is available at Issels Cancer Treatment Centers (and also approved by the FDA for *cutaneous T-cell lymphoma*), this ultraviolet light therapy eliminates cancer cells. A type of white blood cell is extracted, treated with UV light, and allowed to mature, then the patient is given small injections of the mature cells in a regimented dosing over time (290). Issels website is *http://www.issels.com.* Their ph#888-447-7357 (290).

## Fungus Cure Also Cures Cancer, Says Oncology Physician

See chapter 34 of this book for the amazing cancer cure that Italian Oncologist, Dr. Simoncini, is using to cure his cancer patients within just days! Cancerous growths are usually WHITE. He says that they are actually a fungus, which can be killed with a non-toxic soda bicarb solution that quickly alkalizes the tumor for destruction (582).

## A High Dose Vitamin C Regimen Cures Hodgkin's Disease (Also see p. 544 for a new form of vitamin C!)

### Case #1

When Bernard Rimland, Ph.D., was told that his young daughter had terminal Hodgkin's lymphoma, with only a few months to live, he began her on a high dose vitamin C regimen (550). She was given 1000 mg/day of niacinamide, and *40 grams* per day of vitamin C. (He divided the dose throughout the day.) She also received supplements of vitamins and minerals in normal dosages (550). Her father persistently gave the Oncologists documentation on how well vitamin C could work, yet they completely ignored him and never read the material. Though his own daughter improved and completely recovered after receiving the high dose vitamin C regimen, he sadly commented that the Oncologists refused to treat other children in the ward with vitamin C as he had done for his daughter, despite her remarkable recovery (550).

Dr. Rimland believed in high-dose vitamin C for leukemia. Irwin Stone documented many cases of people who recovered from leukemia using this treatment. Though Dr. Rimland's high dose nutritional program saved his daughter's life, and he feels might have spared other children, he could not convince the Oncologists (550).

Note that if you are taking high dose (oral) vitamin C and concerned about the ascorbic acid causing stomach upset, you can obtain buffered C crystals which have an alkaline pH and are less irritating to the stomach, or Ester-C® (calcium ascorbate form). Vitamin C given intravenously (sodium ascorbate form), even in massive doses, will not usually cause stomach upset. There are many websites that offer buffered C crystals. Natural health food stores also carry them. High dose vitamin C is often given intravenously at natural health centers. Taking the liquid C in crystals can be damaging to dental enamel, so use caution. Chewable vitamin C can harm the tooth enamel, yet many C manufacturers distribute these chewable C vitamins for use by children. If your child is seriously ill, and you are interested in a new oral form of vitamin C that is more potent than the intravenous C, refer to page 544 in this book.)

## Case #2

Another human success story using megadosing of intravenous vitamin C therapy was described at website: *http://www.seanet.com/~alexs/ascorbate/197x/stone-I-orthomol_psych-1976-v5-n3-p183.html*, in a paper by Cameron et al, 1975 (571a). This was back when Dr. Irwin Stone, Cameron Campbell, Linus Pauling, and others, believed in using megadose vitamin C to cure their cancer patients (571a). A 42 year-old man with *malignant lymphoma* had planned for "conventional treatment," but due to a set of circumstances and delays, he was given ascorbate "10,000 mg a day intravenously for the first 10 days and then 10,000 mg a day orally thereafter" (571a). He continued with the same oral dose for *five months*. He had recovered so rapidly, he no longer had an "enlarged liver or spleen." For unknown reasons, the daily *10,000 mg* oral *ascorbate* was stopped and he relapsed to the point where he was sent back to the hospital. He was then "given 20,000 mg a day of ascorbate, intravenously, for two weeks and then 12,500 mg a day orally thereafter." Within six months, he was well and back to heavy employment [and] continues to take ascorbic acid 12,500 mg a day and has no evidence of active disease" (571a). See page 544 for information on an exciting new oral form of C.

## Andrographis & Non-Hodgkin's Lymphoma

Andrographis is a plant that has been used for medicinal purposes for many years in Asia. Conclusive studies have shown it to be effective **(with very low toxicity)** against several different forms of cancer, including *non-Hodgkin's* lymphoma. Very rarely, andrographis may cause heart fluttering, light-headedness, or a mild to severe allergic reaction (20). Andrographis can be purchased in a tablet form called *Androtech*, which is standardized and produced by BioTherapies. In their tablet, they also use *enchinacea and zinc* (20).

## Ashwagandha, E. S., & Black Seed (Black Cumin or Nigella Sativa) for Dalton's Ascitic Lymphoma

Dalton's lymphoma is a cancer of the T-cells. These are cells which keep the immune system healthy, some directly killing pathogens and mutants. (If you get an organ transplant, these are the cells that will do their best to reject it.) The herb, Ashwagandha, was tested on mice with Dalton's ascitic lymphoma. The mice receiving the ashwagandha had longer life spans and fewer cancers (542). Another herb that fights this type lymphoma is the leaves of *Elephantopus scaber* [abbreviated as E.S. above]. According to the *Indian Journal of Pharmaceutical Sciences,* in animal studies, the herb extended lifespans. The injections halted the spread of the cancer cells (531). Black seed, sometimes referred to as *black cumin,* has also demonstrated anti-cancer activity against Dalton's lymphoma cells. This herb contains essential fatty acids, carotene, and many nutrients. True black seed is also known as *Nigella sativa,* and is a very common spice in middle-eastern countries. It should not be used during pregnancy, nor without first consulting your physician or Naturopath.

## Aspartame (aka *Nutra-Sweet* & *Equal)* Linked to Several Cancers, Including Leukemia & Lymphomas

Thousands of food items now contain aspartame sweeteners, including drinks and diet foods. A seven year animal study showed a definite link between "high rates of lymphomas, leukemias, urinary tumors, tumors of certain nerves and other cancers in rats" (25). In spite of all this, the substance continues to be put into diet drinks, sodas, foods, and treats for our children. Why? You can walk into any major grocery store chain and find soft drinks advertised as "diet drinks" containing aspartame. No one has acted to voluntarily remove them from store shelves; not the merchants, not the FDA (unless they move to do so after this book comes out in print). Why? Are YOU ingesting diet soft drinks and treats (e.g., pudding, jello, ice cream, yogurt) with aspartame in them? Well, now you know that they have been linked to the above types of cancer. The question is: will YOU continue to ingest them and give them to your children, knowing this?

## Beta-Glucan & Stage IV Non-Hodgkin's Lymphoma

Beta-Glucan is a polysaccharide, a cultured extract derived from baker's yeast (286). At website: *AboutBetaglucan.com,* a victim of Stage IV non-Hodgkins T-cell lymphoma credits survival to beta-glucan supplements, after his physicians had considered him hopeless. This was after giving him chemo for three years and a failed *stem cell transplant* (286). He reversed his cancer using beta-glucan and simple dietary changes (286).

Beta-glucan supplements are available at natural health food stores and some internet sites. Another website that promotes oat beta-glucan is: *www.cancertreatments.net/cancer.html* (221). According to this website, there is now available an even more potent beta-glucan taken from *baker's yeast* (221). Also, see related website: *www.cancer-prevention.net.*

## Burzynski's Antineoplastons CURE Lymphomas & Other Cancers WITHOUT Toxic Side Effects!

Maryjo Siegel was diagnosed with fatal non-Hodgkin's lymphoma in 1991. She was completely cured using non-toxic antineoplastons developed by Dr. Stanislaw Burzynski in Houston, Texas. She is still alive and well (as of an email from her in June 2009), living a normal life, and has never had a reoccurrence of cancer). You can send her an email at *maryjo@siegel.net,* and she will tell you about her experience with antineoplastons. She testified before the U.S. House of Representatives Government Reform and Oversight Committee on February 4, 1998. Below is that testimony:

### Testimony Before the US House of Representatives Government Reform and Oversight Committee on February 4, 1998

> Seven years ago, I was stricken with a fatal cancer, non-Hodgkin's lymphoma, for which no conventional cure yet exists. This disease is treatable for periods of time with chemo-therapy and/or radiation, but the outcome is always death.
>
> My husband Steve and I were devastated by my prognosis, but determined to find a cure. Our research took us to top lymphoma specialists at esteemed medical institutions like UCLA, USC, Stanford, and the Dana Farber Cancer Institute in Boston. All the experts confirmed our worst fears: with existing therapies, my disease was incurable.
>
> At Dana Farber, a ray of hope emerged with the recommendation that I undergo an autologous bone marrow transplant. This highly controversial procedure would require that I receive extremely high-dose chemotherapy and as much radiation as people who were within 1 mile of "ground zero" at Hiroshima. I would lose my hair, experience severe nausea and vomiting, and the threat of bacterial and viral infection would keep me in complete isolation for 6 weeks. My quality of life after treatment would be drastically diminished. From the chemotherapy, I would become sterile. There would be damage to my heart, lungs, liver, kidneys, and bladder. Collateral radiation damage would affect my eyes, salivary glands and

thyroid, with a greater than 50% chance that I would develop leukemia if I were lucky enough to survive just 10 years. I was frightened and suspicious because only a handful of patients had survived this procedure with good long-term results. One such person was the late Senator Paul Tsongas, who eventually died of complications caused by the procedure.

Fortunately, we discovered the work of Stanislaw Burzynski MD, PhD, who was treating patients who have advanced cancer with a gentle, nontoxic therapy he had discovered. As I began Dr. Burzynski's antineoplaston treatment, my lymphoma had progressed to a stage IV (there is no stage V). Malignant tumors were growing throughout my body. My bone marrow was infiltrated, and there was a large tumor growing on the side of my neck. After only 3 weeks on this medicine, that tumor disappeared! Subsequent scans performed at UCLA showed continued reduction in tumor size.

During antineoplaston treatment, my quality of life was excellent, virtually free of side effects. I was an active and involved mother, an absolute necessity when you are raising three teenagers. More importantly, the drug stopped my supposedly terminal cancer. Within 12 months I was pronounced in remission, not by Dr. Burzynski, but by the same lymphoma expert at UCLA who had originally diagnosed me and told me I faced certain death from this disease. I went off treatment and remained in remission for 2 years, when a follow-up scan revealed a possible return of the disease. Immediately, Dr. Burzynski prescribed a regimen of antineoplaston capsules. Within 5 months, I was once again in remission and have remained cancer-free to this day.

That's the end of the good news. The tragedy is that our government, namely the FDA, has been keeping what author [of The Burzynski Breakthrough] Tom Elias calls "the century's most promising cancer treatment" from becoming widely available to cancer patients. The agency has spent untold millions of taxpayer dollars in a systematic attempt to harass, discredit, stonewall, and even imprison Dr. Burzynski.

As incredible as it sounds, in November 1995, the FDA indicted Dr. Burzynski on 75 criminal counts, most having to do with alleged technical violations of the Interstate Commerce Act and none having to do with his practice of medicine or the effectiveness of his drug. Dr. Burzynski had been legally treating patients under Texas State law for some 20 years, and not one patient in all that time had ever filed a complaint. If Dr. Burzynski had been convicted on all 75 counts, he could have been sentenced to 290 years in a federal prison.

Are antineoplastons effective? Ask the FDA. Apparently, the FDA believes the answer is "Yes," because it fought tenaciously to keep the question of the effectiveness of antineoplastons out of the trial. Dr. Burzynski tried to make it a part of the trial. Apparently, both the FDA and Dr. Burzynski believed he could prove the drug works. The FDA also fought to keep the full truth from the jury by preventing Dr. Burzynski's patients from testifying, while Burzynski asked the judge to allow the patients to tell their stories.

In the end, Dr. Burzynski was acquitted on all counts. But I ask you in Congress, and particularly my representative, Mr. Waxman, how you can allow the FDA to squander taxpayer money in an idiotic prosecution, the success of which would mean the deaths of hundreds of cancer patients? The FDA was unable to find even a single patient to testify against Dr. Burzynski!

Peter Barton Hutt, a former FDA Chief Counsel, has said "If you beat the FDA in court, you have an angry FDA that is willing to slit your throat." Indeed, although the FDA lost the courtroom battle against Dr. Burzynski, it continues to wage war against him and his patients. The agency interferes in his practice by telling him whom he can and cannot treat. With many types of cancer, the FDA requires patients to have failed not one but two rounds of chemotherapy before they can be treated with antineoplastons. In many cases the chemo has so ravaged their immune systems that they literally have nothing left to fight with, and they die. The FDA forbids the use of steroids in the treatment of Dr. Burzynski's lymphoma patients, even when they are needed to temporarily shrink tumors and relieve pain, as in my own case. Because I was on treatment prior to the FDA taking over his practice of medicine, Dr. Burzynski was able to inject me with Medrol to relieve the pain and tightness in my neck caused by the tumor. Now, however, the FDA is not concerned with patient comfort, rather, their twisted logic dictates that good data collection outweighs humane medical treatment.

The FDA demands that Dr. Burzynski's patients with lymphoma stop treatment if they have not achieved 50% tumor reduction within 6 months. The absurdity of this typically arbitrary FDA requirement became clear when one Burzynski patient — Frances Langham — was to be forced off treatment because she had only a 44% reduction after 6 months! She is lucky to be from Arkansas and politically connected. She received a "special dispensation," allowing her to continue treatment. But the FDA removed her from the clinical trial, meaning that even if cured in the future, the FDA will count her as a "treatment failure" in determining how effective antineoplastons are! These treatment "restrictions" are only applied to Dr. Burzynski's clinical trials, whereas lymphoma patients involved in Idec Pharmaceutical's C2B8 and Elan Pharmaceutical's phenylacetate trials, do not have to meet these same treatment criteria. Is it possible that FDA has a bias against Dr. Burzynski and his patients have to suffer as a result?

Who gave the FDA the right to play God? Was it the intent of Congress to give the FDA the kind of power it exercises over life and death decisions with no accountability? By denying terminally ill patients with cancer access to antineoplastons, this agency literally decides "who shall live and who shall die."

I have had to watch as children and adults suffer and die as a result of FDA intransigence. Patients plead to be allowed into antineoplaston clinical trials; however, the FDA says "No. You don't qualify." Shouldn't it be the doctor, in concert with the patient, making these important medical treatment decisions, rather than an FDA official who does not even know the case? Clearly, the FDA is denying these patients their freedom of medical choice. Because conventional FDA-approved remedies have failed to work for the majority of Dr. Burzynski's patients, often their only choice is antineoplastons or death!

It has been 26 years since President Nixon declared the War on Cancer. Public expenditures now exceed $30 billion, and private research and development funds must total at least 10 times that amount, yet the death rate continues its relentless climb. It is time for a new approach to treating cancer. The only way this will become a reality is by allowing patients with cancer expanded access to new, experimental, and innovative treatments. Until we have a cure, all treatments, conventional and alternative, are experimental!

Dr. Nicolas Patronas, Chief of Neuroradiology at the National Cancer Institute, testified under oath that antineoplastons are the most effective treatment for brain tumors he has ever seen. Top oncologists have lauded Dr. Burzynski's work, including those at the University of Washington and Georgetown University. Doctors and scientists around the world eagerly await the approval of antineoplastons. [In 1991] Dr. Michael Friedman, [past] commissioner of the FDA, wrote that "Antineoplastons deserve a closer look...the human brain tumor responses are real." So why is the FDA so determined to impede the progress of a drug with such promising results?

Congressmen, we implore you to restore the right to choose our own health care. You have the power to give us back our freedom. Mr. Waxman, as your constituent I know you staunchly support both the FDA and a woman's right to an abortion. But can you really condone a government policy which grants a mother the right to choose death for her fetus, while denying a dying cancer patient one last hope for life?

In his March 29, 1996, press conference, President Clinton announced new initiatives to expedite the approval process for innovative new cancer drugs like antineoplastons. Since then, the FDA has bluntly stated that the President's initiative has changed nothing. It is time for congressional oversight to ensure that this mandate is carried out. Patients with terminal illnesses deserve the chance to win their personal War on Cancer, and it is up to Congress to ensure they have the weaponry with which to fight.
Thank you.

Submitted by Mary Jo Siegel to the Burzynski Patient Group website (562).

Also, see chapter 14 in this book for more information on the non-toxic therapy of antineoplastons, which have brought many hopeless, inoperable cancer patients into total remission, even those with lymphomas and so-called *terminal* brain cancers, many of them children! Maryjo also sent a letter to Ted Kennedy about antineoplastons after he was diagnosed with a brain tumor. The Burzynski Clinic website is at *www.burzynskiclinic.com.* Also, see the story of a woman with fatal non-Hodgkins lymphoma who was cured with antineoplastons at website: *http://www.burzynskiclinic.com/patient_resources.php?table=patient_resources&pag*

*e=8*. When she was diagnosed, she was not expected to live. That was more than seven years ago. Antineoplastons are given intravenously and orally in a form called PBs or sodium phenylbutrates. The FDA has finally approved the oral form of antineoplastons (PBs) for off-label use, and antineoplastons A10 and AS2-1 were recently given orphan drug status for use on human brainstem gliomas.

## Burzynski's Antineoplastons Cure Nurse With Non-Hodgkin's Lymphoma

For another case of a patient, an RN who was completely cured of Non-Hodgkin's lymphoma through Dr. Burzynski's clinic, see website: *http://burzynskipatientgroup.org*.

## Chlorella & Bone Cancer

Refer to other chapters in this book for more details on the benefits of chlorella. Dr. Joseph Mercola of *www.mercola.com* says that cancer patients have taken *30 grams of chlorella* a day, and he knows of a *bone cancer* patient that had remarkable improvement after using chlorella *(20 grams...per day)* for just *6 months* (485). Be sure that you are under the care of your physician or Naturopath when taking this, or any supplement.

## Cholesterol Drug for Sarcomas - No Toxic Side Effects (Including *Osteosarcoma, Chondrosarcoma & Malignant Fibrous Histiocytoma*)

For details on a new cancer-treatment regimen that includes combining "low-dose interferon with lovastatin," so far used in melanoma (but also being considered for other cancers like sarcomas, doctors saw tumors start to regress, often in *a few weeks)* (76a), see website *www.neoplas.org*, and chapter 34 in this book. The treatment has no toxic side effects like those found in chemo and *radiation* (76a). Just be aware that statin drugs can strip CoQ10 out of your body. If you choose this treatment, let your doctor know this so that they can advise you on CoQ10 supplementation. Some physicians are not aware of this problem with statin drugs.

## Essiac Tea for All Cancers

See chapter six for more information on this healing herbal tea. You can obtain Flor-Essence® at many natural health food stores in an already prepared drinkable form, or a powdered form that you brew yourself. Rene Caisse, a Canadian nurse, healed hundreds (possibly thousands) of people of every imaginable cancer using her amazing herbal tea, many of whom came to her after conventional medicine considered them incurable and hopeless. One of the most amazing books describing the effectiveness of this tea and how it was suppressed by the health industry in Canada is called: *The Essiac Report Canada's Remarkable Unknown Cancer Remedy*, by Richard Thomas, who claims that Flor-Essence® is the original (drinkable) formula that Rene Caisse used (580).

Note that there is some competition between the tea produced by Resperin Canada Essiac® and Flor-Essence® Essiac tea. Both companies claim that they have the original Essiac formula (the drinkable formula, not the injectable) that Rene Caisse used in treating her cancer patients. See later in this chapter for the story of a young boy who was cured of lymphoma using a natural program that included Essiac® Resperin Canada's tea formula and 714X injections. A website that has Essiac® Resperin Canada is also given. Though 714X injections are not gentle or natural, they are included because they were used in conjunction with Essiac in this particular case.

## How Flax Healed Hodgkin's Lymphoma & Bone Cancer

Some amazing, even miraculous cancer cures, have been attributed to flax seed oil. Website, *www.healingcancernaturally.com*, gives the case of an eleven year-old boy, Timmy G., who was diagnosed with Hodgkin's disease. After failure to respond to multiple doses of radiation, he was declared incurable with only months to live (99). Someone sent an article to his mother that led her to the use of the Budwig flax oil diet. Within only days on the diet, her son began breathing normally "for the first time in almost two years." He eventually returned to school and is now 18 years of age and credits his life to Dr. Budwig's formula (99). The Budwig diet is very simple. The two main ingredients are flax oil and cottage cheese:

> For each tablespoon of flaxoil, add 2 tablespoons of low-fat cottage cheese (or quark) or 6 tablespoons of yoghurt. The flaxoil/cottage cheese or flaxoil/yoghurt mixture

> should be fully blended until no traces of oil remain visible, proving that the highly unsaturated fatty acids have become water soluble (a hand-mixer or a blender works well) (99). [Quark is a pasty type of white cheese.]

See Chapter 18 of this book for more information on the healing powers of flax oil and details of the Budwig diet. (It is also discussed in greater detail in chapter 14 because of its success against brain cancer.) Website, *www.curezone.com,* relates the story of the Budwig formula being used for a hopeless cancer of the bone, however, the patient used larger amounts of flax oil a day than the official diet calls for. He started out with 4 tablespoons of flax oil a day (plus the cottage cheese) (40). A few days later, he increased it to 8-10 tablespoons of flax oil a day, combined with the cottage cheese. Three months later, all of his lab work came back negative, his cancer CURED. His physician was so incredulous that he ordered tests three times, thinking there must be some mistake. There was no error. The patient, an elderly grandfather, was in complete remission (40).

See chapter eight of this book for more information on natural treatments and cures for leukemia and multiple myelomas. If using dairy, always go with organic, or if you live near a farmer who has healthy herds, practices very sanitary dairy farming, and can provide you with raw milk products and other dairy, use these with the Budwig diet, otherwise, avoid dairy altogether. (See chapter 26.) If raw milk is not produced by herds from scrupulously clean dairy farmers, it can be full of harmful bacteria.

## Fruits & Vegetables Reduce Non-Hodgkin's Lymphoma Risk

Multiple human studies have been done to show that eating more fruits and vegetables reduces the risk for many types of cancer, including non-Hodgkin's lymphoma.

## Ginger & Willow Bark for Lymphoma

Ginger has apparent anti-cancer effects due to its immune-boosting power. It fights cancerous cells and thins the blood (122). One of the many components (out of hundreds) in ginger is geraniol. Geraniol is found not only in ginger, but rosemary as well. Apparently, it only took very minute amounts of the geraniol to produce the desired effects (122).

Another herb that does this is willow bark, from which aspirin is derived (387). Be aware that you should discuss any new herb with your physician or Naturopath first, before ingesting.

## Graviola

See chapters five and six of this book for information on the curative and healing properties of the herb, Graviola.

## Green Tea Fights Non-Hodgkin's Lymphoma

Green tea helps prevent abnormalities in DNA and, in animal testing, cut non-Hodgkin's lymphoma occurrence in half (59). A very popular chemotherapy drug, *Cyclophosphamide,* was also given to lab animals, but it simply could not duplicate **the same results as the green tea in the animals.** Researchers discovered that those cancers responding best to green tea were throat and gastric, melanoma, respiratory (lung), liver, and breast cancers (59). Green tea has also been found, in animal testing by Israeli researchers, to actually regenerate brain cells, something hitherto thought impossible (169).

## Guacatonga & Andiroba - Two Herbs That Fight Sarcoma

Sarcomas are malignant growths that arise in body tissues and bone cells. Ewing's sarcoma, for example, though usually found in bone, can be found in nearly any other part of the body (112). **Guacatonga** *(Casearia sylvestris)* also known as *wild coffee,* and a host of other common names, is a small bush or tree that grows in the Amazon and several Central and South American countries (141). Multiple chemicals have been extracted from the leaves and stems, all showing impressive anti-cancer, anti-tumor properties. It appears that, in some cases, it takes very small amounts of the herb to kill cancer cells. Guacatonga also contains *lapacho,* a component found in pau d'arco tea (141). Lapacho has blood-thinning properties. Japanese researchers discovered an extract from the leaf of guacatonga that was very active, in animal testing, against sarcomas. There are no reported drug interactions or adverse effects in using this herb (141), but always check with your physician before doing so.

**Andiroba** *(Carapa guianensis)* is a tree from the rain forest that produces an oil-rich nut. Researchers reported in 2002, that the oil could fight the type of abnormal cells of the cervix that change to cancer. In laboratory tests, several parts of the tree could restrict sarcoma cells. The oil is used to treat skin disorders, including skin cancers, parasites, rashes, and fungi (19).

## 714X—Gaston Naessens

Gaston Naessens was a researcher who developed a very powerful microscope that allowed him to visualize living organisms in the blood. Gaston believed that diseases are not caused by germs, but that they come about because of disease processes. He believed that the human body (with a healthy-functioning immune system) will not produce diseases. From his work with *somatids*, Naessens later developed enzyme 714X to enhance the body's immunity. 714X, a combination of "camphor and nitrogen, is given by hypodermic needle right into the lymph system" (505). Though 714X is not *natural, gentle,* or *painless*, it is included here for informational purposes, and because of its success treating various cancers without the side effects seen with chemo and radiation.

714X has been credited with many remissions for those with HIV and cancer (505). For details on the amazing story of a young man who used 714X, Resperin Canada Essiac tea®, and nutritional changes to cure his **Hodgkin's lymphoma**, see website *https://www.billybest.net/order Essiac.htm* for *Billy's Story*, as told by his parents, Sue and Bill Best. You may recall seeing Billy on the news. In 1994 he was "diagnosed with Hodgkins Disease...[at] 16 years old" (345). His parents explained that: "Not knowing any better, we took the advice of the oncologists and Billy started chemotherapy in July." He was treated until October, when he left home, leaving his parents a note telling them that he refused to continue the chemo. He felt that it was "killing him" (345). Eventually, the news media picked up the story and it aired on two prominent TV shows in 1999. Once Billy came back home, diagnostics at Dana Farber Cancer Institute in Boston determined that the chemo had not helped him and his cancer was growing and worsening. When his parents decided to opt out of any further chemo, radiation, or conventional treatments, the hospital actually attempted to have his parents declared as "unfit," and have him removed from their custody, however, the hospital lost, because the state refused involvement (345). (Does any of this sound familiar?)

The parents began alternative treatment, including nutritional changes (e.g., no sugar, dairy products, or carbonated beverages, and no red meats), plenty of "fresh, organic produce...distilled water...[and]

unprocessed natural foods." He was also taking "8000 mg of vitamin C" daily and other nutrients such as beta-carotene. It was not a vegetarian diet, because he did eat poultry and *fish*. They began using Resperin Corporation's Essiac® tea "nine ounces daily…for about six months…" (345). Billy also used 714X "for 6 months," which is available from Canada at *www.cerbe.com*. Two and-a-half months later (after he began the dietary changes and the 714X injections), Billy's cancer had completely disappeared "(that was March 1995)," and he has had no reoccurrence. That was fourteen years ago. (He did continue to use the 714X for a total of 6 months.) He remains on the dietary changes, takes 4 ounces of Essiac daily, and occasionally does a "booster 21 day cycle of 714X" (345). His parents have this to say about chemo and radiation: "Chemotherapy and Radiation are man made and kill the body's immune system" (345).

You can read Billy's entire story at *www.grand-strand.com/suebest/boy who.htm*, and see photos there as well. His parents were so impressed with Resperin Essiac®, that they began taking it too and are now distributors for the tea. You can order Resperin Essiac® from their website above. For those interested, 714X can be obtained from *www.cerbe.com*. The Centre expérimental de recherches biologiques de l'Estrie inc. (C.E.R.B.E. Inc). See chapter six (in this book) for more detailed information on Essiac tea.

Note that there is some competition between the tea produced by *Resperin Canada Essiac*® and the brand known as *Flor-Essence*® Essiac tea. Both companies claim that they have the original Essiac formula (the drinkable formula, not the injectable) that Rene Caisse used in treating her cancer patients. You can get Flor-Essence® in most health food stores and many internet sites. You can obtain Resperin Essiac® at some health food stores and internet sites, such as *https://www.billybest.net/order Essiac.htm*. There are other brands of Essiac on the market, but these are the two I see most.

## Hodgkin's Disease & Hydrazine Sulfate

Though hydrazine sulfate is not what is considered a natural substance, it is embraced by many who promote alternative medicine, simply because of its effectiveness at treating so many forms of cancer (including lymphomas) without toxic side effects, and it is being included in this chapter for that reason. Joseph Gold, M.D., of Syracuse, New York, tested and promoted the use of hydrazine sulfate as a cancer treatment (505). Dr. Gold tested hydrazine sulfate extensively on animals before

**human** testing. He found that with optimal dosing, he could kill cancer cells with very few adverse reactions. Not long after he published the results of the animal testing (while lecturing on the drug), a physician approached him asking for permission to use hydrazine sulfate on one of his patients whom he estimated had 3-4 days to live. Shortly after receiving the formula, the woman improved remarkably and was soon living a normal life (505). This substance has been used in treating over a thousand cancer patients.

Sloan-Kettering gave the drug to some of their *chemotherapists* for testing, however, someone apparently dropped the ball. After the start of the study, Gold said that no one corresponded with him on the results. He went unannounced to Sloan-Kettering and looked at records of some of the patients who had received the drug. The results were promising, but a controversy arose (505). Gold claimed that the protocol given was inadequate and the entire testing was not conducted as he had recommended (505). He said that the study was flawed because dosing was not correct. Patients were either given double or triple the amount he ordered or they were given a few milligrams, when the prescription was written for ten times as much, making it impossible to measure outcomes. Eventually, SKI published a report saying that none of the patients responded effectively to the drug and the whole thing was shelved, however, in spite of all the opposition that Gold experienced, his discovery was curing cancer (505).

The story of a cancer patient who used H.S. and suffered fatal liver damage was given much publicity recently, however, when you study the facts in cases like this, there is always missing information that is never given. For example, it is unknown whether or not the patient was ever told that H.S. is a MAO inhibitor. If not, and he ingested any medicines or foods that are strictly prohibited with MAO inhibitors, this could explain what happened. Also, you need to be sure that you are using reliable sources for any alternative therapies. If using H.S., be sure that you are seeing a reliable licensed natural health physician for this therapy, rather than trying to self-medicate.

When the FDA raided suppliers of *hydrazine sulfate*, taking the drug as well as all the files connected with it, Gold was referred to as a *well-meaning zealot* who had used the discovery for twenty years in a lucrative manner (505). The drug is very inexpensive, however, as it retails for about *$5.00 for 25 tablets*, so the treatment is hardly lucrative, as claimed (505)!

For an excellent article on the truth about this substance and Dr. Joseph Gold who developed it, go to website *http://www.hydrazinesul*

*fate.org* and read the article*: THE TRUTH ABOUT HYDRAZINE SULFATE DR. GOLD SPEAKS*, from July 14, 2004 (last amended Oct. 13, 2007). Also, see the link there: *MedTruth A commentary on truth in medicine.*

The entire story of Hydrazine Sulfate and the activity of the FDA in seizing the drug are reminiscent of others who butted heads with conventional medicine (e.g., Harry Hoxsey, Dr. Burzynski, Max Gerson, Gaston Naessens, and Rene Caisse), who have spent a good part of their lives being constantly harassed and ridiculed by the current cancer industry, which is apparently upset that non-toxic treatments have been curing cancer cases without the toxic chemo drugs and radiation being promoted and forced onto the public. After all, why should they embrace natural, non-toxic cancer cures when doing so would mean certain death to their drug monopoly and the millions pouring into the pharmaceutical companies that many in the FDA hold stock in?

If you don't think that toxic treatments are being forced on the public, just refuse to allow your young child chemo drugs for cancer and see what happens! The state will do their best to take over custody of your child to force chemo on them whether you like it or not! If you have a young child, just diagnosed with cancer, and you have no desire to see them go through chemo drugs, you'd best be making plans to head for Canada or Mexico where parents can still protect their children from American drug tzars, who promote poisons (and forced immunizations) via pharmaceutical drug lords. If you don't believe this, check out the recent news story (05-20-09) of a young boy with Hodgkin's lymphoma and his mother, who ran from authorities because the AMA wanted to force him to take chemo without his or her consent! All they wanted was to pursue alternative medicine! He has Hodgkin's lymphoma, and I have a detailed history of a woman in this book who was CURED of this same cancer without ever using chemo or radiation! (See this chapter.)

As described at website, *www.diagnose-me.com*, about 50% of the recipients who are given hydrazine sulfate in correct dosages, when treated early, demonstrate excellent results, including tumor shrinkage, as well as "immediate weight gain and reversal of symptoms; in some instances the tumor eventually disappears" (296). The cancers that appear to respond most favorably to this therapy include: "recto-colo cancer, ovarian…prostatic…lung (brochogenic)…Hodgkin's disease and other lymphomas, thyroid cancer, melanoma, and breast cancer" (296). Other cancers that do not occur as often also respond to this treatment. Dr. Gold's clinic is located at Syracuse Cancer Research Institute, Inc.,

Presidential Plaza, 600 East Genesee St., Syracuse, N. Y. 13202 (296). Your health care practitioner can reach them at ph #315-472-6616.

## Hoxsey Formula & Lymphoma

Harry Hoxsey developed an herbal tea that helped many people regain their health, yet he too was relentlessly hounded by the AMA and FDA. It is noteworthy that his herbal tea, "which contains red clover, buckthorn bark, stillingia root, barberry bark, chaparral, licorice root, cascara amarga, and prickly ash bark, along with potassium iodide...." has had good results against "lymphoma and skin cancer" (519). More details on Harry Hoxsey and his tea formula are given in chapter 19 and other chapters of this book.

## LifeMel Honey for Cancer Patients

This amazing honey is also discussed in chapter 29 and other chapters of this book. It is a special honey, developed in Israel, that is produced from the nectar of 40 herbs, including *Echinacea, Siberian ginseng,* and *Uncaria tomentosa,* with other natural ingredients. Two teaspoons per day (one in the morning and one in the evening) are recommended (614). This special honey has been able, in **human** testing, to prevent the neutropenia (serious white blood cell drop) caused by chemotherapy and to lower the risk of severe platelet drop (thrombocytopenia), often found in chemo patients (614). You can find out more about this remarkable honey at website: *http://www.lifemel israel.com* (614).

## Magnesium & Iodine for Cancer Prevention

These minerals are critical for cancer prevention. Animal studies have shown that magnesium deficiencies can lead to lymphosarcoma. It is also important in preventing leukemia, prostate cancer, and stomach cancers (566). Also, see page 129 and page 400.

## New Nanotechnology Kills Lymphoma

Researchers from Texas are studying ways to kill cancer cells by using *cancer-seeking antibodies* (in the form of *monoclonal antibodies*) attached to *tiny carbon tubes* which *heat up* when they are then *exposed to near-infrared light* (300). Once the light hits the cancer cells where the *nanotubes* are clinging, the heat from the light basically fries the cells (300). More and more testing is being done using nanotechnology. Before widespread human testing is carried out, *nanomaterials* must be deemed safe and feasible for humans (300). Some scientists are using magnetic nanoparticles to fight cancer cells.

## Poly–MVA for Lymphomas & Sarcomas

See chapter 14 for more information on this amazing, nontoxic nutritional formula that many cancer survivors (who were told they were *hopeless)* are crediting with their complete recovery, many of them without ever resorting to chemo or radiation. Their main website can be found at: *www .polymva.net.*

## Psoralea Seed & Osteosarcoma

Osteosarcoma is a malignant bone tumor. The herb, psoralea (*Psoralea corylifolia),* contains compounds that may be important in stopping lung cancer cells and osteosarcoma cells from multiplying, and may help prevent *secondary lung cancer.* Psoralea seed can be found in capsule form. This compound causes an increased sensitivity to sunlight, so stay out of the sun if you are using psoralea. If the herb causes slight abdominal discomfort, ginger tea is recommended (184).

## Reishi Mushroom & Green Tea Combo Kills Sarcoma

Scientists in Beijing, China, recently made an amazing discovery during animal testing with sarcoma cancer. They discovered that they could combine nutrients from the reishi mushroom and green tea, and dramatically slow the growth of sarcoma tumors, as well as increase the life span in the animals receiving the treatment (112a).

## Rexin-G™ for Pancreatic Cancer & Metastatic Cancers

Rexin-G™ has been undergoing clinical trials at Mayo Clinic, M.D. Anderson, and a few other facilities. It is a drug for cancers that have spread, and those types of cancer that conventional medicine says do not respond to chemo drugs (256). Human clinical studies, thus far, have had good results. In the very first human trial, 83% of the patients experienced tumor shrinkage. The patients all had spreading pancreatic cancer (256).

Good responses were also achieved in human studies involving several other types of metastatic cancer. Due to the reports, this drug is now used for treating all forms of *solid tumors* in the Philippines that are resistant to conventional therapy (256). The U.S. FDA has given the drug its *orphan drug status* (meaning it can be used for rare diseases) for use with pancreatic cancers in the US, as well as other types of cancer metastases, so testing will continue (256). It is given intravenously, so isn't exactly natural or painless, but could be considered gentler than older chemo drugs because it is said to be a non-chemo drug, showing itself in **human** clinical trials, not to have the adverse side effects normally associated with chemo drugs (256). You can get more information on this drug at *epeiusbiotech.com/rexin_g-factsheet.asp*. Epeius Biotechnologies are the producers of Rexin-G™ (257).

## Scutellaria Fights Lymphoma, Leukemia & Myeloma

A mint herbal remedy used in Chinese medicine, *Scutellaria baicalensis* [sometimes referred to as *skullcap*], in laboratory testing, was shown to prevent the growth of lymphoma, myeloma, and ALL (acute lymphocytic leukemia) cells (459).

## Selenium & Vitamin C Heal a "Fatal" Lymphoma

Selenium and vitamin C are crucial in treating severe lymphoma. Dr. Abram Hoffer, M.D., Ph.D., in writing about the importance of these two supplements, believes that selenium has been much maligned in the medical community and that higher levels are not toxic as has been claimed (431). He recounts the experience he had in treating a patient from Chile, who was told that he had fatal lymphoma. The patient had surgery, but the cancer returned. **He received radiation and still the cancer returned**. He was told that he had just a few months left (431). Dr. Hoffer started him on 600 **mcg** of selenium a day. However, the patient, on return visit, admitted that he was not taking 600 mcg per day, but 2,000 mcg per day! Dr. Hoffer was alarmed about such a huge dosage of selenium, and recommended that he decrease his dosage at least by half. The patient went into total remission and survived many years without further trace of cancer (431).

Dr. Hoffer uses selenium, zinc, vitamins E, beta-carotene, the B complex vitamins, and mega-doses of vitamin C. He is convinced that the most vital ingredient for fighting cancer is vitamin C. In his experience, he says that doses of *12 grams per day (sodium ascorbate or calcium ascorbate)* can be tolerated. He starts his patients off with a *teaspoon three times per day*, then has them increase the dose until they develop diarrhea, at which point, they cut back just below the dose that caused the diarrhea (431). You will sometimes hear this being described as the *bowel tolerance level* (431). You can get powdered vitamin C in health food stores.

## Shark Liver Oil & Hodgkin's Lymphoma

Shark liver oil has helped those with advanced Hodgkins lymphoma. Do not use the supplement unless the vitamin A and vitamin D is taken out. If not, you will get overdoses on these fat-soluble vitamins. Use the supplement that is *30-40 percent AKGs* (386). (Note that shark cartilage and shark liver oil are two entirely different supplements.)

## Thymus Extract Successfully Treats Lymphoma

In an article at *cancertutor.com*, the results of a remarkable controlled study, involving the use of *calf thymus extract* on humans with *fatal lymphocytic* tumors and "lesions (Letterer-Siwe disease, Hand-Schuller-Christian disease and esinophilic granuloma)," were reported from the *New England Journal of Medicine* (127). It was noted that 17 of the cancer participants in the study were injected on a daily basis with the *thymic extract.* The control group, on the other hand (a total of 20 patients), received standard conventional treatment (chemotherapy). Of the 17 people who received the extract, ten were in "full remission after one year" (127). *Cancertutor.com* says that "Seven" either did not respond or worsened after nearly a month, and the extract was halted. This *remission* rate *was* found to be exactly the same in those who received chemo, with ONE big difference. Those receiving thymus extract had **absolutely NONE of the side effects experienced by the group receiving chemo** (127).

Thymus extract from calves is not a natural substance, and though I recommend natural substances over those that are synthetic or animal in origin, **whenever possible**, if I knew someone with terminal lymphoma, I certainly would not tell them to avoid this extract, especially in comparison to immune-destructive chemo drugs and radiation.

## Ukrain for Many Types of Cancer

There are several chapters in this book that discuss the remarkable ability of Ukrain therapy to bring about total remission in some cancer patients.

2009 update: note that because Ukrain is not authorized in Austria, the Ukrain website has been changed and is now called *Nowicky Pharma.* You can read information about Ukrain now in the book*: Anti-Cancer Agent Ukrain—The Crime Story of an Obstruction* by Eleonore Thun-Hohenstein. See *www.ukrin.com* for more information. Also, for pictures of how Ukrain works, website: *http://www.ukrain-drug.net/webspeed/index. htm.* Ukrain is a safe, non-toxic substance.

For details of a case study on a young girl successfully treated with Ukrain for Ewing's sarcoma of her right femur, see the National Institutes of Health and U.S. National Library of Medicine NCBI PubMed website. The ID of the study is PMID 10190081. The child was given hyperthermia treatment and Ukrain therapy. The disease had stopped within six weeks, and after two more treatment sessions, *no negative changes could be detected* (335). For a laboratory study which showed that the effects of Ukrain on Ewing's tumor are very similar to that of the common chemo drug, *Etoposide*, see the detailed study from U.S. National Library of Medicine and National Institutes of Health at: PubMed, NCBI website under PMID 17001175 (462).

## Vitamin C & Ewing's Sarcoma

Dr. Abram Hoffer has also used high dose vitamin C, in combination with large doses of niacinamide, to cure a case of Ewing's sarcoma. His teenage patient had already been scheduled to have her arm removed due to the presence of Ewing's sarcoma. When she followed Dr. Hoffer's simple daily regimen of *1000 mg* of *niacinamide* and *1000 mg* of *vitamin C* after each meal, she rebounded completely, did not need the amputation, and went on to lead a normal life (432). If you decide to take a powdered form of ascorbic acid (that you mix with water), ascorbic acid taken this way is very hard on your teeth enamel. Another reason why you may not want to give your children chewable vitamin C. (You can get empty vegetarian gel capsules at the health food store and put the powder in the capsules and swallow them to bypass the teeth.)

Dr. Hoffer has also had great success treating schizophrenia patients with niacinamide and other vitamins and minerals. (See his webpage at *www.islandnet.com/~hoffer* for more information.) Note that niacin causes your skin to flush because of its ability to open up the capillaries in the body, increasing blood flow. You may also experience some itching with the flush, but this is all temporary and not harmful. It is actually good for the body. Niacinamide does not cause the flush, but neither will it open up the circulation like niacin does. Niacin also has the ability to lower harmful cholesterol levels. Do NOT ever take niacin or niacinamide in the *timed-release* form. (You can take a baby aspirin or two about twenty minutes before taking niacin to prevent the flush, but many people take it for the positive flush-effect.) It temporarily dries out the mouth as well!

Dr. Hoffer also reports that, as far back as the eighties, scientists knew the benefits of niacin in cancer prevention, and it was discussed as a cancer prevention in a Texas 1987 conference. Human cancer cells receiving sufficient amounts of niacin were 90% less likely to develop tumors as those who did not receive adequate amounts of the B vitamin (432). Dr. Hoffer says that in some individuals (though rare) niacin may cause a type of liver problem with jaundice. As soon as the niacin is stopped, the problem clears (432). If you are a physician, see his book: *Orthomolecular Medicine for Physicians.*

## Zapping B-Cell Lymphoma, Lupus, Rheumatoid Arthritis, Sjogren's Syndrome & Dermatomyositis Safely

For information on patients who had all their signs and symptoms of B-cell lymphoma reversed through using only one ingredient, low dose Naltrexone, see the National Library of Medicine's PubMed website at PMID #17761642 and the article by B.M. Berkson, D.M. Rubin and A.J. Berkson entitled: "Reversal of signs and symptoms of a B-cell lymphoma in a patient using only low-dose naltrexone." (Website is: *http://www.ncbi.nlm.nih.gov/sites/entrez*) (344c). For the successful use of ALA (alpha lipoic acid) and low-dose Naltrexone to reverse lupus, rheumatoid arthritis, Sjogren's Syndrome, dermatomyositis and other auto-immune disorders, enabling the patients to go off all their prescription meds, see the article by Dr. Joseph Mercola at *www.mercola.com* entitled: "Alpha Lipoic Acid One Powerful Antioxidant" (483b)! Dr. Mercola explains this gentle treatment in his video at *http://blogs.Mercola.com/sites/vitalvotes/archive/2009/04/27/alpha-lipoic-acid-one-powerful-antioxidant.aspx* (483b). Check with your health care practitioner because the Naltrexone may need to be obtained at a compounding pharmacist for your unique dosing.

# CHAPTER 17

# GOD'S GREAT GRASSES

*"But he was wounded for our transgressions, he was bruised for our iniquities: the chastisement of our peace was upon him; and with his stripes we are healed." (Isaiah 53:5)*

## Barley Grass Used to Heal Carcinoma

Researchers from Japan isolated a compound, *P4-D1,* from the juice of barley which appears to shield cells from sun radiation. Using chlorophyll (such as that found in barley grass) as therapy, has actually prevented people from having their limbs amputated (e.g., Ann Wigmore), and one of the greatest advantages to using chlorophyll, is that there are NO toxic side effects (386).

Another example is that of a woman who was treated with a rare skin carcinoma by drinking a barley juice from Japan known as *bakuryokuso.* The woman opted out of chemo and radiation and instead mixed a teaspoon of the dried barley powder in either water or her favorite juice, and took it with her meals. Her cancerous skin condition began clearing up in less than two months (386). Realize that surgery can often completely eliminate skin cancers before they spread to other sites.

The power of green grasses has been attributed mainly to their chlorophyll content (386). Chlorophyll is such a speed healer, that D. H. Collings proved that wounds took less time to heal when patients were taking this nutrient, than when using sulfa drugs, *penicillin,* or nothing at all (386). It has also been used to treat G.I. conditions, such as ulcers and inflammation of the pancreas, and has been used for those with *endocarditis.* Remember that wheat grass juice comes from the young green leaves of the wheat berry, so even those with *gluten allergies* can safely consume the juice (386). Chlorophyll thins the blood, and this helps to balance out the effects of vitamin K in green foods, which thicken the blood. The two complement each other.

## Chlorella for All Cancers

Chlorella *(Chlorella vulgaris)* is an algae found in fresh water. It is a one-celled organism containing more chlorophyll than any other green plant, including spirulina (426). This is reported by C. M. Hawken in *Green Foods: "Phyto-Foods" for Super Health*. Due to its high level of chlorophyll, chlorella is good for the body (426). Nutrient-dense foods, such as chlorella, as well as fresh fruits and vegetables, can counter-attack free radicals and their insidious effects, thus wiping them out before they can harm us. Chlorella can remove dangerous heavy metals from the body, and many studies have been done to show that chlorella can boost the immune system (426). Chlorella can also halt the formation of abnormal cells and restore them to normal, since it raises the body's levels of *interferon* (426).

Chlorella and other green grasses enable the body to maintain a state of alkalinity, rather than acidity. A high acid environment generates free radicals and causes the leaching of calcium out of the bones to alkalize the blood. Keeping the body in a state of alkalinity fights free radicals and prevents this calcium leaching from the bones, thus preventing osteoporosis and other degenerative diseases. Chlorophyll—found in all green plants—soothes the colon and rebuilds damaged intestinal cells, prevents the build-up of harmful microbes in the intestines, helps heal gastro-intestinal problems (such as ulcer formation and colitis), purifies the liver, and keeps the colon healthy (426). Remember that there are many other "grasses" that are part of what we consider *green* foods, all of which are not discussed in detail here. Some of these include: sprouts, seaweed, the cruciferous vegetables, leafy greens, and many others (426).

## Wheat Grass - The Miracle Nutrient

Ann Wigmore was so impressed by the health effects of fresh wheat grass juice on her life that she not only wrote books about it, but she founded the *Hippocrates Health Institute* in Boston, where her guests were treated to a life of natural health living with a strict raw foods regimen. For years, many people came to the *Wigmore Mansion* as it was called, some with terminal illnesses. Many left, cured of their illnesses, including Eydie Mae Hunsberger (a patient discussed earlier in this book in chapter four), who cured her breast cancer while on the Wigmore program.

Ann Wigmore healed her own body of many ailments (caused she said by ingesting an American diet for two decades), by ingesting instead, fresh wheat grass juice. She discovered that within *a few weeks* of starting on *wheat grass juice* (as well as using *sprouts and greens*), she was healed of *colitis* (600). Though she felt that a vegetarian diet of raw foods was very beneficial for health maintenance, she considered wheat grass juice the greatest healer for the *body's immunity* that exists (600). Wheat grass juice is very rapidly assimilated into the body when taken. It does not need 30-60 minutes to go through the digestive process, since the nutrients are almost immediately absorbed into your cells. If you are fighting a debilitating illness, you need nutrition that is immediately available and not taxing on your body.

## Wheat Grass Regimen Used Successfully To Treat Primary Peritoneal Cancer in 89-Year-old Woman

For an amazing case study from Guisseppi A. Forgionne Ph.D., about an 89-year-old woman who experienced total remission from advanced peritoneal cancer using an alternative nutritional approach, see website: *http://www.cancerlynx.com/peritonealcase.html* (400). After having surgery, she refused chemo. According to the article, her nutritional regimen included *2 grams of wheat grass* per day (which she started taking a week after her surgery), then *100 mg* of *CoQ10* a week after that, and within 2 more weeks, the addition of *9 grams of bovine cartilage*/day. *Nine months* later, her CoQ10 was changed to *150 mg per day* (400).

See chapter seven for information on a new test from LabCorp for early ovarian cancer detection that they claim is highly accurate.

## Benefits of Purchasing a Juicer

For those of you who *are* already ill, one of the first and most important things you can do is to purchase a juicer. Be sure that you obtain a juicer that has the capacity to juice not only fresh vegetables and fruits, but green foods like spinach, broccoli, wheat grass, celery, kale, and others. Some juicer manufacturers will claim that their juicers can juice wheat grass, but they do a very poor job of it. The juice will come out very foamy and warm, so that it has oxidized nearly all of its vital enzymes during the process.

## Types of Juicers

There are many good juicers on the market that will juice wheat grass as well as fresh vegetables and fruits. Four very good choices that juice wheat grass, vegetables, and fruits are the *Samson* juicer, the *Green Star,* the *Green Power juicer,* and the *Omega 8003* juicer. These type juicers can sometimes be found at natural health food stores, or they can be ordered on the internet. If your local health food store does not have the model you desire, they can usually order it for you. (The first large juicer I purchased was a *Champion.* I read on the internet that it did not do a good job of juicing grapes, but mine juiced grapes wonderfully, however, it juiced everything wonderfully, EXCEPT greens!)

There are manual juicers that juice wheat grass only that are very economical, as well as electric juicers made just for juicing wheat grass; however, if you buy one of these, you will need another juicer for your fruits and vegetables. An excellent manual juicer is the *Miracle* manual wheat grass juicer. *Miracle* also makes electric wheat grass juicers, but as stated earlier, if you get this type, you will need a separate juicer for your fruits and vegetables.

If you juice citrus fruits (e.g., oranges and grapefruits) in your main juicer, you will need to peel them first, or you can obtain a very inexpensive citrus juicer for about twelve dollars just for oranges, grapefruits, lemons, and limes at your local department store or pharmacy; then, your main juicer can be one that does vegetables, other fruits (such as berries, apples, grapes, cantaloupe, etc.) and greens. Good choices of juicers that do it all are the ones I listed above (except the *Champion*). They will juice greens as well as veggies and fruits (without oxidizing the enzymes out of your greens), and the *Omega 8003* is supposed to take just five minutes for cleanup.

A good rule of thumb is that the softer the fruit you are juicing, the thicker the juice will be. You will get a much thicker juice from soft pears than hard pears. Strawberries, pineapples, and berries will give you a very thick, mushy-type juice. You can dilute it with water and other juices and drink it, or freeze it into popsicles. A general rule of thumb is that one pound of produce will give you approximately 6-8 ounces of juice. If you want an eight ounce glass of carrot juice, for example, be prepared to purchase about one pound of carrots; however, yield will also depend on the type juicer you choose as well. Some juicers extract more efficiently and you get more juice from your produce. The drier the pulp that comes out, the more juice you are getting. The 6-8 ounce rule does not apply to juicing greens. Yield depends on many variables, such as the type of greens you are juicing and the type juicer you are using. The *Norwalk* juicer is said to give one of the best yields, but it is very expensive—about $2,000. I have heard users complain that it takes 30 minutes to clean after each use, but it gives an excellent yield and quality of juice, possibly 50% higher yield than less expensive models. It is often used at health institutions, and you can order it on the internet.

## What to Juice

If you are seriously ill, purchasing a juicer that provides you with fresh wheat grass juice, vegetable and fruit juices, is one of the most important **first steps** you can take for your health. You can also use green powdered drinks. If you want to boost your immune system and prevent sickness in the first place, juicing is not an option, it is a lifestyle that you will need to incorporate, along with fresh air, exercise, sunshine, and other tenets of health, as described in this book. You will soon find that investing in a juicer has priceless benefits that far outweigh your initial cost. Fresh wheat grass juice detoxifies the body so rapidly, only small amounts can be tolerated at a time. Start out consuming more than an ounce or two at a time and you will become nauseated or dizzy, simply because of the quick detox effect. You can gradually work up to larger amounts as needed. The same applies for beet root juice. Also, remember that raw foods (even those that are organic) must be washed thoroughly. You do not want to juice for health and end up with an e-coli or salmonella infection!

Wheat grass and other green juices are excellent sources of calcium and chlorophyll. Many people have been led to believe that we must get our calcium from milk, dairy products, and supplements. This is not true. Even carrot juice is higher in calcium than milk! The best source of calcium is the SAME place that the cows and goats extract it! They get it from the soil—green plants in the soil. Your very best and most natural source of calcium is **green foods.** And you don't have to worry about whether or not your body is going to absorb the calcium when you ingest it in this format. The cells literally inhale it. (They know a good thing when they see it coming!) You can often purchase fresh wheat grass in trays at your health food store, or kits where you can try growing your own. It is also available in frozen cubes that you thaw and use as needed in some health food store freezers.

Grasses, such as wheat grass, are rich in 17 amino acids (including the 8 *essential* amino acids), as well as dozens of different enzymes. They are also rich in many vitamins, minerals, trace minerals, and essential fatty acids (600). Because of this rich supply of nutrients, green foods and fresh juices are excellent for women who are pregnant, however, let your doctor know your dietary trends. It has been proven, in many cases, that cancer can be induced in laboratory animals by simply depriving them of specific minerals, vitamins or enzymes. Is it any wonder that fresh wheat grass juice with its multiplicity of nutrients is so beneficial to the immune system?

## Green Powder Versus Fresh Green Juice

A word about green powders. There are some excellent green powders on the market. If you do not have the time to juice before leaving the house in the morning, powders are an acceptable alternative, but try not to resort to them 100% of the time. You can even take the powdered drinks with you and mix them during the day for a healthy alternative to coffee and soda. Dee Simmons' company, *Ultimate Living,* produces *Green Miracle*, an excellent green powder choice. Her green powder is advertised as *pharmaceutical grade pure,* containing 80 ingredients including: kamut, wheat grass, barley grass, spirulina, chlorella, flax seed, bee pollen, apple fiber, astragalus, reishi, papain, bromelain, curcumin, lutein, lycopene, carrot, beet, pepper powder and many others. You can find Dee's popular health food products at her website: *www.ultimateliving.com.* Green *Kamut*® is a powdered wheat grass juice, while *Just Barley*™ organic green juice, and *Barley Green*™ contain barley only. Many green powdered drinks on the market, such as *Green Miracle*, not only contain green grasses, but medicinal mushrooms, minerals, spirulina, chlorella, vitamins, enzymes, herbs, and fibers that you would not get merely consuming powdered barley, algae or alfalfa.

When possible, try to consume grasses (like wheat grass) in their most natural state while they are alive. Doing this in combination with an excellent green powdered drink will boost the immune system and ensure optimal health. (Note that whole-leaf dried wheat grass actually has more chlorophyll than the fresh juice. This is because, once powdered, it is more concentrated.) A few of the health food stores in the area where I live have fresh juice bars. You can order an ounce or two (or six ounces if you want) of fresh-squeezed wheat grass, and they will make it for you in minutes, while you wait. They also juice fresh carrots, celery, beets, and smoothie mixes. Many people who cannot invest in the time and expense of a juicer, obtain their fresh juices at a juice bar, though after a period of time, you will spend enough at a juice bar to pay for a juicer.

When using fresh wheat grass juice, it is best to consume it within ten minutes of the time it is juiced. After that amount of time (unless it is frozen), the living enzymes begin to oxidize rapidly. The same is true of any fresh-squeezed juice. This is one reason why store-bought canned and bottled juices are no comparison to fresh-squeezed. By the time they are bottled, canned, packaged, homogenized or pasteurized, all of the LIVING enzymes in them have been zapped. You may get a few benefits from the Vitamin C (if it hasn't all been killed by heat), but the syrups, sugars, food colorings, and preservatives that may also be added, provide empty calories and possible carcinogens. You can find bottled juices at health food stores that have no added sugars and preservatives. There are some brands that are even *flash pasteurized*, but you have to check the expiration date; they have a short shelf-life. There are even a few commercial juicers that are finally getting the message that we don't want additives, food coloring, preservatives, and sugar put into our juices, no matter how pretty the color, and a few of them are coming out with better quality juices.

There is ONE exception when it comes to consuming wheat grass immediately after juicing. The late Dr. Virginia Livingston-Wheeler, who successfully cured many cancer patients at her clinic, used a "vaccine…based on abscisic acid" [an ingredient in wheat grass juice], and according to her, "the hormone abscisic acid (ABA) is 40 times more potent **4 hours** after cutting the wheat grass than it is at the time of cutting" (319). As *cancertutor.com* website asks: "what do you do, eat it immediately or 4 hours after you cut it? Perhaps both." They suggest that when juicing the wheat grass, consume most of it right away. Set the rest aside and drink it after 4 hours (319). In this manner, you are getting the benefit of live enzymes (as advocated by Ann Wigmore) in consuming the juice within ten minutes of making it, and you are still getting large amounts of the abscisic acid 4 hours later. Fresh-squeezed juices are also excellent for children, however, before giving them to young children, check with their pediatrician. Infants and very young children do not have the intestinal maturity to assimilate many of the nutrients in raw juices that older children are capable of.

**Never give honey and other bee products to children under two years of age**. (Some pediatricians will let children over one year-old take honey products.) The spores found in honey cannot be assimilated by young children and babies. The result can be the formation in a child's intestines of **infant botulism,** a deadly toxin.

Sea grasses or *sea vegetables,* as they are sometimes called, belong to a family of *grasses* that will be discussed later in this chapter. Some of the sea vegetables recommended by Ann Wigmore were "arame, dulse, hiziki, kelp, kombu, nori [and] wakame" (598). She recommended covering and soaking sea veggies for twenty minutes in "warm water…until they are soft enough to slice," then to pitch the salty water when you are done (598). Because of the high iodine content of sea vegetables, if you have thyroid problems, check with your physician before consuming them.

## Seaweed for Detox

Seaweed (sea grass) is consumed in large amounts in Asian countries, but Americans rarely touch it. There are many different types of seaweed. The next time you pull up to a sushi bar, you may find your sushi covered with seaweed (495). There are also *brown* alga (or seaweed), including: *kelp*, *wakame*, *arame*, and *kombu*, and a red seaweed known as *nori*. Research has shown that there are ingredients in seaweed that may inhibit cancer formation (495). Scientists believe that these substances prevent cancer by boosting the immune system, and that they can help prevent and halt the progression of abnormal cells, lower cholesterol levels, and act like magnets, pulling many dangerous heavy metals out of the body (495). Restaurants often put wakame in their salads (495).

Researchers conducted a study (in 1974) which revealed that kelp could not only be used as a breast cancer preventative, but it halted the spread of tumors (in animal testing), putting more than half of them into remission (520). It is believed that a chemical in kelp, *fucoidan*, contributes to its cancer-preventative effects, but seaweed also has very powerful *antibiotic* effects, which means it may help fight cancerous colon cells as well (520). You can now get fucoidan supplements at health food stores and on the internet.

As described by J. E. O'Brien, author of *The Miracle of Garlic & Vinegar*, research done at the University of Hawaii School of Medicine revealed that "a dried version of...wakame" when *injected* into test animals, helped cure their lung cancers (520). Scientists have shown that an ingredient in seaweed has blood pressure lowering effects. It appears to work like an "antidote to excess sodium consumption..." and could be important in warding off *strokes* (520). (Check with your doctor before supplementing with seaweed products.)

## Spirulina - Chelator & B12 Source

Spirulina is another green food that, when taken as a supplement, is still considered a *whole food* because the entire plant is used during production, not merely an extract of the plant (571). An ingredient in spirulina (known as *Phycocyanin)*, gives it the characteristic deep bluish-green it is noted for. In animal testing, it had the ability to fend off viruses, cancer, and anemia by increasing the production of *red blood cells* in the body (571).

Spirulina can act like a chelator in removing heavy metals from the body, and has been used for helping diabetic patients, as well as those fighting high blood pressure and elevated blood fats (571). Spirulina is helpful in the intestines since it ensures survival of good *bacteria*, and it is given to children in third world countries for the prevention of *blindness* (571). There are no known adverse effects from ingesting this green wonder food. Even those with gout can take spirulina, and it is an excellent source of vitamin B12 (571). Spirulina can boost the immune system (426), and may be especially beneficial to those who are fighting blood disorders such as leukemia, anemia, and multiple myelomas.

You can also take vitamin B12 as a sublingual tablet that dissolves under the tongue, or injections from your physician. Another excellent source of B12 is chlorella. Just be sure to get the broken cell-wall chlorella. Chlorella has the highest concentration of chlorophyll of any green food.

You may want to check out Dr. Andrew W. Saul's recipe for a nasal delivery form of B12 at *http://www.doctoryourself.com/nasal.html*, and Dr. Mercola's website for a new mist spray form of B12: *http://products.mercola.com/vitamin-B12-spray/?source=nl.*

## Spirulina & Mouth Cancer

Spirulina has also proven useful in the treatment of mouth cancer. When researchers gave *tobacco chewers,* who had abnormal pre-cancerous cells in their mouth, a gram of this green food every day for a *twelve month* period, nearly 50% of the participants receiving the spirulina had significant *improvement*, which did not happen in those not given the spirulina (571).

## Sprouts - Tiny Seeds That Pack A Punch

Ann Wigmore was so convinced of the high nutritional value of fresh sprouts that she not only grew them for her clients, she incorporated them into her meals on a daily basis and wrote a book called *The Sprouting Book*. She believed that sprouts were an excellent way of ridding the body of toxins (599). Sprouts are so nutritious and easily digestible, that Ann Wigmore believed that when consumed, they are nearly capable of digesting themselves! They are very high in beneficial enzymes that aid digestion, amino acids (plant proteins), and many vitamins (599). The human body has the ability to manufacture 14 essential amino acids, but there are eight which must be obtained through outside sources, and sprouts have all eight (599). In *The Sprouting Book*, Ann Wigmore said that, unlike living foods, such as raw fruits and vegetables whose nutrient value begins going downhill as soon as they are picked or cut, sprouts keep their nutritional level until consumption (599).

Ann Wigmore also believed that you can triple the amount of vitamin E in your diet by relying on wheat berry sprouts, rather than wheat, since sprouting increases the vitamin E content, and this natural form of vitamin E has a tenfold greater absorption within the cells than the man-made E supplements (599). She reported that one of the highest sources of calcium is fresh sesame sprouts, which have more calcium than *cow's milk*. Other sprouts, such as those from *sunflower* seeds and *chick peas,* are also high in calcium (599). Sprouts are very high in chlorophyll, the benefits of which were discussed earlier in this chapter. They are so nutrient-dense that they enhance the immune system. Be sure that if you grow or purchase sprouts that you always buy organic. Sprouts can get contaminated with bacteria if not grown, handled, and washed properly.

## Wheat Grass & Alkalinity

Wheat grass is very alkaline. Ann Wigmore said that it had been used to treat digestive problems, "ulcerative colitis…itchy or scaly scalp," sore throat, sore gums, sick pets, as an external poultice for skin problems, and a disinfectant, and for many other chronic health problems. It is high in chlorophyll (598). Did you know that most of the expensive mouth washes and breath fresheners sold in your dentist's office merely use chlorophyll to kill the bacteria that cause bad breath? Chlorophyll is one of the most important nutrients in fresh green juices like wheat grass.

Ann Wigmore advocated in her book, *The Hippocrates Diet And Health Program*, raw fresh foods, fruits, vegetables, fresh juices, nothing cooked. (This was a total vegan diet—no meats—and no dairy products allowed) (598). Some cancer patients are so weak and debilitated that they cannot tolerate a totally raw diet. It is easier for them to gradually convert to a totally raw diet over a period of time, however, in most cases, the sooner they make this transition, the better off they are. When facing a terminal illness, time becomes a precious commodity.

Stephen Blauer, author of *The Juicing Book*, considers chlorophyll an energizing blood *cleanser* and *tonic* (350). It is so much like the *hemoglobin molecule*, it has been discovered that animals can change "chlorophyll into hemoglobin…," and some scientists believe that we humans may have the same capacity (350).

What an amazing ability! Perhaps one day, patients needing blood transfusions will simply be drinking chlorophyll products instead, thus eliminating all the potential complications related to receiving blood products. Is it any wonder that green drinks are so beneficial to leukemia patients and those with *anemia* and other blood disorders?

## Wheat Grass Has Anti-Oxidants That Fight Many Types of Cancer

See website: *healingcancernaturally.com/barley-green-powder-medicine.html*, which has more information on the healing properties of wheat grass juice, which can be taken in fresh or powdered form (352). Wheat grass juice is not a panacea or *silver bullet* cure-all, though it may be close! Restoring health after a devastating illness depends on many factors. Nutritional juicing is just one of those factors. Wheat grass is an amazing boost for the immune system. Cancer and auto-immune disorders happen when the immune system is ill. As many cancer patients described in this book have discovered, heal your immune system and it will get you well!

## Vitamin D, Lupus Connection & Alfalfa

Though not a *grass,* alfalfa has nutritive value comparable to *cereal grasses* because it contains many of the same minerals and vitamins. Alfalfa sprouts are especially nutritious. They are rich in minerals such as phosphorus, contain twice the calcium of lettuce, and are a great source of all the *essential amino acids* (426). Individuals with a diagnosis of **lupus** should **avoid alfalfa products**, as alfalfa may cause a flare-up.

Studies have shown that lupus patients have abnormally low levels of vitamin D, indicating that supplementation may be needed (309), and they may also be low in magnesium, vitamin C, and CoQ10. Lupus is an auto-immune disorder. Auto-immune disorders are symptoms of a sick immune system. Your body is being attacked, not because of an immune system that is too strong, but one that is SICK. When the immune system is ill, it becomes confused, attacking indiscriminately, causing debilitating diseases. Many of the items in this book can help heal the immune system.

# CHAPTER 18

# FLAX & OTHER MIRACLE OILS

*"Thou lovest righteousness, and hatest wickedness: therefore God, thy God, hath anointed thee with the oil of gladness above thy fellows." (Psalm 45:7) "But my horn shalt thou exalt like the horn of an unicorn: I shall be anointed with fresh oil." (Psalm 92:10) "Is any sick among you? Let him call for the elders of the church; and let them pray over him, anointing him with oil in the name of the Lord." (James 5:14)*

## Flax Seed Inhibits Cancer

Flax seed has been in use for thousands of years. Studies were done in 1986 in Canada on flax seed, showing its power at fighting cancer and harmful fats in the blood. Flax is rich in lignans, nutrients that fight cancer, especially breast cancer (550). Two other essential fatty oils that could destroy several types of cancer (in laboratory testing) without harming normal cells, were *evening primrose oil* and *borage oil* (550). Many physicians also recommend flax oil (gel caps) to their patients who have problems with dry eye syndrome, psoriasis, and other skin disorders.

The wrong kinds of fat not only depress the immune system, they transport cancer-causing chemicals into and throughout the body. Avoid the use of anything that is *hydrogenated* or refined, including margarines. *Hydrogenation* creates millions of free radicals that strip vitamins, especially *vitamin E* from the body (550). Obtain organic, unrefined oils from natural health supply stores. Even the FDA has recognized flax seed oil as a cancer preventative (550).

Cold-pressed organic olive oil is also a good choice. (Note that most of the onion rings, french fries, fried chicken, and other fried foods that are found in today's fast food restaurants, are cooked with unhealthy oils.) Some states are finally wising up and passing laws to eliminate the use of unhealthy fats in restaurants. You will see more of these type laws go into effect as consumers become more and more aware that the unnaturally high fats that Americans consume in popular fast food dishes are a primary cause of cancer. Dietary fats are needed, but the RIGHT kind of fats. Processed vegetable oils are contributing to the deterioration of the health of millions of people! See information later in this chapter (and others) about a brilliant German scientist's fight with margarine manufacturers to disclose their harmful substances to an unwary public! Her name is Johanna Budwig.

Flax seed has been called *the ideal survival food* because all the anti-oxidants in flax are enclosed in a small, shell-like structure that keeps the seed from spoiling for years. Once the outer shell is cracked or crushed, the oil inside begins to deteriorate as it is mixed with oxygen, and will eventually spoil if not used within a short period of time. Refrigeration will retard the spoilage process, but not indefinitely (415). In his book, *Fantastic Flax*, Siegfried Gursche lauds the many benefits of flax seed as a healing food and nutraceutical, and says that adding these seeds to the daily diet will help with all sorts of digestive disorders, including constipation. He says that it will also help those with high triglycerides, blood pressure problems, circulatory, and degenerative diseases (415).

The importance of maintaining the body's alkalinity was noted earlier in this book and in chapter 30, which is devoted to that concept. Mr. Gursche explains that flax can assist with sustaining a healthy state of alkalinity as it is *very alkaline*. It is a good preventative for *heartburn* and excellent for promotion of a correct acid-alkaline balance. It forms thick *mucilage* in the stomach, thus providing a protective coat for those with ulcers and inflammation (415). Essential fats are healthy. In normal amounts, they do not make people fat. It is all the non-essential fats that are being ingested that are causing the problem of obesity in America. Mr. Gursche described Dr. Johanna Budwig as "a pioneer in the field of health and nutrition research" (415).

Flax contains *lignans,* which are nothing more than natural estrogens from plants, yet these powerhouses play a vital part in fighting degenerative diseases and cancers of the "breast, prostate, uterus and colon," says Mr. Gursche. They also keep bones healthy, and because they bind with *bile acids*, they help prevent *gallstones* (415). He describes flax seeds as being so rich in lignans that they "contain 75 to 800 times more [lignans] than wheat bran, oats, millet, rye, legumes soybeans…" and many other foods (415). They are important cancer-fighters because they block the growth of cancers by causing **"excess estrogen" to be driven "from the body."** They also prevent existing fat cells from producing more estrogen (415). (What this means is that all your cells have receptor sites where harmful estrogens can attach themselves and be absorbed. Lignans from flax take the place of the harmful estrogens, thus preventing them from being absorbed into your body.) Flax is also high in fiber and protein.

When combined with cottage cheese or yogurt, as in the Budwig diet, flax becomes a complete protein. There are several varieties of flax seed—either brown or golden, but there is little difference between the brown flax and the golden. If you buy the gold flax seed, you will get more protein and less oil than the brown flax. You may also pay more for the golden (415). Do not buy flax that has already been ground, unless it is in a sealed package and once opened, you can keep it refrigerated and use promptly. It is preferable to purchase the flax seed whole, then grind in a coffee grinder the amount you need as you use it. This will prevent the flax from going rancid (415). Once rancid, it will do you more harm than good.

When using flax oil, or flax seed **never heat it,** and be sure to purchase organic flax from a reputable health food store (415). I prefer flax oil in salads, juices, cold dishes (such as chopped salads or avocados), or poured over a baked potato. (Just be sure the potato is not burning hot as flax oil should never be heated.) If using fresh flax seed, take 2 or 3 tablespoons of the seeds, grind them in a coffee grinder, mix them with 8 ounces of water, shake and drink for a breakfast drink. Or you can add the crushed (or cracked) seeds to cereals or salads. However, if adding to a drink, you must drink it quickly, because it thickens very fast! You may need to follow it with more water since it is rather gritty.

## Dr. Johanna Budwig & the Margarine Battle

Dr. Johanna Budwig, a six times Nobel prize nominee, famous for her work in isolating and identifying fatty substances in the blood, was appalled at the way margarine manufacturers took and transformed *good unrefined healthy oils* "into processed and hydrogenated health-endangering margarine," and she was very vocal about saying so (415). In *Fantastic Flax,* author Siegfried Gursche says that the government, the margarine producers, and conventional medicine basically ganged up on her to prosecute her for claiming that margarine and all such hydrogenated fats are like giving poison to the human body (415). The margarine producers were wealthy and had a lot of clout behind their lawsuits. (Does any of this sound familiar?) Johanna said the following about margarine: "[T]he process of artificially hardening liquid vegetable oils (hydrogenation) creates life-threatening fat molecules—the trans fatty acids" (415). The margarine industry brought legal action against Johanna. "She fought twenty-eight court cases," winning every single one of them (415). We see warnings everywhere today about the dangers of trans-fatty acids (like those in margarine) that contribute to all forms of chronic illnesses and cancer (415), and of course, we now know that it was the margarine manufacturers who were lying and not Johanna! Perhaps this makes you wonder about other warnings that are currently being issued by natural health advocates—warnings against using homogenized/pasteurized milk; warnings against immunizations; warnings against the deadly effects of chemo and radiation to the immune system; warnings against aspartame; warnings against fluoride and chlorine in drinking water, and warnings against amalgam fillings—that are currently being ignored by conventional medicine, the FDA and big business. How much longer do you think it will take for these warnings to finally be accepted? How many times has history vindicated people like Johanna Budwig and Rene Caisse, in spite of the fact that they were swimming upstream at the time?

Organic butter is actually better for you than margarine. We can thank Johanna Budwig for exposing the truth about margarine and margarine manufacturers. One of the richest sources of *omega-3* is *flax oil.* Be careful in purchasing flax oil that you check the label for the words, *cold expeller-pressed* and *unrefined,* and check the expiration date on the container (415). (Butter also contains natural lecithin, an ingredient that lowers bad cholesterol, margarine does not.)

Always keep flax seed **oil** refrigerated. Once opened, use it by the expiration date given, or at least "within three weeks after opening" (415). You can use the flax seeds in baking if you soak them "in water for at least an hour before using them" (415). Dr. Budwig also authored several books on flax oil. One in particular, *The Oil-Protein Diet Cookbook*, has many of her recipes for a variety of ways to incorporate the Budwig diet into your menus.

## Flax Prevents Many Diseases—Helps the Heart, Kidneys, & Those with Lupus Nephritis, M.S., Diabetes, Colon Problems & HIV

Research studies have found that flax seed has an anti-cancer effect comparable to that of some chemotherapy drugs, but minus the toxic side effects. It is a well-known fact that women having the highest levels of omega-3-fatty acids (such as those found in fish and flax) are the least likely to develop breast cancer. Flax has also been very effective at treating skin disorders, and it is possible that it could extend the lives of patients with lupus who are fighting nephritis (caused when the lupus attacks their kidneys).

Flax seed and its oil can help in the prevention and treatment of many forms of cancer, including those of the female reproductive tract, intestinal tract, and prostate cancers, and offer some help for those suffering with digestive disorders, including Crohn's, colitis, and bowel irregularities (571). One physician in particular, *Dr. Roy Swank*, has shown that multiple sclerosis responds to a diet that is *low in saturated* fats, but high in *essential* fats (e.g., flax oil) (571). (If you have any of these disorders, or are taking prescription medications, be sure to consult with your licensed health care physician for appropriate amounts to take.)

Essential fatty acids help to metabolize dangerous blood fats, preventing them from accumulating in blood vessels and tissues. Other sources of omega-3 oils (besides flax) are leafy greens, *cold water fish* (551), and krill oil.

Borage oil is high in omega-6. One researcher has discovered that the GLA in borage oil helped reverse some diabetic health complications, "especially retina problems" (551). (Another excellent source of essential fatty acids is the avocado.) Researchers have shown repeatedly that omega-3 fish oil (the same type oil found in flax oil), in animal testing, shrank tumors and halted their spread. It helps suppress colon cancer and breast cancer in humans (386). Krill oil also has omega-3, and is even healthier than fish oil, and much more potent. Chia seeds also contain omega-3.

Studies reveal that within just a few weeks, pre-cancerous polyps in the colon could be halted by greater than half—if men would take fish oil supplements every day (386). GLA and fish oil supplements were shown to greatly increase (by as much as double) the *life expectancies of* people fighting the HIV virus (386). These essential oils have also been used to treat rheumatoid arthritis. GLAs work by enhancing the body's ability to increase immune cells that kill pathogens and other mutant cells in the body. Good sources of GLA are *borage oil* and *evening primrose oil,* as well as *black currants* (386).

Flax is rich in *vitamin F*, and as described earlier, it provides very nutritious and healthy *mucilage*, which helps detoxify and clean the colon (344). Selene Yeager, author of *Doctors Book of FOOD REMEDIES,* says that flax is so high in lignans that you would have to eat 5 dozen "cups of fresh broccoli or 100 slices of whole-wheat bread to get the same amount of lignans that are in ¼ cup of flax seed" (604). Research showed that tumors that are estrogen-positive could be reduced to half their size, in animals given flax seed, in less than two months. As described earlier in this chapter, lignans apparently have the power to counter-attack the harmful effects of synthetic estrogen in the cells, estrogens that cause cancer (604).

Heating oils to extreme temperatures changes their molecular structure, making them unfit for human consumption. Fats that are artificially hardened, the fats that are bad for you, will be labeled *as "hydrogenated, modified, fractionated or partially hydrogenated...avoid all products that contain these dangerous fats"* (416). You will find these fats in processed foods, in fast foods, and in many items in your grocery store. Butter is actually better for you unless you burn it. Burning butter completely ruins it. Never eat anything cooked in butter that has been burned. It has become a harmful fat and will flood your body with dangerous free radicals (416). Refined oils are considered by Siegfried Gursche, in his book, *Good Fats and Oils,* to be a *dead food*—meaning that they are completely empty of nutrients. These are the oils you will find on supermarket shelves, including the refined safflower and peanut oils. Avoid even the so-called *light olive oils.* Some oil manufacturers try to fool the public into believing that their oil is olive oil. A good example is a canola oil that is called *olivera.* These are the high trans-fatty acid oils that are unhealthy (416). The same can be said of margarine and vegetable shortening. Some processors are now removing trans-fats from their oils.

Organic cold-pressed extra virgin olive oil (unrefined) can be purchased at your local health food store. Another good oil (if organic, unrefined) is pumpkinseed oil (which has been shown to prevent prostate enlargement), but beware, some oils are watered down (416). Mr. Gursche says: "one drop of genuine pumpkinseed oil on a lettuce leaf will remain a solid drop..." (416). If it has been *mixed* with another oil, it will run (416). Be a label-reader.

Pumpkinseed oil is famous for boosting the health of the *urinary tract* as well as the prostate (416). Look for other good oils (unrefined, cold-pressed) such as natural organic *coconut oil*, *walnut,* and *almond* oil (416). (Organic perilla oil, krill oil, and black seed (*nigela sativa*) are also a good source of healthy oils.)

## The Famous Budwig Flax Oil Diet

Johanna Budwig combined flax oil with cottage cheese as part of her anti-cancer program. I do not recommend cow's milk simply because many dairy products in this country are so tainted with hormones, pesticides, and herbicides, and because cow's milk has been linked to juvenile or type I diabetes and sometimes carries leukemia and lymphoma cells. If you do use dairy products, such as cottage cheese, I would recommend that you use only organic or better yet, if you have a nearby farmer who can provide you with raw milk and dairy (providing he or she practices scrupulous farming methods and has a healthy disease-free herd).

There is so much controversy about soy, especially the GMO or genetically-modified soy products, you are better off without soy, unless it is fermented soy. (See chapter four in this book for details on the amazing fermented soy drink, Haelan.) In the Budwig diet, you can use yogurt, but again, see the note above about organic and raw products. Milk is not for children. It is for baby cows! Some studies indicate that giving cow's milk to babies under one-year-old causes milk allergies, and may be the culprit in Type I diabetes. I do encourage the use of the Budwig flax oil diet in anyone battling cancer, such as brain cancer or some other type of cancer, and as stated earlier, it can be done with organic, or better yet, raw dairy products. As described at *www.healingcancernaturally.com*, ingredients are combined as follows:

> For each tablespoon of flaxseed oil, add 2 tablespoons of low-fat cottage cheese (or quark) or 6 tablespoons of yoghurt. The flaxoil/cottage cheese or flaxoil/yoghurt mixture should be fully blended until no traces of oil remain visible, proving that the highly unsaturated fatty acids have become water soluble (a hand-held mixer or a blender works well) (99). [Quark is a pasty type of white cheese.]

## Flax Oil & Malignant Cancers

The type of GLA found in flax seed, as well as *evening primrose oil and borage oil*, in laboratory testing, was able to destroy *alpha-cell chronic lymphocytic leukemia cells*. As a matter-of-fact, their anti-tumor effects have been demonstrated against many types of cancer, including deadly brain cancers (351). See chapter 14.

Essential fatty acids work by protecting the walls or membranes of the cells. The membranes work by allowing nutritious elements to enter, while blocking out harmful scavengers. This is why flax seed is such an important anti-oxidant. It works to fight inflammations and pathogens, and it contains naturally-occurring plant estrogens also called *phyto-estrogens* (288). According to *The Healing Power of Vitamins, Minerals, and Herbs*, by the Reader's Digest Association, flax seed and flax oil have been used to treat many health disorders, including gastric problems, *shingles* and *lupus*. It can also help the body in preventing (and dissolving) gallstones (288).

The Budwig diet works by making important oils and lipoproteins easily available to the body at the cellular level, elevating oxygenation and energy. There is one website, in particular, that describes a new omega oil product known as *Omegasentials*™ that it says is already *water-soluble* and works much the same way that the Budwig diet works. You can find more information on *Omegasentials*™ at website: *www.mnwelldir.org/docs/cancer1/budwig.htm,* or you can email them at: *info@integritydirectinc.com* if you want to try the product (171). I have never tried their product, nor can I attest to its integrity. This is for informational purposes only.

## Oxygenation & Flax Oil

Dr. Otto Warburg won *the Nobel prize in 1931* when he discovered that, unlike normal cells in the body, cancer cells do not use oxygen—meaning that they are *anaerobic*—and they cannot thrive in a highly oxygenated environment (171). See website: http://*www.mnwelldir.org/docs/cancer1/budwig.html*, which explains that this resulted in the advent of many types of cancer therapies for increased tissue oxygenation, such as using *ozone* for blood oxygenation, the use of *hyperbaric oxygen*, and doing exercises (such as walking on a treadmill) while breathing in pure oxygen (*EWOT* or *Exercise With Oxygen Therapy*) (171). This is probably one reason, among many, that regular exercise lowers cancer risk; it increases oxygenation at the cellular level.

It was this principle of increasing oxygen to the body at the cellular level that interested Dr. Budwig, and was part of the rationale behind her flax seed oil/cottage cheese combination. Dr. Budwig assisted many terminally ill patients in regaining their health through her simple diet of flax seed oil and low-fat cottage cheese. She was known as *Germany's premier biochemist* with "a Ph.D. in Natural Science" (601). She was also trained in *pharmaceutical science* and many other fields. Those in Germany, who were producing margarines and other solid shortening, bitterly attacked her in order to silence her and keep her from exposing the truth about their harmful hydrogenated fats (601).

Some websites vary the Budwig diet slightly by allowing the addition of fresh ground flax seed. Oncologist, Dr. Dan C. Roehm, studied the Budwig diet recently and said that, "this diet is far and away the most successful anti-cancer diet in the world" (601). Dr. Budwig claimed that the diet not only prevented disease, but cured disease as well. She believed that the total lack of *linol acids* in the diet is the reason for the rampant epidemic of cancer and other diseases, especially in the West (601).

Apparently, Dr. Budwig cured cancer by discovering that cancer patients were always deficient in essential fats, which are critical for controlling cancer cells (601). What she found in her research was a completely natural way for people to obtain the missing ingredients they needed (601). Many testimonials have been given of patients brought back from terminal illness to amazing health by Johanna Budwig's diet. One example is that of Sandy A, who was told he was terminal after he developed bleeding from a brain tumor. He was told that nothing could be done for him, and sent home to die. He started on Dr. Budwig's formula and said that he recovered so rapidly, he was able to resume his job part-time. That was over *ten years* ago, and he said that his amazing healing has been described in many prestigious health periodicals (601).

The parents of 11-year-old Timmy G. were told that he had *Hodgkin's disease*. He was given just a few months to live, after failure to respond to 24 conventional *radiation treatments* (601). His mother was told of the Budwig diet, which she gave to her son. She marveled that less than one week later, he was, "for the first time in…two years," breathing normally. He eventually returned to school and is now more than 18 years of age and credits his life to Dr. Budwig's formula (601). Website *www.curezone.com,* documents the case of a person diagnosed with a terminal osteosarcoma using the Budwig diet; however the patient used larger amounts of flax oil a day than the official diet calls for. He started "out with 4 tbl. [tablespoons] of flax per day," plus the cottage cheese. A few days later, he increased it to "8-10 tbl [tablespoons] of flax [oil] per day" with the cottage cheese. Three months later, all his lab work came back negative. His cancer was CURED. His physician was so incredulous that he thought there was some mistake and ordered his tests repeated **three times**. There were no errors. The patient, in his eighties, no longer had any traces of cancer (40).

Be aware that there are other components involved with the Budwig flax oil diet, besides the oil and cottage cheese. For example: no processed sugar is allowed. *Grape juice* is used as a juicing sweetener. All processed fats and *animal fats* are forbidden. Processed and *preserved meats* are not allowed. *Fresh-squeezed* juices are encouraged, as are teas, with *honey* used as a sweetener (601). Every day, those on the diet are to drink either a glass of [organic] *sauerkraut juice…before breakfast*, or a *glass of acidophilus milk*. On the first day of the diet, nothing is taken except for "250 ml (8.5 oz) of Flax Oil with honey plus freshly squeezed fruit juices" (no sugar added) (601). Note that many people skip that 8.5 ounce flax oil dose on day one and proceed to the main diet (601). (That much oil would be in divided amounts.) Just be sure (if using the Budwig diet) that you are getting two to five tablespoons of the flax seed oil daily with ½ to 1 cup of organic yogurt, or cottage cheese, thoroughly blended until no traces of the oil can be seen. If you do not care for the taste of the flax oil, you can add fresh fruit to the mix, or cinnamon and other spices, which hides the oily taste, however, don't add fruit or cinnamon until after the oil and yogurt are thoroughly mixed. You may want to eat the fruit as a side dish.

## Flax Versus Fish

Many nutrition experts will tell you that fish is the healthiest form of omega-3, but studies have shown that this may not be the case. FLAX may be the best! For one thing, many of our coastal waters are dangerously polluted. There is much documentation available on mercury poisoning in fish. Even if you are able to get untainted fish, while some fish may be good, eating it more often may not be best. When researchers completed a **human** study that lasted 30 years and involved 2000 male participants, they discovered that those eating more than "8 ounces of fish a week," had greater risk of *stroke*. While the Japanese do eat a large amount of fish in their diet, it is also true that they have high statistics for stroke (604) in their population.

During research studies, when mice received fish oil, flax oil, or corn oil, and were then injected with cancerous breast cells, the only oil of the three that successfully retarded the growth of the cancerous tumors and their spread was the flax oil (504).

## Krill Oil - Potent Source of Omega-3

A high anti-oxidant marine oil that also provides omega-3 fatty acids (perhaps one of the best new sources), proteins, phospholipids, and astaxanthin carotenoids, is the oil from the shrimp-like creature known as the *Antarctic Krill.* This oil can also help alleviate arthritic pain, PMS, seasonal allergies, auto-immune disorders, and high cholesterol levels (553). The amazing health properties of the oil of this little sea creature are described *in The Healing Power of Neptune Krill Oil,* by Tina Sampalis, M.D., Ph.D. Be certain if you obtain supplements, that you use the Neptune Krill Oil (NKO™) patented formula that has a proprietary process to keep the oil potent. For PMS, they recommend 600 mg/day; to lower high cholesterol 1000 mg/day; to maintain good cholesterol 500 mg/daily; and for "joint pain and inflammation 300 mg krill oil" daily

(553). Of course, consult with your physician if you are lactating, pregnant, have shellfish allergies, blood clotting disorders, or have chronic health problems, or are awaiting for or just had surgery.

## Oil of the Green-Lipped Mussel

Another form of oil that should be considered for those fighting diseases, such as cancer and arthritis, is the oil from the green-lipped mussel from the country of New Zealand, known as *Lyprinol*®, an anti-inflammatory that some say is equivalent in potency to Celebrex, but without the side effects associated with Celebrex. This is a rare type of omega-3 that has an anti-inflammatory affect on the body. It is described at website *http://www.primohealth.com/PILyprinol.a.html,* and is said to have hundreds of times the potency of salmon oil, evening primrose oil, or flax oil. The damaging gastric side effects of NSAIDS, over-the-counter (and some prescription) drugs is well known, yet Lyprinol® is without toxic side effects, and exerts a protective effect on the GI system. As a matter-of-fact, when it was given at the rate of *50 capsules* a day to those who were very ill, no toxic effects were experienced (182). It has been used for everything from arthritis to asthma, and even given for CFS or *Chronic Fatigue Syndrome* (182). This supplement is marketed at the above website. Even those with severe *rheumatoid arthritis* have had tremendous results using Lyprinol®.

Another supplement made from the oil of the green-lipped mussel is a *concentrated superfood* from New Zealand known as *Moxxor* (327a). Many people are using Moxxor to rid themselves of the painful inflammation caused by arthritis, without the side effects of NSAIDS and other drugs. Many researchers believe cancer is an inflammatory process. This oil fights inflammation (327a). Testing on this supplement is currently underway. You can purchase it at website: *http://www.mymoxxor.com/productListPage.aspx?ID=consumerwellness* (327a).

## Perilla Oil & Salba

Perilla oil and salba are other healthy sources of plant-based oils. See Life Extension's website: *http://www.lef.org/magazine/mag98/nov98_perilla.html* and *http://www.allhealthtrends.com/salba-information.html.*

# CHAPTER 19

# ANTI-CANCER HERBS & FOODS

*"And God said, Behold, I have given you every herb bearing seed, which is upon the face of all the earth, and every tree, in the which is the fruit of a tree yielding seed; to you it shall be for meat." (Genesis 1:29)*

## Our God-Given Wonderful Varieties

God has provided many healing herbs for our use. The herb, graviola, is one of them. It has already been discussed in chapter five and six, as well as *Essiac* herbal tea, for their anti-cancerous benefits. Many herbs that we call *grasses* (barley, alfalfa, wheat grass, kelp, etc.), have also been discussed earlier in this book, as well as garlic, saw palmetto, and dozens of important preventative and curative herbs. However, there are many other herbs and herbal remedies used effectively in cancer prevention and/or treatment. Only a few of them are covered in this chapter. There are so many medicinal herbs provided by our great Creator God for our benefit, it would be impossible to include them all in a book of this size, and new remedies from herbs are being discovered every day!

Carl C. Pfeiffer, M.D., Ph.D., a pioneer in researching the biochemical relationship of natural substances and their relationship to mental illness, believed that for each drug designed to benefit humanity, nature has already provided a natural ingredient that accomplishes much the same purpose, but without adverse effects. Quite a profound belief coming from a physician born in 1908. I believe this is true because God's word declares that he has freely given us every herb (as noted in the quote at the beginning of this chapter). Below are just a few of those amazing herbs. I have taken what I believe to be some of the most important herbs related to cancer prevention and treatment and—either listed them in this chapter—or covered them elsewhere in this book in cancer-specific chapters. (Be aware that some of these herbs have not yet undergone extensive testing in humans.)

If you are interested in pursuing more in-depth information about herbs and herbal remedies, a good book to begin with is *The Scientific Validation of Herbal Medicine,* by Daniel B. Mowrey, Ph.D., and of course, the internet has a glut of information on herbs. There are also several very informative herbal books noted in my reference section, such as: *Earl Mindell's Herb Bible*, by Dr. Earl Mindell, R.Ph., Ph.D; *The Herbal Drugstore*, by Linda B. White, M.D., and Steven Foster; and *Healing Power of Herbs*, by John Heinerman, as well as many informative herbal websites, such as: *herbs2000.com, rain-tree.com, planetherbs.com,* and *iherb.com.* Remember that you should never give herbs or herbal preparations to children without consulting their physician, nor should you take them yourself without doing the same, especially if you are on prescription medications, are pregnant or nursing, or have a health condition that requires close monitoring. Prescriptions and even over-the-counter remedies may have adverse effects when combined with certain herbs or herbal remedies. (Even simple kitchen spices that may not affect you, may have an adverse effect on your baby if you are nursing or pregnant.)

## Actinidia Root & the Common Kiwi Fruit

This herb, common in Chinese folk medicine, was discovered by research scientists, to contain an extract capable of halting the growth of cancerous liver cells in test animals (470). The rate at which some tumors were stopped was nearly 90% in one type of cancer, and 50% in another (470). An extract from a Japanese fruit very similar to kiwi (in laboratory testing), was able to suppress leukemia. Note that the common **KIWI fruit found in your grocery store is a type of actinidia, however, it is** *Actinidia chinensis* (not the same as the above root). Kiwi fruit has amazed scientists because it appears to be able to help prevent free radical (oxygen) damage to DNA at the cellular level (173).

According to website *www.whfoods.com*, studies on nearly nineteen thousand young children in Italy revealed that common store-bought kiwi fruit (not the root mentioned above), high in anti-oxidants, could help prevent respiratory-related illnesses in the children who consumed at least half-a-dozen or more servings weekly (173). They report that the fruit is high in fiber and may offer some help for fighting asthma. Kiwi also thins the blood and helps normalize high lipids (173). Be aware that if you are taking blood-thinning medications, preparing for a surgical procedure, recovering from surgery, or have a chronic disorder (e.g., a blood dyscrasia), you should not eat excessive amounts of this fruit. If you are already taking an aspirin regimen, do not substitute the fruit for aspirin without first consulting your physician. Do not consume excessive amounts of kiwi if you have a tendency to develop kidney stones or gallstones, since it is a high oxalate food (173). High oxalate foods can cause stone formation in some individuals.

## Aloe Vera

Aloe is a medicinal plant that has been used for thousands of years for many purposes, including skin disorders (psoriasis), "Sunburn… Wounds…Hemorrhoids…Infections…Jellyfish, Stinging Nettle…Ulcers [taken internally]…Arthritis…Asthma…[and]…Sore Throat," as well as "digestive problems" (567). According to Max B. Skousen, in his book *The Ancient Egyptian Medicine Plant Aloe Vera Handbook,* "There are many reports of total elimination" of skin cancers, simply by the topical application of aloe (567).

Be aware though, if you have a suspicious-looking skin lesion, you need to seek professional medical attention immediately. Also, if you have problems such as ulcers, abdominal cancer, Crohn's or IBS, seek your physician's advice about using aloe products internally. Aloe has been used to treat leukemia, and it is sometimes used to help increase the absorption potential of green juices and to soothe the intestinal mucosa. (Dee Simmons uses an aloe-papaya preparation with her nutritional products. Her website can be found at *www.ultimateliving.com.)*

Note that papaya enzymes can have blood-thinning effects. This is one reason you should always discuss any new herb or nutrient you are considering with your physician. Your physician will be able to tell you if aloe or papaya might interfere with current medications you may be taking, such as anti-coagulants, and of course, the same applies if you have any sort of chronic disease or condition, or if you are a transplant patient. Be certain that when you use the drinkable form of aloe vera jel juice, that it is organic cold-pressed. The label should give you this information.

## Artemisinin

Artemisinin, extracted from the wormwood plant, is gaining a reputation for being able to hunt down and destroy *breast cancer cells* without harming normal cells (460). In laboratory testing, the herb killed (within 16 hours) every single breast cancer cell it came in contact with. Researchers used it on a dog so riddled with osteosarcoma, that he was barely able to walk. Within less than a week after receiving the treatment, the dog made a total recovery. No trace of the tumor could be found. At last check (two years later), the dog is still alive and well (460); however, artemisinin has been used by the Chinese (in **humans**) for many centuries for treating malaria, but because of recent testing, is emerging as a potential treatment for tumors, especially those of the breast (460). Recent reports show that it can (in lab testing) kill leukemia cells.

Dr. Hulda Clark used wormwood as one of her parasite-killing remedies, which is discussed later in this book in chapter 28. Much research is being done on cancer being caused by fungus and parasites. When you consider the high amount of processed sugar that is in the average diet, this is not hard to understand. Wormwood is not recommended for those who are pregnant or nursing. Human testing is still being conducted.

Researchers from the University of Washington recently discovered that they could outfit wormwood (artemisinin) with a *homing device* that sends the substance to cancer cells only, keeping normal cells unharmed (75a). The substance gets inside the cells and acts like a *bomb inside the cell*, as described by Professor Tomikazu Sasaki. It works against the high iron content found in cancer cells (75a).

This herb should not be taken on an empty stomach. Be sure to consult with your physician before taking artemisinin, especially if you are on radiation, or have recently been treated with radiation therapy.

## Ashwagandha

Ashwagandha belongs to the tomato family of plants and can be found growing abundantly in several countries. Extracts from the herb have been known to cure cancer. This herb is also known as "*winter cherry*" and "*Indian ginseng*," and has the ability to boost the body's natural immunity and help in fighting stress (542). Substances from the leaves inhibited several types of cancer cells, including those of the *breast*, *colon*, and *central nervous system* (542).

If choosing this herb, be sure that you get an extract *standardized with anolides* (26) (542). It is usually found sold as a *capsule*. Do not use the oil from ashwaganda as this is a facial toner only, and avoid using the berries which can be harmful if ingested (26). Do not use this herb if you are on seizure meds, nor if you are being treated for *anxiety* or *insomnia* (26). Dr. Sahelian's website has standardized ashwagandha herbal supplements available. For those interested, see website: *www.raysahelian.com* (542).

## Bromelain

Though not usually considered an herb, *bromelain* is a protein substance found naturally in pineapples, and it is being included here because it is often added to herbal remedies for digestive disorders, and to treat arthritis sufferers (571). In the results of a **human study on** bromelain ingestion, a dozen people received *600 milligrams* every day for a time span of *6 months* to *several years*. The bromelain helped dissolve tumors (*ovarian and breast*) (571). Tumor cells are wrapped in a type of casing composed mostly of protein. This casing acts like a camouflage, making it difficult for cells from the body's natural immune system to recognize the cancer cell and destroy it. It is believed that the bromelain enzyme dissolves this disguise so that the body's immune cells can recognize the cancer cells and destroy them (409). Bromelain is not for those with ulcers or blood disorders, nor for those who are allergic to pineapples.

## Bupleurum for the Liver

Bupleurum *(Bupleurum chinense)* is a wild herb that has been used in the orient for more than two millennia for liver health, working much like milk thistle (50). *Sakosides* in this herb are very liver-protective, helping to enforce the liver and may be helpful for those who are battling auto-immune diseases. It has been used to treat liver diseases (e.g., *hepatitis*), as well as *bone cancer* (50). This herb should not be used if you are running a temperature or if you are on prescription *antibiotics*. It can cause epigastric discomfort, in which case your herbalist or natural health practitioner may need to lower the amount that you are taking (41). It may also cause swelling, and should not be combined with other medications.

## Cascara Sagrada for Cleansing

Cascara Sagrada *(Rhamnus purshiana)* is known as an anti-oxidant and colon rejuvenator. When you check the labels of some laxative medications, you will find cascara sagrada among the ingredients (333). According to Marie Nadine Antol, in *Healing Teas,* it may help fight intestinal disorders, such as colon inflammation and *diverticulosis*, as well as liver problems, *gallstones* and *leukemia* (333). It has been used for years to rid the body of parasites and increase the normal forward movement (*peristalsis*) in the colon. It also helps strengthen the walls of the colon. Just be sure if buying the herb, advises Ms. Antol, that you purchase the *sacred bark*, not the "purging buckthorn, *Rhamnus cathartica*," which is so much stronger in action, it can be harmful! Taking excessive doses of cascara can result in loose stools and cramping in the bowels (333). Don't give to children.

## Cat's Claw

Cat's claw (also known as *Uno de Gato)* is discussed in many cancer-specific chapters in this book. See chapter 20 for instances when you should not take this herb.

## Chinese Asparagus

Chinese asparagus *(Asparagus cochinchinensis)* grows near the ocean and can be found in several oriental countries. It is also known as *Tian Men Dong*, and is used to fight infections, excess fluid buildup, *congestion, diptheria, tuberculosis*…and other ailments. In animal testing, it blocked tumor formation (75). It is currently being investigated for use in fighting cancer cells in the lungs, as well as *lymphosarcoma* (75).

## Cilantro, Natural Chelator & Blood Purifier

Cilantro is a mild herb that gets little attention, but it is powerful. The herb acts like a chelating agent to remove toxic substances (e.g., *heavy metals*) from human cells (78). (I.V. chelation therapy is common in alternative medicine as a way to get toxic metals, such as aluminum, cadmium, mercury, and other free radicals out of the body.) One physician in particular, Dr. Omura, discovered that using *fresh cilantro* could cause the body to excrete these toxic metals within 14 days, and this is one chelation agent that you can take orally, rather than intravenously (78), without toxic side effects.

## Ciwujia, Ginseng Cousin for CFS

Ciwujia (*Acanthopanax senticosis…or Siberian ginseng*) has been tested in **humans**. It can be found in a supplement known *as Endurox*™, as well as by itself. It has strong *ginseng-like effects* that, in animal studies, protected the heart from dangerous arrhythmias (583). In **human** studies, according to K. Gilbert Udall, author of *Immune and Stamina Booster Cordyceps Sinensis*, ciwujia extract strengthens the body's immunity. It is also being used to treat "chronic fatigue syndrome in humans" (583).

## Cranberry, Protectant Fruit

It is believed that cranberries protect against bladder infections by either acidifying the urine, destroying pathogens, or by facilitating the flushing of parasites and bacteria out of the body (494). It is important to drink unsweetened cranberry juice, because the bottled type of commercial juice found in your grocery store is usually loaded with sugar (corn syrup), and other additives. You may want to opt for supplements or extracts from cranberries at health food stores, which have fewer calories and may be more powerful than drinking the juice (494). Some health food stores have unsweetened cranberry juice available, or you can always juice your own when cranberries are in season, using a natural herb, such as *Stevia,* for sweetening purposes. It will take a lot of stevia, depending on personal taste, because fresh cranberries are usually extremely tart. The berries are rich in anti-oxidants that can boost the immune system.

You may want to check out Dr. Mercola's website at *www.mercola.com* for *D-Mannose* supplement. *D-Mannose* is a nutrient extracted from peaches and berries (such as cranberries), which is said to maintain urinary tract health without giving you the high sugar dose that is found in most bottled cranberry juices. Cranberries can also help fight leukemia.

## Curry Versus Curcumin (Turmeric)

Many curry products sold on supermarket shelves have potentially toxic amounts of artificial color additives that have been associated with attention deficit disorders. One such additive is known as *tartrazine* in the U.S. (You may see this listed in the ingredients section as *FD&C Yellow No. 5.)* This additive is derived from coal tar, and can be harmful to the body's metabolism (140). You will be shocked to see how many products you pick up at your local supermarket that list *FD&C Yellow No. 5* on them. They are found in makeup, lotions (where they are absorbed into the skin), candles, perfumes (where you and your children are inhaling them everyday), frangrances, chips, cake mixes, candies, soft drinks, and many other products that are in grocery stores. Is it any wonder that our food supply is being completely poisoned and that so many adults and children are being diagnosed daily with cancer and debilitating diseases? This is yet another additive that the FDA has determined is *safe* for human consumption. Do NOT use curry powder! Get your curcumin from organic turmeric at natural health food stores. Curcumin is discussed in more detail in several cancer-specific chapters of this book. See chapter 20 for instances of when you should not use turmeric (curcumin).

We have also been led to believe that artificial sweeteners like aspartame are safe. Avoid all aspartame products, which are sold under various brand names like: *Nutra-Sweet*™, *Canderel*™ and *Equal*™. By now, you should realize that the FDA treats humans like guinea pigs. Many studies have shown that aspartame truly is a *sweet poison.* Though the FDA has not removed it from shelves, it has been known to cause grotesque tumor formation in animals, as well as migraines, seizures (in some individuals), visual disorders, heart palpitations, asthma, panic attacks, dizziness, mental problems (e.g., memory loss, personality changes, and depression), insomnia, and many other ailments in humans!

If you want to see an excellent laboratory study that was done on the effects of aspartame sweetener, see website *myaspartameexperiment.com.* You have to check some products that are advertised as *sugar-free* closely to see exactly WHY they are *sugar-free.* Many of them contain aspartame, but you have to read the SMALL print to find this out! Many food processors have figured out that people **don't want** aspartame in their food, so they are putting it in the ingredients in such tiny print that you need a magnifying glass to read it, or disguising it under various names. Be a label-reader! If the label has the above sweeteners in the list of ingredients, do not use them! They may also be referred to in the label of ingredients as: *aspartyl-L-phenylalanine*, *APM*, *aspartic acid*, *methanol* (which is wood alcohol) or the label may tell you that there are *phenylalanines* in the product, or a word similar to this. AVOID them!

## Echinacea, Wonder Herb

According to Dr. D. B. Mowrey, author of *The Scientific Validation of Herbal Medicine,* this herb (sometimes called *purple coneflower*) is used by some people for battling colon cancer. It also has a popular history of treating "typhoid, meningitis, malaria, [and] diphtheria…" and is still being used for this purpose in modern times (510). It helps boost the immune system by increasing white blood cells. It also protects the body's reserves of hyaluronic acid, a critical substance that helps the cells ward off germs (510). Echinacea has an *anti-inflammatory* effect, stimulates the lymphatic system, and protects against viruses like "herpes, influenza, canker sores, etc" (510). Dr. John Heinerman, author of *The Healing Power of Herbs*, says that the best form of echinacea is not the one most popularized, *echinacea angustifolia*, but the one known as ***echinacea purpurea,*** as this form of the herb increases the immune system's ability to fight diseases (428).

## Ginkgo Biloba, Anti-Oxidant for Circulation

Ginkgo, another herb that has enjoyed prominence in China for several millennia, is the subject of intensive research throughout the entire world. It is excellent for overall circulation, so much so, that people have credited it to the prevention of these disorders: dementia, abnormal clotting, circulatory problems, e.g., "phlebitis and diabetic peripheral vascular disease" (494). It also has blood pressure lowering effects.

## Ginseng Fights Cancer & Cholesterol

In his book *Cancer Therapy,* Dr. Ralph Moss describes several different types of ginseng: the *American* variety known as *Panax quinquefolius*; Siberian ginseng (*Eleutherococcus senticosus);* [and] oriental ginseng: "Chinese or Korean—*Panax ginseng*" (504). The Chinese have been cultivating and using it for thousands of years. Japanese researchers found that consuming ginseng caused bad cholesterol levels to drop in test animals that were purposely fed a high-fat regimen, and it raised good or *HDL cholesterol* (494). Recent studies revealed that ingredients from oriental (*panax*) *ginseng* could halt cancer cells, and even revert them back to *normal* (494). The big issue with cancer cells is that they do not differentiate. A cancer cell in the liver won't normally become a liver cell. If it did, it wouldn't be a cancer cell. The fact that this type ginseng actually caused the cancer cells to differentiate and turn back into normal cells is most remarkable!

Recently, scientists found that a ginseng isolate could help reverse *melanoma* (504). Note that more than 5 to 10 grams of panax ginseng a day can cause nervousness and over-stimulation, as well as problems with hypertension and *headaches* (494). Women who have already gone through menopause may find, after using panax ginseng, that they have developed *vaginal bleeding*, but this side effect is highly unusual. Do not take Vitamin C at the same time you take ginseng. Space them apart by at least two hours for best assimilation by the body (494). As explained in Dr. *Earl Mindell's Herb Bible,* the only difference between red and white ginseng is that the red variety is more highly prized, since it is "steamed with a solution of herbs," and the white is not (494).

## Gymnema Sylvestre & Banaba Leaf for the Pancreas

Gymnema is another herb that has been tested on **humans.** The herb has been in use for many years for helping those with *diabetes…arthritis and gout,* and (in animal testing) was not found to be toxic (545). Research was also done in India on **humans** with type II diabetes on a substance isolated from the leaf of this herb (545). During this period of time, those taking the gymnema were able to cut dependency on oral blood-sugar-controlling drugs, and the most amazing thing of all was that this herb may help the beta cells of the pancreas to repair themselves in Type II diabetes) (545). No toxic effects were noted. More research on gymnema sylvestre confirmed that it was capable of beta-cell regeneration in the pancreas (142). Another herb that is gaining popularity for lowering blood sugar, widely used in the Philippines, is **banaba leaf.** Also, be sure that you are getting sufficient levels of the mineral, vanadium.

## Hoxsey's Famous Tea

Harry Hoxsey developed an herbal tea that he used in fighting cancer. He was very much against the cancer establishment and even had his own radio program where he boldly proclaimed a very "anti-AMA message" at every opportunity. He successfully operated several *clinics* until the federal government moved in and closed them (504). The Hoxsey Formula is still being used at his Mexico clinic, and a Hoxsey tincture list of ingredients can be found at website *www.naturalopinion.com* (189), as well as other internet sites.

Hoxsey was ridiculed, made to look like a *snake oil salesman*, harassed, and finally run out of the country when he claimed that his formula was curing cancer patients. This is nothing new and often happens when someone uses a cancer remedy that defies the golden calf of the cancer industry (chemo and radiation). They do not take kindly to physicians that buck their system. In the years that followed his death, research into Hoxsey's herbal formula revealed that many of the compounds Hoxsey used have powerful anti-cancer effects (504). Some of the herbs (e.g., the pokeweed root and the burdock) can be dangerous if taken in excess amounts or improperly prepared. Burdock contains a substance that, as reported by WHO (*the World Health Organization*), can fight HIV, and another Hoxsey tea compound, known as barberry, can help fight cancer (504).

The treatment that Harry Hoxsey received at the hands of the AMA was nothing short of criminal, and is described as a 25-year-battle between the AMA's Morris Fishbein and Hoxsey, with Hoxsey winning, though the FDA eventually moved in and closed his U.S. clinics (526).

The Hoxsey formula is still available at their clinic in Tijuana, Mexico. They can be reached at: Bio-Medical center 615 General Ferreira, Colonia Juarez Tijuana, B.C. Mexico. Tel: 011-52-664-684-9011/Fax: 011-52-664-684-9744.

## Iscador (Mistletoe)

Iscador is actually a type of mistletoe. It is used as an alternative cancer therapy in Europe, but not widely promoted or used in the U.S. It was given a flash of notoriety back in 2001 when an American celebrity announced to the world that she had opted out of chemotherapy for breast cancer and was using iscador treatments instead. Many people in the mainstream medical establishment criticized her immediately as though she had done something vile and unforgivable. Of course to them she had. After all, she was kicking their untouchable golden calf in refusing chemo, so naturally the entire medical establishment had a cow!

Human studies, reported as recently as December of 2008, show that iscador can help extend the life span of those with cancer, most notably, those with ovarian and cervical cancers (197a).

## Jiaogulan

Jiaogulan (*Gynostemma pentaphyllum*), is a liver-protective herb that also fights cancer by increasing natural killer cells in the immune system. The herb is a natural anti-histamine and has been used for years in Chinese medicine. You may hear it referred to as *Southern ginseng.*

## Licorice for Gastric Ailments & Estrogen Reduction

Licorice *(Glycyrrhiza glabra)* is soothing to the gastric system and has been used in treating ulcers. According to Marie N. Antol in *Healing Teas*, it is also used for soothing the colon and stomach, and works to expel mucus from the body and fights inflammation (333). It has even been successful in treating topical *herpes simplex*, says Ms. Antol, however, it is important if you choose to use this herb, to obtain the *DGL (deglycyrrhizinated)* form (333). Licorice that has **not** been *deglycyrrhizinated* can cause water retention, loss of potassium, and hypertension, and should not be used if you have heart or kidney ailments, nor if you have hypertension, palpitations (333), glaucoma, or other health disorders, without checking with your physician. Licorice also has the unique ability to normalize the body's use of estrogen (333), a very important activity, since **excess estrogen in the body has been linked to breast cancer.**

## Milk Thistle for the Liver

Milk thistle is so important in liver health and cleansing, it is discussed in detail in chapter nine of this book for its use against liver cancer and some forms of hepatitis. See the report in that chapter on the patient whose ***terminal*** liver cancer completely disappeared while he was taking this common, nontoxic herbal treatment.

## Olive Leaf Extract for Healthy Immunity

Olive leaf not only boosts energy, but the immune system as well, by enhancing the ability of white blood cells to destroy viruses and bacteria. It can also enter cells that are already infected and help halt the growth of viruses (60). This nutrient, in supplement form, has been used in treating many health disorders including *meningitis…shingles* [and] *HIV*…(60).

## Oregano for Overall Health

Oregano is another herb that has been used for centuries for many purposes, including toothaches, as an antiseptic, for candida, indigestion and ringworm. Wild oil of oregano has also demonstrated the ability to kill bacteria, parasites, fungi, athlete's foot (when used topically), and a myriad of other uses. Research using potent extracts from oil of wild oregano revealed that it even exerts some capacity at suppressing melanoma. I have used a drop or two to clear up an earache, however, it should never be used if eardrum perforation is suspected, or in very young children, without consulting their physician.

## Parsley, Cleanser & Blood Purifier

Parsley *(Petroselinum crispum)*, long known as a diuretic, is an anti-oxidant and cancer preventative (235). One of the ingredients found in this herb was shown to suppress cancer formation. It should not be used by women who are pregnant or nursing since it can cause premature uterine contractions and interfere with the *milk supply* in those who are nursing. Do not use it in the presence of an infectious process of the kidneys (235). If you purchase dried parsley for tea, be aware that tea made from the root is going to be much more potent than if it comes from the leaf. ***Parsley oil*** can cause skin irritations and is highly toxic (228). Fresh, organically-grown parsley (used in small amounts) is best.

## Red Clover for Immune Health

Red clover is a favorite morsel for wild rabbits, but packs a punch when used as a tea. It can help boost the immunity in those with cancer, HIV, and other ailments (428). You can find red clover tea in many health food stores. It contains naturally-occurring plant estrogens, and is often used as an herbal alternative for the treatment of *osteoporosis*, combined with other herbs like *Horsetail* [and] *stinging nettle* (597).

Naturally-occurring estrogens in plants (such as red clover) lock onto estrogen-receptor sites on the cells, thus preventing the **harmful, toxic forms of estrogen** from being transported into the cells (597). Be aware that red clover has blood thinning properties, so should not be used without consulting your physician or Naturopath, especially if you are on prescription medications. Never use any form of **fermented** red clover. Toxic forms of estrogen come from the environment and synthetic estrogen (man-made). Even plastics (and some shampoos and cosmetics) contain toxic, synthetic estrogens.

## Rose Hips, Powerful Anti-Oxidant

Rose hips are important simply because they are an excellent source of natural vitamin C, and vitamin C is critical in fighting cancer. There are as many types of rose hips as there are roses! They are many times more potent in vitamin C content than *oranges* (235). They contain *bioflavonoids* that enhance the effects of vitamin C, and are also rich in several other vitamins and minerals. They help purify the blood and ward off *infections*, especially those of the urinary tract. As described by Marine Nadine Antol in *Healing Teas*, check roses—once they have bloomed and faded and start dropping petals—you will see little *pods* that appear. These are the *rose hips* (235). Many vitamin C supplements are made from rose hips (235). Use organic only, as they are free from pesticides and herbicides.

## Wolfberry for Health, Longevity & Fighting Cancer

Recently publicized in the West, though it has been used for hundreds of years by locals in Mongolia, where it is also known as the *Chinese wolfberry* and *goji berry* (606), it was found that many of the peoples consuming this berry are centenarians who have never had the type of debilitating diseases found in the West. It is a very mild berry without known toxicity. Researchers in Beijing analyzed the nutritional components of the wolfberry fruit and found that it contained a greater concentration of amino acids than bee pollen; higher amounts of beta-carotene than carrots; dozens of trace minerals, B vitamins, vitamin E; and had *500 times* more vitamin C than oranges! The *fruits and pedicels* of the berry were able to boost the immunity and were found to be liver-protective with blood pressure lowering capacities (606). When an alcohol extract of the fruit was tested (in animal studies), it cut cancerous growths by greater than half, and had a hypoglycemic and fat metabolism effect (606). Recently, goji berries are said to have appetite-suppressing abilities.

In another study (using **human** cancer patients), the wolfberry increased killer immunity cells in the body. It was also discovered that the berry may be useful in treating *Epstein-Barr* and *Chronic Fatigue Syndrome,* and that it may help fight genetic deformities in the DNA of cells (606).

You can find a bottled wolfberry juice that uses not only wolf-berries, but other berries and fruits (like pomegranates) at website *www.aromanotes.com/87/berry-young* (32). The drink is called *Berry Young Juice*, and apparently, is so high in anti-oxidants, that producers say you only need an ounce a day (32). Note that pomegranate juice is said to have three times as many *anti-oxidants* as *green tea* (32).

## Xi Shu - The *Cancer Tree.*

Xi Shu *(Camptotheca acuminata)* is also known as the *Cancer Tree...Happy Tree,* and *Tree of Joy.* It is a Chinese herb used for medicinal purposes to treat digestive organ diseases and *leukemia*, from which its name was derived (323). The FDA has approved two derivatives from this herb for treating cancer. The two drugs are *Topotecan* and *Irinotecan* (323). It is interesting that both of these drugs created by pharmaceutical companies are **toxic to normal cells,** having a variety of adverse side effects. Amazing that an herb safely used for centuries by the Chinese, once synthesized into chemo drugs by pharmaceutical companies, **becomes highly toxic to the immune system!**

# CHAPTER 20

# MORE CANCER-FIGHTING SUPER ANTI-OXIDANTS

*"Heal me, O Lord, and I shall be healed; save me, and I shall be saved: for thou art my praise." (Jeremiah 17:14) "For I will restore health unto thee, and I will heal thee of thy wounds, saith the Lord;" (Jeremiah 30:17)*

## I. Some of the Best Anti-Oxidants

### Acai Berries

There has been much recent publicity about *acai* berries, and many new health foods and drinks that are on the market today, claiming that they are high in acai berry content. Acai is an anti-oxidant berry taken from a palm tree in the Brazilian Rain Forest. This berry is said to have twice the anti-oxidants found in blueberries and ten times more than those found in grapes. There are many websites that market acai berry juice, and you can find it at local health food stores, pharmacies, and chain grocers. It is also available in capsules, as a supplement.

### Alpha Lipoic Acid

This important anti-oxidant has great protective benefits, especially for the liver. Dr. Ralph Moss, author of *Anti-oxidants against Cancer,* reports that Europeans have used alpha lipoic acid for years to fight the deadly effects of poison mushrooms (507). It also protects against dangerous blood clots, *heart disease and cataracts*, increases glutathione in the body, and even works much like glutathione (507). Does your family have a genetic disposition toward some types of cancer? Dr. Moss explains that alpha lipoic acid has the unique ability of being able to help fight genetic forms of cancer without harming normal cells (507). Scientists are not sure why, but research proved that cancer cells in humans and animals take in large amounts of ALA, and when lipoic acid was given to lab animals with cancer, their lifespan increased (507).

This vital nutrient is made by every cell in our body when we are children, then as we age, we produce less and less of it, however, the older we get, the more we need ALA to stay healthy (344). It appears to work by preventing cellular damage, and when taken in normal supplemental doses, it is non-toxic (344). It has a health-promoting effect and helps treat many diseases, such as leukemia, liver problems, cancer and diabetes (344).

## Alpha Lipoic Acid & Liver Transplants

Dr. Burt Berkson, author of *The Alpha Lipoic Acid Breakthrough*, describes treating several of his *hepatitis C* patients with ALA—patients who were told that they would die unless they received a new liver. After treatment with ALA therapy, all of his patients *except one*, were back to normal (344). He believes that before anyone contemplates going through a *liver transplant*, their physicians should first try this valuable nutrient. His treatment regimen also includes a nutritious diet, information on the importance of coping with stress, supplementation with *vitamins*, an *exercise* workout, and of course, milk thistle (344). ALA is also discussed in chapter nine of this book for its importance in treating liver cancer. A few natural food sources of ALA include: spinach, potatoes, brewer's yeast, and broccoli, but it is difficult to get adequate dietary amounts without supplementing.

## Blueberries Fight Cancer Growth in Youngsters

Recent studies from Ohio State University have shown that a substance from blueberries may help shrink tumors that are commonly seen in young children and babies.

## Cat's Claw - Pycnogenol® Source

Another source of *pycnogenol®* is an herb known as ***cat's claw***. Though it is not as high in OPCs as grape seed extract and pine bark, cat's claw is emerging as an important anti-oxidant in the treatment of a vast array of disorders, including *cancer…Crohn's…Lupus…*viruses, and many others (393). Scientific research on cat's claw showed that it can help the body fight *leukemia* (393). Thus far, as described by website *herbs2000.com,* there have been no reported harmful side effects for the normal use of cat's claw, however, it is not recommended for those with "auto-immune illness [though it has been used for Crohn's and lupus], multiple sclerosis, and tuberculosis," nor should it be given "with hormonal drugs, insulin, or vaccines," nor taken if you are pregnant or lactating (67).

## Coenzyme Q10 - Miracle Worker

Cardiologist, Dr. Stephen Sinatra, M.D., F.A.C.C., in his book, *Coenzyme Q10 and the Heart,* considers this super anti-oxidant miraculous, and says that he would not even think of practicing cardiology without it (565). Though he says that this nutrient is a great remedy for heart disease, he states that most physicians have no idea it exists (565). I can understand where he is coming from. When I had a relative hospitalized for heart disease and took CoQ10 to her physician, and asked him to put her on it, he asked me what it was! He had no idea. He was a cardiologist, and this was four years ago. He refused to allow it. It was not on the formulary.

CoQ10 is useful for many degenerative disorders, such as hypertension, cancer, gum disease, diabetes and many others (565). Even more amazing is the fact that the discovery of CoQ10 was accidental.

Apparently, cancer cells absorb substances in a different way than normal healthy cells. According to Dr. Ray D. Strand, author of *What Your Doctor Doesn't Know About Nutritional Medicine May Be Killing You,* normal cells only consume the nutrients that they need, whereas cancer cells don't know when enough is enough. They keep on absorbing nutrients even when they are not needed, as though they haven't the sense to stop (573). In a nutshell—the right nutrients can kill them! Perhaps this accounts for why anti-oxidants like CoQ10, lycopene, resveratrol, beta-carotene, quercetin, and ellagic acid are so powerful. It may also explain why Johanna Brandt's grape cure was so effective. Cancer cells thrive on sugar. The grape diet requires a few days of fasting before starting. Then when you start drinking the grape juice, the cells suck it up very rapidly in their hungry state. In the case of the grape diet, you are using a type of nutrient (high in resveratrol) that will kill the cancer cells, because they absorb more nutrients than they need, and in so doing, they also absorb excess anti-oxidants, sealing their own doom.

Anti-oxidants destroy free radicals, sometimes by giving up one of their own electrons in the process. Another way of looking at how anti-oxidants work is to remember that a molecule of oxygen is made up of 8 *electrons* (443). Because of everyday stress (e.g., toxins in the environment, lack of sleep, vitamin/mineral deficiencies) and the normal aging process, the oxygen molecule loses an electron and the result is a *free radical* (443).

This new renegade goes about trying to steal an electron to substitute for the one that was taken. Once it succeeds in stealing an electron from another molecule, another *free radical* forms and a vicious cycle begins (443). This stealing of electrons starts to weaken the cell membrane and eventually the cell begins to deteriorate. After this happens, as explained by Lynn Keegan, Ph.D., R.N., in *Healing Nutrition*, the cell is then left open and vulnerable to attack (443).

Anti-oxidants can enter cellular tissues and willingly donate an electron, but they do so without attacking healthy cells. This puts a stop to the vicious cycle of electron theft, says Ms. Keegan, and the chain reaction comes to a halt. The cell wall is saved from destruction (443). (Note that not all free radicals are bad. Some are essential to normal bodily processes.) Ms. Keegan further points out that no cell in your body is over "7 years" old, and that you have "no blood cell…that is more than 14 days old." Your own body is able to "rebuild a new heart every 30 days" (443). This means that at least once a month, you get a new chance to turn any bad habits around and provide your body with the nutrition to re-energize and regain your health (443). I believe that super anti-oxidants, such as CoQ10 and others discussed in this book, can help you to do just that. Simply think of it this way: the quality of many of the cells that you have a month from now will be the result of **what you are eating today!**

## CoQ10 & Cancer

One major factor present in nearly all cancer patients (discovered by the late Dr. Karl Folkers) has been a profound deficiency in CoQ10, as well as B6. It appeared that the lowest levels of CoQ10 were found in those having cancer of the breast (564). Dr. Folkers was also credited with the discovery of vitamin B12, the vitamin that prevents pernicious anemia.

For optimum health, CoQ10 should be taken in conjunction with selenium, because (in animal testing) being deficient in selenium reduces liver levels of this nutrient, as well as cardiac levels (507). Selenium can be found in many food sources, including leafy greens, garlic, and Brazil nuts (507); however, if the soil that produced them is selenium-poor, there is no guarantee you will profit from eating them. Most adults will find it difficult, if not impossible, to get an adequate amount of CoQ10 daily without supplementing.

Current research conducted by the Leonard M. Miller School of Medicine in Miami, under Niven R. Nerain, revealed that CoQ10 has the ability to kill cancer cells without damage to healthy cells. Not only that, but the National Cancer Institute acknowledged in 2005 that CoQ10 can extend the lives of those with breast cancer and other cancers. Issels Treatment Centers use CoQ10. Their phone #888-447-7357 (290).

For one of America's largest alternative health care centers, the Whitaker Wellness Center, which is in Newport Beach (4321 Birch Street), California, see this link: ***http://whitakerwellness.com/about_us/medical_team.*** Dr. Julian Whitaker, who runs this health care center, has written many books on alternative healing. He has an excellent website with a great deal of helpful information. They use many of the alternative health treatments that I have mentioned in my books, including chelation, hyperbaric oxygen, and various intravenous therapies.

## CoQ10 & Congestive Heart Failure

One of the largest research studies involving the effectiveness of CoQ10 to treat heart disorders (e.g., heart failure), was an Italian study using more than 2500 people with the disease (565). It is described by Dr. Stephen T. Sinatra, M.D., author of *Coenzyme Q10 and the Heart.* All participants in the study were suffering with congestive heart failure and were given daily doses of CoQ10, most of them *receiving 100 mg daily.* After three months of taking CoQ10, patients experienced very dramatic decreases in all their congestive heart failure symptoms (565).

One of Dr. Sinatra's patients was an elderly woman, so severely affected with CHF, that she was struggling to breathe and her weight had plummeted. She had a dysfunctional valve, and her heart's pumping capacity was barely enough to get her out of bed for short periods of time (565). (EF or *ejection fraction* is a measurement of the heart's pumping ability. Normal is 70-80%, and the patient's was **15%.**) Dr. Sinatra started her on "30 mg of CoQ10 three times a day (90 mg/day)," however, she continued to deteriorate until something amazing occurred (565). Her son accidentally bought his mom "100 mg capsules instead of the usual 30 mg…" She was taking 100 mg three times a day without realizing it (a total of 300 mg). Within a month, she had improved so dramatically that she was kept on the higher dose of CoQ10, and several months after starting on the increased dosage of CoQ10, she was out and about with friends. As a result of this case, Dr. Sinatra feels that if patients do not respond to CoQ10 at low dosing, physicians should give larger doses, especially in those who are most severely ill, until they do respond (565).

Is it such a profoundly simple solution that mainstream medicine cannot grasp it? Apparently so. It is also a fact that CoQ10 cannot be patented, thus big pharma has no interest in promoting this nutrient (565). There are very few problems associated with the long term use of CoQ10. In a study of 5000 patients using the supplement, very minimal effects of gastrointestinal upset, diminished "appetite… Nausea… Diarrhea… Elevated LDH (rare)…[and] Elevated SGOT (rare)," were reported (565).

Dr. James F. Balch, M.D., in his book, *The Super Anti-Oxidants,* discusses the story of Gina F., whose experience with CoQ10 was aired on a national news broadcast in a nutrition series. Gina was only 24 and dying from heart failure (337). She was so ill that doctors had given her only a few days to live. Her physicians were ready to give up, having already tried various powerful pharmaceutical drugs that were not helping. Finally, they suggested she try CoQ10 supplements (337). A month later, Gina was still alive. Her heart had improved so dramatically that she called the nutrient her *lifeline* (337). The mystery is why more physicians don't recommend CoQ10 to their patients.

Dr. Ray D. Strand, M.D., also questioned this in his book, *What Your Doctor Doesn't Know About Nutritional Medicine May Be Killing You.* A transplant is costly, involving hundreds of thousands of dollars. This, in comparison to a CoQ10 supplement, that will cost about seven to ten dollars a week (573).

Although CoQ10 can be found in foods like *eggs, rice bran,* and *wheat germ,* Dr. Ralph Moss says that you cannot get enough of it without supplementing (507). A few other natural sources of CoQ10 are "…mackerel, peanuts, salmon, sardines, and spinach" (411).

If you are taking any type of statin (cholesterol-lowering drugs), studies show that one of their dangerous side effects is that they strip the body of CoQ10. Patients on cholesterol-lowering drugs are sometimes plagued by weakness. It is because they are losing all the CoQ10 from their cells. Ask your physician or Naturopath about placing you on CoQ10 with your cholesterol-lowering medication. There are many natural ways of lowering blood cholesterol (discussed in this book) that are just as effective as drugs, but without any side effects.

## Curcumin (Turmeric) Fights Many Cancers

This common table spice was shown, in animal testing, to have the ability to fight many types of cancer, including breast cancer and multiple myeloma. Turmeric is discussed in several other chapters of this book because of its amazing anti-cancer properties. You will find more curcumin in turmeric than you will in curry powder. Use organic turmeric rather than curry. If you want a turmeric capsule that is free of magnesium stearate additive, see *Nature's Way*® brand.

Turmeric can thin the blood. Do not use turmeric without first checking with your physician, especially if you have gallbladder problems, are pregnant, on blood-thinners, contemplating or just recovering from surgery or transplant, or if you are breast-feeding (571). If you want your body to absorb turmeric more easily, eat it with pineapple or supplement with bromelain. (Yellow mustard is very high in turmeric.)

## Eggplant Blocks Cancer From Spreading

Eggplants, also known as *aubergines*, are rich in substances known as terpenes, which block enzymes desperately needed by cancer cells (55).

## Ellagic Acid & Tangeretin

Ellagic acid, abundant in berries, grapes, cherries, pomegranates, pecans and walnuts, fights the formation of cancer cells. They can also prevent harmful DNA changes. One of the richest sources of ellagic acid is raspberries (571). Pomegranates are also a good source of ellagic acid. Tangerines contain a powerful anti-oxidant (*tangeretin)*, which suppresses cancer spread (571). Ingredients in tangerines also help fight brain cancer cells. See other cancer-specific chapters in this book for more information on these anti-oxidants, for example, the amazing prostate cancer prevention ability of raspberries, as described in chapter five.

## Glutathione & Glutamine

*Glutathione* helps protect the brain and gastric wall (against toxins) and enhances the body's immunity (507). If you do use glutathione supplements, it is best to combine them with *selenium and vitamin B2.* They enhance its function (507). Milk thistle also raises glutathione levels in the body and vitamin C preserves it. Even better, use natural sources of glutathione, such as raw veggies of every color (e.g., carrots, tomatoes and spinach). Just remember that cooking and freezing food kills glutathione. This is also true of canned foods (148). This is another reason to consume your veggies and fruit raw, their most nutritious state. Eat tomatoes, both cooked and raw. Cooking appears to increase their lycopene availability, but eating them raw means more glutathione.

Animal studies show that several spices and plants can raise glutathione levels in the body. Scientists concluded from their studies that these phyto-compounds can help play a role in the prevention and suppression of cancer, e.g., the next time you bake bread, you may want to add some poppyseed or flax seed. Flax seed can be used for cooking, if you soak them "in water for at least an hour before using them..." (415).

Avocados are very rich in glutathione. They are also high in beta-carotene and a better source of *potassium than bananas*, and they may be important in protecting the liver, as well as fighting *viral hepatitis* (62). Avocados are also high in lutein. Another excellent source of beta-carotene, which is also high in lutein and other carotenoids, is chlorella. Just be sure to get the broken cell-wall chlorella. Chlorella has the highest amount of chlorophyll of any green food.

An amino acid nutrient, known as *glutamine,* is essential for the human body. Tumors feed on glutamine to grow (507). They seem to need excessive amounts of this amino acid, and they absorb it to the extent that the patient's own body is depleted of the nutrient, causing the patient to waste away, a disorder commonly found in cancer patients, called *cachexia* (507). Glutamine appears to boost immunity. Rats with tumors had a remarkable decrease in cancerous growths after just *seven weeks* of "glutamine supplements" (507). Beans, fish, and whey protein contain glutamine. This amino acid is also available in supplement form at health food stores.

## Grape Seed Extract—Pycnogenol®

*Pycnogenols*, also known as *OPCs* and *proanthocyanidins*, for the purposes in this chapter, will include those found in grape seed and pine bark. They have been used to reduce inflammation, maintain the integrity of the joints, and prevent circulatory problems in the legs, as well as helping in the overall strengthening of the walls of blood vessels (457). According to James D. Krystosik, D.C., in his book, *Nature's Prescription for Over 60 Diseases—Grape Seed and Pine Bark Extract,* they are also used for many other ailments. If you are bothered with restless legs at night, you may want to try this extract before resorting to a drug that might have potentially harmful side effects. Grape seed and pine bark also help in fighting vein inflammations and variscosities, as well as *retinopathy* in those with diabetes. They are a natural anti-histamine and help to rejuvenate the skin. Studies show that they also help stroke victims recover their memories. Because of their anti-oxidant effect, they fight stress (457).

Pycnogenols were probably first discovered when French explorers in Canada developed scurvy (rotting gums, swollen legs, bleeding and grotesque discolorations of the skin) due to a lack of *fresh fruits and vegetables.* It was not until they lost 25 fellow explorers to scurvy that a *Quebec Indian* saved the rest of them, sharing a tea he steeped with "pine needles and bark of the 'Anneda' tree," and within days, the surviving French explorers recovered (457).

It was much later in history that a discovery was made linking citrus fruits to the prevention of scurvy (457). Scientists discovered an ingredient in citrus fruit skins that could fortify *blood vessels* and prevent the fatal bleeding found in the dreaded disease. They isolated the nutrient and called it *vitamin P* for *permeability*. Dr. Krystosik further notes that this nutrient enhances the work of vitamin C. Since these bioflavonoids are found in all plants and trees, obviously the tea from the pine needles and bark cured the explorers (457).

Dr. Krystosik says that it was not until several centuries after the Cartier expedition that the nutrients were identified as "pycnogenols (pronounced pick-na-gen-nols)," and the best sources were found to be "grape seed extract and pine bark," though they can also be found in "peels, skins, pits, seeds, bark, and the leaves and blossoms of woody plants," usually the parts of the food that we humans pitch in the trash (457). They also help to lower harmful fats in the blood, and have been linked to the reason why moderate amounts of wine were found to be heart-protective. You may want to discuss pycnogenols with your physician (as an alternative to aspirin) for preventing heart disease (457).

It is their fearsome ability at destroying free radicals that make grape seed extracts so important. Dr. Krystosik says that there is very little difference in the potency of the pycnogenols found in pine bark as opposed to grape seed extract, except that *grape seed* is a little higher in "anti-oxidants," while *pine bark* extract is higher in "antihistamines" (457). (In most cases, you will find that pycnogenol® from pine bark is much more expensive.) Do not take grape-seed extracts at the same time that you take Vitamin C. Research suggests that taking them at the same time may raise blood pressure in some individuals.

A recent **human** study (on 38 people) showed that pine bark pycnogenols, taken with bilberry, may help lower eye pressure in those fighting glaucoma. The study, which was headed up by Dr. Robert Steigerwalt, Jr. (University of Chieti-Pescara in San Valentino, Italy), used a substance which had *standardized bilberry and French maritime pine bark,* known as *Mirtogenol* (423a). For dosage details, see website: *http://www.nu*

*traingredients-usa.com/Research/Bilberry-and-pine-bark-combo-wards-off-glaucoma-study* (423a).

It is interesting that animals are able to manufacture their own vitamin C (something humans are not capable of), giving them greater blood vessel integrity than we humans have, and they usually consume the parts of plants we throw away (high in OPCs), such as peelings, pits and seeds. This is one reason why animals don't usually have heart attacks and strokes—only humans (457).

## Pomegranates

Pomegranate juice is very high in anti-oxidants that fight free radicals. One brand describes their juice *(POM Wonderful Pomegranate Juice)* as being very high in anti-oxidants (1). You can find *POM Wonderful Pomegranate Juice* in the refrigerated section of most grocery stores and some natural health food stores. For more information, see their website at: *www.pomwonderful.com* (1). The juice of pomegranates (as well as the seeds) have been shown to kill parasites. For a report on a phase II study of the benefits of pomegranate substances for men with prostate cancer, see their website: *http://www.pomwonderful.com/pdf/Clinical_Cancer_Research.pdf.* Recent studies have also shown that substances in pomegranates work much like anti-inflammatories, helping arthritis sufferers.

## Quercetin

Dr. James Balch, in *The Super Anti-Oxidants,* says that this nutrient helps prevent the damage that free radicals can do to the entire cardiovascular system, and keeps blood platelets from gumming up, thus protecting against "clots, strokes and heart attacks" (337). **Statistics from both animal, and human testing as well, reveal that quercetin suppresses cancer.**

Quercetin is one of the strongest anti-cancer agents known. This anti-oxidant not only blocks the formation of cancer, but existing cancerous cells (552). It is found in large amounts in red onions and very small amounts in the white variety (551), in apples (440), *cayenne…green tea* (551) in berries, some nuts and seeds, and broccoli. See cancer-specific chapters in this book for more information on quercetin's powerful role against cancer.

# II. Nutrition & Disease

## ALD

*Lorenzo's Oil* was the name of a movie in 1992, the true story of a child battling a rare disease, *ALD (Adreno-leukodystrophy),* which is described by the National Institute of Neurological Disorders and Stroke (NINDS) at website: *http://www.ninds.nih.gov/disorders/adrenoleukodystrophy/adrenoleukodystrophy.htm,* as a hereditary disorder affecting the brain's nerve cells (315). Those suffering with this disorder have difficulty using fatty acids, thus, these fatty acids accumulate in the body and cause damage. Parents may not be aware that their child has the disorder until they exhibit memory problems, symptoms of social withdrawal, and problems such as deteriorating grades in school (217). The National Institute of Neurological Disorders and Stroke says of Lorenzo's oil that it is composed of "a mixture of oleic acid and euric acid," and that it "can reduce or delay the appearance of symptoms" (217).

According to website: *www.jr2.ox.ac.uk/bandolier/booth/neuro/lorenz.html,* Lorenzo's oil is thought to help reduce the damaging build-up of fatty acids in the body (179). Lasting effects of the oil are uncertain. The main problem with the oil is that it cannot enter the brain, so it does not "replace the very long chain fatty acids in the brain" (179). Though it can "delay onset of symptoms," it does not appear to be able to reverse them, nor prolong them indefinitely (179).

## Anti-Oxidants Not Merely for Cancer Prevention & Treatment

Anti-oxidants not only protect against debilitating and deadly diseases like cancer, they also protect the rest of the body and its vital functions, for example, the xanthophylls, such as zeaxanthin and lutein, and also bilberry, which protect valuable eyesight from free radical damage. Be aware that bilberry can thin your blood, much like garlic does.

According to Beth M. Ley, Ph.D., author of the book: *Bilberry & Lutein,* studies show that people having high dietary amounts of "lutein and zeaxanthin—abundant in spinach, collards, and other dark, leafy greens—had **57% less risk** of developing macular degeneration" (467). Bilberry has also been used for protecting the eyes (e.g., preventing cataracts). Researchers in Italy have identified a "dried leaf extract" of bilberry which helped lower blood sugar in laboratory animals (467).

Bilberry, says Ms. Ley, has even been used to lower harmful "LDL cholesterol…reduce hypertension…alleviate symptoms of diabetes…as a remedy for diarrhea and indigestion," and in treating ulcers (467).

## Help for Down's Syndrome Children

For parents with Down's syndrome children, Maureen Kennedy Salaman suggests calling (504) 769-TRIS. She says that you may also want to check into *live cell therapy*, which has been effective with some of these children (551). *Contreras Oasis Hospital in Tijuana, Mexico,* practices live cell therapy (Their ph# (800) 700-1850), as well *as Claus Marten's Four Seasons Clinic and Health Resort* at Fareerweg, Rottach Egern, W. Germany, phone: 80-222-6780-24041 (551).

If you have a child with Down's syndrome, you may wish to check the new research on proteins NAPVSIPQ and SALLRSIPSA (NAP- and SAL-) that may help these children. You can read about them on several internet sites, for example, here is one article from the National Institutes of Health website: *http://www.pubmedcentral.nih.gov/articlerender.fcgi?artid=2001299.*

## Help for Muscular Dystrophy

As described by website Alternative Health & Herbs *(http://www.healthherbs.com/conditionitem.php?id=192,* muscular dystrophy was produced in rabbits by giving them insufficient amounts of choline (one of the *B vitamins),* as well as insufficient vitamin E (201). The website also contains a sample dietary outline for those with MS. Natural sources of *choline* are: some of the cruciferous veggies, *egg yolk…[and] Wheat germ* (411). One of the highest sources is *bottle gourd* (388).

This is a disease where muscles in the body deteriorate, causing extreme weakness. It differs from multiple sclerosis (MS) in that *nerves* deteriorate in MS, and in muscular dystrophy (MD), the *muscles* deteriorate. CoQ10, a powerful anti-oxidant, has been very effective in helping those with MD (551). As noted by Maureen Kennedy Salaman in *All Your Health Questions Answered Naturally,* a study in Sweden showed that improvement in adult muscular dystrophy occurred with supplements that contained the mineral *selenium,* as well as *vitamin E* (351). Not only that, but keeping the muscles healthy requires the essential fatty acids, as well as other essential minerals and amino acids (551). Ms. Salaman has an easily absorbable, good tasting liquid mineral drink that I use and highly recommend, called *Mineral Rich*®. You can find it at her website *www.mksalaman.com,* and in some health food stores, along with her many other excellent nutritional products and books.

Note that some research has shown that the gamma-tocopherol form of vitamin E could be more powerful at cancer prevention than the alpha-tocopherol, though the alpha is more easily used by the body. If the alpha-tocopherol is the only kind you are able to find, at least be sure you use the d-alpha tocopherol and not the **dl**-alpha tocopherol which is more difficult for the cells to absorb. Just remember not to use the form with the **l** after the d (meaning it is synthetic, not natural).

Good natural sources of vitamin E are: wheat germ oil, olive oil, sunflower oil (and seeds); dandelion greens, spinach, broccoli, turnip greens; almonds and other nuts; eggs (411) (492), kiwi, and mangoes; fortified cereals and fresh sprouts; especially wheat berry sprouts.

## Help for Multiple Sclerosis, Down's syndrome & ALD

More and more research is pointing to the fact that diseases like multiple sclerosis and muscular dystrophy are preventable as well as treatable, through nutrition. For Dr. Frederick Klenner's MS protocol, see website: *http://www.seanet.com/~alexs/ascorbate/198x/smith-lh-clinical_guide_1988.htm.*

## MS Patch - Prokarin™

During a phone conversation with me on May 26, 2005, Elaine DeLack, a registered nurse, told me that she was diagnosed with M.S. in 1988, though her symptoms actually began in 1984. She said that when the symptoms first began, she would wake up in the middle of the night and could not move her left leg. After her son was born, the symptoms extended to her left hand. Initially, she was in denial until the day that she was carrying her young son and her left leg gave out on her, causing her to fall. She consulted with a physician in her home town, who sent her a prescription for vitamin B12 and *adenosine monophosphate* injections. She improved and was able to finish nursing school. Ms. DeLack did a great deal of research and felt that histamine should be added to the vitamin B12 and adenosine monophosphate. The end result of her research was a treatment for multiple sclerosis, a histamine patch known as *Prokarin*™, that she says has even enabled some M.S. sufferers to leave their wheelchairs behind.

The actual formula for Prokarin™ is proprietary information. Ms. Delack has had amazing success treating herself with this product. She said that she has remained symptom free while taking Prokarin™. This is remarkable when you consider that her symptoms began over 23 years ago. Although the FDA has not approved Prokarin™ for treating MS, your physician can still write you a prescription for Prokarin™, but you have to request it. Studies are continuing on the compound.

## Nutrition & MS

A physician by the name of Hinton D. Jonez used nutrition to bring about incredible results with MS patients. You can find his book, *My Fight to Conquer Multiple Sclerosis*, on the internet.

See chapter six, earlier in this book, for the amazing results obtained by one physician when he merely placed his M.S. patient on a nutritional supplement program. Also, see website: *http://kinsman.epix.net/water/Multiple.htm*, for the story of M. Fox, who claims that all her symptoms of M.S. disappeared when she went on Dr. Batmanghelidj's *Water Cure*. His water cure is also discussed in chapter 23. Vegetarian diets and low fat diets significantly reduce the risks for M.S. Research has also shown that curcumin may be beneficial in fighting M.S., because it appears to have a protective effect on nerve cells. See earlier in this chapter for instances of when you should not use turmeric (curcumin). Also, see p. 488 for new research showing a link between MS & vitamin D deficiencies.

## ORAC Rating

Dr. Guohua Cao was part of a team that developed a way to measure the anti-oxidant potency of foods in the early part of the 1990s. It is known as the *Oxygen Radical Absorbance Capacity test (ORAC)*. Each substance on the list was compared in potency to that of a "standardized amount of vitamin E" (507). Of course, the greater the ORAC value, the higher the anti-oxidant power of the food. If possible, try to get at least 10,000 or more ORAC points per day from the ORAC list (especially if you are struggling against cancer or some other life-threatening illness), and this is not hard to do. Eating just 3.5 ounces of prunes, raisins, red grapes, kale, and onions in one day, will give you OVER 11,000 ORAC points.

Various nutrient-rich drinks are being promoted that are high in ORAC content. One in particular is called *7 Essentials*. Their producers claim that one serving of their drink contains a whopping 21,010 ORAC units. As explained in an email from them, this "value was determined by Brunswick Laboratories according to the Tufts University method of rating."

If you are interested, *7 Essentials* is marketed at *www.healthy-living.org/html/essential_seven.html* (267). Besides the ORAC-rich drink discussed above, some foods that are naturally very high in their ORAC rating are raisins, blueberries, raspberries, and prunes. Most berries are high on the ORAC scale, as are green leafy vegetables, and it does not require a large serving, about 3-4 ounces at the most. Our Creator God made it possible for us to greatly benefit from small servings of fruits and vegetables!

## Soy Products

There is a great deal of controversy about soy, and even more so with the advent of genetically-modified soy products, the negative effects on humans (and animals) of which may not be known for decades yet to come! Fermented soy is fine. The harmful substances are removed in the fermentation process. Scientists are experimenting with soy products because of their role in halting and even reversing abnormal cells "back to their original precancerous state" (371). I would avoid soy, unless fermented. Fermented soy products, such as Haelan, may help remove harmful estrogens from the body in estrogen receptor-positive cancers.

For information on Haelan, see the company's website at *www.haelan951.com.* Information on Haelan's Research Foundation's website was accumulated from clinical studies performed on fermented soy beverages manufactured by Haelan Products, Inc. of Woodinville, Washington. The Haelan fermented soy beverages are sold in the United States, without medical claims, and are available directly from the company or one of their distributors (143).

# CHAPTER 21

# CURING WITH CAROTENOIDS & OTHER HEALING FOODS & NUTRIENTS

*"Now ye are clean through the word which I have spoken unto you." (John 15:3)*

## I. Carotenoids—What Are They?

Carotenoids give fruits and vegetables their wonderful colors. They are what give the deep oranges, blues, reds, and greens to vegetables and fruits. Jack Challem, in his book, *All About Carotenoids Beta-Carotene, Lutein & Lycopene,* reports that there are actually "600 different plant pigments" included in this group, yet very few of them are known to be important to our health (366). Although there are dozens that we ingest "only fourteen have been identified in the bloodstream," meaning that the body does not absorb all of them. Even though some of the others are not absorbable, they may play vital health roles that we are not yet aware of. All of them are *fat-soluble,* meaning that they should be eaten along with some form of fat, such as olive oil or flax oil, rather than water (366). What all this means (in a nutshell) is that if you are eating a fresh veggie salad with lettuce, diced tomatoes, peppers, onions, summer squash, broccoli, and carrots, your salad dressing should be oil-based. (A good choice would be organic flax oil or olive oil, or dice up an avocado and include it in the salad.) Mr. Challem has a new book out: *Stop Prediabetes Now,* with co-author Ron Hunninghake, M.D. Also see his new book*: The Food-Mood Solution.* For more information on both books, see website: *http://www.thenutritionreporter.com.*

## How Carotenoids Fight Cancer

Beta-carotene makes the monocytes (white blood cells that hunt for and kill cancer cells and pathogens) more powerful at what they do. According to Jack Challem, in order to be able to identify an abnormal cell, such as a cancer cell, our immune system has a type of sonar alert called *MHC II.* As soon as this warning system suspects an abnormal (intruder) cell, the *MHC II* sends an SOS signal to related immunity cells, which rush to the scene, surround and zap the intruders! If the monocytes are deficient in these sonar proteins, cancerous cells slip by undetected, then begins the full onslaught of this disease (366).

David A. Hughes, Ph.D., and fellow researchers at the Institute of Food Research in England, discovered that they could boost the body's MHC-II warning system, simply by giving "15 mg…supplements…[of] beta-carotene" to a group of *healthy men* for one month, which caused a dramatic increase in these sonar proteins. He also discovered that the men taking beta-carotene had an increase in *TNF-a*, an important immune substance that kills abnormal cells, such as cancer. The control group received a placebo and did not have the same results (366).

Mr. Challem, in *All About Carotenoids,* also discusses research showing that beta-carotene has reversed *precancerous* mouth lesions (in **human** tests). Vitamins A, E, and beta-carotene were all able to fight, and even help *reverse* a type of precancer of the mouth known as *oral leukoplakia* (366).

Organized medicine, in their bias against alternative cancer treatments, will now admit (after years of denying it) that good nutrition can prevent cancer, however, they will not admit that it can reverse cancer, though there are many case histories (e.g., some of which are documented in this book) that prove this to be true.

Numerous research studies have been done to prove that beta-carotene can protect against many types of cancer, including those difficult-to-treat, such as pancreatic cancer. Mr. Challem explains that a prolonged deficiency in beta-carotene may contribute toward such debilitating diseases as lupus and rheumatoid arthritis (366). This nutrient also helps asthma sufferers, prevents visual problems, reduces the risk of heart disease, lowers cholesterol, and protects against sunburn (366). When it comes to taking beta-carotene, it is best to take natural, rather than synthetic beta-carotene. As described by Mr. Challem, natural beta-carotene can be found in "lettuce, parsley, sweet potatoes, apricots… asparagus, broccoli, cantaloupe, carrots…kale…pumpkin, spinach, watermelon," and many other foods (366). Another excellent source of beta-carotene and B12 is chlorella. Be sure to get the broken cell-wall chlorella. Chlorella has the highest concentration of chlorophyll of any green food.

While synthetic vitamin A can be toxic in large doses (because it is stored in the liver), beta-carotene in natural form (e.g., carrot juice) converts into natural vitamin A in the body, in a slow process that prevents system overload. According to H. Winter Griffith, M.D., in *Vitamins Herbs, Minerals & Supplements*, the liver normally stores "a 2-year supply" of vitamin A. Once that supply is gone, deficiencies will show up as "Night blindness, lack of tear secretion…eventual blindness…dry, rough skin…poor bone growth, weak tooth enamel, diarrhea…acne, insomnia, fatigue," and a host of other health problems (411). If you have any of these health problems, get a physical from your health care provider. You may be severely deficient in vitamin A.

## Exotic Fruits & Their Drinks

Besides other high anti-oxidant fruit drinks mentioned in this book, you may also see health food stores selling such fruit supplements or drinks as starfruit (carambolas), mangosteens, durians (with the reputation of being the *stinkiest* fruit in the world), Asian pears (or nashi), persimmons, baobab pod fruit, sharons, kakis, ugli fruit, plantains, bignay, gandaria, Indian jujube, lychee, olallieberries, Malay apple, hogplum, mammey apple, otaheite gooseberry, biriba, mammey sapote, peach palm, rambutan, rose apple, breadfruit, sansapote, surinam cherry, mountain soursop, sea grape, star nut palm, jackfruit, velvet tamarind, akee, bael fruit, champedak, custard apple, Ceylon gooseberry, sala, cherimoya, morinda, nangka, soncoya, santoli, jaboticaba, ketupa, sweetsop, star nut palm, araza, black sapote, calabash, Barbados cherry, kepel, loquat, sapodilla, monkey bread, feijoa, chalta, wood apple, lucuma, rambai, voavanga, cannonball, genipap, Philippine roseapple, tree tomato, pitachaya, sweet grenadilla, nance, ita palm, medlar, goumi, cherimoya, giant grenadilla, clementine, kumquat, mandarin, minneolas, tangelos, satsuma, cashew apples, and many others—some having multiple names for the same fruit—depending on the country where you find them.

## Gac, Mangosteen, Goji & Seabuckthorn

Besides the fruits mentioned earlier and high ORAC health drinks, such as MonaVie™, you will find some strange-sounding, unusual-tasting fruit drinks now in health food stores. Gac-Chi™ (which comes from the gac fruit) is a liquid drink which is said to have 70 times the content of lycopene as tomatoes, and 10 times the beta-carotene found in carrots. Gac is an odd-looking, spiny-covered fruit. This drink also contains seabuckthorn berry, goji berry, rosehips and a proprietary blend of other juices, including roselle, pear, grape, apple, aronia, acerola, and cranberry.

Mango-Xan® is a drink that comes from the mangosteen fruit with an ORAC rating at 2466. It is a proprietary blend of several ingredients, including the juice of red grapes, pear, sour cherry, blueberry, cranberry, pineapple, starfruit, and lychee.

Goji-Zen™ is made from goji berries, rosehips, and seabuckthorn berries, along with grape seed extract, juice from pears, apples, cranberries, grapes, and aronia in a proprietary blend.

Seabuck-7™ is another high anti-oxidant drink you will see in health food stores. It is made from seabuckthorn berries and other fruits, such as mango, pineapple, apple, grape, red sour cherries, pear, rosehips, and cranberry in a proprietary blend. Other exotic fruit blends may contain pepinos, cherimoyas, cape gooseberry, physallis or Chinese lantern, breadfruit, jujube (or black sapote), Chinese dates, wampee, jakfruit, loquat, pummelos, bilimbi, canistel, feijoa, jaboticaba, nashi, quince, caperberries, olallieberries, huckleberries, miracle fruit berries, mamey sapote, camu-camu berries and many others. (The olallieberry is a cross between loganberries and youngberries.) Organic muscadine grapes (and their juice) are also becoming popular as a natural health food.

## Papaya, PawPaw & Guavas

Papaya has important enzymes that are useful in treating cancer, but without toxic side effects. Scientists have been studying the effects of enzymes like those found in papaya for the treatment of illness for nearly twenty years. In his book, *Papaya The Healing Fruit,* author Harald Tietze says that many people with cancer have successfully healed themselves using a papaya leaf concentrate (581).

In modern times, the use of papaya for cancer treatment has documented scientific research in support of it. Studies have shown that cancer cells contain a *fibrin* disguise so that the immune cells cannot see them, thus their insidious attachment to the walls of blood vessels (581). Dr Wolf, described as "The founder of modern enzyme therapy," taught that victims of cancer are deficient in *proteolytic enzymes*, which work by splitting up the fibrin that allows the cells to hide themselves, thus exposing them (581).

Harald Tietze tells the story of a Swiss homeopath's experience in 1996 using a concentrated form of papaya on a woman who had metastasizing cancer, and was told she had only days to live. The patient began improving after she started taking the papaya. Her physicians were baffled. Within months, her symptoms had nearly disappeared and she had returned to work (581). This was almost a year after doctors had given her *two weeks* to live! Mr. Tietze also reports that "papaya leaf concentrate [and] Kombucha-papaya extract" have been used for fighting *skin cancer.* Papain itself proved effective when half the test animals in a research study were "given papain [and] survived a normally lethal dose of radiation" (581). Be aware that papaya enzyme preparations can thin the blood. If you are taking blood-thinners, your physician should know if you plan to use papaya enzymes. You can get proteolytic enzymes at health food stores, but you should not take them if you are allergic to papaya, pineapple, or pork.

Papaya not only tastes good, it is very nutritious, and as stated by Mr. Tietze, has "more vitamin A than carrots and more vitamin C than oranges" (581). It fights cancer of the breast, cleanses the body by removing toxins, and increases metabolism. Every part of the plant is useful. Hens are even fed this fruit to give egg yolks a deeper color (581). The next time you consume a meal high in protein, remember that papaya has important enzymes that help digest proteins. It is actually more nutritious for this purpose when the flesh is mature, but still a little on the *green* side. When fully mature, most papayas are yellow.

There are teas available that are made from the leaves of the papaya plant. If you see a tea called *Dried Paw-Paw Leaves* from *The Kombucha House in Australia,* this is actually a papaya tea (581). There is a pawpaw found in New Zealand, as well as Australia, called *Carica papaya,* which **is** a true papaya. Just be aware that if something is called *pawpaw,* it may not necessarily have anything to do with papaya. Check the label of contents (581). It is noted that the carotenoids in papaya are life-saving, with higher amounts of anti-oxidants than many other fruits and vegetables (604).

The papain found in papaya is very much like the digestive enzymes that occur in the gastric juices, making papaya an important digestive aid for eating raw with your meals, or immediately after them. Selene Yeager in her book, *Doctors Book of FOOD REMEDIES,* says that it may also be important as an anti-ulcer food (604). This was demonstrated when researchers gave test animals large amounts of *papaya for several days,* then fed them acid-producing drugs (604). Those receiving papaya were protected against *ulcers.* Women who are pregnant should avoid any part of papaya that has not fully-ripened (604).

According to website: *http://alternativecancer.us/pawpaw.html,* an extract from pawpaw, "a cousin of the graviola, guanabana, and soursop trees," has ingredients that have anti-angiogenesis properties, which means that they prevent new "blood vessels" from growing, thus cutting off the nutrient supply to tumors (230). This is similar to what shark cartilage does. Also, see information (in chapter 34) on the bindweed plant that is even more powerful than shark cartilage at blocking blood vessel growth (150) (301a).

Pawpaw also slows down "MDR (multiple drug resistance) cells," and nothing is comparable to it, except substances *from trees* that are similar to it in fighting *MDR cells*. About 2% of tumors are made up of MDR cells which remain even after chemo (230). This is one reason why a tumor that initially appears to respond to chemo, often returns a short time later. Problem is, when the tumor returns, all of the cells that make it up will now be MDR cells, and usually no amount of chemo (or radiation) will kill them. **"PawPaw is the only cancer treatment that has shown effectiveness against MDR cells"** (230). (Emphasis mine.)

During **human** testing, when many dozens of people were studied, pawpaw was helpful in 50% of them. Website, *alternativecancer.us/paw,* recommends that you do not take pawpaw at the same time that you take other supplements, such as CoQ10 and SOD. For a full list of the non-compatible nutrients, see their website (230). Check with your health care provider for dosing on the capsules. They are usually taken with food. The above website also has ordering information for the extract, or you can contact any distributor from *Nature's Sunshine* to obtain pawpaw for you. It can also be found in health food stores.

As for side effects, it is recommended that you ingest pawpaw with meals, since it can cause nausea (230). Selene Yeager says that guavas are sometimes mistaken for papayas, but they are very different. The thing that makes guavas significant is that they are much higher in lycopene than tomatoes, plus they are very rich in fiber (604). So, the next time you grab tomatoes for their lycopene content, you may want to add a guava to your cart along with that papaya. Be sure to consult with your physician or Naturopath about pawpaw consumption.

## Peas & Beans

Peas are rich in a substance that is very similar to chlorophyll, which is so unique that it can latch onto substances that cause cancer and stick to them, preventing their use by the cells (604). Beans (legumes) carry nutrients that help fight cancer and regulate serum glucose (an important benefit for diabetics). Besides being fiber-rich, they also contain *protease inhibitors,* which help fight breast and colon cancers (534). This is explained in Charmaine Rivers' book, *Manna from Heaven—Healing Foods From The Bible* (534).

## Other Carotenoids: Alpha-Carotene, Cryptoxanthin & Astaxanthin

A very close relative of beta-carotene, ***alpha-carotene***, is also found in orange foods like pumpkin and carrots, and as described by Jack Challem in *All About Carotenoids Beta-carotene, Lutein & Lycopene,* research conducted by Michiaki Murakoshi, PhD., and others, found that this carotenoid can slow down or inhibit many types of abnormal cells, such as pancreatic, gastric, and brain cancer (366). Another study using human subjects in New Jersey, showed that those men who ate diets high in alpha-carotene, had lower risks for developing respiratory cancers (366).

**Cryptoxanthin,** found in many orange-colored fruits, also has anti-cancer properties. A study that involved thousands of women (over a period of 15 years), revealed that consuming foods high in this carotenoid greatly decreased their risks for cancer of the cervix (366).

**Astaxanthin**, another *carotenoid*, is found in marine animals like *salmon and trout.* Sometimes carotenoids, such as this one, are mixed with the diets of *farm-raised fish*, says Jack Challem, to heighten their color and marketability. This particular carotenoid was better at protecting against harmful UVA exposure than other popular carotenoids (366). See Mr. Challems new books: *Stop Prediabetes Now,* with co-author Ron Hunninghake, M.D., and *The Food-Mood Solution.* For more information on both books, see website: *http://www.thenutritionreporter.com.*

# II. Other Healing Foods & Nutrients

## Apples & Figs

Though apples have natural substances that may be their main weapon against cancer, to get the full benefit, it is best to consume the fruit and the skin. The skins are rich in *pectin*, a type of *fiber* which boosts the immunity, decreases harmful LDH, fights high *blood pressure,* and high glucose levels (534). There are also ingredients in apple peelings that can kill cancer cells.

According to Charmaine Rivers, author of the book, *Manna from Heaven Healing Foods From The Bible*, figs contain *benzaldehyde,* a substance that helps fight cancer. It has been tested on animals and **humans** (534). During human testing, says Rivers, "Of the 55 patients in the test group, seven went into complete remission, 29 into partial remission," and most remarkable of all was that the compound **actually performed better** on the humans than it did on the animal *tumors* (534).

## Artichokes & Asparagus

Research revealed that a compound in artichoke not only inhibits cancer, but it can also help reverse liver damage. As noted by Selene Yeager, et al., in *Doctors Book of FOOD REMEDIES*, the compound is *silymarin*, and in animal studies, helps fight *skin cancer*. Artichokes are merely *the immature flower of the thistle plant* (604). (Silymarin is the main ingredient of the herb, milk thistle. Milk thistle is so important for liver health, it was discussed extensively in greater detail in this book in chapter nine on liver cancer.)

Ms. Yeager further explains that *asparagus* protects against colon cancer and malformations in the spine (during formation in the mother's womb), due to its high folate content (604). It is one of the richest sources available of natural glutathione and also contains vitamin E. In an analysis of dozens of vegetables tested for glutathione levels, researchers placed "freshly cooked asparagus" at the top (604). Asparagus is so alkalizing to the body, it retains some alkalinity, even when it is cooked.

For years the FDA refused to acknowledge that one of the leading causes of spinal birth defects was a deficiency of folic acid during pregnancy (413). Thousands of newborns were sentenced to a life of crippling disability because of the stubbornness of the FDA in refusing to tell pregnant mothers to supplement with a common vitamin known as folic acid. Before they finally caved in and admitted that they were wrong and that a lack of folic acid was causing thousands of spinal birth-defects, they were harassing vitamin-manufacturers for making the exact same claim on their folate supplements (414)! What has the public learned from this blatant cover-up? You cannot trust the FDA. They are in bed with big pharma, and they have no concern for the health of the general public.

## Barley, Buckwheat & Bulgar - Cancer-fighting Grains

**Barley** is an excellent way to get your daily supply of natural tocotrienols, which protect the heart and help the liver cut cholesterol levels. Vitamin E is just one example. Barley is a rich source of anti-oxidants, minerals, *lignans…and vitamin E* (604).

**Buckwheat**, high in flavonoids, as well as *quercetin and rutin*, fights dangerous hormones within the cells. If carcinogenic substances do enter the cells, quercetin and rutin can keep DNA from being injured further.

Rutin inhibits clot formation and can lower total cholesterol levels. Buckwheat is higher in protein than any other grain. Once *roasted*, it is referred to as *Kasha* (604).

As Selene Yeager explains in *Doctors Book of FOOD REMEDIES*, **bulgar** is nothing less than wheat "in its whole form" (604). Nearly everyone is familiar with nitrates (cancer-causing compounds used in sausages, hotdogs, and packaged luncheon meats. Once nitrates enter the body, they are chemically changed into *nitrosamines*, which cause cancer (604). Ms. Yeager further explains that bulgar has a substance known as *ferulic acid*, which prevents the body from changing nitrates into dangerous nitrosamines. It also has *lignans*, notable for their anti-cancer properties (604). Bulgar wheat is important for diabetics because during digestion, its sugar content is not dumped rapidly into the bloodstream, but *released…slowly*, assisting in blood sugar stability. This grain can spoil rapidly, so it should be kept in your refrigerator until used (604).

## Celery Inhibits Tumors, Hypertension & Bad Cholesterol

Celery has the ability to inhibit cancer and fight blood pressure and harmful cholesterol. When a hypertensive patient was told by his physician to cut back on his salt intake, he also started consuming "about four stalks…of celery per day," which caused his blood pressure to drop significantly. Celery does have natural sodium (604), a healthy type of sodium. Celery may cause sun-sensitivity in some people. Usually, this can be countered simply by being sure that the vegetable is scrubbed vigorously before consumption; however, any raw fruit or vegetable should be cleaned completely before consumption (604). Celery also contains anti-cancer ingredients called *acetylenics*, which can inhibit tumors. It is best to consume celery with the leaves, where many of the vitamins and minerals are most concentrated (604). Celery juice could be especially helpful in fighting colon and abdominal tumors.

Another natural nutrient, besides celery, that can help lower blood pressure is rye. Baking rye bread from rye flour, or even purchasing ready-made rye bread and eating it, can help contribute to a lower blood pressure. Be sure, if baking, that you add plenty of limonene-rich (388) caraway seed.

## Chinese Red Yeast Rice, Guggul & Policosanol

Though promoted mostly for its ability to lower cholesterol levels, Rita Elkins, M.H. in her book, *Chinese Red Yeast Rice*, says that this substance helps prevent cancer (397). It is a fermented extract containing valuable compounds, such as "mevinolin, also known as lovastatin," capable of lowering blood cholesterol (397). Even though substances taken from red yeast rice were made into drugs for treating high-cholesterol, some of the extracts are now available in natural health food stores. Ms. Elkins says that during an animal study at a pharmacy college in Japan, the "red yeast rice pigment referred to as *Monascus* pigment," could fight tumor formation (397). It is best to get the Chinese Red Yeast Rice that is combined with guggul for fighting cholesterol, which is available at many health food stores and internet sites. (You may see it as *guggul-lipid*.)

**Policosanol** is another nutrient that can be found in health food stores that some believe fights high cholesterol as well as (if not better than) red yeast rice with guggul, though some red yeast rice products also contain policosanol. Check the label for contents. Niacin also helps lower cholesterol, but do not use the *flush-free* for this purpose, and never use the *timed-release* form of niacin. If you cannot tolerate the flush, some nutritionists suggest that you take a baby aspirin or two about 20 to 30 minutes before the niacin. The flush, however, is supposed to be good for you, opening up the blood vessels. Niacin has been given to workers in the arctic because of its warming effect. Check with your Dr. first.

## Indoles—DIM—The Phytonutrient That Prevents Cancer

DIM *(diindolymethane)* is a plant compound that appears to have impressive anti-cancer effects by blocking harmful estrogens from being absorbed into the body. DIM can be purchased as a supplement at most natural health food stores. This plant nutrient is most abundant in the cruciferous foods (e.g., cabbages, broccoli, brussel sprouts, kohlrabi, watercress, mustard, arugula, cauliflower, collards, kale, turnips, bok choi (tatsoi), wasabai, daikon radish, and others).

## IP-6—Anti-Tumor Pill

IP-6 is a significant nutrient for fighting cancer. It has anti-cancer properties, and is a natural extract derived from soy and grains. Testing, thus far, has shown that IP-6 can suppress cellular mutations better than green tea without harming normal, healthy cells. Many believe that IP-6 can cause abnormal cancer cells to revert back to their healthy state. Studies have shown that the extract can suppress several types of cancer. Many websites and local health food stores market IP-6. See other chapters of this book for more information on this supplement. Check with your physician or Naturopath before supplementing with IP-6, since it can thin the blood.

## Nutrition at the Cellular Level

The advocates of *Orthomolecular Medicine* (discussed elsewhere in this book) use a nutritional approach to disease, stressing the importance of mega-vitamins such as vitamin C, and mega-minerals such as niacinamide, selenium, and amino acids (e.g., lysine). Some natural sources of lysine are: *eggs…and brewer's yeast* (118), as well as fish, avocados, and whole wheat bread. Many people suffer from gluten allergies. If you are fighting disease, you may wish to avoid all wheat and gluten products.

Another devotee in favor of high dose vitamin C supplementation for cancer prevention was Dr. E. Cheraskin, M.D., D.M.D., author of *Vitamin C Who Needs It?* In his book, he discussed a research discovery by the Albert Einstein College of Medicine in New York City, which showed that women who consumed higher amounts of vitamin C in their daily diets (greater than 30 mg) were able to cut their risk of cervical dysplasia, a precursor to cervical cancer, tenfold (367).

See chapters eight and sixteen of this book for an amazing account of how a teenager was healed (of what her father was told was a fatal Hodgkins disease) with a high dose vitamin C regimen.

Chapter eight also explains how people are sometimes misdiagnosed with leukemia when they don't have leukemia at all. What they have is scurvy, or dangerously low vitamin C levels in their body; levels so low that they can't even be measured. Sometimes they have dangerously low levels of B12 and/or folic acid (550).

## Oils for Cancer Prevention (& A.D.D.)

Evening primrose oil is a rich source of gamma-linolenic acid, discussed earlier in this book. It has been used with some success in treating diseases like multiple sclerosis, and it demonstrates aggressive anti-cancer properties. The late Dr. David Horrobin (notable for his studies involving essential fats), believed that GLA could help children with ADD

(Attention Deficit Disorder) (110). In fact, as detailed at website *www.absolutelythepurest.com,* the American Journal of Clinical Nutrition (Oct. 1995) reported that tests on dozens of children with ADD showed a lack of sufficient EFAs (*essential fatty acids*) in their brain cells (110). Dr. Horrobin's research also demonstrated the importance of GLAs in cancer prevention. He and his colleagues believed giving GLA to cancer patients might help the body reverse abnormal cells (504). He suggested using it in malignant cases considered terminal or hopeless. When scientists tested his theory, they found (in test tube experiments) that *GLA supplements* dramatically halted cancerous liver cells (504).

Dr.Ralph Moss in his book, *Cancer Therapy,* says that the studies carried out by Dr. Horrobin and his fellows showed that GLA could kill "breast, lung and prostate cancer cells" without harming *normal* cells (504). Dr. Moss believes it is possible that GLA works by increasing the production of *free radicals* in tumor cells, thus killing them (504).

A new very tasty source of EFAs is the CHIA seed. You can buy the little seeds in bulk (add a scoop to water) let it thicken and drink at your convenience (but stir first)! It is great for supplying omega-3 and omega-6, but also as a healthy support for bowel health & regularity. It coats the stomach and colon in a thick protective mucilage, similar to flax.

For those parents concerned about high fructose corn syrup added to processed foods (in spite of all those commercials promoting it), the next time you go to your grocery store to buy maple syrup for your kids, thinking that you are getting real maple syrup, check the label of contents. Most store-bought bottles of maple syrup in this country have no actual maple syrup in them!

## Vitamin D for Cancer & Multiple Sclerosis Prevention

Scotland has more MS sufferers than any other country. These alarming statistics promoted a study at Oxford (headed up by Professor of Neurology, George Ebers), which found that not only is vitamin D important in prevention of cancer and autoimmune disorders, but in prevention of MS as well. It was revealed that the disease rarely afflicts those in warmer countries, where people get more vitamin D from sunlight exposure. It was also found that children who develop MS all seem to have one thing in common – they are seriously deficient in vitamin D (532b). Recommending supplementation to children and pregnant moms is on the horizon (532b).

# CHAPTER 22

# PRESCRIPTION HRT - CANCER CULPRIT VERSUS BHRT

*"And his fame [Jesus'] went throughout all Syria: and they brought unto him all sick people...and he healed them." (Matthew 4:24)*

## Deceiving the Public Trust

There are several different forms of estrogen, however estrogen is merely the name of a group of similar hormones (466). These different types of hormones are described by the late Dr. John R. Lee, M.D., et al., in *What Your Doctor May Not Tell You About Menopause.* One form of estrogen known as *estriol,* is actually a natural estrogen hormone found in nature. He explained that synthetic estrogen, created in the laboratory and dispensed by pharmaceutical companies, is either *estradiol* or *estrone* (466). (There is night and day difference between natural estrogen and synthetic estrogen.) Natural hormones, as opposed to synthetic prescription hormones, are exactly like the natural hormones that the body produces! These natural hormones are now commonly referred to as ***bio-identical hormones.***

There are also plant estrogens that behave like human estrogens, but weaker in action. Since they lock onto the body's estrogen receptor sites and compete with synthetic, harmful estrogens, they can often block the harmful forms of estrogen from getting into the cells (466).

Other types of estrogens are the *Xenoestrogens*, harmful estrogens that come from toxins and pollutants in our environment, and they have powerful hormone effects, but they are detrimental to the health (466). Are you aware that estrogen is even being put into hair products, such as shampoos? As noted at website *alkalizeforhealth.net*, Dr. David Williams discussed the shocking fact that babies are growing pubic hair from the shampoos their mothers are using on them, due to their estrogen content. If you see the words *placenta....estrogen...estriol* or *natural hormones* on the label, do NOT USE these shampoos! The same is true for skin softeners, conditioners, makeup, lotions, and other products (266). Many moisturizers contain estrogen! Always check the labels before using them. Be a label reader. Even some products that you purchase at health food stores may have questionable ingredients. I have seen many vitamin supplements with titanium dioxide and magnesium stearate additives in them, ingredients I try to avoid. When you are looking for supplements, always check to see what ELSE is on the label. It does you little good to take a supplement for bone health when it contains potentially harmful dyes and additives.

The late Dr. John Lee left behind a remarkable achievement in his studies and contributions, including several health books that he authored and co-authored, clearly pointing out the dreadful after-effects that women are facing from synthetic HRT (hormone replacement therapy). He, along with David Zava, Ph.D., and Virginia Hopkins, M.A., discussed the safe estrogen, the estrogen that occurs in nature (known as *estriol)* in their book: *What Your Doctor May Not Tell You About Breast Cancer* (465).

This found-in-nature-estrogen (*estriol)* has about the same benefits of the pharmaceutically-created *estradiol and estrone*, however, it does not have the toxic adverse effects on the body. It is very common for physicians in other countries to give their female patients natural estrogen (465). Yes, there is a form of natural bio-identical estrogen made by our great Creator that does not have the toxic side effects of the freak-of-nature synthetic estrogen created by pharmaceutical companies—and most conventional doctors know next to nothing about it, or when asked about it, they will parrot what the pharmaceutical companies tell them: *that natural estrogen is absorbed into the skin in unreliable amounts, therefore, use the prescription form*—of course! (Guess who loses in this deal!?) BHRT or bio-identical hormone replacement therapy uses NATURAL hormones exactly like those found in the body, rather than prescription drugs that the body cannot recognize, which can cause a horrible array of potentially life-threatening side effects.

## Synthetic Estrogen Replacement - A Double-Edged Sword

As noted above, there are vast differences in the types of estrogen on the market today. Dr. Lee believed that it is possible that so-called estrogen-deficiency is untrue. His studies and research revealed that most women are *estrogen dominant* rather than estrogen deficient (466). This is because, as he explained, estrogen is manufactured in fat cells. Women naturally have a higher ratio of fat cells than men, and the more fat cells a woman has, the more estrogen she produces (466). Not only that, but most Americans consume a lot of meat. It is no secret that our meat (including poultry) and dairy supply is tainted with hormones, herbicides, antibiotics, and pesticides. Also, many women have received estrogen in prescription form (466). Dr. Lee believed that the main culprit in *estrogen dominance* is the prescription form that they received from their physicians. He also believed that it is the main culprit in causing cancer of the breast, especially for women in their fifties (465). For women who are pre-menopausal, too much estrogen will show up in them as the inability to ovulate.

The problem with *estrogen dominance...a term coined by Dr. Lee*, is that regardless of a woman's estrogen level, even if her estrogen levels are low, if she has no progesterone in her body, she will still be *estrogen dominant* (465). There are many symptoms of this excess estrogen. A few of these include mood swings, uterine fibroids, thinning bones, heavy periods, migraines, heart disease, lumps in the breast, uterine cancer, and many, many others (103).

Synthetic estrogen replacement hit a snag as far back as 1975 when it was discovered that women taking it had up to *eight times* higher the incidence for uterine cancer over those not taking the substance (466). A main problem of this excess estrogen, explained Dr. Lee, is that once there is too much estrogen in the body, progesterone levels are too low and the estrogen actually becomes *toxic* (466).

According to Dr. Ray D. Strand in his book, *What Your Doctor Doesn't Know About Nutritional Medicine May Be killing You,* drug companies convinced physicians that their patients needed HRT despite the hazards, including a 40 percent greater incidence for cancers of the breast in women taking these prescription hormones for more than five years. What was the reply of the drug companies to these reports? Their pat answer to many such reports: "the benefits of HRT far outweighed the risks" (573). The benefits to whom, I wonder? Certainly NOT to the women using them! And WHO is taking the risk here?

Research also shows that, contrary to earlier belief, women do not have to take synthetic hormones for long periods of time to increase their risks. As reported from the website: *www.natural-progesterone-advisory-network.com,* in an article by Catherine P. Rollins, that she discusses from the *Million Women Study* that was done, participant risk began within just one to two years of starting on this hormone, and it kept increasing proportionate to longer and longer usage (538).

Do you have a female friend or relative who has died from breast cancer or uterine cancer? Were they on hormone replacement therapy prescribed by a physician? I have an older cousin who was on HRT for many years and developed breast cancer. She was then on Taxol for the breast cancer, and developed uterine cancer (caused by the Taxol) and had a hysterectomy. The cancer later returned and spread to her bones. She opted for chemotherapy and died eight months after starting on chemo.

Dr. Lee et al, in *What Your Doctor May Not Tell You About Breast Cancer,* said that when researchers began pouring over medical charts of thousands and thousands of women, they discovered that those using *combined HRT* were more likely to be diagnosed with difficult and more *aggressive tumors* to treat and detect (537) (538). Estriol, the natural form of estrogen found in nature, is free of the toxic side effects found in prescription HRT. However, *naturally-occurring* estrogen was competing with a prescription drug, *Premarin,* a synthetic estrogen marketed by drug companies and extracted "from pregnant mares' urine" (465). As Dr. Lee pointed out, Premarin had the backing of a pharmaceutical company that had invested millions to study, promote, and market it. Once it was given FDA approval, this meant that a well-equipped aggressive army from the drug company would ultimately use high-pressure sales reps to talk thousands of physicians into using it for their patients (465). Some physicians are finally wising up, and they will no longer **allow** drug reps into their office.

Lest you are unaware of how successful the campaign was to get women on synthetic estrogen, in 1996 alone, doctors wrote more than twenty million Premarin prescriptions. C. Norman Shealy, M.D., Ph.D., in his book, *Natural Progesterone Cream, Safe and Natural Hormone Replacement,* suggests that maybe they should call it "Horse Replacement Therapy" (560)?! Even more alarming is the fact that Premarin causes a **"43 percent increase of breast and/or uterine cancer,"** as well as many other potentially dangerous side effects (560).

## Are You On Prescription Hormone Therapy?

I wonder how many women taking Premarin were told by their physicians: *"This prescription I am writing for you comes from the urine of pregnant horses and, oh—by the way—it can increase your risk of breast or uterine cancer by 43%"* (560)! Do you think this happened? Are you or a loved one taking Premarin? Did your physician ever tell you this? How did this happen? How is it that there is a safe, natural form of estrogen without the toxic side effects of the synthetic form, yet millions of women were never offered the natural bio-identical form, but given instead, the synthetic form produced by a pharmaceutical company that brought with it a deadly cloud of adverse side effects? It is because drug companies have no vested interest in a natural substance like estriol, regardless of its safety status, because natural substances cannot be patented! If they cannot patent a product, anyone can sell it, thus they cannot get exclusive rights to market it and make millions in profits (465).

Synthetic estrogen has many potentially life-threatening risks and side effects besides those already listed. Some of them are listed at http://*www.ninds.nih.gov* (the National Institute of Neurological Disorders & Stroke): "...blood clots, nausea, abdominal pain, breast tenderness, irregular bleeding, headache...hair loss...edema, weight gain, hot flashes, mood swings and acne," and they verify that it can "increase the risk of uterus cancer" (111). Recently, 22 federal lawsuits were filed against the drug manufacturer of a prescription hormone replacement therapy, claiming that the pharmaceutical company knew their product could cause cancer and other serious and fatal adverse effects, yet they continued to actively market and promote their usage.

There were many professionals, however, who realized that natural, bio-identical estrogen (*estriol)* was a safe form of estrogen replacement therapy. Professor Henry Lemon had been advocating this for three decades. Fifty years ago, he said that **natural** estrogen combined with **natural** progesterone could **prevent** breast cancer and uterine cancer (465).

Note that there are some instances when natural progesterone should not be used. (Always check with your health care practitioner.) Do not use natural progesterone if you have rotor syndrome, hepatitis, liver disease, Dubin-Johnson syndrome, jaundice or history of jaundice, or if you are allergic to nuts. Do not use it if you are taking Primulut N, Duphaston or patches that contain progesterone, nor if you are taking contraceptives, the Morning After Pill (check with your physician), nor if you are taking any type of cortisone or steroid treatments. If you are having any sort of abnormal vaginal bleeding that has not been diagnosed, or if you have other health conditions, it is always best to check with your physician about taking natural progesterone or any other ingredients, however, I also recommend that you get the opinion of a Naturopathic physician, because some conventional physicians are against anything that is natural and does not come from a prescription pad.

## Natural Versus Synthetic Estrogen

**Estriol** (NATURAL estrogen), according to Dr. Lee in *What Your Doctor May Not Tell You About Breast Cancer,* is vastly different from the synthetic form—so much so—that it actually helps the body ward off reproductive cancers in women, and it fights osteoporosis and urinary infections, as well as aging skin, yet it does not increase the risk for *blood clots,* one of the potential complications of synthetic estrogen (465). Apparently, the body does not assimilate estriol as rapidly as with other hormones and the topical cream is better than taking it orally (465).

You should not be taking any type of estrogen treatment without consulting with your physician, especially if you have a history of unusual bleeding, any sort of liver disorder, or a history of cancer, nor is it recommended during pregnancy. As always, if you are nursing or pregnant, you should consult your physician about any medication, herb, or hormone you are contemplating. However, if your physician is planning a hysterectomy for you, I would recommend that you read both books by Dr. John R. Lee, et al: *What Your Doctor May Not Tell You About Menopause,* and *What Your Doctor May Not Tell You About Breast Cancer,* as well as Dr. Stanley West's: *The Hysterectomy Hoax* (313). Website, *www.safemenopausesolutions.com,* also has a women's hormone profile test that you can take if you have more questions about natural bio-identical hormone replacement. They explain that many menopausal and premenopausal symptoms can be caused by a deficiency of natural progesterone in the body.

## Natural (Non-Prescription) Progesterone

Dr. John R. Lee called natural progesterone *the great protector,* and for good reason. Natural (bio-identical) progesterone has the opposite effects on the body that are seen with the synthetic hormones (465). Chances are that if you are going through menopause, or even if you are several years pre-menopausal, you may already have excess estrogen in your cells, and in need of natural progesterone, rather than estrogen. It was only after years of putting women on prescription estrogen that the medical profession finally admitted that synthetic estrogen was causing many adverse side effects, as well as being implicated in deaths from blood clots, strokes, heart attacks, and cancer. Studies were done to back up their suspicions. It finally dawned on them that progesterone was needed.

Not to be outdone, it did not take the pharmaceutical companies long to change a molecule (or two) in natural progesterone and develop the SYNTHETIC form of progesterone (known as *Progestin*), just as they had done with estrogen! (Are you smelling a rat yet?) Physicians then began prescribing HRT to their patients, which included both **synthetic** estrogen and **synthetic** progesterone (465). The BIG problem was that the synthetic progesterone (*Progestin)* was also found to have some very ominous side effects (just as synthetic estrogen does), many of which are listed at website: *www.rxlist.com/cgi/generic/medrox_ad.htm,* including blood clots, swelling, weight gain, mood swings, loss of hair, lumpy breasts "...scleroderma, osteoporosis...cervical cancer...deep vein thrombosis," and infertility (244).

There was a glut of HRT being prescribed in the U.S. up until 2000, that is, until the study done eight years ago by the NCI, which revealed that HRT could cause a dramatic rise in the risk for *breast cancer.* Since that data was made public, Dr. Lee said that prescriptions decreased (465).

A study done by "*The Women's Health Initiative*...sponsored by the National Institute of Health...found that women on hormone replacement therapy of combined estrogen plus progestin (PREMPRO)," experienced a staggering increase for blood clots, heart attacks, heart disease, cancers of the breast, alzheimer's (older women), and strokes. See website: *www.safemenopausesolutions.com* (161).

Dr. Marcia L. Stefanick of Stanford University stated that the risk for cancer increased according to the amount of time women used HRT. She explained that women who had been taking HRT the longest were at the greatest risk (161). The website above also has information on how safe, natural bio-identical progesterone can help with male menopause problems.

Dr. Lee believed that it was very supercilious of drug manufacturers to assume that they can change the chemical structure of something like natural progesterone, make a synthetic form, patent it, then presume that the body will assimilate it to accomplish the same purpose as the natural substance (465). Do you see how the public has been duped? There is also a **natural bio-identical progesterone** available, and if you are on prescription hormone replacement therapy, I could win a bet right now that your physician has never told you that natural bio-identical progesterone exists (so does natural estrogen), and it does not have the toxic side effects associated with prescription *progestin!*

Natural bio-identical progesterone has many of the EXACT opposite effects on the body that **synthetic** estrogen and **synthetic** progesterone have. As noted by C. Norman Shealy, M.D., Ph.D., in the book, *Natural Progesterone Cream*, this natural hormone is critical for a developing embryo and for prevention of thinning bones, obesity, mammary cysts, depression, water retention, and out-of-control blood sugars, as well as preventing many other health disorders (560). Since progesterone relaxes the body, **using excessive amounts** of the hormone can cause "sleepiness, depression...[or] digestive problems..." However, using normal dosages is connected with no toxicity, as is found with the synthetic hormones (560). Of course, anyone can have an allergic reaction to a natural hormone, just as they can with any other natural or prescribed ingredient. Any severe allergic reaction to an ingredient should always be a reason to seek medical health immediately. Side effects with natural progesterone only occur with excess dosing and are very extremely rare. Compare this to the deadly array of side effects from the synthetic drug, *Progestin!*

Always check with your physician before beginning any new bio-identical hormone therapy, or any new supplement, especially if you are already taking medications, or have any type of medical condition or allergy. See the instances given above when you should not use natural bio-identical progesterone (BHRT). If you are having any sort of abnormal vaginal bleeding that has not been diagnosed, or if you have other health conditions, it is always best to check with your physician or Naturopath about taking natural progesterone.

Some physicians recommend using natural progesterone with caution in those with migraines, however, Dr. Lee was an expert on natural progesterone (having used it in his own practice for many years), and he used the cream successfully to treat migraines. Be sure in using the natural cream, to follow the label directions and your physician's advice.

Even though natural progesterone is actually developed from Mexican wild yam, it is bio-identical to the progesterone found in nature (human progesterone), so it is considered natural. Being a natural product, it could not be patented. Dr. Lee said that synthetic and natural progesterone are so vastly different that **natural** progesterone protects pregnancy, but the **synthetic** form not only can cause an abortion, but it can produce defects in the developing fetus (465). Natural progesterone can be found in health food stores in a cream form that is applied topically to the skin and absorbed through the skin. It is a very effective mode of delivering the hormone. You should not use natural progesterone cream or any products containing Mexican wild yam if you are allergic to peanuts.

In her book, *How to Renew You*, Maureen Kennedy Salaman says that a research study on HRT was brought to a halt in 2002 (after just one year) because it was discovered that women participating in the study had much greater risks for clots, *breast cancer...and heart attacks* (552). Ms. Salaman's company, *Maximum Living*, produces a natural bio-identical progesterone cream called *ProgestiMax®*. More information on *Progesti-max®* and Maureen's other health products can be found at *www.mk salaman.com*.

If you are wondering where pharmaceutical companies obtain the raw materials to make their **synthetic** progesterone, they manufacture it from NATURAL progesterone. That's right! They purchase NATURAL progesterone (which is derived from Mexican wild yam or soybeans) and then "chemically alter its molecular form" to create their synthetic and potentially deadly hormone (466). Why not just leave it in its natural state instead of changing the molecules? Because, changing the molecular structure was the ONLY way that the pharmaceutical companies could patent it and make a profit! (Do you see how the drug companies operate?)

## Are You *Estrogen Dominant?* (Do You Have Too Much Estrogen?)

If you are a woman who is pre-menopausal and you are having problems with fibroids, lumpy breasts, migraines, mood swings, chronic fatigue, unusual vaginal bleeding, hypertension, difficulty losing weight, or you have been diagnosed with *endometrial cancer* or *breast cancer*, you may very well be estrogen dominant (103). These are ALL problems associated with too much estrogen and a deficiency of progesterone (103). Be aware that you should not purchase products with *wild yam extract* thinking you are getting natural bio-identical progesterone. You will need to read the label of contents. To get natural progesterone, the label must say: ***USP Progesterone*** in the list of ingredients. If you purchase a two ounce container, for example, it will tell you the exact dosage of progesterone you are purchasing. There are many products on the market that contain black cohosh and wild yam, and while some users claim that they can relieve hot flashes and other menopausal symptoms, they may contain no natural progesterone whatsoever. Also, try to use the natural creams which do not contain mineral oil (466).

A few of the many brands Dr. Lee and Virginia Hopkins discussed in *What Your Doctor May Not Tell You About Menopause*, that do contain natural USP progesterone ("400-600 mg. progesterone per ounce...") are:

*"BioBalance...FemGest...Natural Prog...Progest...ProgestaCare...Pro-OsteoAll...Supra-Gest...Endau...[and] ProCreme Plus..."* among others. Check with your health practitioner about the dosage that you will need (466).

Dr. Lee and Virginia Hopkins also noted that excess estrogen problems do not automatically begin with menopause. Here in the U.S., many women who are several years pre-menopausal are experiencing the symptoms associated with excess estrogen, yet their physicians place them on prescription estrogen (466). Women who are menopausal and are placed on HRT for irregular bleeding, hot flashes, insomnia, weight gain, etc., often worsen in their symptoms, going on to develop severe uterine bleeding with clots and lumpy breasts **after** being on synthetic HRT. They are then told that they will need hysterectomies or lumpectomies. No one is putting two and two together and figuring out that it was the prescription HRT that probably CAUSED their excess uterine bleeding and cystic breasts to begin with! Who is going to point it out to them when it is making a gold mine for the surgeons doing the hysterectomies and lumpectomies? What is wrong with this picture? Their bodies are producing estrogen, but insufficient amounts of progesterone. The very last thing that they need is more estrogen, but that is often exactly what they are given! Many of these same women go on to develop severe osteoporosis, degenerative hip disease, degenerative disc disease, and subsequent back pain and disability, and numerous other ailments, when all they ever needed to begin with was progesterone—NATURAL progesterone—and no estrogen.

Natural bio-identical progesterone helps balance the rest of the hormones in the body. If you are having menopausal symptoms, find a good alternative health physician who is knowledgeable about natural progesterone or a conventional medicine gynecologist that believes in natural progesterone, and prescribes it. Natural progesterone will help in the replacement of bone. Estrogen will help slow bone loss, but only briefly, and it does nothing to replace the bone that has already been lost (466). You may also wish to consider supplementing with the natural substance, **ipriflavone,** for its amazing ability at fighting osteoporosis and reversing bone loss. (See Appendix II at the back of this book for help in finding alternative health physicians in your area.)

## It's Never Too Late To Start

It is never too late to begin a natural progesterone regimen. Many elderly women in their eighties and nineties could benefit from using natural progesterone cream for prevention of osteoporosis and for dry skin relief (466).

## Fibrocystic Breasts, Uterine Fibroids, Infertility & Miscarriages

Many women who lack sufficient progesterone also develop fibrocystic breasts and problems with uterine fibroids. Instead of trying them on natural progesterone, their physicians are performing hysterectomies that may be totally unnecessary. Lack of sufficient progesterone has also been linked to problems with infertility and miscarriages. Countless women have been put through needless fertility studies and agonizing months and years of infertility, when all they really needed was a safe, simple regimen of **natural** progesterone. Dr. John Lee treated a number of his patients (complaining of infertility) with natural progesterone, and recommended that when treating infertility, women should be checking their basal body temperature every morning and not use the cream until *after* their monthly ovulation (466).

If you ask your physician about taking natural bio-identical progesterone, some of them have forgotten that there is such a thing as natural progesterone that is delivered topically and has no toxic side effects. They will immediately begin writing you a prescription for SYNTHETIC progesterone. Why? Because most conventional doctors have been trained to serve the interests of a mechanized multi-million-dollar pharmaceutical industry that has no interest in natural substances that they cannot patent and sell for a profit, and many physicians have pharmacy drug reps continuously lapping at their doors, like hungry dogs, and unfortunately, only a few physicians are refusing them entrance.

Your doctor may be very insistent about putting you on prescription *Progestin,* possibly even quoting all the reasons from the fliers that he or she has received from drug companies that brag about the wonderful benefits of their synthetic hormones. This is the time that you need to point out all the toxic side effects of prescription HRT, and the non-toxic effects of NATURAL progesterone.

## How Much Progesterone Do You Need?

Always follow the label directions on the natural progesterone cream you purchase and your physician's advice. Realize that dosing will also depend on your age, whether or not you are currently taking HRT, whether or not you have had a hysterectomy in the past (466), or if you are pre or post-menopausal. Dr. Lee and Virginia Hopkins explained that if you are taking prescription estrogen, you should wean from it slowly, never all at once, however, they had no problem with stopping *Provera abruptly* (466). Remember that when you start taking NATURAL bio-identical progesterone (BHRT), you will no longer need to be on the synthetic form of the hormone. Be sure to discuss this with your doctor and express your concerns about being on synthetic hormones (466).

Many women are apprehensive that if they are menopausal and take **natural** progesterone that they may start having periods again. This usually does not happen; however, if this does occur after you have been taking natural progesterone, this is due to the high estrogen level in your body, and Dr. Lee's recommendation was to discontinue the natural cream for seven days, then resume for *three weeks* (466). The label you receive with your natural progesterone cream should answer many of these questions, as well as your physician resource. Because of the difference in days in the month, sometimes the simplest way to remember is to always go off the cream the last six or seven days of every month, regardless of how many days there are in the month. (This way you would always start using the cream on the first day of every month.) However, you should always check with your licensed health care practitioner to verify proper dosing and advice regarding hormonal creams, as they may have a different recommendation for you. Factors such as age, weight, height, current health, past health history, etc. are also taken into consideration when hormones are given. Your physician may send you to a compounding pharmacist to get a certain dosage of natural bio-identical progesterone or estrogen cream, custom-fit for your own personal requirements.

## Migraines - Natural Progesterone & Other Natural Treatments

Natural progesterone cream has been used successfully to stop migraine headaches. Dr. Lee recommended natural bio-identical progesterone cream for migraines.

As described at website *www.mcvitamins.com/migraine.htm*, research has shown that taking "riboflavin (400 mg a day)" can cut the intensity and occurrence of migraines by more than 50% in patients taking it. Some medical sources, including *The Lancet,* reported that headache relief could be obtained by most people if they would simply abstain from any foods which cause allergic reactions (195). Also, using the supplement lecithin may help prevent migraines. The dosage recommended was "between three and six 1,200-milligram capsules… when they felt a headache coming on" (195). The website above also suggests that you include "exercise…alternative hot and cold showers, and taking [the herbs] feverfew & hyssop," for migraine headache relief (195). Also, see chapter 23 in this book regarding the connection between dehydration and migraines.

Taking niacin may help get rid of migraines, however, you cannot use the *flush-free* niacin for this purpose as it will not work as well. This is similar to what patients are given when they go to the E.R. for an unrelenting headache. They are placed on a histamine drip that opens up blood vessels and causes a flushing effect on the body. Never use the *timed-release* niacin. For a migraine, you may want to begin with a 25 mg dosage of niacin, then proceed to 50 mg, etc., until relief or the flush is obtained. Get your doctor's opinion. Taking a baby aspirin or two 20-30 minutes before taking niacin will reduce the flushing effect, however, with migraines, you want the flush. It is the flush that is opening up your blood vessels. This helps circulation as well.

## Testing for Low Hormone Levels

At his website, *www.johnleemd.com,* Dr. Lee explained that some practitioners are using an article that was published in the *Lancet* (casting doubt on the absorption of topically used natural progesterone cream), to argue that taking the natural hormone in topical cream form was not adequately absorbed by the body (262). However, Dr. Lee called the report in *Lancet erroneous,* because he said that the writers of the article were unclear about the difference between blood levels versus *saliva levels* of natural progesterone (262). Most of the progesterone produced by the ovaries is bound to protein. A minute amount (which is unbound) is the natural progesterone that goes into the *tissues* and the *saliva* (262). Therefore, the progesterone that is found in blood is not the amount the body is going to be using since it is bound up in protein (262). The cream form is absorbed into the skin rapidly, and this progesterone is the amount calculated in the saliva tests developed for that purpose. This is why blood levels are not an accurate measurement, because only very tiny amounts are found in the *serum* (262). (You can order saliva testing kits from Dr. Lee's website: *www.johnleemd.com*, as well as a few other websites on the internet.)

See Dr. Lee's website for more information on saliva testing and normal levels of progesterone at: *johnleemd.com.* Everyone is unique, and your dosage will vary according to your own bodily needs. Find a licensed, alternative health care practitioner, or at least be sure that your conventional medicine physician is up-to-date on natural bio-identical progesterone creams. Many doctors are now recommending this cream.

There are also times when it is beneficial to have higher levels of progesterone in the body, for example, during times of stress when the body produces excess cortisol. Cortisol has the ability to block progesterone from reaching its destination and to prevent it from functioning (466). See website, *www.johnleemd.com,* for more information on using natural progesterone cream for conditions like endometriosis and migraines (93).

## Estrogen Excess & Cancer

Why has there been such a tragic rise in breast cancer in women? Dr. Lee believed that it was probably due to the fact that thousands, perhaps millions, of *menopausal women* were given synthetic estrogen, especially during the past fifty-five years. Even though conventional medicine realized that this practice increased the risks for cancer of the uterus, he said that they simply refused to acknowledge that it was responsible for *breast cancer* as well (465). Think back. How many of your loved ones have died of uterine and/or breast cancer that had a history of taking prescription hormone replacement therapy?

What was the response of the medical community to the rise in breast and uterine cancers? They actually claimed that breast cancer rates were falling and tried to attribute this to the use of Tamoxifen, a chemotherapy agent given to breast cancer patients. However, the late Dr. Lee was very scornful of Tamoxifen due to the potential side effects of causing clots, visual disturbances, and uterine cancer (465).

Do you see how the statistics are manipulated to make chemo drugs look *attractive?* A woman with breast cancer is given Tamoxifen. She develops **uterine cancer (a side-effect of the Tamoxifen)** and dies, but the statistics say that she didn't die from breast cancer, she died from uterine cancer, making it APPEAR that the Tamoxifen HELPED her breast cancer, because after all, the breast cancer didn't kill her, the uterine cancer did—right? Thus, the drug company prints up a lovely rainbow-colored chart for everyone to see how effective Tamoxifen is at curing breast cancer—I mean—just **LOOK at the statistics**! The Tamoxifen cured the patient, course she is dead, but at least she didn't die from breast cancer—right? The exact same thing happens when a patient has liver cancer and they take chemo or radiation therapy. They may develop a severe blood disorder from the chemo (such as leukemia) that kills them. Well, the liver cancer didn't ***kill*** them, so the chemo or radiation must have HELPED their liver cancer, right? Well, that is exactly how the statistics are done, and how drug companies dupe the public into believing that chemo is an effective cancer treatment. **(Can you see the insanity of this type of reasoning?)** This is exactly how some drugs get pushed through quick approval by the FDA, based on statistics that are often manipulated just like this—to make them look successful and favorable. Drug companies often throw out studies on their drugs that show unfavorable results, and publish only those studies that make them appear favorable.

Dr. John Lee received a letter from a 56-year-old woman who had declined the use of Tamoxifen on his advice. She expressed her great appreciation for his boldness in telling her his concerns with this drug when he advised her against using it (465).

Author of *The Breast Cancer Prevention Diet,* Dr. Bob Arnot, was scathingly criticized by U.S. media moguls and made to look like an idiot for even hinting that perhaps a healthy diet could fend off breast cancer (465). If you will recall in chapter four of this book, Eydie Mae Hunsberger and Rita Myers proved **that a healthy diet and lifestyle changes can CURE breast cancer!** There are several examples given in chapter four of breast cancer **CURES** using natural means.

Remember that another major culprit in the cause of all this excess estrogen is environmental factors. For example: the FDA **allows** farmers to inject cattle with synthetic estrogen which makes them gain weight and gives the farmers a better price for their livestock. However, YOU are consuming this extra estrogen when you buy the meat (466). Did you know that most European nations have BANNED the use of estrogen in their cattle, yet the FDA continues to allow it in America?! Teenage acne is now being linked with hormones found in cow's milk.

If you want to see a video of the hypocrisy of Monsanto's activities in their genetically-modified foods, as well as the creation and addition of growth hormone to cow's milk (along with the blatant lies and cover up by the FDA), as well as how many top government officials and FDA officials were in Monsanto's revolving door employment, you will want to see the video for yourself at *http://www.celsias.com/article/the-world-according-to-monsanto.* (Monsanto is the same company that gave us *Agent Orange!)*

At one time, cattle were allowed to freely roam, but many are now often kept in tight, huddled quarters, making them more susceptible to disease. They are given large amounts of antibiotics to fight disease, and these antibiotics end up in the meat (and dairy products) that end up in your food supply! This is one of the many reasons for all the new antibiotic-resistant strains of microbes baffling scientists (466).

The fact that estrogen causes water retention, salt retention, and fat retention has been a *gold mine* for the cattle industry. All they have to do is shoot the cattle up with estrogen hormones, they gain weight rapidly, go to market sooner, bring bigger bucks, and consumers ingest the stuff every time they feast on poultry and beef. Is it any wonder that our teenagers, who consume fast-food hamburgers and other meats, are struggling with acne, insomnia, weight problems, difficulty concentrating, irritability, and—later in life—develop problems with infertility, irregular menses, and high blood pressure? And don't forget that dairy products too, are contaminated with hormones. We are pushing milk on youngsters, not realizing that cow's milk has been linked to auto-immune disorders, insulin-dependent childhood (Type I) diabetes, multiple sclerosis, and a myriad of other ailments to which I have devoted chapter 26 of this book. (Also, see p. 488 on MS & vitamin D deficiencies.)

If you truly want to win the battle against *estrogen dominance*, stay away from meat and dairy products. (If you do keep them in your diet, for your health's sake, use only ORGANIC meat and dairy that has been certified to be free of hormones, herbicides, antibiotics, and pesticides. It used to be safe to substitute soy, but much of our soy has become contaminated and studies show that soy can damage the thyroid. The only soy that some nutritionists recommend now is fermented soy.

We are plagued with companies that think it is perfectly fine to manipulate nature and give us GMO or genetically-modified soy and other foods with no assurance that they are safe. Better to be safe than sorry. Remember this, if it's from nature as GOD MADE IT, you can depend on it. If MAN has tampered with it in any way whatsoever (e.g., changing molecules), it could kill you! Taking natural progesterone to balance out your hormones will be of little benefit to you if you are consuming synthetic estrogen in meat and dairy products every day.

## How Safe Is Natural Progesterone?

In an article by Catherine P. Rollins at *www.natural-progesteroneadvisory-network.com*, she reminds us that no one has ever been sent to the hospital from overdosing on natural progesterone; however, hundreds of thousands of people DIE every year from the side effects of pharmaceutical drugs prescribed by physicians (537) (538).

Ms. Rollins explains that the problem in most women is not enough progesterone in the body to oppose all the excess estrogen. Catherine Rollins is author of *A Woman's Guide to Using Natural Progesterone* and Director of the website above (537) (538).

## Breast Cancer Awareness Month?

What about *Breast Cancer Awareness Month?* Are you aware that *Breast Cancer Awareness Month* (October) is a marketing bonanza that is mostly hyped and supported by the same pharmaceutical company where Tamoxifen is produced (465)? Dr. Lee thought it very ironic that this same company produces chemo drugs that may help cause the disease! There is little emphasis in October on prevention, or using some of the millions collected by concerned citizens for non-toxic, alternative cancer research. The main focus is about being aware of ONLY those breast cancer treatments recognized and pushed by today's cancer industry (465). WHY is this? Because drug companies and the FDA control the media and the medical establishment.

## Natural Progesterone & Auto-Immune Disorders

A lack of sufficient progesterone in the body has the ability to throw the thyroid out of whack, resulting in hormonal disarray with a debilitating effect on the immune system. (How many women do you know on thyroid medication post-menopause?) It is very odd that during the time of their lives when they are most likely to be estrogen dominant, is when women fall victim to auto-immune diseases (465).

This was a troubling fact to Dr. Lee. Patients he placed on natural progesterone often told him that they no longer had symptoms associated with auto-immune disorders, and he wondered if auto-immune disorders could be caused by excess levels of estrogen in the body (465). He felt it was very possible, from evidence with his own patients, that having sufficient natural progesterone in the body could prevent some of these illnesses that are caused by too much estrogen (465). In fact, Catherine Rollins points out at her website (*discussed above),* that recent data shows that women who use HRT with estrogen have a greater risk for *lupus*, and the hormones women get from *birth control pills* increase their risk for auto-

"immune diseases by causing the body to form antibodies to its own hormones" (536). (This ominous trend is especially insidious when you realize that many more women succumb to auto-immune disorders than do men, and the fact that they do not occur in such dismal proportions in areas outside the U.S, where estrogen dominance and HRT are less common.)

When purchasing natural bio-identical progesterone, always look for creams that contain ***USP Progesterone*** on the label, and apply the cream as advised by your physician, and as the label recommends.

Natural bio-identical progesterone cream has been successfully used to treat rosacea and psoriasis when applied topically to the affected areas (466). Be sure when applying the cream, you give it time to be absorbed so that most of it does not end up on your clothing, instead of in you!

## Osteoporosis—How to Prevent It—How to Reverse It

Dr. Lee, in his own practice, proved that natural progesterone had the capacity to dramatically **REVERSE bone loss in patients who came to him with advanced osteoporosis.** He was perplexed by the obstinacy with which the medical system was using estrogen as their main recommendation for osteoporosis prevention, because, as he explained, scientific validation for it does not exist (466). He pointed to an article in the *New England Journal of Medicine* (1995) involving 10,000 elderly female participants and many *years* of research. What Dr. Lee found so disturbing about this study was the fact that even though the participants were all more than 65 years of age and taking estrogen, it did absolutely nothing to protect them from *hip fractures* (466). He discovered and taught that while estrogen may slow down the loss of bone, progesterone turns the bone loss around by actually increasing bone restoration. In his own practice, he observed that combining natural progesterone with correct nutrition *and exercise* was very beneficial in the fight against osteoporosis, and explained that the majority of women have bone thinning a decade or more prior to even going through menopause, yet this is during a time that they are not estrogen-deficient (466).

Many of Dr. Lee's patients came to him suffering with osteoporosis in various degrees of severity. He was soon to discover that their being on estrogen hormone did nothing to stop the progression of their bone loss, nor *reverse* it. Even when his patients supplemented with essential minerals and vitamins and gave up their cigarettes, nothing changed (395). He placed his patients on *natural progesterone* cream and within a three-year-period, their *bone mass* increased by *15%* without adverse *effects* (395). (Eventually, his patients had a return to what is considered normal bone density.)

How serious is osteoporosis? In the book, *Remifemin: Herbal Relief for Menopausal Symptoms*, author Frank Murray explains that millions of people, mostly women, suffer from this disease (513). Osteoporosis has been linked to the cause of "about 1.5 million fractures each year…" (513). (Also, see p. 498 for information on ipriflavone.)

Men can often profit from taking natural progesterone, as well as women (552). For healthy bones, you also must have sufficient vitamin D, calcium, magnesium, and boron. Remember that your best vitamin D source is natural sunlight. Food sources are: *bee pollen…sun flower seeds* (552), cod liver oil, mushrooms, and salmon. If you taking calcium supplements, you should be using a brand that includes magnesium and boron, and if it does not include vitamin D3, you need about ten to twenty minutes of sunshine every day (without sunscreen) to give your body an adequate vitamin D. It is best to get your vitamin D from the sun. (This sun exposure should not be during the hottest times of the day, and not while you are on herbs or drugs that increase sun-sensitivity.) Check with your physician if you or your family members have a prior history of melanoma, or have a greater risk for the disease.)

Be sure that you are not taking excess calcium, which has been linked to clogged arteries. (Also, recall that you can get your **calcium** from the same place the cows and the goats get it—not from milk—but from the soil, in the form of green leafy vegetables.) See the information in this book regarding the high amount of calcium in fresh carrot juice and dried barley grass juice. Another ingredient that is gaining popularity in bone and joint health is the combination of *glucosamine* and *chondroitin sulfate*, commonly used for arthritis patients.

Chondroitin sulfate actually functions in the body much like Heparin (a pharmaceutical blood-thinner), but does not have the potentially harmful adverse reactions that are found in Heparin (552); however, very few physicians prescribe chondroitin over Heparin for this purpose. Recently, there was a Heparin recall due to a problem with one of the main ingredients in the drug.

## Menopause & Weight Gain

It is important to realize that when women become estrogen dominant, they get caught up in a vicious cycle. A high fat diet increases estrogen levels in the body, but fat cells also make estrogen, and as discussed earlier, we consume synthetic estrogens in our diets. We also get toxic estrogens (xenoestrogens) from substances we use everyday. A good example is plastic. If you do not want to get additional estrogen (or dioxin) in your food, avoid plastic containers and pots for your foods, and using plastic wrap in the microwave. There are times this is unavoidable, such as purchasing frozen fruit that usually comes in plastic bags. NEVER heat foods in plastic! Fat accumulates in breast tissue, the body makes even more estrogen from this stored fat, the estrogen causes the body to accumulate even more body fat, and then more estrogen is produced.

Women find themselves caught up in this vicious cycle of finding it not only more and more difficult to lose weight as they get older, but they keep gaining more weight as their estrogen production rises and their progesterone levels drop out of sight. They do not understand what is happening to them, especially if they haven't changed the amount of calories they ingest and they can't account for the weight gain. Many try one fad diet after another, or one exercise regimen after another, only to fail in the end. Regaining a normal hormone balance between estrogen and progesterone is sometimes all that is needed to win this battle.

Note that your physician should be checking your progesterone levels with a saliva test, which gives a much more accurate reading than a blood test, as discussed earlier in this chapter. If you have a conventional doctor unwilling to recommend natural hormone replacement therapy, find a reliable, licensed alternative health care physician, knowledgeable about natural hormones. See the sample list of practitioners at *http://altmedangel.com.*

## Phyto-Estrogens

There are many plants and herbs that mimic the action of natural estrogen in the body. Black cohosh is one of them. These are called *Phyto* or *plant estrogens.* As noted by Rita Elkins, M.H., in her book: *Natural Alternatives to HRT*, these plant estrogens are beneficial in that they can block harmful estrogen levels in the body. They can also help *reduce cholesterol* and prevent *osteoporosis* and *heart disease* (395).

There are many herbs available that contain plant estrogens, such as *Red Clover...Black Cohosh Root...[and] Ginkgo* (395). Red clover and black cohosh root should not be used by children, nor by women who may be nursing or pregnant. Be aware that new reports are surfacing that black cohosh could cause liver problems in some individuals. Always check with your physician or Naturopath first.

You should realize that while these natural forms of estrogen may be beneficial by blocking out harmful estrogens in the body, all the plant estrogens in the world won't help if your main problem is a lack of progesterone, or if you are consuming large amounts of synthetic estrogen in meat and dairy every day. Fermented soy products, such as Haelan, may help remove harmful estrogens from the body in estrogen receptor-positive cancers.

For information on Haelan, see the company's website at *www.haelan951.com.* Information on Haelan's Research Foundation's website was accumulated from clinical studies performed on fermented soy beverages manufactured by Haelan Products, Inc. of Woodinville, Washington. The Haelan fermented soy beverages are sold in the United States, without medical claims, and are available directly from the company or one of their distributors (143).

## Preventing Cancer in Women with Iodine & Magnesium

Both of these minerals are discussed in several chapters of this book. Their importance for women's health should not be underestimated. See pages 129 and 400 for more details. Magnesium and iodine are both critically important for breast and uterine health.

# CHAPTER 23

## WATER, WATER EVERYWHERE, BUT ARE YOU GETTING ENOUGH?

*"But whosoever drinketh of the water that I shall give him shall never thirst; but the water that I shall give him shall be in him a well of water springing up into everlasting life." (John 4:14)*

### If You're Already Thirsty, Is It Too Late?

Chances are you've been thirsty enough at some point in your life to know what it means to crave an icy, cold drink. The problem is, the very **LAST symptom** that your body gives for dehydration is usually thirst. This means that once you hit the actual point where you are physically thirsty, you may already be seriously dehydrated. It is important to make sure that you are providing your body with enough water that you never reach the point of being overly thirsty (apart from unusual circumstances, such as running a high fever, grueling exercise, excess salt consumption, illness, diarrhea, etc). Scientists are only recently making the connection between longstanding dehydration and the onset of chronic, degenerative diseases. Most people drink a few cups of coffee during the day, soda, juice, or tea with their meals, and are convinced that they're getting their quota of fluids. Unless you are drinking 8-10 (8 ounce) glasses of WATER per day (depending on your body weight), you are depriving yourself of water and risking your health. Caffeinated drinks are diuretics—they strip valuable water from your body. If you can't seem to stay away from them, then you will need more water to make up for their dehydration effects on your body.

It is critically important that the water you drink NOT contain fluoride or chlorine. Dr. John Yiamouyiannis, in an article at *website www.health-science.com/fluoride_toxicity.html* on "Fluoride Toxicity," estimates "that 30,000—50,000 people die from flouride (sic) poisoning each year" (605). Author of *Fluoride: The Aging Factor*, he attributes this chemical to harming the body's natural immunity and the destruction of collagen, as well as *genetic damage* (605). It has also been shown by Dr. Takeki Tsutsu, and fellow researchers in Japan, that fluoride is responsible for causing cellular changes within the DNA, including the formation of abnormal cancer cells (605). Research done by Dr. Dean Burk, "former Chief

Chemist of the National Cancer Institute, showed that 10,000 or more fluoridation-linked cancer deaths occur yearly in the United States" (605). Did you know that eating several mouthfuls of toothpaste with fluoride can kill a small child? Do not leave toothpaste out for your toddler to find.

In his very informative book, *Your Body's Many Cries For Water,* the late Dr. F. Batmanghelidj, M.D., insisted that some symptoms (which are actually the body's thirst symptoms) are incorrectly treated with prescription drugs (341). Dr. Batmanghelidj, born in Tehran, Iran, was incarcerated there during the days of the Iranian revolution. It was during this time in prison that he discovered a treatment for stressed inmates who were developing peptic ulcers. The only thing he had to give them was water, which cured their ulcers. The government of Iran was so impressed with his findings and subsequent article, that they published his work in the *Iranian Medical Council Journal* (1982), and he was eventually released in June of that year. His article also appeared in *The New York Times* (341). Dr. Batmanghelidj had successfully used water to treat thousands of his *ulcer patients.* He claimed that "dyspeptic pain is the most important signal for the human body. It denotes dehydration. It is a thirst signal of the body" (341). He also believed that most of the chronic and severe *diseases* in our world can be linked to "Chronic and persistently increasing dehydration" (341).

Just as we have a hunger stimulus when we get hungry, Dr. Batmanghelidj taught that our "'thirst pain' signal in the body'" is called *dyspepsia,* and when treated for long periods of time with prescriptions, the result can be gastric injury and ulceration. He also taught that the continual use of antacids in treating this type of pain "is a...slow poison" (341). It is very alarming that antacids are high in aluminum content. The accumulation of aluminum in the brain has already been linked to an *Alzheimer-type* disease. A good example is from the island of Guam in the Western Pacific (341). At one time there was such a high level of aluminum in Guam's drinking water, the entire population on the island, including "the younger people," were afflicted with a mental "dementia" very "similar to Alzheimer dementia," however, once they figured out what was wrong and cleaned up the water, the statistics for this dementia began to decline (341).

Dr. Batmanghelidj believed that "aluminum toxicity is a secondary complication of dehydration," and that "chronic dehydration" is what actually causes "*Alzheimer's disease.*" He also believed that in most cases of "Colitis Pain...False Appendicitis Pain...[and] Hiatus Hernia..." these are actually "thirst signals," and results of starving the body for water (341).

here is clinical evidence presented in *Your Body's Many Cries For* to link arthritic pain (e.g., *rheumatoid arthritis*), back, neck pain, and , as well as problems with allergies and asthma attacks, to chronic ation, and in some instances, inadequate salt intake (341). Just be avoid drinking water and cold beverages with, or immediately after unless you need them for taking medications or vitamins and other ents.

Also, see the book by Richard Thomas: *The Essiac Report Canada's Remarkable Unknown Cancer Remedy,* where he documents a copy of a letter from Larry H., who was cured of rheumatoid arthritis drinking Flor-Essence® Essiac tea (580). If you are just starting on a detox like Essiac tea, wheat grass, carrot or beet juice—after the first few days—you will feel worse because your body is going through a detoxification process. You will gradually begin to feel better once your body has gone through several days of ridding itself of toxins accumulated throughout your life.

## Help for Asthma Patients

Dr. Batmanghelidj discovered, almost by accident, exactly what causes asthma. He even tried to present his discovery to the American Medical Association in a letter to then President of the "AMA…Dr. C. John Tupper," but Dr. Tupper's response a month later was evasive and non-committal. Basically, he promised to share the information with others, and that was the last Dr. Batmanghelidj ever heard from him. Nothing was ever done with the information he gave them, however, his asthma cure was "aired on June 5, 1995, by Paul Harvey News for the first time" (341). The treatment Dr. Batmanghelidj received by the AMA isn't at all surprising. It is the typical treatment that anyone gets when they promote a natural cure for a disease that is treated conventionally with a whole gamut of *acceptable* pharmaceutical drugs.

How happy do you think it would make all those producers of asthma medications (and inhalers) if the public suddenly realizes that there is a natural, inexpensive treatment for asthma, apart from the use of multiple pharmaceutical drugs? Dr. Batmanghelidj pointed out that adults and children with asthma and allergies have a high level of histamine in the cells of their lungs. In a nut shell, histamine regulates water and "bronchial muscle contraction" (341). Asthma can be caused by years of chronic dehydration. This lack of water causes the body to increase histamine production so that water will be conserved (sort of like an emergency stop-gap in a water crisis). A great deal of water is lost through the lungs every day, just from breathing (341).

Since the body is already starved for water, the histamine tries to conserve what little is left by constricting the bronchioles to keep water from evaporating through breathing. What is the end result? ASTHMA. Choking, suffocating, inability to breathe. This is also the reason for many allergies. Dr. Batmanthelidj very successfully weaned his asthma patients off asthma medication, simply by having them increase their water and salt intake (341); however, he warned that not taking enough water for months or years cannot be compensated for in a day or two. You should increase your water intake if you are suffering from allergies and asthma, but you cannot "overdrink thinking you can undo the damage of many months or years of dehydration by excessive intake of water in a few days" (341). You should take the normal amount recommended ("eight to ten 8-ounce glasses") until such time as the body maintains normal hydration. He did not recommend more than eight to sixteen ounces a day of *orange juice* (especially for asthmatics), due to its "high…potassium content," which can increase the body's *histamine* (341).

## When You Need Extra Salt

For every two quarts of water that you drink every day, you need to add 1/2 teaspoon of salt to your diet (341). Salt plays a crucial role in asthma, because any time your body is dehydrated, it automatically begins to hoard salt. As per Dr. Batmanghelidg: "Salt is a natural antihistamine. People with allergies should begin to increase their salt intake to prevent excess histamine production," if their physician does not have them on a salt-restricted or water-restricted diet (341). In describing what happens with **asthma**, Dr. Batmanghelidg explained that tasting salt with your tongue can deceive the body into thinking you have taken a lot of salt, and this will reduce the asthmatic symptoms by causing a subsequent opening up of the bronchioles (341). He described several case studies in his book, *Your Body's Many Cries For Water*, on the effects of increased salt and water intake for asthma patients. One case in particular, was a young boy who was taking multiple asthma medications (341). After following Dr. Batmanghelidj's advice, the child was able to come off every single one of his asthma drugs, and this was not an isolated case. Another child was able to come off all of his asthma medication after only one month of sufficient water and salt treatment (341).

If you are the parent of a child with asthma, think about this—do you know how much water your child is taking in every day? You cannot include all the pop, tea, juices, coffee, and soups. If, for example, you have a seven-year-old in the second grade and you send them off to school after a breakfast that includes a glass of orange juice, do they go the entire remainder of the day with no water? What about lunch time? What do they drink for lunch? Milk? Soda? Soup? Water? Most school children go their entire 12 years in school chronically dehydrated. Schools have water fountains, but how much water do you think your child gets from a water fountain during the school day, rushing between classes with ten minute breaks? Many people believe that drinking extra water means too frequent trips to the bathroom; however, even though this happens initially when you begin increasing your water intake, once your body adjusts to the extra water, those frequent bathroom trips will taper off.

## Banish Back Pain & Prevent Auto-immune Disorders

Dr. Batmanghelidj authored several books and videos on the importance of water consumption for banishing back pain and auto-immune disorders, such as lupus and rheumatoid arthritis. It is important to realize that much of the degenerative disc disease that we encounter as we age is because of the fact that the discs in the spinal cord are composed mostly of water, and chronic dehydration over many years will shrink the discs, causing degeneration and herniation, resulting in severe back pain and disability (341). Dr. Batmanghelidj pointed out that "75% of the weight of the upper part of the body is supported by the water volume that is stored in the disc core" of the "5th lumbar disc," and it is this disc that is so critical to back health (341).

## The M.S. Symptoms That Vanished

Dr. Batmanghelidj also taught that months and years of starving your body for water can lead to auto-immune disorders ("multiple sclerosis…rheumatoid arthritis…lupus"), high blood pressure, diabetes, and many other ailments (341). At website: *http://www.watercure2.org*, the story of M. Fox, who suffered for five years with multiple sclerosis, is described. All of her M.S. symptoms disappeared after following the water cure. She said that she had been diagnosed with M.S. for several years. She was bed-bound and "retaining fluid so badly," that she was unable to walk (402). She also said that for her height she was overweight, and she even had difficulty talking. She had no idea what was happening to her. She also had chronic problems involving her bladder and bowels, and physicians informed her that she would eventually have to undergo "a colostomy" (402). An LPN for 44 years, she had already been through a trial of several different medications. She did not begin the *water cure* until her disease was advanced. She explained that increasing her water intake totally cured her, and she was able to go off all the prescription medications she was taking (402). According to Bob Butts at the *www.watercure2.o*rg website, "This is the 5th report of a person losing all symptoms of M.S. after going on the WATER CURE. All were ambulatory" (402).

Be aware that vegetarian diets and low fat diets can significantly reduce the risks for M.S. Research shows that curcumin may help fight multiple sclerosis because it appears to have a protective effect on nerve cells. (It also stimulates the digestive system and is a blood thinner.) Also, see p. 488 for the link between MS and vitamin D deficiencies.

## Cancer & Dehydration

As for cancer, Dr. Batmanghelidj believed that people develop tumors from years of starving their cells for water (341). You can find his books and products at his website: *www.watercure2.com*, or from Global Health Solutions, 8472 A Tyco Rd., Vienna, VA 22182, USA. The products and books are also available at many natural health food stores.

## Banishing High Blood Pressure

When the body is deprived of water, it hoards salt, leading to high blood pressure (as well as high cholesterol). Dr. Batmanghelidj believed that many physicians are currently misleading their high blood pressure patients by putting them on salt-restricted, water-restricted diets, since the majority of high blood pressure problems are nothing more than the body's way of trying to compensate for a severe "water deficiency" (341). He explained that the way conventional medicine currently treats high blood pressure is *scientific absurdity*. Due to dehydration, the body is actually trying, in its desperate state—to conserve water—so what do physicians do? They give their patients diuretics to get rid of water! In his experience, Dr. Batmanghelidj said that, "Water by itself is the best natural diuretic" (341). If patients having hypertension, **who have sufficient urinary output**, take in more water, they will not need to rely on *diuretics*. He advises that, in cases of heart failure, this water intake has to be done very gradually (341).

If you are on a water-restricted or salt-restricted diet, discuss this with your physician. You should not discontinue any medications you are taking without consulting your doctor. To do so could be harmful. (I highly recommend Dr. Batmanghelidj's books and videos; information you may want to share with your family and with your physician.)

## Water & Oxygen

Remember, if you are fighting any chronic illness, many diseases (such as cancer) cannot survive in a highly oxygenated environment, and the main component of water is OXYGEN. Starving your body for water = intracellular oxygen starvation and deprivation. Cancer patients are usually dehydrated. Inadequate oxygen at the cellular level promotes cancer formation.

## How Much Water Do You Need?

As noted earlier, most adults need six to eight glasses of water per day, depending on body weight. They also need about "¼ teaspoon of salt in every quart of water" (341). More water is needed during times of illness (e.g., fever, vomiting, diarrhea, stress), or excessive perspiration (341). If your kidneys are not functioning correctly, and you increase your water and salt intake, you will start swelling up. Dr. Batmanghelidj's remedy (if you accumulate fluid in your skin and ankles) is to "Reduce salt intake for a few days, but increase your water intake until the swelling in the legs disappears," and increase your activity (341). However, you should have your regular physician involved at the very onset before you ever begin a new water/salt regimen, or if you experience any type of swelling as noted above. It is best NOT to drink water and other fluids while you are eating because they dilute the hydrochloric acid in the stomach needed to digest food. The exception to this, of course, is when you will swallow vitamin/mineral supplements that go with food, or if you are taking medications that are supposed to go with meals.

## How Pure Is Your Drinking Water?

If you do not have a good filtration system on your home water supply, you may want to consider a good bottled water or distilled water, rather than the fluoride/chlorine water that most city water systems provide. Even re-cycled drinking water can contain pharmaceutical drugs.

## Heartburn & Reflux Disease

According to Dr. John R. Lee and Virginia Hopkins in their book, *What Your Doctor May Not Tell You About Menopause,* despite what you are being told by the manufacturers of antacid chewables and prescriptions, excess acid in the stomach is not always responsible for heartburn (466). It is often the result of the body producing insufficient hydrochloric acid. When you have too little stomach acid, your food begins to ferment and this can result in esophageal irritation or *gastroesophageal reflux* (GERD), another word for "heart-burn" caused by reflux acid (466). If you have too little stomach acid, Dr. Lee suggested "a tablespoon of apple cider vinegar in one-third of a cup of water before a meal." Just be sure you don't take the vinegar while you are experiencing heartburn (466).

You may find digestive help from chewable papaya extracts as well (available in health food stores). Most taste delicious, or you can try eating fresh papaya with your meals. There are also enzyme supplements available that aid in digestion. Maureen Kennedy Salaman has digestive enzyme supplements available at her website: *www.mksalaman.com,* Enzyme Ease®, and Multi-Enzyme. Be aware that papaya enzymes can have blood-thinning properties. (Other natural helps for GERD are DGL, orange peel extract, mint, and blackstrap molasses.)

## Asthma & Mushrooms

See the information in chapter 25 of this book regarding Cordyceps Sinensis mushroom and asthma. (Also, look under ***asthma*** in the **index** for other natural ways to prevent and fight asthma.) Realize too, that use of over-the-counter drugs like Tylenol® (Acetaminophen) can increase asthma problems.

# CHAPTER 24

# PREVENT CANCER WITH OXYGEN, EXERCISE, SUNSHINE & REST

*"For thou art the God of my strength." (Psalm 43:2) "…God is the strength of my heart, and my portion forever." (Psalm 73:26) "In him was life; and the life was the light of men." (John 1:4)*

## Oxygen Therapies for Cancer

The importance of oxygen in cancer prevention was discussed briefly in chapter 23. According to Ann Wigmore in *The Wheat grass Book*, Otto Warburg, M.D., won a *Nobel prize* by showing that cancer cannot survive in a highly oxygenated *environment.* He ultimately saw cancer as a result of abnormal cells taking over, due to severe oxygen deficiencies within the cells (600). Even though Dr. Warburg's discovery was more than five decades ago, it has never been disproven. Healthy ways to increase your cellular oxygen is with hyperbaric oxygen, fresh vegetable and fruit juices, *deep breathing* exercises, adequate water intake, regular physical exercise, and green foods that increase chlorophyll in the body; foods like wheat grass, barley juice, other green drinks (600), chlorella, broccoli, kale, spirulina, and spinach.

One cancer treatment that seeks to get more oxygen into the body at the cellular level is **ozone treatment**. You can purchase ozonators at some health food stores, but they are rather expensive. Ozone is another form of oxygenation, important to all body cells. Hydrogen peroxide is given intravenously for increasing the body's oxygenation. Many patients claim that they have been cured using an intravenous form of hydrogen peroxide given by Naturopathic physicians, even though the mainstream media has presented it as controversial by claiming that ONE patient was harmed with this ingredient. However, there never was any evidence substantiating that this alternative therapy harmed the patient in question. I studied the case. It was just another example of the never-ending bias against Naturopathic practitioners and natural medicine. Though I do not consider this a natural, gentle, or painless treatment (since it is given intravenously), you will see it promoted by some alternative health practitioners, and many people claim that it has brought them into complete remission. Another thing, researchers have discovered, in the last few weeks, that the reason intravenous Vitamin C is effective at killing cancer, is because it creates **hydrogen peroxide** in the body, which increases oxygen levels and destroys cancer cells (329a)! Imagine that!

What we need are T.V. programs highlighting all the THOUSANDS of cases of people who are fatally harmed with toxic chemo drugs and radiation every year, but their family members would have to provide the documentaries, since the witnesses are all dead!

According to Conrad LeBeau in his book, *Hydrogen Peroxide & Ozone*, a health food store proprietor in California said that she was able to shrink a cancerous growth dramatically when she used a **topical** "hydrogen peroxide based gel," and she also reported that her pain had disappeared (463).

See page 544 in this book for information on a new form of oral vitamin C (*liposome-encapsulated vitamin C*) that is said to be more clinically effective than intravenous C.

## R.N. Cures Her Pancreatic Tumor with Dietary Changes & Topical Gel

Also described by Conrad LeBeau, is the story of a registered nurse from Arizona, who had been diagnosed with a terminal pancreatic tumor. She was able to cure her cancer on a *vegetarian diet.* She also used "½ tablespoon of a hydrogen peroxide based gel three times a day. She absorbed about 67 drops of 37% H2O2 into her skin each day" (463).

This was a **topical** application; it was not taken by mouth. (Never take non-food-grade hydrogen peroxide by mouth! It is poisonous!) Her story is extraordinary because her Oncologist had given her only a few months to live. When she showed up at his office twelve months later, diagnostics revealed that the tumor had completely disappeared (463). LeBeau describes another case where a cancer patient was able to shrink a tumor by "mixing 1 part of 35% H2O2 with 5 parts of aloe and applying it directly on the tumor" topically, and he discusses a patient from Ohio who said that she was able to heal her *rheumatoid arthritis* by applying hydrogen peroxide ***externally*** (463). She had been fighting the arthritis for nearly two decades. In a fourth case study, another patient used "Peroxy Gel" to heal herself of *breast cancer* (463). This too was topical, NOT internal! Never take peroxide internally unless you are ordering or purchasing a type of peroxide that is manufactured and sold for oral consumption. If so, it should be clearly stated on the label as **food-grade**.

## Hyperbaric Oxygen Therapy

Hyperbaric oxygen therapy is used to increase oxygen levels in the body. It is often resorted to in cases of severe oxygen deprivation (e.g., *strokes*), and is also finding popularity as an alternative cancer therapy. Orthodox medicine uses hyperbaric oxygen therapy extensively. It is often prescribed after delicate microsurgery for increasing cellular oxygen in cases where fingers or entire limbs have been re-attached after traumatic injuries. (It was not unusual for my patients to receive hyperbaric oxygen therapy when I worked on a hospital surgical floor, and this was several years ago.) In getting more oxygen to your cells, remember that you need FRESH AIR every day. Cancer cells grow faster in stale air.

## Exercise & Cancer

One of the quickest ways to oxygenate your body is with regular exercise. Studies have shown that exercise on a regular basis (at least 30 minutes three to four times per week) greatly reduces the risk of all types of cancer.

Exercise need not be exhausting in order for you to benefit. For example, as described by Valerie Saxion, author of *How To Feel Great All The Time,* walking fast for half-an-hour will accomplish the same thing for you that "15-20 minutes of jogging" will do (555). Research involving 17,000 **human** participants revealed that you can increase your *life expectancy* with exercise; however, pushing yourself to exercise to the point of burning "more than…3,500 calories per week" was described as, "counterproductive" (555), though there is disagreement among professionals about exactly how much time you should spend on weekly exercise. Scientists have found a relationship between routine exercise and cancer prevention. A survey resulting from two decades of data revealed that colon cancer can be prevented with routine exercise. Merely riding a bike or taking walks every day can cut the risk of colon cancer in half. A womens' study also confirmed that regular physical exercise can prevent breast and uterine cancers. The more exercise the women undertook, the least likely they were to develop cancer.

## Adequate Rest Keeps the Immune System Healthy

If you are not getting adequate rest at night, you may be doing significant damage to your immune system. Insuring that you get adequate amounts of sleep can slash your cancer risk. Most of us need about eight hours of sleep every night. A very important hormone is produced by the body during sleep, known as *melatonin.* It is very crucial in regulating the body's rest, sleep cycles (552). It is produced when you are asleep and while it is dark. Levels decrease during the day (552). Because of this wake-sleep melatonin cycle, and the way growth hormone is released in the body, it is most important to get several hours of sleep before midnight. Going to bed at nine pm and rising at five am is much healthier for you than staying up until midnight and getting up at eight am, where all of your sleep hours occur after midnight. (Note that some people require 8-9 hours of sleep every night, rather than the usual 7-8. If you require much more than that, you are either a teenager or pregnant; an infant or young child; breast-feeding; 85-years-old; the parents of a newborn; or you may have a medical problem.)

The only time that human growth hormone (HGH) is produced is when your sleep is at its *deepest* level. You need HGH since it helps your body fight stress and programs how all the other hormones in your body will function. Failure to get adequate rest at night will rob you of much needed HGH (and melatonin), and eventually your overall health will suffer (552).

It is not unusual for physicians, lab techs, nurses, and other health care workers (and industrial workers) who do swing-shifts, to have problems later in life with insomnia when they try to revert to sleeping at night, rather than in the daytime. Many of them don't realize, at the time, that working these odd hours can cause them problems years later when they try to readjust their sleep pattern for nighttime hours. (This has happened to me, even years after working hospital evening and night shifts.) And beware, if you work midnights while you are pregnant, your newborn will keep the same hours!

## Sufficient Sunlight Prevents Cancer

Everyone has been so brain-washed by the health community and news media that sunlight is so bad for you, that there are even cases arising of children with ricketts, a disease where the bones are soft and malformed from vitamin D deficiencies. This is a disease that we thought had long ago vanished in America. What is happening? Parents are over-reacting to the hype about skin cancers and the sun, bundling their children up against **all sunshine exposure**, slathering them with globs of sunscreen and sending them outside to play. Since the best source of **natural**

**vitamin D is SUNSHINE**, children are sometimes suffering from vitamin D deficiencies from not getting adequate sun exposure. When sunshine hits the skin, a chemical reaction occurs that creates natural vitamin D in our bodies. People who live in northern states often have problems with vitamin D deficiencies (more so than those living in the south) because of less sun exposure in colder climates.

Many health articles and physicians (e.g., Dr. Joseph Mercola, author of the *Total Health Programs*—website: *www.mercola.com),* are reporting that inadequate sunlight is putting us at increased risk for cancer (484). A study in the journal, *Cancer,* supports this belief. Researchers found that those suffering from low levels of ultraviolet B-light were more likely to die from cancer (484). It is believed that the body needs ultraviolet B-light in order to produce vitamin D (484). The author of the study, Dr. William Grant, is concerned that people in northern climates (who experience longer winters) may have no opportunity at all for *vitamin D synthesis* (484). The study also found that people with darker skin require as much as "10-20 times" more sunlight for adequate amounts of vitamin D synthesis as those with lighter skin (484). There were 13 different malignant cancers that were affected by this sunlight phenomenon, but the ones most affected were: "breast, colon, and ovarian cancer" (484). Others included: "tumors of the bladder, uterus, esophagus, rectum, and stomach" (484).

Dr. Mercola believes that skin cancers could be linked to an excessive consumption of the "omega-6 fats", which increase cancer risk during excess sun exposure. He says that we can stay out of the sun to cut skin cancer, but in so doing, we run a greater risk for cancers that can be much more lethal (484).

Perhaps you are thinking you will just get your vitamin D from milk and supplements. After all, we see commercials about milk and its vitamin D content plastered everywhere to make us **think** that milk is actually good for us, right? As described in H. Winter Griffith's, *Vitamins, Herbs, Minerals & Supplements,* the vitamin D you find in milk and vitamin supplements is "synthetic…D2...also called *ergocalciferol,*" and it's a poor substitute for the one that comes from natural sunlight "or natural food sources…vitamin D3 or *calciferol*" (411). Other sources of vitamin D (besides sunlight) are: "…Egg substitutes…Herring, Mackerel, Salmon, Sardines… [and] Tuna…" (411). Mushrooms also have vitamin D.

There is no way that mankind, hard as he tries, can improve on what our great Creator God has given us in its natural state. Vitamin D from natural sunshine is one of God's many gifts to us, intended for our well-being. As with any good thing, over-exposure can be harmful.

As described at *www.mercola.com*, vitamin D is critical in promoting supplies of minerals like phosphorus and calcium (484). One reason for the rampant osteoporosis in this country, is because people are not getting adequate vitamin D from sunshine. It regulates our body's absorption of calcium, assisting with the maintenance of a strong skeletal system. Taking all the calcium supplements in the world will not help you if you are deficient in vitamin D. Vitamin D is fat soluble, meaning it can be stored in the body, so overdosing with synthetic forms can be dangerous. This is another reason why getting vitamin D through sunlight (rather than taking supplements) is preferred (484), if you are not at a risk for melanoma. (Also, see p. 498 for information on **ipriflavone**.)

Some researchers believe that Caucasians need at least five to ten minutes of sunlight (without sunscreen) twice or thrice weekly in order to get sufficient vitamin D levels (540). A study revealed that 23,000 people die from preventable cancers every year—preventable by adequate amounts of vitamin D—and this statistic may be much higher (540). One physician in particular, estimated that (in the UK) at least a fourth of those who die from cancer of the breast, do so because they had insufficient amounts of vitamin D, which caused the breast cancer (540). Some sources recommend ten to twenty minutes a day (without sunscreen) for sunshine exposure.

Just consider someone you know that may be elderly, or live in a northern climate with very short summers. How much sunshine are they exposed to every day? What about those who spend their time in nursing homes and assisted-living centers? How much sunshine do you think they get every day—if any—or fresh air?

Professor Holick and his colleagues discovered that there is an essential substance within our colon which helps in the "processing of vitamin D," which also fights colon cancer, thus the reason why vitamin D deficiencies will lead to colon cancer (540).

Sunshine has been proven to boost the immune system, lower blood pressure, and relax the body. Have you had **your** dose of sunshine today? What about fresh air (oxygen) and exercise?

# CHAPTER 25

# CURING WITH SOME AMAZING MUSHROOMS

*"From the end of the earth will I cry unto thee, when my heart is overwhelmed: lead me to the rock that is higher than I." (Psalm 61:2)*

Several different mushroom varieties have already been discussed in this book. There are many others, barely mentioned, with amazing healing properties. This chapter is devoted to some of those. (It is important to note that the only vegetables that contain natural vitamin D are mushrooms!)

## Agaricus Blazeil Murill

Agaricus mushroom (also known as the *himematsukake* mushroom) is described at website: *www.mnwelldir.org/docs/Newsletters/01_Aug.htm*, as "The most powerful chemotherapy in Japan today." According to them, the healing properties of this Brazilian mushroom are amazing, and known for curing many deadly cancers (10). One health provider in Brazil was so impressed with the healing results of the agaricus, that he invited people from anywhere in the world to come stay with him, at his expense, and witness for themselves the curing properties of this mushroom (10). He had very few who took him up on his offer. Apparently, when researchers visited the province where this mushroom grew, they found that the people who lived in the area were free of disease, many of them living over a century. Since that time, it has been discovered that a substance found in this mushroom is "effective against Ehrlich's ascites carcinoma, sigmoid colonic cancer, ovarian cancer, breast cancer, lung cancer and liver cancer as well as against solid cancers" (11).

The School of Medicine at Ehime University in Japan discovered, in animal testing, that ABM (Agaricus Blazei Murill) mushroom can help prevent and fight cancer even when the animals were given LLC or *Lewis Lung Carcinoma* cells (447). Not only did the mushroom prevent the growth of tumors, but metastases as well. The report also showed that the mushroom increased the numbers of *natural killer cells* in the immune system (447). The substance that was extracted from the Agaricus mushroom was *sodium pyroglutamate* (447). There are many websites that provide agaricus or ABM mushroom—some in dried form—some fresh. Also included in fighting cancer are the reishi, mesima, chaga, tinder polypore, and split-gill mushroom (15).

If you need these mushrooms fast, at the very best prices, check website: *www.mitobi.com.* This mushroom is introduced into cooking much like any other type of mushroom. *Wellness Directory of Minnesota*™ website recommends taking vitamin C with your mushroom supplements for better absorption (11). Mushrooms are the only vegetables that contain natural vitamin D.

## Cordyceps Sinensis

Cordyceps sinensis is considered by Chinese medicine experts as their most valuable, powerful mushroom (583). Kate Gilbert Udall in her book, *Cordyceps Sinensis,* says of this mushroom: "It has been helpful in curing asthma and other respiratory ailments" (583). An extract from this fungi, known as *cordycepin* (in a 1989 study), was helpful at fighting HIV. Cordyceps sinensis, says Ms. Udall, can help stop the division of cancer cells and strengthen the immunity (583). Note that the common table spice, turmeric, also inhibits HIV. (You will find more curcumin in turmeric than you will in curry powder. Use organic turmeric rather than curry.)

## Coriolus Versicolor (Karawatake) Mushroom

An important cancer-fighting extract comes from this mushroom, called *PSK,* discussed earlier. This derivative may help extend the lives of those fighting gastric, intestinal, and lung cancers (211). Also, lab studies show that coriolus versicolor can help fight HIV. Further testing is needed to see if it will function the same way in humans. When these mushrooms were used to fight cancer in humans, there were no adverse *effects* (211). Be sure if using coriolus, you use the heat-extracted form. (However, as noted earlier, agaricus appears to be more potent than PSK – try both!)

## Enoki

Research from Japan showed that people consuming enoki mushrooms could reduce cancer risk by 40% (301). You can often purchase fresh enoki in health food stores.

## Hoelen

This mushroom, known as *hoelen (Poria cocos),* can be found underneath some types of tree roots. According to an article at *herbs2000.com,* they are sometimes used in a form of bread known as *tuckahoe bread* (156). They are high in potassium and have been used for the regulation of *blood sugar,* hydrochloric acid, and *kidney* problems (156). An ingredient in this mushroom (*poriatrin*) appears to be helpful for patients struggling with *kidney disease* caused by *lupus.* Best results are obtained from actually ingesting the mushroom, rather than relying on extracts (156).

## Kombucha

You may have tasted kombucha tea, but it's not from a mushroom. *Kombucha* isn't exactly a mushroom. According to *www.drlam.com*, it is actually a "group of yeasts (simple fungi) and bacteria," but it contains many similar substances that heal the body, like those found in mushrooms (461). Kombucha boosts the immune system by increasing the body's amount of *interferon* (461).

## Maitake

Dr. Ralph Moss, author of *Cancer Therapy*, says that maitake mushrooms have successfully halted cancers in animal tests. In one study in particular, ten mice were fed the powdered form of the mushroom for "one month after tumors had been implanted," and 40% of the mice were cured. For the others on the mushroom, tumors decreased *86.3%* (504).

In his book, *Alternative Cures*, Bill Gottlieb says forget the *chicken soup*, because these mushrooms outperform the soup when it comes to combating the common cold (409).

Maitake D-fraction and *beta-glucan* are discussed in other cancer-specific chapters of this book for their ability at reducing the size of tumors in animal tests, and human usage. Most nutritionists recommend cooking mushrooms, because, as noted by Selene Yeager in *Doctors Book of FOOD REMEDIES*, there are *toxins* in the raw fungi that are destroyed at high temperatures (604). Maitake should not be taken by those with *multiple sclerosis.* It can increase a substance that destroys nerve tissue in people with MS (184). Remember to see information elsewhere in my book about newly discovered studies showing that MS may be caused by severe vitamin D deficiencies!

## Morels

Morel mushrooms, in animal testing, not only fought inflammation, but was comparable to the drug *Diclofenac* (an NSAID). The extract was also very potent in fighting tumor cells (516).

## Oyster Mushrooms Versus Shiitake

Oyster mushrooms demonstrated a remarkable ability at halting tumor growth in animals, especially colon and breast cancer cells; however, shiitake appears to be even more potent than oyster mushrooms (508). Extracts from shiitake resulted in even better results. The power of the mushrooms came from complex sugar substances extracted from them (508). Eat both for best results!

## Polyporus Umbellatus

This immune-boosting mushroom is one of ten mushrooms found in Garden of Life's RM-10 product developed by Jordan Rubin (317). His 80-year-old grandmother used the product to heal her advanced ovarian cancer. See chapter seven and website: *http://www.crohns.net/Miva/education n/testimonial_rosemenlowe.shtml* (30). This mushroom, in a test involving 146 **human** participants, reduced by half the reoccurrence of bladder cancer (317). It has also been helpful for those with urinary tract infections, and may help stop the spread of leukemia (317). For information and resources where you can obtain RM-10, see website: *http: //www.crohns.net/Miva/productinfo/whatsin*RM*10.shtml* (317).

## Reishi Mushroom

According to Deanne Tenney, author of *Medicinal Mushrooms*, the reishi mushroom *(Ganoderma lucidum)* comes in several types, each one being a different color. They are "Akashiba (red reishi), Kuroshiba (black reishi), Aoshiba (blue reishi), Shiroshiba (white reishi), Kishiba (yellow reishi), and Murasakishiba (purple reishi)" (576). Studies from Moscow's *Cancer Research Center* prove that this mushroom can enhance immunity and halt tumor progression (576).

Dr. Earl Mindell, popular nutrition author, says that Reishi in Japan is known as *kisshotake* or the *lucky fungus*, and that compounds in reishi boost the immune system, fight dangerous fats and clots in the blood, and act as *antihistamines* (495). As discovered by one researcher, you can greatly enhance the *cancer-fighting* properties of this mushroom by taking it with *vitamin C* (461). Be aware that reishi has blood-thinning abilities. Some people are allergic to mushrooms. Several people have had severe reactions to matsuka mushroom and others.

## Shiitake & Immunity

Shiitake mushroom, already mentioned earlier, increases *interferon* in the body, and helps the body fight cancer. **Human testing** has been done in China on those with leukemia and in Japan on *breast cancer*, using shiitake. The mushroom can also lower blood cholesterol (363). An extract from shiitake, *lentinan,* has been very popular in fighting cancer (604). Scientists discovered that this shiitake extract, in animal testing, halted tumors by *67%* (604). It was during the 1980s that researchers from Japan discovered, in animal testing, that shiitake could stop liver cancer (504). Lentinan injections are discussed in other cancer-specific chapters of this book, and are often given by alternative health physicians.

## Suehirotake & Yamabushiitake Mushrooms

Extracts from suehirotake mushroom (e.g., SPG) are being studied for their effects in fighting cancer, as well as chronic fatigue syndrome. See Chapter 34 for information on MGN-3, which contains several mushrooms, including suehirotake. Yamabushiitake (Lion's Mane mushroom) is also being studied for its potential at stopping the onset of senile dementia.

## Wood Ear Mushrooms

Evidence points to this mushroom, the wood ear or *tree ear,* as having the ability to fight cancer. As with many other mushrooms, this one has a blood-thinning effect, which can help in preventing strokes and cardiovascular ailments. The oyster and enoki mushroom also provide this benefit (202). One must really LIKE this mushroom to eat it. The texture (and taste) is like chewing plastic!

## Yun Zhi Mushroom

Also known as the *zhi,* and/or the *Cloud Mushroom*, yun zhi has been popular in folk medicine for liver ailments, general immunity and energy (438). Studies have shown that *polysaccharides* in this mushroom can increase *white blood cells* in the body, which boosts the immunity (438).

## Zhu Ling, Chicken-of-the-Woods, Enokitake, Mesima, Chaga, Ice Man, Agarikon, Conk, Polypore & Pearl Oyster (Hiratake)

These are other medicinal mushrooms you will see in supplement form that have anti-oxidant, anti-cancer, or anti-viral properties. A few of these are noted above, and are mentioned elsewhere in this chapter and this book. Keep in mind that some mushrooms are called by half-a-dozen different names!

Also, see supplements made by New Chapter®, such as their multiple-mushroom compound called *Host Defense*®, which contains 17 different mushrooms. You can find this brand in health food stores and it is available at their internet site: *http://www.newchapter.com/products/host-defense.* I have also discussed other mushroom supplements in this book.

# CHAPTER 26

# WHAT HAPPENED WITH DAIRY?

*"Beloved, I wish above all things that thou mayest prosper and be in health, even as thy soul prospereth." (III John:2)*

## Are the Risks Worth That Dose of Calcium?

Our culture has been so brainwashed by the media into believing that drinking milk is absolutely essential to strong bones and teeth, most parents are shocked when they are told that cow's milk is actually for baby cows (CALVES), not humans. Though humans do need some calcium, there is controversy about the amounts actually needed and the best sources. "But, doctor, what will happen to my teeth and bones if I stop drinking milk?" is a question asked of Dr. Frank A. Oski in his book, *Don't Drink Your Milk!* His reply? "Nothing. Nothing that wouldn't have happened anyway" (522).

Do you realize that you can get your daily calcium needs from the same place the cows and goats get it? From the soil, via green foods. Food sources of calcium listed by Dr. Oski include: "collards…turnips…rhubarb…kidney beans, broccoli, soybeans, almonds" (522), carrots, and just about any GREEN food you can think of. Wheat grass, barley grass, kale, sprouts, spinach, chlorella, dandelion greens, and celery all have calcium. After all, what do cows, goats, and sheep eat all day? Green foods mostly, that is, if they are left to their choice of grazing out in a field as our Creator intended. Have you ever known of a cow with osteoporosis, brittle bone disease, or heart disease?! (On the other hand, if you really want to foul things up—something we humans are so-o-o good at—just grind up some dead animal parts, add that to the grain you feed your cows, and give them **mad cow disease**, or start manipulating the genes in plants (genetically-modified foods), until you have a world-wide disaster on your hands, but that's another story!

Other excellent sources of calcium, as described by H. Winter Griffith in *Vitamins, Herbs, Minerals & Supplements* are: "Almonds, Brazil nuts…Kelp…[and] Sardines…" (411). Salmon is also high in calcium. Realize that you don't need milk or meats to get your calcium. As noted by Deborah Lee in *Juicing: Your Liquid Nutritional Supplement,* an eight ounce glass of carrot juice will give you more than twice the calcium of the same amount of milk. Besides that, you also get a huge dose of beta-carotene that is much healthier than all those hormones in the milk, given to the cows to increase milk output (464).

If you still aren't convinced that milk is NOT the place to get your calcium, a research study by Harvard (involving 80,000 nurses) showed that consuming milk—the kind you find in your local grocers—raised their incidence for bone fractures (248). Not only that, but evidence showed that drinking milk could increase the incidence of rheumatoid arthritis, multiple sclerosis, and cancer (248). Also, see p. 488.

When an investigation by the *Consumers Union* was done to evaluate milk for "taste, bacterial contamination, and undesirable additives…Their findings should frighten even the milkaholics away from their local dairy bars" (522). Dr. Frank A. Oski, M.D., summarized those findings in his book, *Don't Drink Your Milk!* when he said: "Not only is there very little evidence that cow milk is of nutritional benefit to humans, but it…may be contaminated with bacteria, and can contain substances that are actually hazardous to your health" (522).

Many people think (erroneously) that cow's milk is *sterile* due to the pasteurization process. Nothing could be further from the truth. Even disease-free cows will have *some bacteria*, says Dr. Oski. This comes from *fecal material* that ends up on the cow and goes into the milk. Farmers know this; they are around cows all the time, so they know about cleaning off the cow in preparation for milking in order to remove any traces of fecal matter (522). Are they doing this efficiently? Most of them probably are, but if so, WHERE is all that bacteria coming from? According to the U.S. government, explains Dr. Oski, once milk has been pasteurized, it "should contain no more than 20,000 bacteria per milliliter of milk and no more than ten organisms of the coliform species in each milliliter. (…there are 5 milliliters in a teaspoon…)" (522). Do the math—that comes out to **100,000 bacteria allowed in every teaspoon of milk that you drink.** (I don't know about you, but I think that's a pretty hefty dose of allowable ***bugs!***) So you see, it isn't expected that the milk will be sterile after pasteurization, just that the contamination by bacteria will be at an acceptable level. (Does the word *acceptable* sound familiar by now?) Of course, if the milk isn't kept cold, the bacteria begin to multiply like mad. Dr. Oski reveals that the investigators from the *Consumer's Union* discovered that many of the *samples* contained 130,000 bacteria "per milliliter. One sample had almost 3 million and some had too many to count" (522). Of even greater concern perhaps, was that some of the milk samples tested also had *pesticides* and other harmful toxins; however, realize that "The FDA operates on the notion that a little bit of cancer-producing material won't hurt you" (522). (You do remember the FDA, don't you—from chapter two? You know—that august, designated, staunch, elite government body that is concerned with your welfare, right?)

What did the *Consumers Union* testers have to say about all of this? Dr. Oski summarized their findings: "The Consumers Union expert milk consultant 'considers the milk supply throughout the five-state Midwestern area covered in our tests to pose a potential hazard'" (522). Now **that** should greatly enhance your ability to sleep well tonight—along with that warm glass of milk—right?

## Milk to Die for

One scientist in particular, after being diagnosed with breast cancer, going through chemo, then having it return, found that her cancer completely disappeared when she finally eliminated all dairy products from her diet.

Dr. John R. Lee, et al., in the book, *What Your Doctor May Not Tell You About Breast Cancer*, attributed the hormone given to cows to raise milk production *(rBGH)* as a possible culprit in cancers of the breast, because it causes a rapid rise in IGF-1 growth factor (465). And if that isn't scary enough, if you are a woman, dairy products can also increase your risk of ovarian cancer (551). Dr. Daniel W. Kramer, from Harvard Medical School, rates the type of sugar *(galactose)* found in milk "with an increased risk of ovarian cancer" (551). He wasn't the only one concerned. According to website, *http://www.hsialert.com,* scientists from Stockholm, Sweden, were also suspicious of a connection between milk consumption and ovarian cancer. They studied medical histories of more than **sixty thousand women**, "aged 38 to 76 years who were cancer-free at the outset of the study" (176). They followed the participants for more than a decade. During that time, "more than 260...were diagnosed with epithelial ovarian cancer, and 125 of those cases were considered 'serious'" (176). After compiling all their information, they concluded from their study that milk sugar intake (lactose) was associated with dramatic increases in ovarian cancer (176). Which dairy product posed the greatest risk? MILK! You've seen the ads—you know—the kids (and adults) wearing the cute, little milk mustache? Health Sciences Institute prefaced the above article on their webpage with the title: "One dangerous moustache" (176). As for the cases being considered *serious*, I believe any woman with this diagnosis would consider it *serious*.

Realize that the synthetic vitamin D that is added to milk, is actually nothing more than a hormone, which prevents maximum use of magnesium by the body (15). The majority of the people on this planet are located near the equator. This is an area with a warm climate where people harvest living plants twelve months a year, and they do not consume milk from dairy cows. Most of them have healthier *bones* than people in the more developed countries (466). Not only that, but the now former U.S. Surgeon General, C. Everett Koop, M.D., once told the world: "'Dairy products are bad for you'" (503). **(Why has no one LISTENED to him?)**

## The Calcium Myth

According to Deborah Lee, author of *Juicing: Your Liquid Nutritional Supplement*, don't look to milk for a *perfect food*, it's not. She says that most people have been taught throughout their lives that you need milk for calcium, however, it is not the best source of calcium. As she notes, "Heavy metals, detergents, antibiotics, viruses, and other toxins have been found in milk" (464). Even though we need minerals like calcium for our bones, there is a large imbalance in the proportion of calcium to phosphorus in cow's milk. This unbalanced ratio results in calcium being removed from the bones, increasing the risk for *osteoporosis* (464). In a nutshell, **cow's milk does NOT prevent osteoporosis, and may even cause it!** Ms. Lee also reports that large amounts of an enzyme responsible for heart disease, known as *xanthine oxidase,* is found in your supermarket milk. Homogenization makes it possible for this enzyme to be "absorbed through the" gut and this is what damages arterial walls, leading to coronary artery disease (464).

## Dairy (Milk) Likely Culprit in Causing Acne

The *Journal of American Academy of Dermatology* studied more than 47,000 women and discovered a definite correlation between milk consumption and acne, which they attributed to the hormones in milk, as well as the insulin-like growth factor given to cattle, and the iodine that farmers feed their cows to decrease infections (88).

## How Not To Give Your Child Juvenile Diabetes, Leukemia, Lymphoma, or Multiple Sclerosis

Besides the obvious link to breast cancer, noted above, cow's milk has also been singled out as a potential culprit in the rising statistics of juvenile diabetes in the U.S. Dr. R. M. Kradjian, in a report at *www.notmilk.com*, says that researchers believe that during the "first year of life," infants produce "antibodies…against the milk protein" in cow's milk. Since the milk protein is very similar to the protein in the pancreas cells that produce insulin, those same antibodies that the child has made, attack the pancreas cells, resulting in juvenile or Type I diabetes (452). Do the facts support the theory? YES! Did you know that the biggest consumer of *dairy* in the world is the country of Finland, and they also have the **"world's highest rate of insulin dependent diabetes"** (452). As Dr. Kradjian further notes, Finnish scientists followed '"142 Finnish children with newly diagnosed diabetes. They found that every one had at least eight times as many antibodies against the milk protein as did healthy children, clear evidence that the children had a raging auto-immune disorder"' (452).

Burt Berkson, M.D., Ph.D., author of *The Alpha Lipoic Acid Breakthrough,* agrees that there are problems associated with milk and diabetes, and that nations with higher milk consumption also have more cases of diabetes, both type I and type II (344). He also notes that eating healthy (especially vegetarian diets) can help protect against type II diabetes (344). Dr. Berkson recommends that anyone with diabetes avoid dairy products. (From what I have read, you should be avoiding them to prevent getting diabetes in the first place. Once you already have diabetes, is it then too late?)

Still unconvinced that milk is not for children, or adults for that matter? According to Gabe Mirkin, M.D., at *www.drmirkin.com*, "In Puerto Rico, almost all babies get cow's milk. In Cuba, almost all babies are breast fed. Puerto Rican babies are **10 times more likely to suffer juvenile diabetes,"** than babies in Cuba (Emphasis mine) (498). Now, it doesn't take a rocket scientist to add two and two together to get the big picture here, does it?

This is human babies we are discussing, not animal studies; however, Dr. Mirkin says that even animal testing bears this out: "Among animals bred to develop diabetes, infant animals given cow's milk have a much higher incidence of diabetes" (498). The only exception was baby calves fed raw, unprocessed, unpasteurized milk from their mother cow, but then again, baby calves are supposed to drink cow's milk!

Are you aware that the virus that is responsible for *bovine leukemia* turns up in "more than three of five dairy cows in the United States? Dr. Kradijian explains that this involves about 90% of dairy herds" (452). He says that random sampling showed that "the bovine leukemia virus was recovered from two-thirds" of the raw milk (452). Do the statistics show that states having the highest incidence of leukemia in humans also have the highest incidence of bovine leukemia? Yes. These states in the U.S. are: "Iowa, Nebraska, South Dakota, Minnesota and Wisconsin." It is also true, says Dr. Kradijian, that leukemia statistics are higher in *dairy farmers* (452).

Not only may cow's milk promote juvenile diabetes, but according to Dr. Russell Blaylock, author of *Natural Strategies For Cancer Patients*, milk often contains *leukemia and lymphoma* viruses (351). In the U.S. alone, more than half of the dairy cows tested were positive. Research has even shown a statistical rise of ALL (*acute lymphoid leukemia*) in human populations where the herds are also highly infectious (351). Even though *pasteurization* is supposed to destroy many of these viruses, Dr. Blaylock emphasizes that the milk will still contain a large amount of *white blood cells,* and it is these cells that the viruses live within (351). He even advises mothers against drinking milk while they are pregnant, since they can transfer these viruses to their baby (351). (Ever wonder about the rising statistics of young children developing leukemia and lymphoma? Why are so many **very young children** coming down with leukemia and type I diabetes? I know of parents who have to give insulin to babies and toddlers.)

When researchers followed more than a thousand participants for over a decade in Norway, Dr. Kradjian says the results revealed that consumers of "2 or more glasses of milk per day had 3.5 times the incidence of cancer of the lymphatic organs" (452).

It isn't just diabetes, T.B., leukemia, and lymphoma that we need to be concerned about. As noted at website: *http://ezinearticles.com/?6-Risk-Factors-for-Multiple-Sclerosis&id=782577* (and many other articles), giving your infant cow's milk may increase their risk for multiple sclerosis (412).

For you moms-to-be, new research shows that getting adequate sunshine while you are pregnant (for vitamin D production in the skin), may also help prevent your child from developing multiple sclerosis (310). (Also, see elsewhere in this book for new studies which show that MS may be caused by severe deficiencies in vitamin D.)

## To Homogenize or Not to Homogenize

Many people are unable to digest the lactose sugar found in milk. There are entire ethnic populations that are born with lactose-intolerance, however, this intolerance isn't the major problem. Besides killing pathogens (something it is supposed to do), homogenization and pasteurization of milk may have some very undesirable effects most of us are not aware of. Retired veterinarian, Earl D. Smith, D.V.M., discovered, to his horror, that when he tried to use pasteurized, homogenized milk for his baby calves, they died from diarrhea. Turns out that the baby calves could not digest the processed milk. Rather than *curding* in the gastric juices as their mother's milk did, the milk went into their intestines very quickly, causing what Dr. Smith diagnosed as *toxic enteritis* (568). Dr. Smith learned to counter the problem by providing the baby calves (without feeder cows) goat's milk. Goat's milk forms a larger *fat globule* that does not pass as rapidly into the intestines, thereby eliminating the enteritis and saving the baby calves (568).

Dr. Smith also discovered that when drinking raw milk on his farm, he had no problems, but after going off to college and using processed milk that he bought in the local supermarket, he developed severe systemic problems. He has had no such problems with raw, unpasteurized, unhomogenized milk (568). Naturopathic physician, Dr. Robert Morse agrees with Dr. Smith. He writes in his book, *The Detox Miracle Sourcebook*: "What happens to a baby calf if you feed it pasteurized milk instead of its fresh, raw mother's milk? It dies" (503). Ask yourself this question: **if pasteurized, homogenized milk kills baby calves when they drink it, what in the world are we doing giving it to our children to drink?**

## What About Unpasteurized & Unhomogenized (Raw) Milk?

Raw, unprocessed milk from healthy cows is probably your best bet if you want to ingest milk. The only way to get it in the U.S. is to live near an organic farmer who practices meticulous farming, has disease-free cows, and can sell you raw milk that is free of bacteria. Since cattle can carry lymphomas and mylomas, as well as leukemia, you must verify that the herd is disease-free. Raw milk is growing very popular in the UK where it is much easier to purchase. It does have more of the omega-3 fats that have not yet been destroyed by heat treatment. Those who drink raw milk will usually find that they have no lactose-intolerance, because raw milk contains the enzymes that are needed to digest it—enzymes which are destroyed in pasteurization and homogenization, and raw milk is alkaline.

Raw milk does have some of the *good* bacteria (such as acidophilus and lactobacillus) needed for healthy intestines. It also does not contain synthetic vitamin D which is found in pasteurized and homogenized milk. The synthetic form is put in milk after it is processed, yet it is a type of Vitamin D that can be toxic to the liver! (Your best source of Vitamin D is natural sunlight.) Raw milk also contains a natural butterfat that has one of the best sources of naturally-occurring *Vitamin A* (248a).

Can you see why people living three-hundred years ago did not have the health issues we face today? Their food was natural. They did not have to be concerned about herbicides, pesticides, hormones, and other poisons in their water and food supply. They ingested unpasteurized and unhomogenized goat and cow's milk and dairy products from raw milk, and their crops were toxin-free and genetically pure.

## The Mucus Myth

Dr. Robert Morse also attributes much of the upper respiratory ailments we suffer to dairy products, due to the fact that they cause the body to produce excess mucus, resulting in respiratory problems, tonsillitis, influenza, constipation, and possible other health issues (503). Are your kids plagued with constant ear infections, colds, sore throats, tonsillitis, and sinusitis? You may be able to rid them of these type problems, simply by taking them off all milk and dairy products.

Dr. Don Colbert, M.D., in his book, *What You Don't Know May Be Killing You*, agrees that dairy products cause many childhood ailments. As soon as he takes his young patients off dairy, their upper respiratory disorders and other conditions often disappear (373). He also reminds us that no other *species* consumes milk when they are full-grown, except for humans (373). Do you have children getting tubes in their ears because they have incessant ear infections and are plagued with colds and tonsillitis? Try taking all dairy products out of their diet. Ask their pediatrician about substituting organic rice milk. There is so much controversy about soy, you may want to consider eliminating soy from your diet, though fermented soy is fine.

Cooking milk, heating it in the pasteurization, homogenization process, also raises acidity and reduces alkalinity, which can cause kidney stones, gastric irritation, and *muscular weakness,* as well as many other health disorders (373). Milk is naturally alkaline until it is heated!

## Pass Me the Hormones n' Cream, Please

Dr. Gary Null believes that it is best to avoid dairy products completely if you want to cut your risk of disease. In his book, *The Complete Encyclopedia of Natural Healing,* he explains another risk in drinking milk, one that women in particular should be concerned about: cattle are injected with estrogen pellets. Estrogen causes the dairy herds to increase their milk production and weight. He believes that this may account for the dramatic difference in breast cancer rates between U.S. women and those in Japan. Milk simply is not a major component of the diet in Japan. Not only that, but he says milk has toxins (e.g., dioxin), as reported by the Environmental Protection Agency, which can cause birth defects, cancers, immune disorders, and fertility issues (519).

Neither are excessive amounts of hormones healthy for men. Dairy products have been linked to prostate cancer. If you are wondering about the addition of hormones (found in cow's milk) consider this note in *The Milk Letter: A Message To My Patients,* from Dr. Robert M. Kradjian, M.D., at website *www.notmilk.com:* "Fifty years ago an average cow produced 2,000 pounds of milk per year. Today the top producers give 50,000 pounds! How was this accomplished? Drugs, antibiotics, hormones, forced feeding plans and specialized breeding; that's how" (452).

## Who Put the Hormones in the Milk Supply?

If you want to see a video of the hypocrisy of Monsanto's activities in their genetically-modified foods, as well as the creation and addition of growth hormone to cow's milk (along with the blatant lies and coverup by the FDA, and how many top government officials and FDA officials were in Monsanto's revolving door employment), you will want to see the video for yourself at website: *http://www.celsias.com/article/the-world-according-to-monsanto.* Yes, you can thank Monsanto and the U.S. FDA for the hormones in our milk supply. Consumers who do drink milk are getting the picture and demanding hormone-free milk. I saw a recent ad from Wal-Mart where some of their stores are now carrying hormone-free milk. Why aren't all stores demanding hormone-free meats and milk?!

## Mother's Milk

Everyone knows by now that breast feeding provides the best milk for human babies; however, if you are convinced that "mothers' milk is pure," guess again (452). Dr. Kradjian discussed a large study revealing that "human breast milk in over 14,000 women had contamination by pesticides." What was the source of this contamination? "Meat and—you guessed it—dairy products" (452). Interestingly enough, a smaller group study of breast feeding moms who were "vegetarian" revealed 50% less "contamination" levels in their milk (452), but the toxins were still there.

# CHAPTER 27

# ORTHOMOLECULAR MEDICINE, MACRO-BIOTICS, PROBIOTICS, MOLASSES & SEED FOODS

*"Trust in the Lord at all times; ye people, pour out your heart before him: God is a refuge for us. Selah." (Psalm 62:8)*

## Orthomolecular Medicine

Orthomolecular Medicine uses huge doses of vitamins and nutrients to heal the body. This type treatment is responsible for many complete cancer cures, but is not given the publicity that it deserves. Many cancer patients are never informed about this safe, non-toxic, alternative treatment for cancer. Dr. Abram Hoffer, M.D., Ph.D., and Linus Pauling, Ph.D., in their book, *Healing Cancer—Complementary Vitamin & Drug Treatments,* attribute most disease processes to metabolic problems that can usually be overcome via nutritional excellence and supplements, whereas pharmaceutical chemicals are foreign to the body. Drugs basically confuse the body because they are unrecognizable, and the body does not always know what to do with them (433).

I highly recommend *Healing Cancer* for anyone wishing to pursue Orthomolecular Medicine and/or complementary treatments. Dr. Hoffer has authored many books that deal with Orthomolecular Medicine, including: *Putting it All Together: The New Orthomolecular Nutrition, Orthomolecular Treatment for Schizophrenia*, and *Vitamin C & Cancer: Discovery, Recovery, Controversy.*

See chapter ten, earlier in my book, for the case of a lung cancer patient who was cured with Orthomolecular Medicine. Also, see chapter twelve for the story of a patient completely cured of pancreatic cancer using this therapy, as well as chapter sixteen for information on a teenager who was miraculously cured of Hodgkins lymphoma with mega-dose vitamin C therapy. Be aware too, that mega-dose vitamin C therapy has been used successfully in curing polio, shingles, and other diseases. Also, see Dr. Robert F. Cathcart's website at: *www.orthomed.com,* for his opinion on how vitamin C might be useful in treating other deadly immune-threatening diseases and illnesses (e.g., the ebola virus, and West Nile).

Perhaps it might even help in the fight against newer bugs like SARS, Bird Flu, Hanta, Bartonella, and others (e.g., anthrax). See page 544 for information on an amazing new oral form of vitamin C – *Lypo-Spheric*™.

## Macrobiotics

The word *macrobiotic* means *long life*. The macrobiotic diet was popularized by Michio Kushi (504). Cancer and other diseases were basically blamed on the unhealthy *Western diet* and lifestyle, and macrobiotic followers believe that cancer is the body's way of retaliating against errors that we make in our dietary and lifestyle choices (504). Though many people with cancer have claimed that this diet cured them, it is also true that there are some cancers that have a hereditary link.

Lynn Keegan, Ph.D., R.N., author of the book, *Healing Nutrition*, explains that macrobiotics is a combination of "low fat, high…complex carbohydrates and fiber, and nearly cholesterol free…" (443). Those on the diet are basically trying to use the right foods to create a balance essential to the body for good health. Those who follow the diet try to get natural, organic food whenever possible, avoiding refined carbs and dairy (443).

Macrobiotics is also based on Chinese philosophy and harmony within nature. The diet allows many natural grains, fresh vegetables, soups, tofu, certain fish, and some teas. Animal foods are not allowed in the diet, or at least extremely discouraged. Foods should be natural and organic as much as possible. There are reams of books in health food stores on macrobiotics.

Gary Null, Ph.D., in *The Complete Encyclopedia of Natural Healing*, says that advocates of macrobiotics claim that many terminal cancer patients following this diet have gotten well (519). This is understandable, because of the many anti-oxidants provided by this diet. It is also based on a low fat diet which has been linked to lower risk for all cancers. Dr. Null also says that: "Best results with the macrobiotic diet are seen with endocrine-related cancers, such as cancer of the breast, prostate, pancreas, uterus, and ovaries" (519).

As a Christian, I do not support some of the philosophical tenets promoted by those who use macrobiotics, especially oriental astrology, or any type of astrology. I do believe that you must have harmony in your life for healing (see chapter one), but this is not the harmony promoted by Eastern philosophies. It is the harmony that comes from trusting in God (the Lord Jesus Christ), and having the right attitude, proper rest, diet, exercise, fresh air, and a natural concern for others. Just be aware that if you are a Christian, many promotions for oriental diets are steeped with mysticism, astrology, Buddhism, and other "isms" that you may wish to steer clear of.

## Probiotics

You can eat the healthiest foods in the world, but if your intestines are sick and unable to digest and absorb the nutrients from that food, it will do you little good. As described by Dr. Joseph Mercola in, "The Benefits of Probiotics 9/29/04," we humans are host to trillions of bacteria in our intestines that carry out critical bodily functions and are considered helpful or *friendly* (486). These good bacteria should flourish in the intestines, unless they've been zapped with harmful enemies (e.g., antibiotics and processed sugars). As explained by Dr. Mercola, sufficient amounts of these beneficial bacteria in the intestines will help in preventing common health disorders, including bowel diseases and disorders, allergies, vaginal infections, bladder, and ear problems (486). Killing these vital organisms, or keeping the body in a state that prevents their survival, can create havoc. Just restoring the body's natural flora can bring about maximum wellness and banish disorders such as Crohn's disease, ulcerative colitis, and irritable bowel syndrome (IBS). Dr. Mercola has a wide variety of health products available at his website: *www.mercola.com*. His website also markets *Primal Defense*™ probiotics.

If you wish to make your own probiotic cultured cabbage juice, just do an internet search for cultured cabbage juice and you will find several websites with recipes. *Http://www.molocure.com*, of Molo-Cure Research in Florida, developed *A.M.P. Molo-Cure*® "(Aloe Mucilaginous Polysaccharide), a…highly concentrated healing agent extracted from the aloe vera plant," which has helped in the healing of many people with intestinal disorders and other ailments (77). Aloe vera has long been popular as an aid in establishing and maintaining healthy intestinal flora. Be sure to discuss an aloe regimen with your physician, and just be certain that when you purchase aloe vera jel juice, it is cold-pressed. (A raw foods alkaline diet, including green foods, wheat grass juice, barley grass juice, chlorella, and other nutrients promote colon health.)

Diane K. wrote a letter to the manufacturer's of Flor-Essence® Essiac tea that all her husband's worst symptoms of ulcerative colitis, which he had suffered with for several years, disappeared after he began drinking the famous herbal tea (580).

## Molasses

Molasses, particularly blackstrap molasses, is being mentioned here because it is one of the few sweeteners richer in nutrients than it is in calories, and because of its anti-cancer properties. According to Cyril Scott and John Lust, Naturopath, in their book: *Crude Black Molasses, The Natural "Wonder Food,"* A physician known as Dr. Forbes Ross "drew attention to the value of Molasses in connection with cancer…" prior to WW I. It was he who noticed that "workers on sugar-cane plantations who were constantly sucking the crude sugar, seldom if ever were known to suffer from that dread disease [cancer]." He believed that it was due to the high level of "potassium salts in unrefined sugar-cane," and he believed that cancer was primarily due to a potash deficiency (559).

Authors Cyril Scott and John Lust also describe an account of James Persson, over sixty-years-old, from New Zealand, who was incapacitated with a bowel growth, heart disease, bronchial congestion, digestive problems, "pyorrhoea, sinus trouble and weak nerves…" (559). He was also "losing weight, and his hair had turned white" (559). When he discovered that a neighbor of his had been sent home to die with a terminal colon cancer and cured himself completely by drinking crude black molasses, he decided to do the same. As a result, the bowel growth disappeared, along with his other health problems, and he claims that his hair regained its original color (559). The authors of the book also state that many other cases of cancer have been treated and "cured solely by Molasses-therapy," including "growths of the uterus…breast…intestinal growth…[and] numerous cases of growths of the tongue, diagnosed as malignant" (559). Another patient had been diagnosed with breast cancer and was told she was terminal. She began taking molasses and completely recovered, with no reoccurrences (559).

It is recommended that molasses be taken "before meals…one teaspoonful" dissolved in a few ounces of warm water, then add enough "cold water to equal a total of 2/3 cup. Drink it warm. For children, half the dosage" (559). For those with tumors, not only is the molasses taken "during the day [but] last thing at night and on rising," as well (559). There is night and day difference between processed white sugar and molasses. So much so, that processed white sugar is acid-forming, while crude black molasses is alkaline. Besides being high in potassium, this thick-syrupy liquid is high in several other minerals and vitamins (559).

## Seed Foods

Jean Carper, author of *The Food Pharmacy*, reports that substances in seeds can help fight malignant cells, especially those of the intestines and breast (363). Researchers were unable to promote skin cancers in mice, even when they treated their skin with carcinogens, as long as they added *protease inhibitors* as well (363). There are many seed foods: sunflower seeds, grape seeds, poppy seeds, some spices (e.g. dill seed), flaxseed (one of the best), mustard seed, pumpkin seed, coriander, celery seed, onion seed, chia, all manner of sprouted seeds, nuts, and others. Even dried beans are considered seeds. When you eat pomegranate fruit, you are actually eating seeds. Try chia seeds for bowel regularity and omega 3.

## Toxins, Deadly Dentistry & New Liposomal Vitamin C

As noted by Dr. Thomas Levy in his books and in his speech at the *Cancer Control Society* in September 2007, he says that a "root canal is highly toxic," even if you just have one in your mouth. He says that the "root canal treated tooth is the number one…cause of cancer and of heart disease, period" (466b). It is "…the king of toxins," and you simply "cannot overcome, with any degree of vigorous supplementation, the chronic electron-robbing activity of a root canal" (466b).

Dr. Levy describes a new form of vitamin C that is vastly superior to any yet developed, and it is taken orally. It is known as "liposome-encapsulated Vitamin C," and he says that a mere "5-6 grams…is much more effective clinically than 50 grams of vitamin C intravenously" (466b). This is a form of vitamin C that is clinically superior to that given intravenously and is absorbed 100%. He does recommend for those who are ill, it is best to take both the *liposome-encapsulated C* and the intravenous C. Dr. Levy's website is at *http://tomlevy.com* and *www.peakenergy.com.* You can find this new liposome-encapsulated vitamin C at website *livonlabs.com* under the brand ***Lypo-Spheric***™ Vitamin C.

Dr. Levy says that high doses of vitamin C will "neutralize botulism" toxins, "heavy metals," and the toxins found in "snake bites" (466b), and said that he used only "10-12 packets of Liposomal Vitamin C" to cure a woman with hemorrhagic dengue fever (466b). For Dr. Frederick Klenner's clinical guide to vitamin C, see *http://www.seanet.com/~alexs/ascorbate/198x/smith-lh-clinical_guide_1988.htm.* High doses of vitamin C have been used to cure acute viral hepatitis, polio, and many other diseases.

# CHAPTER 28

# FLUSH THE BUGS

*"Seek the Lord, and ye shall live;" (Amos 5:56). "Seek him that made the seven stars and Orion, and turneth the shadow of death into the morning." (Amos 5:8)*

If you still think that your tap water is safe to drink, and you do not believe that getting infested with parasites is very alarming, consider this: several victims of a parasite found in common drinking water lost their kidneys and ended up on the kidney transplant-waiting-list, after the organism attacked and destroyed their kidneys.

## Cancer & the Parasite Connection

If your immune system is sick, it will not be able to fight off parasites, yet there are some physicians who believe that cancer itself may be caused by parasites. The late Dr. Hulda R. Clark, Ph.D., N.D., believed and taught this. In her book, *The Cure For All Cancers,* she believed that cancers are caused by a parasitic fluke within the human intestines, and that killing parasites will kill the cancer (369).

If you are a citizen of the United States or another industrialized nation, you may have been brainwashed into believing that we don't get parasites in the developed nations. This isn't true. Do you own a pet? Do your children keep hamsters for pets? Mice? Guinea pigs? Parrots? Lizards? Fish? Cats? Dogs? If you own a pet, you probably have parasites, plain and simple. Even aquariums contain parasites. You can take your pet to the vet and get shots to fight parasites, but they never get ALL of them, especially if you have animals that run about outdoors (e.g., dogs and cats), or if you work around cattle and poultry. Even indoor cats scratch around in dirty litter boxes that are full of parasites. Raw food, such as undercooked meat, is full of parasites. If those fresh vegetables you are eating have been fertilized with cow manure, and they have not been thoroughly cleaned, they will be full of parasites! (This is one excuse the FDA is giving to take control over the entire food supply by irradiating food! Irradiation of food will ensure that all the enzymes, vitamins, and nutrients in our food are dead before they ever leave the store! This is a great concern! None of the cancer-killing plant enzymes will be left alive when the FDA gets finished. People will get sicker and sicker, having to rely on (you guessed it!) pharmaceutical drugs to stay alive, until these kill them as well! Let your representatives know that you do not want your food irradiated!)

Soft cheeses and processed lunchmeat can also become infected with parasites. If you are eating at a restaurant, the food you eat is only as safe as those who are preparing it. If the workers are not washing their hands, especially after bathroom trips, they could be serving you parasites with dinner. And don't think you are any safer dining at a fancy restaurant as opposed to a fast food joint. Whenever you eat out, you may want to carry a few capsules of milk thistle, cinnamon, garlic, and 3-4 cloves to chew on or some Magnascent iodine drops. This will help, but may not give you a full jump on some bug that you ingest along the way, depending on what it is and how many there are. Some people sip wine with meals, which may help kill parasites; but unfermented grape juice will do this too. Neither one is a total guarantee. Have you or a loved one ever been hospitalized for an ailment such as dehydration from diarrhea? A very common lab test your physician will order is called a test for *O & P*, which stands for *Ova and Parasites!* When your physician orders this test, **he or she is checking you for worms and their eggs.**

According to Dr. Hulda Clark, the intestinal fluke does not cause cancer in the intestines, but if it travels, for example to another organ (e.g., the liver) and burrows in, it causes cancer. As long as it just stays in the intestines, you may end up with an intestinal disorder such as "colitis, Crohn's disease, or irritable bowel syndrome," or you may be unaffected (369).

Dr. Hulda Clark also linked many of our health issues, such as arthritis, cancer, and auto-immune diseases, to the metal dentistry that we allow in our mouths. Have you ever noticed that when you have a mercury filling removed from your mouth, your dentist will very carefully put it in a *hazardous* materials waste box, yet tell you that when it is inside your mouth, not to worry, that it won't harm you? (369). All polymers and metals eventually deteriorate and begin seeping—dental ingredients and appliances are no exception. Not only that, but clostridium bacteria may get into dental fillings and caps (369). If you don't believe this, the next time a cap comes loose from a tooth and you take it back to have it replaced, before you do, have it cultured at a local laboratory. It may be swarming with clostridium bacteria. Because of all the dangerous chemicals that can leach into our bodies from plastic and metal dental fillings and teeth, Dr. Clark believed that we are giving ourselves diseases (like cancer), due to the way that these chemicals suppress our immune system. She suggested that, for anyone who is bound in a wheelchair for disability that has no *reliable diagnosis*, try this: get a dentist who knows what he or she is doing and have all the metal taken out of your mouth (369).

If you are interested in the dangers of metal in dentistry, a very good book on the subject is by Dr. Frank J. Jerome, D.D.S., *Tooth Truth—If You Want to be Healthy Don't Metal With Your Mouth.* Other good books are: *Root Canal Cover-up* by George E. Meinig; *Elements of Danger: Protect Yourself Against the Hazards of Modern Dentistry*, by Morton Walker; and *Dentistry Without Mercury*, by Sam Ziff and Michael F. Ziff, D.D.S. If you ask your dentist not to put a mercury (silver amalgam) filling in your mouth, he or she will usually tell you that it is perfectly safe and harmless, that the mercury is bound up with other chemicals which cannot be broken down, exactly what the dentistry profession has been telling us for years. There are some dentists, however, who are speaking out and telling the truth about these hazards (see the article below).

## FDA Finally Admits That Amalgam (Mercury) Fillings Could Be Harmful—AFTER They Have Been Put Into the Mouths of Millions of People!

After decades of denying that mercury fillings were potentially harmful, the FDA has finally admitted (in 2008) that mercury fillings could be hazardous to your health! In response to a *legal settlement*, the FDA *agreed to release* a statement to alert consumers about *potential related hazards* of mercury fillings (193). They are finally admitting that amalgam (mercury) fillings not only *release mercury vapour* in the mouth, but that *mercury vapor* is also released *during chewing*, and these fillings could have "neurotoxic effects on the nervous systems of developing children and fetuses..." (193).

Why has it taken them this long? How do you think that all the baby-boomers with a mouth full of amalgam fillings are going to feel about this ruling? They have admitted that these fillings can give off mercury, which can cause problems for those women who are *pregnant* and people with *kidney disease* (193). How many people are aware that amalgam fillings have already been banned in *Sweden and Norway* (193)? For more details, you can google "FDA and amalgam fillings" on the internet to see many related articles, such as the very informative article found at website: *http://www.c*

*bc.ca/consumer/story/2008/06/05/dentalamalgam.html (193).* Also, see below for results of **human** studies involving thousands of people with amalgam fillings!

According to Sam Ziff and Michael F. Ziff, D.D.S., in *Dentistry Without Mercury,* it takes very little mercury to make you seriously ill. Even minute amounts can adversely affect every single vital organ in the body, including damage to the blood, hormones, and immune system (613).

These dentists have a survey that was done showing 221 patients who had all their mercury fillings removed, and as a result, the majority of them were cured of many of their ailments, including: allergies, blood pressure problems, fatigue, migraines, multiple sclerosis, insomnia, memory loss, skin disorders, and thyroid problems, to name a few (613). Even Alzheimer's has been linked to mercury fillings.

Though some dentists still claim that the mercury in amalgam fillings is in a *dead* state where it cannot *escape* into your mouth or into the environment, thousands of studies have been done on **human** saliva, showing that those people who have more mercury fillings in their mouth have correlating higher amounts of mercury in their saliva (613). In their book *Dentistry Without Mercury*, Doctors Sam Ziff and Michael F. Ziff, D.D.S., discuss 1995 German research involving more than 17,000 people, which showed that saliva levels of mercury in those people with amalgam fillings was anywhere from 10-100 times the "acceptable" level (613), yet many dentists will still argue that mercury is bound in a non-toxic compound when it is used for fillings. A word of caution though! If you decide to have all your metal fillings removed, if not done properly, it can cause you more harm than good, including severe heart damage.

Dr. Hulda Clark not only blamed parasites on dentistry metal (as well as pets), but isopropyl alcohol. She recommended that once you rid yourself of parasites, stay away from isopropyl alcohol, because once it gets into the body, it enables flukes to multiply in some people. She also recommended getting all toxic chemicals, cleaners, etc, out of your home environment; because we are often inundated with toxins in the everyday cleaners, shampoos, soaps, sprays, and even toothpaste that we use. Each item alone may have little effect on your health, but if your immune system is already compromised, the combination of all of them can be overwhelming, especially for those already fighting a chronic illness. Realize that chemicals, such as benzene, can cause leukemia.

For information on using a form of *calcium bentonite clay* to detox your body from mercury, see the article: "New Safe Detox for Mercury Amalgam Fillings" at website: *http://www.naturalnews.com/023652.html.* This clay has also been discussed elsewhere in this book for its ability at killing MRSA.

## Getting Rid of the Bugs

Dr. Hulda Clark, Ph.D., N. D., recommended three main items (taken in combination) in her de-parasitization program: *"Cloves, black walnut, and wormwood"* (369). All of these items can be obtained at local health food stores (and at various websites), but she says that you must be sure in purchasing black walnut hull tincture, that it is still pale GREEN. Once it turns from green to black, it has lost its effectiveness (369). She provides instructions in her books for making your own tincture if you happen to have a black walnut tree in your back yard. Dr. Clark has an informative website at *www.drclark.net.* Also see *website: http://www.drclark.net/esp/products_devices/vitamins/coenzyme.php.* Her clinics are found in California and Mexico. I have heard much criticism, as well as much praise, for Dr. Clark. She has certainly been controversial, to say the least. There are many testimonials of cancer cures at her website, *www.drclark.net,* as well as many professionals that also use her therapy, or parts of her therapy, that you can read and judge for yourself. She also uses an electrical frequency generator device that she says can eliminate pathogens.

Wormwood comes from the artemisinin herb and has been discussed in chapter 19 of this book for its use at fighting cancer, especially breast cancer. If cancer can be caused by parasites, as Dr. Clark believes, this would account for artemisinin's effectiveness. It isn't unusual for parasites to be found in tumors that have been removed from patients. Dr. Clark has an 18-day program for taking the clove, wormwood and walnut hull. Her "Parasite Cleanse Handy Chart," showing exactly how to combine these three ingredients can be found on her website at *www.drclark.net/info/p_chart.htm*, as well as on page 23 in her book, *The Cure for All Cancers.* Be sure if you are using cloves, they are freshly ground, or they will not work at killing parasites. Once the cloves are ground up, the compounds released kill the parasites. In order for the wormwood, cloves, and walnut hull to be effective, Dr. Clark says that they must be taken together (369).

Artemisinin (wormwood) herb should not be taken on an empty stomach. Be sure to consult with your physician before taking artemisinin if you are on radiation, have recently been treated with radiation therapy, are on prescription drugs, or have other health problems. It should not be taken by those who are pregnant or breast-feeding, undergoing surgery or transplant.

I have discussed the role that parasites may have in causing cancer in other areas of this book. Some researchers are convinced that many cancers develop due to fungal or parasitic infestations. An excellent way to fight yeast is by ingesting chlorella and other chlorophyll-containing greens every single day. Soda bicarb also kills yeast and fungi. It is extremely alkaline. (See chapter 34 for info on killing cancer with soda bicarb due to the high alkalinity of the bicarb.) Also, see page 544 for information on the dangerous toxins from root canal fillings, which one physician in particular believes causes not only cancer, but heart disease.

## Where Do All The Bugs Come From?

There are many reasons for the increase in parasitic infestation in the U.S.—citizens traveling back and forth to third-world nations, child care centers, treaties allowing more and more international foods to come across borders, prolific use of antibiotics, spread of communicable diseases, and pets—some of which are left to wander the neighborhood—sniffing up every parasite that they come across (406).

To help get parasites out of the digestive tract, Ann Louise Gittleman, in her book: *Natural Healing For Parasites,* recommends using items such as "psyllium husks, agar-agar, flax seeds…beet root…citrus pectin and papaya extract…" (406). Also, in order to kill parasites and keep them from coming back, there are many natural substances that she recommends, such as chewing on the seeds of "papaya, pumpkin and lemon…" The lemon seeds are supposed to be "crushed and taken with honey once a day for five days…[repeat] in two weeks" (406). She recommends fruits that are fresh, such as the "pineapple and papaya…" and suggests that you eat one handful of raw or roasted [pumpkin] seeds…twice a day for one week…Repeat in two weeks" (406).

Other foods that fight parasites are: garlic, parsley, *ground almonds, kelp and fig extract* (406). There are also many herbs and herbal teas that kill worms and parasites. One example, described by *herbs2000.com,* is *Aspilia,* also known as *Wild Sunflower* (27). Not only does this herb kill parasites, but it fights infection as well as *breast* and *lung* cancer (27). There are many other herbs, nutrients, and spices that have parasite-killing abilities. A few of these are: cinnamon, pomegranate juice, honey, grape juice, cayenne pepper, wine, wild oil of oregano, ginger, curcumin, parsley, barberry, buckthorn, cajueiro, gentian, horseradish, cascara sagrada, slippery elm, violet, marshmallow, golden seal, dandelion, catnip, chickweed, coptis, pau d'arco, quassia, sage, Swedish bitters, glutamine, myrrh, and grapefruit seed extract. (Grapefruit seed extract is so potent at killing pathogens that some hospitals use it in their respirator equipment.)

A T.V. program announced not long ago, that "a homoelytic parasite (blood parasite) was found in all cancer patients. It was so tiny, the announcer said, that many hundreds could live in a drop of blood" (455). According to Hanna Kroeger, Ph.D., N.D., an excellent way to fight such parasites is with *Calmyra figs*. She said that these figs contain a substance inside them that destroys the worms by tearing off their skins (455). Most health food stores sell organic, calmyra figs. Remember that if you keep your immune system healthy, it will help destroy parasites in your body before they can take over.

For more amazing information on how an Italian Oncologist has successfully cured many of his patients of cancer, which he says is a fungus, and information on Dr. Mark Sircus' viewpoint in fighting cancer with soda bicarb taken by mouth, see chapter 34 in this book.

Dr. Sircus' book, *Iodine Bringing Back the Universal Medicine,* discusses how a simple food-grade iodine can destroy parasites, flu viruses, diseases (like malaria), and help prevent many virulent ailments (566a). To find the type iodine he discusses, see websites: *www.magnascent.com* and *www.magneticclay.com.* Realize that the build-up of heavy metals, parasites, and toxins in the body increases acidity, which drives out oxygen and increases yeast overgrowth.

See page 544 for more information on the dangers of dental toxins put into the mouth. Dr. Thomas Levy has spent many years telling people that root canal fillings are toxic to the body's immunity (466b), causing not only cancer, but heart disease as well. He discusses a new oral form of vitamin C known as *liposome-encapsulated Vitamin C*, which he used to cure a woman of *hemorrhagic dengue fever.* He said that *5-6 grams* of this type C taken by mouth is clinically more effective than *50 grams* received intravenously (466b). It is available in a brand known as *Lypo-Spheric*™ C. It is absorbed 100% by the body *at the cellular level* (466b).

Vitamin C has been used to kill many viruses, including polio and acute viral hepatitis.

# CHAPTER 29

# HEALING FROM BEES

*"The fear of the Lord is clean, enduring for ever: the judgments of the Lord are true and righteous altogether. More to be desired are they than gold, yea, than much fine gold: sweeter also than honey and the honeycomb." (Psalm 19:9-10) "My son, eat thou honey, because it is good; and the honeycomb, which is sweet to thy taste." (Proverbs 24:13)*

Be advised that if you have severe allergies, are an asthma sufferer, or have other chronic illnesses, consult with your physician about using honey, bee pollen, apis, propolis, or related products. There are cases of individuals who have had severe reactions to these products. Never give them to children under two. If giving to older children, consult with their physician for advice on dosages beforehand, especially if they have asthma, allergies, or other respiratory ailments. Do not take bee pollen supplements if you are allergic to bee stings, without first checking with your physician or Naturopath.

## Apis & Bee Pollen

Bee pollen, as well as honey, has been used as a medicinal for thousands of years by nearly every civilization on the earth, yet not until modern times are scientists discovering exactly why these ingredients are packed with such healing power. The pollen bees gather accumulates in tiny specks as they flit from flower to flower. The insects will gather only the best for their hives, passing up inferior pollen (590). Human testing using bee pollen has brought some amazing results. Apis is a naturopathic remedy used for bee stings.

As noted by author Carlson Wade in the book, *Carlson Wade's New FACT BOOK ON Bee Pollen and Your Health*, some health problems that were found very responsive to bee pollen, often when other remedies failed, were: "chronic constipation…colonic infections…[and] chronic diarrhea" (590).

If you have allergies or asthma, note that there is daylight and darkness between the pollen you inhale that is irritating, and the bee pollen collected by bees (590). Mr. Wade says that bee pollen has actually been used to strengthen breathing, "heal and even prevent allergies. By taking one teaspoon of bee pollen daily, resistance to wind-carried pollen is slowly built up and the sensitivity to allergy is reduced" (590). Just be sure to test the pollen first (see below). Your naturopathic physician can assist with the test. The property of bee pollen to be able to "immunize the body against allergies," was noted several years ago in the "*Florida Farmers Bulletin* (October 15, 1969)," from the article: "Doctors Recommend Raw Honey Treatment for Allergies" (590). The popularity of honey and bee pollen has since grown.

Dr. Mark Stengler, N.D., author of *The Natural Physician's Healing Therapies,* admits that though he had been able to help his own allergy-suffering patients, when he developed severe allergy problems himself one Spring, nothing worked for him (571). When some of his patients and friends told him that they had been relieved or even cured of problems with allergies using bee pollen, he started taking "8 capsules daily" (571). He explained that before a week was up, he was nearly free of most of his allergic misery (571). He continued to take the pollen, reducing the dosage. Later, he says that the problem did not return. He does not, however, recommend bee pollen for anyone allergic to bee stings. He recommends that you start slowly, placing a very tiny bit of the pollen "powder on your tongue," and if any type of allergic reactions occur—discontinue immediately (571).

As described by Jean Carper in her book, *Miracle Cures*, it took many years of taking antihistamines before a Senator from Iowa found a better treatment for his hay fever. With a friend's suggestion, he tried bee pollen and said that he was later cured of his allergies (364). (I have seen the product that he used on the internet, spelled *Aller-Bee-Gone*.)

The power of bee pollen in cancer prevention isn't new. As explained by Carlson Wade, it was known at the turn of the prior century, before the 1900s. An article in the *Journal of the National Cancer Institute* (October 1948) described a study where bee pollen was tested on animals exposed to cancer. The scientists were surprised to learn that bee pollen significantly affected the growth of tumors (590). Scientific studies on animals given "standardized pollen extract [revealed that] mice with lung carcinomas survived almost twice as long" as those not given the bee pollen (358). C. Leigh Broadhurst, Ph.D., in *Health and Healing with Bee Products*, explains that it was believed that the pollen worked by boosting the body's natural immunity (358). Bee pollen has also been shown to prevent liver injury, and to "reduce pain, inflammation and the risk of prostate cancer" (358).

According to Carlson Wade, there are many medical reports of patients not responding to antibiotics for inflammation of the prostate, who were helped with bee pollen supplements (590). (See precautions given earlier in this chapter.) Carlson Wade also describes bee pollen as the *perfect food* (590). This is because it is considered a *complete food,* having "every nutrient required to sustain life in addition to substances added by the bees…" (590). Researchers have determined that the human body is capable of existing for long periods of time in good health consuming just water and bee pollen (590).

In her book, *Bee Pollen Royal Jelly Propolis and Honey,* Rita Elkins, M.H., says that honey may even prove to be a new weapon in the fight against ulcers caused by *H Pylori bacteria.* Laboratory research showed that honey outperformed many other parasitic-killing substances (392). It is actually sweeter than sugar and a healthy alternative. The best honey is organic honey found at health food stores (358). Be sure you check with your physician or Naturopath about using bee products, especially if you have allergies and/or diabetes. Diabetics cannot safely consume large amounts of honey or royal jelly.

Researchers are discovering that it isn't necessarily just bee pollen that inhibits cancer. Animal testing in Croatia showed that everything from honey to bee venom could halt the progression of cancer. The venom produced best results when it was given by hypodermic right into the cancer growth (517).

In *Health and Healing with Bee Products,* C. Leigh Broadhurst, Ph.D., says that the *caffeic acid* in propolis (in lab studies) helped fight colon and skin cancer cells (358). Substances in propolis and other bee products are strong anti-oxidants, helping to rid the body of toxins and prevent abnormal cells from flourishing (358). Never give honey or honey products to children two and under.

Recall that in chapter three, caffeic acid is also found in grapes.

## Honey – New Formulas that Heal

Honey is also effective at killing bacteria and is often used for packing wounds just for this purpose (363). It will help relieve asthma and diarrhea, and it is often combined with other substances to control coughing (363). A surgeon in Great Britain appalled his fellow physicians when he admitted to them that he had often used honey to pack wounds after cancer surgeries (363). He explained to them that the wounds (e.g., *vulvectomies*) healed quicker than those on which he had used antibiotics. His fellow physicians were amazed when they did an experiment using honey (in laboratory testing), and found that every single pathogen, without exception, was destroyed by the honey (363). See the article, later in this chapter, on Manuka honey from New Zealand, popular for fighting diabetic ulcers. Also, see info on *Dermomel Honey* (below).

Ms. Carper further describes a human experiment at the University of Natal, Durban, South Africa, which proved honey's effectiveness against gastroenteritis diarrhea caused by bacteria. Half the children with the ailment were given a sugar concoction, while another group received honey. Those children with the diarrhea who received the honey, got well nearly twice as fast as those not receiving the honey (363).

You will find many types of honey in supermarkets and health food stores. There are honeys made locally, avocado honey, clover honey, and just about any other type of honey you can dream up, made from the nectar collected by honey bees from different flowers. There is even a honey that was developed specifically for treating pressure sores (bed sores) in the elderly, by the name of *Dermomel Honey*, developed in Israel, by Zuf Globus. See the article at: *http://www.israel21c.org/bin/en.jsp?enDispWho=Articles%5El1933&enPage=BlankPage&enDisplay=view&enDispWhat=object&enVersion=0&enZone=Health.*

Be certain that you **never** give honey or other bee products to babies and children under two years of age. Always check with their physician. There are spores in honey that can cause deadly botulism in very young children, due to their immature digestive systems.

## Life Mel Honey

A special honey that is produced from the nectar of 40 herbs, including *Echinacea, Siberian ginseng,* and *Uncaria tomentosa* (with other natural ingredients), was also developed in Israel. Two teaspoons per day (morning and evening) are recommended (614). This special honey has been shown, in **human** testing, to prevent the neutropenia (dangerously low white blood count) caused by chemotherapy and to lower the risk of severe platelet drop (thrombocytopenia), often found in chemo patients (614). You can find out more about this amazing honey at website: *http://www.lifemelisrael.com* (614). It is often said to be the most expensive honey in the world.

## Manuka Honey

A very potent honey, as far as bacteria-killing ability, is the honey made from the pollen of flowers that are found on the manuka plant. Honey that comes from the pollen of this plant, which grows prolifically in New Zealand, has the capacity to kill deadly staphylococcus aureus germs (and many other pathogens), and is becoming a popular treatment for diabetic sores and leg ulcers. Many health food stores carry manuka honey. (Also, see *Dermomel Honey*, above.)

## Propolis

In *Bee Pollen Royal Jelly Propolis and Honey,* author Rita Elkins calls propolis *Nature's Penicillin,* because it works like a natural antibiotic. There is no insect, besides the bee, that has been discovered to be "free of bacteria" (392). Apparently, propolis helps to keep the hive from being contaminated, probably one reason why it is sometimes effective at fighting bacteria that has become resistant to mainstream antibiotics, yet without the side effects that antibiotics bring with them (392).

In *Health and Healing with Bee Products*, C. Leigh Broadhurst, Ph.D., reports that honeybees collect propolis-rich resins from plants and use them like a cement to reinforce sections of their hive, as well as to *mummify* insects that have been killed trying to invade them (358). When used *topically*, she says that propolis has powerful healing properties, and is such a potent anti-inflammatory that it is often effective in the treatment of "arthritis, boils, acne, asthma, dermatitis, ulcers… inflammatory bowel diseases such as Crohn's disease, irritable bowel and chronic diverticulitis…." though some conditions may require "six to ten capsules of propolis per day…" (358).

Propolis works against cancer, possibly due to its content of caffeic acid. In **human** studies, participants in Romania were given propolis, which caused them to go into remission from their cancers. Another recent study suggested that propolis may inhibit colon cancer (392). Be sure that in purchasing propolis, you do so from a reliable organic health food provider to ensure that you are getting a pure product untainted by toxins (e.g., heavy metals, pesticides, and herbicides).

## Royal Jelly

Royal jelly continues to be an enigma to researchers, who find it so complex that they cannot duplicate it, nor thoroughly analyze it (392). Although honey, if stored in a sealed container, will not spoil, royal jelly will spoil. Mixing it with honey will preserve it (392). Dr. Paul Niehans discovered that this complex nutrient can dramatically replenish the body's glands (392).

# CHAPTER 30

# ALKALIZE FOR HEALTH

*"I am come that they might have life, and that they might have it more abundantly." (John 10:10)*

## Alkaline is Best

Undoubtedly, the reason that the organic raw foods diet is so successful at cancer prevention and cures, is because it keeps the body in a state of correct acid balance, on the side of alkalinity. If you've ever owned a fish aquarium, you know that once the water gets acidic, the fish sicken and die, unless you change it periodically to restore its alkalinity. We humans cannot tolerate an acid system in our body either. Chronic, degenerative diseases—and even cancer—can be traced to a body that has high levels of toxic acid. Cooking foods increases their acidity. If you eat a diet primarily of cooked meats and few raw vegetables, your body's acidity will increase as the foods are digested. This may account for the fact that cancer is less common in vegetarians than it is in meat eaters. In their raw state, **most foods** are more alkaline than they are acidic, so eating a raw foods diet will help keep your body in an alkaline state, which is optimum for health. This does not mean that you eat meat and fish raw! You should never eat raw or undercooked meat, poultry, or fish. In speaking of *raw foods*, in this book, it only applies to fresh fruits, vegetables, and seed foods. Some grains (like oatmeal) are used in raw food recipes.

Worms, parasites, bacteria, molds, yeasts, and fungi are more apt to attack and take up residence in a body that is highly acidic, rather than alkaline. In the low carb diet, the emphasis on meat and other high protein food, leaves the body in an acid state. This is why adherents to this diet check their urine for acidity levels. According to the diet, if the urine is acidic, you are burning fat, however, you are also losing valuable calcium from your bones (as well as other minerals) in the process. When your blood is acidic, the body tries to balance it out the best way it knows how and that is to rob your bones of calcium. The calcium raises the pH—but remember this—the body does not care WHERE it takes the calcium from in order to raise the pH of the blood; it will scavenge it from anywhere it can get it. Other minerals that your body will rob (usually from your bones) to alkalize the blood are: potassium, magnesium, and sodium.

(See other chapters in this book, especially chapter 34, for the oncology physician, Dr. T. Simoncini, who believes that cancer is simply a fungus, and can be treated effectively with sodium bicarbonate, which totally alkalizes the tumor and surrounding area, killing the cancer. He has cured many of his patients of massive tumors within six or seven days, simply by giving them sodium bicarb infusions.)

## What Causes Excess Acidity?

According to Dr. Theodore A. Baroody, N.D., D.C., Ph.D, C.N.C., in his book, *Alkalize or Die*, foods have different minerals in them that, once they are incorporated into the body's system, they either produce residual matter that is acidic or alkaline, and these substances can be found in the urine (340). Dr. Baroody also has an excellent ten-day detox drink that you can use to quickly alkalize your body (see pp. 217-218 of his book), which he refers to as the *Lemonade Diet* by Stanley Burroughs (340). You mix 2 tablespoons of fresh-squeezed lemon juice, 2 tablespoons of maple syrup and 1/8 tspn cayenne pepper into 8 oz of water. Drink as often as needed to maintain energy. Follow for a ten day period, but eat and drink nothing else (340). (See directions in chapter 35 of my book about coming off a fast gradually!)

A healthy saliva and urine will measure 6.4 (340). The pH scale goes from 0 to 14. Seven is neutral. If your blood pH is below seven, you are getting acidic. If it is above seven, you are alkaline. If you have **blood** drawn by your physician, they like to see a serum pH of 7.35—7.45. When your pH starts dropping, your oxygen levels also decrease. This is why your physician may start you on oxygen if you are in the hospital and your lab tests show a high acid level in your blood. He or she will be doing other diagnostics to determine the cause. Sometimes the cause is quite obvious, for example, someone having an asthma attack with wheezing and difficulty breathing will very rapidly develop dangerous blood acidity. Remember that cancer cells cannot thrive in an oxygen-rich environment. Constantly having a high blood acidity in your body means you are starving yourself for oxygen.

This process is described by Robert Young, Ph.D., and Shelley Young in their book, *The pH Miracle Balance Your Diet, Reclaim Your Health* (607). Once your blood is overloaded with too much acid, it begins dumping the "acid…into the tissues for storage," and it often ends up right back where it started, in the bloodstream (607). This draws out essential minerals and not only puts a taxing load on the liver, but the kidneys as well (607). Unfortunately, excess acid leads to many chronic disorders, such as the pain of arthritis from the acid build-up in the joints and tissues. It also invites other conditions, e.g., candida infections, fungus, parasites, and worms as noted earlier (607). Raw, vegan foods are better for the joints, however, realize that if you consume foods that you are allergic to, this sets off an auto-immune reaction that releases chemicals into the body, causing inflammation which also damages tissues and joints.

In order to keep your body in a healthy state that keeps the blood alkaline, Dr. Baroody suggests that you "follow the rule of 80/20 – which means to eat 80% of your foods from the alkaline-forming list and 20% from the acid-forming list" (340). Some examples of alkaline foods are: grapes, kelp, and asparagus, as long as they are eaten raw. Once they are cooked, they become more acidic. White rice, other rices, and corn are *acid-forming*. Asparagus is the only vegetable that does retain high alkalinity once it is cooked (340), as long as it is not over-cooked.

There are many nutrition books on the market that list the pH values of foods. Dr. Baroody provides such a list in his book, *Alkalize or Die,* as do Robert Young and Shelley Redford Young in *The pH Miracle*. If you keep your body in an optimal state of alkalinity, you are much less likely to get cancer and chronic, degenerative diseases.

There have been many cases of people curing their cancer by **reversing** their body from acidic to alkaline. Many have done this simply by changing their diet. This is what happened with Eydie Mae Hunsberger, Rev. George Malkmus, Ann Wigmore, and others discussed in this book who were able to cure their cancers by a change in diet and life style. Remember too, that it is not only food that determines your body's pH. Stress will increase the acidity of your body. It is also possible to become too alkaline, which can be just as dangerous as high acidity, but is usually much more rare.

## How Raising pH Cured a Stage III Bladder Cancer

In *The pH Miracle*, Dr. Robert Young and Shelley Young related the story of a bladder cancer patient diagnosed with advanced bladder cancer, who cured his cancer by reversing his body's acidity (607). The malignant bladder tumor had already cut off one of the patient's *ureters* (607). After he underwent chemo (which did nothing to decrease the size of the tumor), his physicians recommended complete surgical removal of his bladder. The patient came to see Dr. Young, who found his blood to be highly acidic, which the patient said was from years of eating the wrong kinds of foods (607). He refused surgery and completely changed his diet, beginning with a "ten-day fast, with vegetable juices and soups" (607). Within a *three month* period, the cancer had nearly disappeared. Though doctors still wanted to do a radical bladder removal, the patient chose minor surgery, which left all of his organs intact (607).

This may seem contrary, but it is possible for highly acidic foods to increase the body's alkalinity. Harald Tietze explains why in his book, *Papaya The Healing Fruit.* He says that limes are a good example (581). Though they are very acidic, with a pH of 1.9, consuming them has an *alkaline effect* on the body. The same is true of lemons. Not only is it important to know which foods are alkaline and acid-forming, but also to know how the body reacts to certain foods (581).

The best way to stay alkaline is with raw foods and juicing. Keeping your body in a state of alkalinity will increase oxygen at the cellular level. Also, see information in chapter 24 of this book, including oxygen treatments, which are being given to cancer patients to increase their oxygen levels, and see chapter 23 on water drinking. Remember that water is mostly composed of oxygen. When you rob your body of water, you are cutting off a major oxygen supply for your cells. The reason a vegetarian diet promotes alkalinity is because most raw vegetables and fruits are alkaline and alkaline-forming, with a few exceptions. All MEATS, including raw meats and processed dairy are acidic. Processed, packaged foods, white sugar, and flour are also acid-forming.

## Juice-Fasting

One of the best ways to restore your body's proper alkalinity is with a juice-fast. While fasting is discussed in chapter 35 in greater detail, juice-fasting is being mentioned here simply because it is very important for establishing alkalinity and detoxifying the body.

Dr. Don Colbert in his book, *Toxic Relief,* explains that even though a total fast (taking in water only) will detoxify the body, using fruit and vegetable juices during a fast will help detoxify the body and result in alkalinity. Juice-fasting will help fortify the liver and maintain your energy level, something water-fasting will not do (372).

See chapter three in this book for more information on the grape juice diet, which brings the body into alkalinity and is very detoxifying.

Remember too, that with any type of fasting, your body still needs water. I never recommend a total fast where even water is not permitted. You should never go for days without water. A total fast (without water) is dangerous! The reason green juices are extremely alkalizing is because they contain chlorophyll and chlorophyll contains magnesium and most of the world's population is severely magnesium-deficient.

## Ume Plums

This Japanese fruit (*Prunus mume*) is said to be highly anti-oxidant. It is often pickled into what is referred to as *umeboshi,* which is usually very alkaline. Ume is used by the Japanese to treat everything from muscle cramps and high blood pressure, to atherosclerosis. You may find natural health food stores selling this fruit as *Japanese plum balls.*

## Uncovering & Neutralizing Yeast

Dr. T. Simoncini has cured many of his cancer patients simply by exposing their tumors to an alkaline solution using soda bicarb. He has been able to rid many people of cancerous growths within six or seven days with his method. He says that cancers are caused by yeast and yeast is WHITE. When cancers are removed, they are usually white in color. So convinced was he with his own research, that he wrote a book entitled: *Cancer Is A Fungus* (582). He suggests that cancer patients be given *sodium bicarbonate*, a non-poisonous substance, directly into the cancerous tissue (582). If you are interested in more specifics on his treatment, see website: *http://www.cancerisafungus.com/cancer-fungus-content.html* (582). You can order his books at his website: *http://www.curenaturalicancro.com.* Apparently, he has been very successful in using this therapy (582). He has reports of patients "using sodium bicarbonate at five per cent solution," to heal *lung* cancers, cancers of the mouth, head and neck, *liver,* gastric and *intestinal, prostate, stomach, pancreas, spleen,* and many others (582). He treats many of his patients with intravenous soda bicarb; however, Dr. Mark Sircus, author of *Sodium Bicarbonate Rich Man's Poor Man's Cancer Treatment,* says you don't need to travel to Europe for an IV bicarb to cure your cancer, not when you can take soda bicarb by mouth (566c)! See chapter 34 for more details.

Also, realize that not only will soda bicarb alkalize the body very rapidly, but so will lemon juice, lime juice, and apple cider vinegar, and without the high salt content that is found in soda bicarb.

# CHAPTER 31

## SPICES TO PREVENT & CURE

*"I have heard thy prayers, I have seen thy tears: behold, I will heal thee: on the third day thou shalt go up unto the house of the Lord." (II Kings 20:5)*

There are many spices that fight cancer. Several of them, such as turmeric, garlic, cloves, and cayenne pepper, have already been discussed in this book. Some are what we consider our most popular seasonings and spices. Those discussed in this chapter are powerful anti-oxidants that help boost immunity to fight cancer and other illnesses and disease.

### Basil

According to Selene Yeager in the *Doctors Book of FOOD REMEDIES*, there are several compounds in basil that are responsible for its ability to, not only ease nausea, but lower your risk of developing cancer (604). Animal testing revealed that basil in the diet raises enzymes in the body that neutralize cancer-causing substances. Basil also contains *eugenol,* which alleviates painful *muscle spasms* (604).

### Cinnamon

This is one spice that doesn't just enhance the flavor of food—it may one day save your life! Studies reveal that it functions as a food preservative, as well as a tasty additive to many dishes and treats. In an experiment done by researchers at Kansas State University, when testing various ingredients for their effectiveness in killing E.coli type 0157 bacteria, a deadly food poison, they discovered something truly amazing—putting cinnamon in apple juice (that had purposely been dosed with e.coli) could kill 99.5% of the harmful bacteria without needing refrigeration, and this was accomplished within 72 hours (239). They also discovered that cloves and garlic had this same ability at killing e.coli (239). Other researchers found bacteria-killing substances in wild oil of oregano, as well as oils derived from coriander and basil (239).

What does all this mean? The next time you and your family eat out and you are concerned about getting food poisoning (and well you should be), it might behoove you to take a small spice jar with some cinnamon, garlic, ginger, and/or cloves with you to add a bit to your food. (Cinnamon can help lower blood sugar in some individuals.) You may also want to include a milk thistle capsule, or cloves to chew on.

## Cloves

When cloves are ground up or chewed, the substance that is released from them is very powerful at killing worms and parasites. (See chapter 28.)

## Ginger & Willow Bark

Ginger is a very healing, protective herb with many advantageous properties, including fighting pain and diabetes. It also helps prevent blood clots, inhibits ulcers, supports the body's immunity, kills pathogens, and suppresses tumor formation (557). It is such a powerful anti-inflammatory that Paul Schulick, in his book, *Ginger Common Spice & Wonder Drug,* describes the account of a *rheumatoid arthritis* patient who began consuming "fifty grams of fresh ginger daily after light cooking along with vegetables and various meats" (557). After following the above ginger regimen for 3 months, he "was completely free of pain, inflammation or swelling," and he maintained his demanding work "as auto mechanic without any relapses of arthritis for the last 10 years," as reported by Dr. K. C. Srivastava from Denmark (557). (I have also known people to use fresh ginger successfully for their migraine headaches.) Realize that ginger can thin the blood, something to consider if you are already taking blood thinning medication.

Mr. Schulick also notes the failure of conventional medicine's treatment of *crippling* arthritis (557). Ginger offers tremendous hope to these individuals. He talks of "two clinical trials conducted in Denmark [where] ginger actually reversed many of the subjects' arthritic symptoms and did so without side effects" (557). (These were **human** trials.) Many other clinical trials have been done showing ginger to be superior to aspirin and NSAIDS as an anti-inflammatory. According to Dr. K. C. Srivastava, consuming ginger was superior to pain relief over NSAIDS, even using it for *colds*, fever blisters, gastric problems, and to alleviate *constipation* (557). (Raw pear juice is also good for constipation!)

Mr. Schulick also reports that ginger has apparent anti-cancer effects due to its immune-boosting power. When cancer-stricken lab animals were fed ginger, they had longer lives (557). Ginger also prevents dangerous clots by slowing platelet formation. Platelets are responsible for producing substances (*growth factors*) that support the growth of cancer. By inhibiting this process, ginger may play an important role in halting cancer (557).

Ginger also has the power to protect the digestive tract from ulcers, hardly good news for the pharmaceutical giants when you consider that in one year alone *$2.8 billion* worth of their antacids*: Zantac, Tagamet and Pepcid,* were sold to the public. As Mr. Schulick concludes from all this: "It is easy to understand why these drug companies would prefer the benefits of ginger to remain in the books or databases" (557). One of the many components (out of hundreds) in ginger is *geraniol.* Geraniol is found not only in ginger, but rosemary and "corn and peas," and apparently, according to website *www.earthnotes.tripod.com*, it only requires tiny amounts. In animal studies, those with tumors who were given only *0.1% of Geraniol,* lived longer (122).

There is another herb that does this, and James Duke, Ph.D., and Michael Castleman describe it in their book, *The Green Pharmacy Anti-Aging Prescriptions;* it is willow bark (388). Aspirin is made from willow bark. It can be used for fighting pain, cancer, and *heart attack* (due to its ability to thin the blood and prevent dangerous clots (388). If you are on prescription medications, awaiting surgery, or just recovering from surgery, be sure to check with your physician before using ginger or willow bark. The same holds true for those who are pregnant, transplant patients, or breast feeding, or suffering from a chronic illness.

## Horseradish & Grapefruit Seed Extract

Horseradish *(Armoracia rusticana)* root, described at *herbs2000.com*, is a very pungent herb (or spice) that has long been considered a medicinal treatment in many cultures. A popular folk medicine treatment for hay fever is shredding horseradish onto a sandwich (157). It is also used for fighting viruses and the common cold (157). The horseradish root is very potent. It is not for small children or pets. Excessive amounts of the root have caused digestive upset (*vomiting*) and copious perspiration, and it should not be consumed by those with thyroid problems. Consuming too much horseradish can inhibit thyroid hormones and cause the gland to enlarge (157). As always, check with your physician or Naturopath.

Fresh horseradish, grated up with cooked beets (also grated) is a concoction that spices up many European dishes. I have been able to kill a cold within 72 hours just by eating a few tablespoons a day of horseradish sauce (with meals) for 3 days in a row. I wouldn't recommend it on an empty stomach though, nor for those with serious thyroid problems. Always take with food.

Another ingredient that quickly kills germs is grapefruit seed extract (GSE), which can be found in pill supplements, drops, or even in a nasal spray. If you are fighting sinus infections that keep recurring, you may want to try this germ killer. GSE nasal spray can be purchased at health food stores. The spray and supplements are used to help kill colds.

## Miscellaneous Spices

Researchers found that many different spices can increase the body's glutathione levels, one of our most valuable anti-oxidants, helpful in protecting against cancer. Some of those tested were common everyday spices used in cooking (e.g., basil and cinnamon). The best advice when cooking is to use a variety of spices for their anti-oxidant effects. Some foods, like avocados, are high in glutathione. Many other vegetables and fruits contain this nutrient. Taking alpha lipoic acid will also raise your glutathione levels. When glutathione levels drop, the results are devastating to the overall health of the body.

## Oil of Oregano

This pungent spice has also been discussed earlier. As noted at website *www.cancertutor.com*, "Greek investigators, publishing in the *Journal of Agriculture and Food Chemistry*," reported that this spice could destroy "human cancer cells" (224). From my own experience, I have found oil of wild oregano to be an excellent earache remedy. Just a drop or two of oil in the affected ear has very quickly cleared up earaches. Do not use for children unless you have consulted with their pediatrician, especially if there is the possibility of eardrum perforation or allergy to this herb. Do not use for yourself if there is eardrum perforation. I use only organic wild oil of oregano, which is available in a small dropper bottle at most natural health food stores. (Some people dilute it with olive oil.)

## Paprika

Paprika may be significant for cancer prevention. It is derived from a carotenoid-rich red pepper. Researchers discovered, in laboratory testing, that this popular spice helps prevent cancer and kill viruses. It suppressed not only skin cancer, but lung cancer as well.

## Rosemary in Small Amounts

Rosemary contains a compound that, in animal testing, stopped cancer formation. Apparently, it blocks a substance that promotes the formation of cancerous breast cells. Do not use this herb excessively. It can raise blood pressure.

Using rosemary in baking wheat bread, for example, slashed the cancer-causing acrylamides by greater than half (361). Very minuscule amounts of rosemary, as low as *one per cent of the dough*, was able to neutralize acrylamides (361).

## Saffron Destroys Cancer Cells

Some spices appear to be able to destroy cancer cells on contact. Saffron is one of them (604). Lab testing showed that ingredients from this common herb could halt the growth of leukemia cells without harming normal cells (604).

## Spices & Herbs (Miscellaneous) That Inhibit Cancer

Many herbs and spices have anti-cancer effects. Ginger and fennel help suppress colon cancer; cumin and fennel inhibit prostate and bladder cancers; coriander fights breast and liver cancers; and mint is high in limonene, a cancer-fighter.

Caraway seed is one of the richest sources of limonene (388).

## V8® Juice & Other Vegetable Juices

If you have little time for juicing, but you want to enjoy the benefits of beets, carrots, celery and other nutrients in a ready-to-drink beverage, try the LOW SODIUM V8® juice that is currently on the market. Do not use regular brand that is high in sodium! Always be sure that the label says **LOW SODIUM V8®**. Just remember that the juice is not said to be "organic," and it is also pasteurized, which removes some of the nutrients.

# CHAPTER 32

# THOSE AWESOME TEAS!

*"Hear, O my son, and receive my sayings; and the years of thy life shall be many." (Proverbs 4:10)*

Several teas with healing, curative powers have already been discussed in this book, including *Essiac* tea and *Hoxsey* tea. There are so many other teas that can be important in boosting immunity and fighting cancer, they cannot all be discussed in a book of this length, however, a few of them are mentioned here. Sometimes you will be told that the NCI, FDA, or some other institution has tested compounds (for example those in pau d'arco), and flatly announced that they do not help cancer. However, what you sometimes are not told is that when a tea is tested, it isn't always the entire tea with ALL of its components that are tested by them. They will extract one or two compounds from the tea and use that extract to test it, then claim that the tea is ineffective. This does not always work because teas (e.g., Essiac, pau d'arco, green tea) usually need to be taken as a whole, without breaking them up into ten different compounds, using only one or two of their main ingredients for the test. There are times, however, when individual extracts taken from teas DO kill cancer cells.

## Black Tea, Cancer Fighter & Anthrax Fighter

For years scientists have agreed that tea, green and black, help boost the body's natural immune system. A new study from Cardiff University and the University of Maryland has revealed that black tea (and it has to be black tea) could be important in warding off anthrax; however, don't be too quick to add a dash of milk to that *cup of tea,* because the milk eliminates the *antibacterial* effect against the anthrax (89a).

## Chaparral Tea

Dr. Ralph W. Moss in his book, *Cancer Therapy*, describes an ingredient in chaparral tea known as *NDGA (nordihydroguaiaretic acid),* which prevented abnormal colon growths in animal tests. It also arrested the formation of cancers in the breast. Lab testing of NDGA blocked leukemia, as well as a type of brain tumor known as *glioma* (504).

There was one report, from Canada, of a consumer harming her liver many weeks after she began ingesting a product known as *Chaparral Leaf* (504). As mentioned earlier, the FDA reported a total of four cases of liver toxicity from this tea. It was taken off the market, but many people still make their own chaparral tea, as it grows wild in some states.

In a **human** study done by scientists in the western U.S., Dr. Moss tells of a patient with melanoma who enjoyed a near total remission after taking chaparral tea. Research conducted by the NCI revealed chaparral tea to be very helpful in fighting cancer (504).

In another remarkable case, an elderly man with skin cancer on his face, who had opted out of surgery, began self-treating with chaparral tea. The patient came back to his physician after several months, having had remarkable reduction in the melanoma (504). I would never advise someone with melanoma not to have surgery, because sometimes surgical removal alone will cure melanoma, depending on how far it has advanced.

## Dandelion Tea

Marie Nadine Antol, in her book *Healing Teas*, reports that this herbal tea cleanses the liver and blood and helps many inflammatory conditions, including gout and those of the liver. It has also been used for cancers of the breast (333). Dandelion has diuretic properties, so using too much can cause dehydration. Also, be aware that dandelion herb and dandelion greens can promote bile secretion and increase gastric acid, something to consider if you have gallstones, billiary disease, ulcers, or other digestive problems.

## Essiac Tea

See chapter six for details on this amazing healing tea. You can find Essiac in several brands. Two major competing brands are Flor-Essence® and Resperin Canada Essiac®. (There are a few others.) You can obtain Flor-Essence® at many natural health food stores in an already prepared drinkable form, or a powdered form that you brew yourself. Essiac® from Resperin Canada can be purchased at several websites, including *https://www.billybest.net/orderEssiac.htm.* Rene Caisse, a Canadian nurse, healed hundreds (possibly thousands) of people of every imaginable cancer using her remarkable herbal tea, many of whom came to her after conventional medicine considered them hopelessly terminal.

For an excellent book describing the effectiveness of this tea and how it was suppressed by the health industry in Canada see: *The Essiac Report Canada's Remarkable Unknown Cancer Remedy*, by Richard Thomas. He claims that Flor-Essence® is the original (drinkable) formula that Rene Caisse used (580). Mr. Thomas' book contains several pages of documentation from physicians and patients who successfully used the Flor-Essence® tea to cure their cancers, in spite of the incessant, underhanded attempts by the Canadian government's health department to discredit and destroy the formula. I highly recommend this book to those interested in Essiac.

Note that there is some competition between the tea produced by Resperin Canada Essiac® and Flor-Essence® Essiac tea. Both companies claim that they have the original Essiac formula (the drinkable formula, not the injectable) that Rene Caisse gave her patients.

See chapter sixteen, earlier in my book, for the story of a young boy who was cured of lymphoma with a natural program that included Essiac® Resperin Canada's tea formula and 714X injections. A website that has Essiac® Resperin Canada is also given in that chapter.

## Ginger Tea

In Dr. *Earl Mindell's Food As Medicine*, ginger tea isn't just for stomach upset, morning sickness, and motion sickness. A human study showed that women given ginger capsules after they had surgery, experienced less nausea and vomiting than those given prescription drugs. Not only that, but they recovered without any need for other meds. This herb has also been under close investigation because of its ability to fight cancer cells (493). I have known of people who successfully used fresh ginger for their migraine headaches. See the story (in chapter 31 of this book) about a rheumatoid arthritis patient who began ingesting fresh ginger with his meals, which totally eliminated his pain and arthritic symptoms. He has been pain-free for the last ten years and credits his recovery to ginger.

## Green Tea

Drinking several cups of green tea a day may be the most important thing you can do to prevent and fight cancer.

In a human research study described by Dr. James F. Balch in *The Super Anti-Oxidants*, this tea was able to reduce pancreatic cancer by 50% in participants consuming the tea. More and more data is supporting the use of green tea as a major preventative in all forms of cancer, including those of the G.I. tract, blood (leukemia), and liver (337). Research also showed that this tea could help kill certain types of leukemia, such as myeloblastic (337). Green tea could be one of the most important developments in fighting leukemia. In the research, it caused premature death in the abnormal cells (337).

If you see *Golden Green Tea* at your local health food store, it is merely green tea combined with *lemon grass*. Research shows green tea can even prevent dental caries and halitosis (235). Green tea has also been found, in animal testing by Israeli researchers, to actually regenerate brain cells, something hitherto thought impossible (169). I would recommend decaffeinated green tea since caffeine can be dehydrating, however, some believe that it does not fight arterial plaque as well as caffeinated tea.

## Kombucha Tea

Kombucha tea *(Fungus Japonicus)* is derived from a popular fungus that resembles a mushroom. According to Marie Nadine Antol in *Healing Teas*, kombucha can help boost the immunity, attacking the HIV virus and abnormal cancer cells. It helps normalize blood lipids, neutralize toxins, stabilize *blood pressure*, attack acne, reduce wrinkling, promote hair growth, relieve arthritis, energize the body, and even help restore hair color in some individuals (333). Speaking of hair color, if kombucha does not give you the shade you desire, there is a vegetable-based hair color (that contains no ammonia and no resorcinal), which you may wish to try that is available in natural health food stores. It is called ***Naturtint®.*** Always be sure to do the patch test on these products to check for allergies.

## Liver Tonic Tea

See the last chapter in this book for my liver tonic tea recipe. When using teas for health and tonic, if you get prepared teas, some of them contain licorice. Do not use undeglycyrrhizinated licorice if you have estrogen abnormalities, blood pressure, or eye pressure problems. Always consult with your physician first. If you take licorice, also add *potassium* to your diet on a daily basis (178). You can purchase DGL licorice in health food stores. If you get the chewable wafers, they taste much like coffee beans.

Also be aware that some of these herbs have blood-thinning properties. You should not take them if you are already on prescription medications such as Coumadin, nor if you have not yet discussed them with your physician. If you are a transplant recipient or waiting for a transplant, a dialysis patient, or you have any type of illness, never start a new herbal, vitamin, mineral, or hormonal regimen without consulting with your doctor.

## Oolong Tea

Oolong tea is said to increase fat metabolism quicker than any other tea. (135). A favorite in China, it is partially fermented and is high in anti-oxidants, but has half the caffeine of green tea. If using oolong tea, sip with food, rather than drinking it on an empty stomach.

## Parsley Tea

Marie Nadine Antol in *Healing Teas*, describes parsley as a natural diuretic, overall cleanser, important anti-oxidant, and health promoter (333). Scientists have recently discovered a substance in parsley that fights cancer. If you buy it dried, be sure to find out if it came from the **leaf or roots**. Tea made from the roots will be much more potent than leaf tea. Parsley tea can help the body in prevention and dissolving of stones (e.g., gallstones), provided that they are small enough. Once they enlarge, it may be too late (333). It can also cause uterine contractions, so should not be used during pregnancy, nor during nursing. It should not be used during any type of infectious process, says Ms. Antol, "especially if the kidneys are involved" (333).

## Rooibos Tea

Rooibos tea is harvested in South Africa and is quickly gaining popularity in the West. It is high in anti-oxidants and flavonoids, such as rutin and quercetin, and some claim that it demonstrates greater anti-cancer activity than that found in green tea. You can purchase rooibos in fermented form, which has no caffeine, or the unfermented rooibos. There are many internet sites and health food stores that carry this tea.

## Sir Jason Winters' Tea

Sir Jason Winters was diagnosed in 1977 with a huge, visible neck tumor. He went the conventional medicine route, but refused major surgery. Nothing happened to the growth. He was sent home with a diagnosis of *terminal*, given a few months of life at the most (602). As described at his website, *www.sirjasonwinters.com*, what happened next is nothing less than miraculous! He traveled to three different continents and developed a tea blend containing red clover, herbalene (a Chinese spice), and Indian sage, that he combined and began drinking religiously. The cancer began shrinking, until it disappeared completely (602). The tea that he used is now called his *Classic Blend Tea.* When it "was tested by Dr. Ian Pierce of England, it was said that the Herbalene acted as a catalyst to make the other two herbs in the tea 27 times stronger" (602). According to their website above, "Hashimoto, the former Prime Minister of Japan, considers Jason Winters Tea to be THE HEALTHIEST DRINK IN THE WORLD" (602). Jason Winters' book, *Killing Cancer,* is available at his website, along with his *Classic Blend Tea*, and several other teas that he offers. His website reports that he has "won awards from six foreign governments and the U.S…for his work in the health field" (602). I would certainly recommend *Jason Winters Tea* for anyone fighting cancer. He has since passed, but not from cancer.

## Tarragon Tea

Tarragon tea can help boost the immune system and fight cancer. It is rich in caffeic acid (284). I have discussed the benefits of caffeic acid in other chapters of this book.

# CHAPTER 33

# THE TRUTH ABOUT CLINICAL TRIALS & NATURAL PRODUCTS

*"My son, attend unto my wisdom, and bow thine ear to my understanding." (Proverbs 5:1)*
*"With him is wisdom and strength, he hath counsel and understanding." (Job 12:13)*

## I. Clinical Trials - Purpose

Clinical trials are used to test new treatments and drugs. There are several phases, with people enlisted in all phases of the trials. Phase I trials have a few human participants, and the purpose of the trial is to get a correct dose for the drug, determine if the drug is indeed safe, and the route via which the drug is to be given (312). Phase II trials include larger numbers of people, concentrate on further testing of the drug and safety issues, such as dosage levels. Phase III trials may involve hundreds or thousands of people, and usually each phase III trial will have two groups (312). One group is normally given a placebo, and the other group is given the actual drug (or treatment). None of the participants know for certain whether they are taking a placebo or the real thing.

It is not my intention in this chapter to debunk all clinical trials. Some of these trials are performed very honestly and effectively—others are completely biased—and you will understand why after reading this chapter.

## How Drug Companies Influence Trials On Their Own Products

In an article by David Gutierrez at *naturalnews.com*, he explains how some pharmaceutical companies are involved in every step of the research on their drug, then regularly "solicit academics to put their names on the final papers," so that no one knows that it is the drug company involved in the entire study. The practice is described by Author Sergio Sismondo as *ghost management* (420).

You can read about a massive coverup involving the drug maker, Merck, in a scheme to take their own company authors and *disguise* them in such a way that the FDA and public thought they were *independent* and *unbiased* (327). How was the cover-up unraveled? Only because of litigation from private citizens who said that pharmaceuticals from Merck harmed them. We now know that Merck lied about their research on Vioxx®, and did so intentionally. Could it be because, in one year alone (per a Senate investigation), Vioxx® brought them 2.3 billion dollars in profits? This one drug could be responsible for the deaths of more than 50,000 U.S. citizens and many thousands more that have also experienced heart attacks (327). Can you think of anyone else in this country—private or commercial—who would still be allowed to stay in business and escape the death penalty, after they were responsible for 50,000 deaths? Yet the FDA will try to convince YOU that they want to control the sale and distribution of all vitamins and natural supplements to keep YOU safe (327), of course! And what happened to those who lied about the research on this drug? Are they doing prison terms? Should this not be considered murder, or at the very least, manslaughter? Do YOU have a loved one who died as a result of taking Vioxx? Who is being held responsible? Who went to jail, or prison for this crime? How many other people running companies in the U.S. would escape prison terms after being responsible for the deaths of 50,000 people?

## II. Double-Blind, Randomized, Placebo-Controlled Clinical Trials—The *Gold Standard*

### Going for the Gold

There are many alternative therapies for cancer, with new ones being discovered every single day. Some of them are supported by clinical trials on humans, and of course, some are not—and that is one of the big arguments that organized medicine gives against alternative therapies, but there is something you should know about the *gold standard* of the modern medical profession. *Double-blind, randomized, placebo-controlled clinical trials* ARE their gold standard; however, the results of clinical trials are often manipulated by those doing them and some are simply lied about, or the results are concealed. For example, if a drug company is in a hurry to get their promising new drug approved by the FDA (and they usually are), there are subtle ways (and some not so subtle!) that they can make sure that the results of their *clinical trials* come out favoring their drug! This is done in a variety of ways:

- For example, if you want to be sure that the participants testing a new blood pressure drug have excellent results, be sure that all the people in your group using the new drug do not have multiple co-morbidities (other sicknesses besides high blood pressure), and choose participants in your placebo group that do! That way it will ensure that those on your new drug are more likely to stay healthier than the control group, making your drug APPEAR to be very beneficial. Also, your new drug testers won't die off and the drug get the blame. (Even though the drug might be responsible for their deaths, the sicker placebo group should have a higher death rate!)
- If someone using your new drug drops dead from heart failure, for example, just replace that person with a live body, or dismiss the death as *unrelated,* so it does not show up as one of the adverse effects when you are reporting results of the study to the FDA. Or, just shelve the old trial, start a new one, and don't report the negative trial.
- Conduct three trials and only turn the two most favorable trials into the FDA when getting the drug approved. You are living in *la-la land* if you think that this isn't being done. It's done, all right, and on a regular basis.
- Get the drug approved for treating one illness, but have the drug reps PUSH physicians to prescribe it for *off-label* usage for a dozen other problems, e.g., it is approved to treat hypertension, but convince the docs that it is also good for insomnia, anxiety, edema, and gastritis, thus expanding the sales and profits for the drug company. This push to use a drug for *off-label* use is what happened with the drug Propulsid. It was supposed to be for adults, but ended up being prescribed to babies. Over 300 people, many of them infants, died before this one was forced off the market (385).
- Admit (in very fine print) on the drug label, that the drug's effectiveness has not been fully determined through clinical trials, so it is important that doctors prescribing the drug routinely determine whether those patients who are to receive it will benefit. (Oops! Did you see how that one was done? You are left hanging out on a limb this time! Suddenly, the responsibility for evaluating the new drug's effectiveness falls in the lap of—you guessed it—your friendly, neighborhood physician.) Six months go by and ten people die from taking the drug, and the drug manufacturer points the finger of guilt at your physician for not conscientiously evaluating the drug's effectiveness! (Nothing like passing-the-buck, is there?)
- Pay an outside investigator to conduct the trials for you. If they do five studies for you and only two studies favor the drug you want approved, bury the three studies you don't like and ship the other two to the FDA with your new drug application. (Yes, there are many loopholes around the system, and you can be sure that most drug companies have figured out every single one of them.) Drug companies have been caught lying about unfavorable clinical trial results, or simply covering them up.

As noted by Dr. Thomas A.M. Kramer, M.D., in "Understanding Clinical Trials in Context," "[M]ost clinical trials are six weeks long. Most patients take their medication considerably longer than that. Who is to say that what is true in 6 weeks will remain so" (453)?

Drug companies often put the worst adverse effects of the drug in very **tiny** microscopic print in the drug warning label on line 153, in complex technical jargon that even a trained doctor can't decipher, ensuring that no physician (in his or her right mind) is ever going to read it, understand it, or warn their patients about it.

Every day it seems that some new revelation is coming out about a drug that has injured or killed hundreds or thousands of people.

Because of the uproar over the antidepressant drugs—the fact that they increased the likelihood of suicide in young people taking them—and the cover-up involving those side effects, congressional *committees* were forced to order the FDA to disclose their records on the drugs that they approved (561). Isn't this amazing? Especially when you consider the pompous claims that many drug manufacturers display on their drug commercials! Yet, let a health food store owner try to make similar claims about a natural herbal remedy that has no toxic side effects, and the FDA will scream *FOUL* and shut them down! In Canada, Rene Caisse suffered constant surveillance and harassment when she said that her herbal formula was curing cancer without toxic side effects, yet the U.S. FDA is no different from the system in Canada. They will remove an herb from American shelves, classifying it as dangerous and harmful, because four people (out of 70,000) had adverse reactions to it, and in the same breath, tell you that it is entirely safe to give your child (with brain cancer) a chemotherapy drug that has already killed 70,000 people! Perhaps they died a little slower, but they are still dead. This is sanity? Well of course it isn't, but think about it, because our entire medical system of treating cancer is based on this type of REASONING, and it is pure insanity! As a matter-of-fact, if your physician wants to give you or your loved one some new chemo regimen, do this: **ask him or her to first provide you with the studies showing how many people were CURED or had their lives extended significantly (e.g., 8 - 10 years) after taking the same drugs that they are wanting to give you!**

## Who Conducts the Trials?

If you still have doubts about the objectivity of clinical trials, consider **who** it is that does most of these trials. According to Dr. Thomas A.M.

Kramer, M.D., many of them are conducted and/or paid for by the very same drug companies that are trying to get the drug approved (453).

If you want to see a video of the hypocrisy of Monsanto's activities in their genetically-modified foods, as well as the creation and addition of growth hormone to cow's milk (along with the blatant lies and coverup by the FDA, as well as how many top government officials and FDA officials were in Monsanto's revolving door employment), you will want to see the video for yourself at *http://www.celsias.com/article/the-world-accord ing-to-monsanto.*

In view of all this, just remember the above when you are considering a safe, non-toxic, alternative therapy and someone (who thinks that they know something you don't) tells you that the therapy you are contemplating is not backed up by ***scientific, double-blind, randomized, placebo-controlled clinical trials!*** Just smile, shake your head, and ignore them completely. They are wasting your valuable time! It was claimed that Vioxx® was supported by *scientific, double-blind, randomized, placebo-controlled clinical trials,* and thousands of people are dead from taking Vioxx®. So much for the clinical trials on THAT drug!

## III. The Opposition to Alternative Cancer Treatments

There is much opposition to alternative cancer treatments, most notably by the AMA, the FDA, some insurance companies, medical schools, many cancer research and treatment centers, and the pharmaceutical industry. As soon as a new alternative therapy with much promise is publicized, it is usually immediately attacked by organized medicine. As a nurse, I do realize that there are always going to be unscrupulous characters promoting their own contrived inventions with unfounded claims that they cure this or that; however, I also know that the powers that be (the cancer industry) have grown into a beauocratic monstrosity with tentacles reaching everywhere, making millions by marketing chemotherapy drugs, radiation treatments, and diagnostic and surgical procedures. They do not like it a bit when someone or something comes along that threatens their wallets. All you have to do is read about Essiac tea, Burzynski's antineoplastons, Hoxsey tea, Ukrain, or Dr. Joseph Gold, to realize that this is true.

Did you know that one of the AMA board members who tried to shut Hoxsey down, eventually became one of his patients (160)?

## Websites That Attack Natural Medicine

There are websites on the internet dedicated to criticizing and defaming every alternative cancer therapy that does not advocate the use of toxic drugs or radiation as part of its regimen. One such website even criticizes *The Grape Cure* diet, saying that there is very little actual nutritional value in grapes, however, current scientific research has already made a liar out of them. Grape juice (including the seeds of the grapes which Johanna Brandt recommended), besides resveratrol, also contain significant amounts of "ellagic acid, catechin, quercetin, oligomeric proanthocyanidins (OPC)… pycnogenol… selenium, lycopene, lutein, laetrile (amygdalin or vitamin B17)…beta-carotene, caffeic acid…" and many other nutrients! This is described in detail at *www.cancertutor.com* (355).

For an excellent 58-page study that was done on resveratrol's role in fighting cancer, see website: *http://www.agrawal.org/PDF/ACR-Resveratrol1.pdf,* which was conducted by M.D. Anderson Cancer Center, and the UCLA Center for Human Nutrition (346). Resveratrol is also being touted as a way to fight obesity, as well as high cholesterol levels, since it keeps the body from storing fat. Other sources of resveratrol, besides purple, red, and black grapes are: pomegranates, blueberries, and cranberries. You can also obtain resveratrol supplements in health food stores. (Cranberries also cut the risk for ulcers and bladder infections, and help fight leukemia (22.)

Another website critical of alternative medicine, expresses total disbelief in the possibility that any type of cancer treatment or diet can enhance the body's immunity—even in light of the fact that the American Cancer Society is now putting on their printed literature—information that a diet high in fruits and vegetables and low in fat can reduce your risk for cancer. Apparently, the alternative medicine critics at this particular website have never read anything of the 1997 *JAMA* article either (noted by Dr. Ralph Moss in his book, *Anti-oxidants against Cancer),* which says: "The era of nutrient supplements to promote health and reduce illness is here to stay…There is overwhelming evidence of immunological enhancement following such an intervention" (507).

This same website has a writer's forum where those who feel that they have been victimized by alternative therapies can submit complaints. There is one case of a patient with a breast tumor that visited an alternative practitioner who charged her thousands of dollars up front before she could be seen. This should have set warning bells off in anyone with an ounce of sense; however, it should be mentioned right about now, that if you are going to a conventional medicine physician to get a bone marrow transplant, or a solid organ transplant, or even another type of major surgery, most of them won't even look at you until they know for sure that you (or your insurance carrier) are going to be able to PAY them the several hundreds of thousands of dollars that some of these transplants and surgeries cost! How many doctors' offices have you visited lately that wanted their co-payment OR the entire office visit payment *up front* before they would even see you? How many of them want the percentage of a scheduled procedure that your insurance isn't going to pay (e.g., 10, 20, or 30%) up front BEFORE they will do the procedure? If they are charging you $3,000.00 For a ten minute diagnostic procedure and your insurance pays 80%, until they get that 20% (not paid by your insurance) up front, many will not even make an appointment with you. If you don't have the money, or your insurance won't cover it, forget about a transplant. It won't happen. (Some people have fund drives to pay for transplants, etc., but the transplant still isn't done until payment is made.) They want to be sure that they will get paid. The U.S. health system has become terminally ill! When a family has to sell their home and everything they own to pay for a medical procedure, there is something very sick about the health care system that supports this travesty!

Another writer to the same website, complained about a doctor who was promoting an alternative cancer cure (because the doctor herself was living proof that it worked). The writer said that this particular doctor was promoting her cure with a television marketing program and thereby profiting from the suffering of other people. How ludicrous can people get?! Did you know that a recent issue of a *Reader's Digest* magazine with 204 pages in it (excluding the back cover), had **THIRTY-EIGHT pages that were FULL PAGE ads by pharmaceutical companies?** WHOSE suffering do you think they were profiting from? Where do you think pharmaceutical companies get the kind of money to put 38 FULL PAGE ads in a major monthly magazine?

Another writer to the site already had metastasizing cancer to the liver and was going through another round of chemo. This writer voiced the opinion that they had complete confidence in their physician. And my question to this writer is: ***why would you place complete confidence in your physician? Why would anyone?*** Granted, you should have some amount of confidence in your doctor—or be looking for another one—but you should never place complete confidence in any physician, because you could be in for a BIG disappointment. You should be questioning your doctor routinely, especially if you have uncertainties about any of their treatments. There are a lot of people who had complete confidence in their physicians, who would still be alive today if they had not placed complete confidence in their physicians and asked a few more questions before they took Vioxx®, Rezulin, and Baycol!

If your doctor puts you on a new prescription, do you research it before you blindly take it? Do you read about the potential side effects and interactions with other medications and foods? Do you check to see if the drug can be toxic to your kidneys or liver, or do you just gulp it down, without question? Does your doctor volunteer to inform you of the side effects of the medication?

Another writer said that they believed the ability to create pharmaceutical drugs and medicine was wisdom given by our great Creator to those who make them. While I believe that our Creator does impart wisdom and knowledge to individuals for the development of medicines and herbal remedies that will benefit mankind, there is a mighty big difference between making aspirin for headaches, or insulin for diabetics, and making a chemotherapy drug that you know will kill the patient, lying about the clinical trials, and purposely withholding evidence of negative results so that you can get the drug approved faster and make a huge profit at the expense of human lives! In going along with the type of bizarre reasoning that the above writer used, I am sure that all the family members of those patients who died with heart attacks while taking Vioxx® will certainly be comforted to know that, according to the above writer, it was God who was responsible for the brains behind the drugs that killed their loved ones!

We've also been given the **wisdom** (and I use the term very loosely here) to develop alcohol, crack cocaine, heroin, highly efficient ways to commit abortion, and pornographic videos, so what are we to do? Blame God for the moral decay and suffering that these developments have caused? What ridiculous reasoning!

Make no mistake about it—conventional medicine and alternative medicine are in constant competition. There are even websites promoted and maintained by agents of pharmaceutical companies, completely dedicated to making the public think that they are impartial reporters, however, their entire website is dedicated to taking everything used for natural cancer cures and making them appear to be total quackery. Their entire facade is dedicated to making you believe that **they** are expert authorities and that they are really concerned about your welfare by revealing what they call—all the *horrors* of natural medicine.

I have visited many such websites, most of which are 99% lies and 1% truth. Some of the people writing on these sites will even use titles like M.D., or *doctor*, before or after their name to make you THINK that they are medical physicians, when in fact, they are not. When you check further, you will find that some of them are not even practicing medical doctors, nor have they ever practiced medicine! Some are retired psychiatrists or have degrees in fields other than medicine.

## Deadly Cover-Up at MERCK Causes Death of Thousands

How many people are aware of the fiasco that went on behind closed doors when MERCK trid to keep VIOXX on the shelves even when it was killing people? See Dr. Mercola's website article if you doubt this: *http://articles.mercola.com/sites/articles/archive/2009/04/23/Drug-Company-Had-Hit-List-for-Doctors-Who-Criticized-Them.aspx* (483c). MERCK actually developed a "hit-list" of doctors who criticized their billion-dollar a year drug market! Dr. Mercola said that he even "criticized the drug a year before it came on the market" (483c), and added that "Fortunately I did not have any funding from Merck, but there are strong suspicions that they and other drug giants fund organizations like **QuackWatch** that openly seek to discredit me and other natural health care professionals" (483c). How far exactly was MERCK willing to go to silence their opponents so that they could continue to push Vioxx? Well, Dr. Mercola says that: "'The company is alleged to have used intimidation tactics against researchers, including dropping hints that the company would stop funding their institutions, and possibly even interfering with academic appointments" (483c). He added that: "The international drug company Merck had a **hit list of doctors who had to be 'neutralized' or discredited because they had criticized the painkiller Vioxx**, a now-withdrawn drug that the pharmaceutical giant produced. **'We may need to seek them out and destroy them where they live'** (483c), a Merck employee wrote, according to an email excerpt read to the court'" (483c) [emphasis mine]. Did YOU READ that last sentence? Seeking out doctors and scientists who were critical of them and "destroying them where they live..." (483c). Dr. Mercola himself was wondering exactly "how FAR" this drug company "would have gone...had Vioxx not been pulled from the market" (483c). What did they mean by **"neutralizing" their opposition?** Don't cringe please, when you read other instances in this book of when I tell you how much power these drug tzars have and how they are ruthlessly using it! This is no GAME with them – it is all about profits and big bucks! [**Emphasis, mine.**]

# CHAPTER 34

# MISCELLANEOUS ALTERNATIVE CANCER THERAPIES

*"Seek the Lord, and ye shall live." (Amos 5:6) "Thou shalt show me the path of life: in thy presence is fullness of joy; at thy right hand are pleasures forevermore." (Psalm 16:11)*

Some of the alternative therapies given in this chapter have cured cancer, others are preventatives only, or they may promote the health of certain organs, such as the liver. Some are not *gentle*, *natural,* or *painless,* since they may be given through injection or other invasive means, however, the majority of them (with a few exceptions) do not involve the use of toxic chemo drugs and radiation therapy, and many have helped cancer patients to survive the disease and extend their lives. A few are considered conventional therapy, but with fewer side effects than normally found in common chemo drugs and other conventional treatments. They are being included here for informational purposes only. Whether choosing alternative or conventional therapies (or a combination of both), the choices you make will ultimately have to be your own decision.

## I. Old & The New

### Acupuncture

Many advocates of acupuncture claim that it has definite immune-boosting effects for all types of cancer. It is not described in detail in this book.

### Cancer Testing & Diagnostics

An article at website, *http://www.alternative-doctor.com/cancer/ca_advanced.htm,* describes two tests to let your physician know if and how well your body is fighting cancer (9). These are the *AMAS* test and the *teleomerase* test. AMAS is an antibody that fights cancer. Oncolab, Inc. holds the patent rights to the test, and it is FDA approved. It is said to be highly accurate, even having the ability to find *cancer* before you've had other diagnostic tests, such as scans or x-rays (9). Teleromase is a substance that is normally found in human blood, but decreases as we age. It prevents DNA damage, but cancerous cells *contain 10-20 times* [greater than] *normal levels* (9). Though other conditions, such as inflammation and infection, can cause an increase in teleromase, if you are fighting cancer and your levels of teleromase are drastically dropping, your body is successfully fighting the cancer (9). Also, see cancer-specific chapters in this book for diagnostics aimed at those cancers.

## ALA - Alpha Lipoic Acid

This nutrient was discussed earlier, especially in relation to liver detoxification and health. It is a very powerful anti-oxidant and occurs normally in the human body in small amounts. When Dr. Burt Berkson, M.D., Ph.D., was asked to treat two victims of acute mushroom poisoning (from the amanita or *Death Angel mushroom),* he did not actually see them until a day after they had ingested the toxic meal, because they had been misdiagnosed, but not by him (344). Because of their lab results, he knew that both patients already had acute liver poisoning. The hospital told him that there was no way for them to survive. He treated them with ALA (alpha lipoic acid) infusion. He obtained the ALA from a physician at NIH (National Institutes of Health), who shipped it to him within a few hours. Both patients recovered completely (344).

Seven days later, the exact same thing happened; another couple came to the hospital with the same diagnosis, their livers in worse shape than the previous victims had been. Dr. Berkson said that the hospital demanded that he not treat them with *ALA* (344). He ignored the order, used the ALA that was leftover from the prior weekend, and within a few days, both patients were recovering, eventually to be discharged home. This, in spite of the fact that he was told it was too late to help either patient, exactly what they told him the weekend before (344). Dr. Berkson was vindicated when he was given an award by the FDA, an "investigational drug permit for intravenous ALA therapy" (344). Even so, the hospital that had ordered him not to use the ALA was enraged (344). Dr. Berkson did not identify the name of the hospital—I'm sure due to legal ramifications—but I can assure you, if I ever found out who they were, I would never go there, nor recommend them to anyone. (Would you?) Do you think what happened to Dr. Berkson in the above story is an isolated incident? It is an excellent example of what happened to Dr. Burzynski, Dr. Koch, Harry Hoxsey, and Rene Caisse. The circumstances regarding Dr. Berkson is actually only two cases, but it is a microcosmic example of the big picture of our modern U.S. medical system of treating cancer, which says to cancer patients—in essence:

***We could care less that this new treatment is non-toxic and will cure cancer. If it isn't approved by our system, or on our hospital formulary, you can't use it! You can only use these drugs for your cancer, because WE approved them—Oh—and never mind the fact that they are so toxic that they may kill you before your cancer does!***

ALA is available in supplement form. Most natural health food stores carry this nutrient. Many vegetables are natural sources of alpha lipoic acid; however, you would have to eat impossible daily amounts to get the ALA equivalent of one 100 mg supplement capsule.

## Autohemotherapy

In this type therapy, a compound is given to the cancer patient that is prepared from blood taken from their own body, with the intention of strengthening their immunity. You can find autohemotherapy at Issels Treatment Center (their website is *http://www.issels.com* and ph# 888-447-7357). Issels has developed their own vaccine taken from the cancer patient's blood, which stimulates the immune system, known as *Issels Autologous Vaccine* (290).

For one of America's largest alternative health care centers, also see the Whitaker Wellness Center, which is in Newport Beach (4321 Birch Street), California. Their website link: ***http://whitakerwellness.com/about_us/medical_team.*** Dr. Julian Whitaker, who runs this health care center, has written many books on alternative healing. He has an excellent website with a great deal of helpful information. They use many of the alternative health treatments that I have mentioned in my books, including chelation, hyperbaric oxygen, and I.V. therapies.

## Avanex 7-1037 for Colorectal & Other Tumors

A new drug that, in animal testing, was able to destroy colorectal and other tumors without the harmful effects that most chemo drugs cause, Avanex 7-1037, is undergoing further testing (29). More information on this drug can be found at *anavex.com* website. Additional studies are being done in France (29).

# B-17—Laetrile - Resurrecting?

There is still much controversy about laetrile and probably will be for some time to come, possibly because so many people were cured of deadly cancers taking laetrile. Some researchers believe that insufficient amounts of B17 in the diet are responsible for diseases such as sickle cell anemia and various cancers. Though B17 has never been given the FDA's kiss of approval as a vitamin (and possibly never will), the body still needs it in small amounts, nonetheless. Some reports even claim that cells can take B17 and make their own supplies of B12, thus preventing certain forms of anemia. (B12 injections can also be given by your physician, or taken as sublingual tablets under the tongue.) You may want to check out Dr. Andrew W. Saul's website at *http://www.doctoryourself.com/nasal.html,* for his recipe on a nasal delivery form of B12. (It is also now possible to get B12 patches where the vitamin is absorbed directly into the skin.)

Animals seem to have instincts that we humans could learn from. When a deadly tsunami killed thousands of people in Asia (December 2004), it was reported that very few animal bodies were found. The animals, sensing something amiss, scrambled for higher ground, saving their lives. Animals often know what is best for them, even when it comes to choosing their food (if they are out in the wild). God gives imparted knowledge to animals to help them survive, something we call *instinct.*

When Maureen Kennedy Salaman's pet cat developed a fatal type of cancer, she says in her book, *Nutrition: The Cancer Answer II,* that she mixed laetrile into her cat's food (550). She also gave him a nutritious diet, and within *six months*, she was told that her cat was cancer-free. He died several years later of old age (550). Ms. Salaman recommends that you should watch what your pet does when they are ill. Many times they will stop eating altogether, or they will scrounge around in your garden and start nibbling plants. Watching what animals eat when they are ill is one way that scientists have been able to select plants we now know to be disease-fighters (550).

Indians from New Mexico include amygdalin (B17) in their daily diets in the form of nutritious foods (e.g., apricot kernels), and they rarely get cancer (551). If using the kernels, a person weighing 100 pounds would need 10 apricot kernels per day; a 200 pound person would require 20 (551) (see next paragraph). Though apricot seeds are one of the richest sources of B17, sweet potatoes also have this nutrient, as well as many other foods and seeds (551). If using the seeds, follow your natural health practitioner's advice on dosing.

Ms. Salaman believes Amygdalin B17 to be the major component in a cancer-fighting protocol. The amygdalin should be taken immediately after you eat, while you still have some "food in the stomach" (550), a total of "...six to nine 500 mg amygdalin tablets should be taken daily" (550). She explains that the best tablet found in the U.S. is *Laevalin.* Others may not be reliable. With the tablets, she also recommends "10 to 15 (apricot) kernels a day to...enhance the action of the Laevalin" for patients who are fighting acute cancer, as well as eating the kernels routinely for cancer *prevention* (550).

Ms. Salaman explained that in one of the published reports from Kanematsu Sugiura, M.D. (a researcher on this substance in animal studies at Memorial Sloan-Kettering Cancer Institute), it was found that giving B17 could stop the growth of breast cancers and spreading lung tumors. In another animal study, the vitamin halted breast cancer in the majority of the test subjects, putting nearly half of them into remission (550); however, Sloan-Kettering hushed the report, saying that the findings were unimportant (550). Insiders though, *leaked* the news to the press. Proponents of B17 argue that it is high in *cyanide* and therefore, dangerous; however, the FDA has admitted that B17 is non-toxic to animals and humans (550).

Interest was sparked in B17 foods when a group of people living in isolation in the Himalayas were discovered. The late Hanna Kroeger, in her book, *Free Your Body of Tumors and Cysts*, said that regardless of age, they appeared very healthy (454). They were also young in appearance for their respective ages. It was revealed that the diet of this tribe "consisted of lots of apricots, vegetables, millet and other grains" (454). Their diet was very high in nitrilosides—B17. It was also discovered that they "cracked the seeds of the apricots," eating the kernels (454). The use of laetrile in the U.S. for cancer treatment was popularized in the 1970s, but conventional medicine worked very rapidly to discredit it, spinning it into a whirl of controversy (504). It was becoming a serious threat to the thriving chemo and radiation industry.

As for the cyanide found in laetrile, the body dissolves and excretes it harmlessly from the system. Realize that small amounts of cyanide can also be found in many berries and seeds, yet people aren't poisoned eating them. You can sometimes purchase bags of apricot kernels in natural health food stores. They are also sold on the internet. If interested in purchasing Laetrile (B17), you can do so from American Biologics, 1180 Walnut Ave., Chula Vista, CA 92011 (360). Taking B-17 with pineapple, as well as turmeric (with food), enhances its absorption by the body. If taking bromelain supplements, use the bromelain with the highest gelatin-dissolving units, at least 2000 or more GDU.

## Beres Drops Plus®

Dr. Josef Beres, a native of Hungary, developed minerals known as Beres Drops Plus® that do not exceed US RDAs (504). Website, *www.cancer tutor.com,* says that Beres tested his mineral drops on 235 people, who were told that their cancer was terminal. After taking the drops, tumors shrank in *one-third* of them (31).

## Bindweed *(Convolvulus arvensis)* Herb Fights Cancers

A common field weed, that you may find sold as *VascuStatin/Angioblock*, or under the name *PGM* or *MPGC,* is being used successfully by numerous health practitioners for fighting several forms of cancer, including ovarian and pancreatic cancers. (See the chapters in this book on breast, liver, pancreatic, and ovarian cancer for more details on using bindweed.) It is said to be non-toxic and "100 times stronger than shark cartilage" at preventing the growth of new blood vessels, a property known as anti-angiogenesis (150). This, as noted at website *http://www.springboard4health.com/notebook/health_bindweed.html.* They remark that a patient taking bindweed extract would only need "2 capsules per day," a much smaller dose than "the equivalent of 200 capsules of shark cartilage per day" (150). Anti-blood vessel forming herbs such as this should not be used for those about to undergo surgery or just having had surgery, nor cardiac patients and those who are pregnant or breast-feeding (150). As with any herb, always consult with a physician first. Bindweed should never be taken from the field and used. Before the cancer-fighting substance is extracted, the weed can be toxic (150). In animal testing, the bindweed extract was found to stimulate the immune system, prevent the growth of new blood vessel formation (which cancer cells must have in order to thrive), and was not found to be toxic (150). Many physicians are giving this herb to their cancer patients. See the website above and *springboard4health.com/store/more_arg_bindweed.html* for more details, and for information on how to obtain *VascuStatin/Angioblock* (150). The MPGC has also been helpful for those with other ailments, such as gum problems, *HIV*, *chronic fatigue* [and] *chronic infections...*(150) (301a).

## Binzel Nutritional Program

For a record of 20 cases of cancer survivors *(long-term)* of nearly every cancer imaginable, including cancer of the colon, breast, bladder, abdominal, myeloma, lymphoma, ovarian, uterine, brain, lung, lymphatic, melanoma, and pancreatic cancers, see *website http://www.brave-souls.com/learn-from-others/Binzel.html.* The site gives a description of the nutritional program of Dr. Philip Binzel Jr. Also see his book *ALIVE AND WELL,* which can be found at website *www.realityzone.com.* Dr. Binzel advocates the use of pangamic acid (vitamin B15), vitamins, B17, mega-doses of vitamins C and A, enzymes (including proteolytic enzymes), and other nutrients (5).

## BioCancell

This is a *targeted therapy* which is said to be free of toxic side effects (34a). It may be useful for those with a *high expression…of the H19 gene*, which can include cancer of the pancreas, ovaries, *liver, lung and colon.* For more details, see their website: *http://www.biocancell.com* (34a).

## Blue Light for Shrinking Tumors, LEDs & Velscope

Scientists from the Medical College of Georgia have discovered that the blue-violet light that dentists commonly use to *harden…fillings* in the mouth produces a *free radical* that actually kills oral cancer cells. It is being considered as a possible adjuvant to current cancer therapy (39). Also, check with your dentist to see if they are using the *VELscope System*, a painless diagnostic procedure for early detection of mouth cancers!

Light-emitting diodes (LEDs) are being used to treat the mucositis, mouth sores, and throat ulcers patients get from chemo and radiation.

## Breuss Total Cancer Treatment

Breuss cancer treatment involves taking a diet rich in nutrients—but in liquid form only—for a total period of 42 days. It is detailed in Dr. Rudolf Breuss' book: *The Breuss Cancer Cure* (47). This diet is based on the premise that you can literally "starve cancer cells…by not providing any solid food proteins" (47). The diet uses raw juices as well as teas. It is described in detail in the book and at websites such as *www.cancertutor.com.* It consists of juicing mostly beets, *celery*, and *carrots* with small amounts of radish and raw potato. They say that the potato isn't necessary, unless you are fighting *liver cancer* (47).

I can certainly understand why this diet would be effective, as well as very detoxifying to the body, with its use of nutrient-dense juices. The Breuss diet is a type of liquid fast. Cancer cells thrive on protein and sugar and this diet reduces protein intake dramatically, as well as processed sugars. Many people believe that fasting will make you ill—if done right—it won't. What usually makes people ill, is food. (Eating too much of the right kind or wrong kind.) Someone who is severely ill may not be able to tolerate a juice-fast. They should always discuss a new diet plan with their physician, and they may be best doing so with a Naturopathic Doctor, because some conventional medicine physicians are totally against anything that hints of alternative therapy. Others are using both!

## Burzysnski's Antineoplastons

Discussed in more detail in chapter 14, antineoplastons were developed by Stanislaw R. Burzynski, M.D., Ph.D., who discovered a substance (*antineoplastons*) missing in the blood of cancer patients. He found a way to isolate the substances and use them for cancer patients, but the FDA has fought him the entire way!

Dr. Burzysnski said that that when he gave oral antineoplastons to some of his patients with *prostate cancer* (who had failed standard treatment), they were in total remission within months. When he was ignored by fellow scientists in the U.S., other countries around the world published his important findings (550).

A few insurance companies are actually beginning to cover antineoplastons, but only under strictly limited circumstances. These substances have been very successful alternative cancer treatments. You can reach the Burzynski clinic through website: *http://www.burzynskiclinic.com/ph/index.html.* Antineoplastons are discussed in much greater detail in chapter 14 and 16 of this book, due to their tremendous success with terminal brain cancer patients and those with lymphoma. (Note that antineoplastons are not to be confused with a group of chemo drugs known as *antineoplastics*. They are **not** the same.) The FDA has finally approved the oral form of antineoplastons (PBs) for off-label use, and antineoplastons A10 and AS2-1 were recently given orphan drug status by the FDA for use on human brainstem gliomas. Some individuals can have side effects from antineoplastons, but they are mild and quickly reversible, unlike toxic chemo drugs that often cause fatal adverse reactions.

## CDA-II

This is a type of nutrition therapy combined with a urine therapy that was studied extensively in Taiwan by Dr. Ming C. Liau, who also spent 14 years working with Dr. Burzynski in Houston, Texas. Clinical trials were done at Anhui Medical University showing that this treatment was effective and safe. According to website *http://www.brave-souls.com/learn-from-others*, the only adverse effect was vein irritation and rarely, a potential for venous thrombosis. It is sometimes combined with B17 and vitamin C with very good results. This particular website discusses a patient with non-Hodgkin's lymphoma and another with lung cancer (who also used radiation with the CDA-II) (468), and successfully treated their cancer.

## Camu-Camu

This Brazilian fruit is also known as *rumberry, mijo* and other names. According to *http://www.wholeworldbotanicals.com/info_royalcamu.html*, it has "30 to 60 times more vitamin C than an orange" (320). Just realize that if you get the juice bottled, it is probably pasteurized, which kills much of the vitamin C, so the best way to consume the fruit is via supplement form or fresh. High in many anti-oxidants, this fruit helps to boost the body's natural immunity and refresh the liver. The website also explains how to purchase camu-camu (320).

## Cancell (Protocel)

This substance, also called *Cantron* and other names, has several ingredients. It was developed nearly 80 years ago and tested in the late 70's, 80's, and early 90's by the NCI. Testing was discontinued because they felt that it was not effective against cancer, though you can find many testimonials on the internet of people who have used it, and claim that it has helped them cure their cancer. Some used it alone, others used it in conjunction with chemo and other therapies.

# II. Is Cancer A Fungus?

## • Candida & Cancer – Oncology Physician Believes Cancer is a Fungus

Italian oncology physician, Dr. Tullio Simoncini, believes that cancer is actually a fungus, namely *Candida.* So convinced was he that he wrote a book entitled: *Cancer Is A Fungus* (582). He suggests that cancer patients be given *sodium bicarbonate*, a non-poisonous substance, directly into the cancerous tissue (582). If you are interested in more specifics on his treatment, see website: *http://www.cancerisafungus.com/cancer-fungus-content.html* and this site as well: *http: //www.cancerfungus.com* (582). You can order his book at his website: *http://www.curenatural icancro.com,* which also has a great deal more information on him and his treatment of cancer. Apparently, he has been very successful in using this therapy (582). He has reports of patients "using sodium bicarbonate at five per cent solution," to heal *lung* cancers, cancers of the mouth, head and neck, *liver,* gastric and *intestinal, prostate, stomach, pancreas, spleen,* and many others (582). If you go to his website: *curenaturalicancro.com,* he has a great deal of information and detailed *instructions* for using this *non-toxic, inexpensive* therapy (582). You can also watch a video showing before and after cancer growths treated with sodium bicarb at website: *http://articles.mercola.com/sites/articles/archive /2008/08/05/fungus-causing-cancer-a-novel-approach-to-the-most-common-form-of-death.aspx?source=nl.* When you consider the SAD (Sad American Diet), which is so conducive to high acid levels and promoting fungal infections, Dr. Simoncini's approach makes a great deal of sense.

Dr. Simoncini says cancerous growths are usually white, the same color as most fungus and yeast. What does the soda bicarb do? It turns the entire cancerous area alkaline and allows more oxygen to get to the cancer cells and, as noted in several other parts of this book, cancer cannot survive in a high oxygen, alkaline environment. Dr. Simoncini says that today's fungal drugs don't work because they only fight the top layer of the yeast, and besides that, the fungus simply adapts to the drug in just a few days (582). He says that soda bicarb is absolutely the strongest anti-fungal substance you can use. He uses a port-a-cath to target tumors directly, going through a nearby vessel in, for example, reaching liver tumors or pancreatic tumors; however, in cavity tumors (those in the abdomen or peritoneal area), a peritoneal catheter can be used to deliver the sodium bicarb. In bladder cancers, you can simply use a urethral cathether to deliver the soda bicarb (582). The treatment is non-toxic and can be used to cure most solid cancers in days! Dr. Simoncini also says that other disorders, such as MS, ALS, and psoriasis are caused by a fungus. He uses a soda bicarb wash for tumors in the colon (582). Is it possible that curing a disease so deadly can be this simple? How many alternative medicine physicians have been telling the public for years that cancer cannot thrive in an alkaline environment? Because of his exclusive non-toxic treatment of cancer, shunning chemo drugs, Dr. Simoncini has had his license revoked by the conventional medicine, pharmaceutical monopoly in his country. (Sound familiar?)

It is interesting that the very first patient Dr. Simoncini cured was an 11-year-old boy with leukemia who was already in a comatose state (582). For brain cancers, he uses *selective arteriography*, via the carotids. He says that the only cancer that isn't easily reached are those in the small bones found in the ribs and vertebrae due to the sparse arterial blood flow into these areas (582). (Dr. Sircus disagrees, see below and see chapter 16.)

For a complete list of individual protocols that Dr. Simoncini uses in his treatment of various cancers, see website *http://www.curenaturalicancro.com*, and click on the tab that says: *Treatments With Sodium Bicarbonate* (582). Dr. Simoncini has used his treatment on many types of cancer. He uses a 5% or 8.4% soda bicarbonate solution fed via a special catheter in order to make direct contract with the cancer (582). As for side effects of this natural substance, they are few and generally mild, such as a feeling of thirst or *temporary tiredness*, and says that some patients who have multiple tumors may experience a temperature rise after beginning treatment (582); however, see below for safer, oral use of soda bicarb.

## • Physician Says ORAL Soda Bicarb Just as Effective for Killing Cancer as Intravenous Bicarb

Dr. Mark Sircus, author of *Sodium Bicarbonate Rich Man's Poor Man's Cancer Treatment*, says you don't need to travel to a European physician for intravenous soda bicarb; not when you can take it orally for best results, and you can find it at your local grocery store for pennies a pound in the form of *Arm & Hammer*® baking soda, with directions right on their box for rapid alkalizing (566c). He discusses the strange and bitter irony that is happening in the conventional cancer establishment – the fact that chemo drugs are so toxic, soda bicarb must be hung alongside them to keep them from killing the patient, and he questions this: are physicians taking credit for healing cancer with toxic chemo drugs when what is really happening is that the soda bicarb is actually doing the healing (566c)? Does the patient even need the chemo? Why not just give them the soda bicarb, which alkalizes the body? Alkalinity kills cancer. This is why cesium works so well, but cesium must be monitored closely and can be dangerous. Soda bicarb is non-toxic. How strange isn't it - that when cancer chemo victims develop mouth sores from chemo, doctors often tell them to use a soda bicarb rinse to heal their mouth (566c)! Soda bicarb users should check with their doctors simply because it is so high in salt. Dr. Sircus says that "Not only is it good for diaper rash it can also kick the teeth out of just about any cancer given a chance," and that "it is as safe as chicken soup and probably more effective than any other single element in any cancer protocol and it can be taken simply through oral administration…" (566c). However, Dr. Sircus also points out that soda bicarb has limits. Many people are deficient in "magnesium, iodine and selenium," and the importance of water and sunshine (vitamin D) in fighting cancer (566c), as I have repeatedly pointed out in this book in several chapters. Also, see Dr. Sircus' excellent books on Iodine and Magnesium described in Appendix II (and my reference section), as well as sources of transdermal magnesium and a superior form of gentle, food grade iodine.

If you want to read about a substance that promoters claim will destroy candida in the body (THREELAC™), see website *www.ghthealth .com*. They also promote many other health products.

## • A "Country Doctor" Claims He Has Made an Amazing Substance that Will Cure Just About Any Cancer.

The 75 year-old former truck driver has no medical background, but those loyal to him, claim that he is a "miracle worker" (377a). 64 year-old Ian Rodhouse with lung cancer was given *six months to live.* He used "Dr. Jim's" preparation. His cancer was gone *within two months* (377a). "Dr. Jim," as his friends call him, has "dispensed his mixture to more than 200 patients diagnosed with terminal cancer" (377a). He says "of that number, 185 lived at least 15 more years, and nearly half" went into complete remission" (377a). Of course, state medical experts are already calling him a "quack" and threatening "to arrest him for practicing medicine without a license" (377a). (Sound familiar? Remember Rene Caisse?) After all, should we not make sure that this terribly natural maple syrup and baking soda doesn't HEAL anyone's cancer without being sure that they have FIRST gone through the toxic chemo and radiation approved and ACCEPTED by the FDA? RIGHT?

Well, of course, you would always consult with your doctor about any new regimen, but should you have more questions: "here…is Dr. Jim's recipe:

> Add one part baking soda with three parts maple syrup in a small saucepan. Stir briskly. Heat for five minutes. Take one teaspoon daily, as needed. Be sure you use ALUMINUM-FREE baking soda and 100% maple syrup (no synthetics) Use organic (obtain from your health food store) (377a). [Do not use an aluminum pan.]

Remember that cancer cells THRIVE on sugar and suck it up rapidly, then the baking soda, which is very ALKALINE, is carried into the cells by "the maple syrup," and "removes the microbe inside the cancer cell" (377a). Remember that cancer cannot THRIVE in an alkaline-environment. (One person who uses this formula says you only need to heat it until it foams.)

According to Dr. Mark Sircus, you can use this formula with honey or blackstrap molasses and it does not need to be heated, and you can probably use it with the maple syrup without heating, as well (566c).

# III. More Cancer Fighters

## Canelim Capsules—Chinese Remedy

Canelim is a compound consisting of four Chinese medicinals, which may be helpful in fighting several types of cancer, including abdominal, throat, lung, and breast cancer. It is not recommended that the remedy be taken with stimulants or cold beverages (65).

## Carctol - Herbal Treatment From India

Dr. Rosy Daniel claims to have seen this Indian herbal preparation perform miracles in curing cancer. Formulated in India by physician, Dr. Nandlal Tiwari, Carctol is composed of eight herbs and has its origin in Hindu medicine (423). The herbal remedy is used in conjunction with consuming huge quantities of water daily, and an acid-free diet. The preparation seems to be more successful in digestive tract cancers. Nearly 2000 patients in India have used the therapy (423). Dr. Daniel admits to having prescribed it to 860 people. Some doctors have given it before and after chemo. See website *carctolhome.com,* for a list of several British physicians that also use this treatment (423). Dr. Daniel believes the treatment works, based on the inability of cancer cells to flourish when the body is alkaline. He prescribes the remedy for two months, then discontinues use if there is no benefit (423). The remedy is controversial, as there is disagreement about its effectiveness (423); however, it is true that cancer cannot thrive in an alkaline environment.

## CellFeed Medical

This therapy uses a *low-charge electrical field* to make cancer cells more able to absorb chemo drugs (128). The cells are first stimulated electrically, then exposed to chemo, with the result being that the chemo is absorbed more efficiently. It is being developed by Tel Aviv University professor, Yona Keisari and associates (128). It is being mentioned here for informational purposes only because the electrical stimulation itself is painless and non-toxic, but it is often combined with toxic chemo drugs.

## CellQuest™ Dietary Supplement

This dietary supplement comes from an extract of a *musaceas* plant, *a banana* or *plantain,* which, in lab testing, seems to help *boost* the natural immunity of the body (69a). It can be used in a gel form that you apply on the skin, or a liquid that you drink. See their main website at *www.cellquest.com* (69a). It is actually "the world's largest herb…a member of the grass family" (69a). It is high in potassium and other minerals and low in salt (69a). The company makes no claims as far as curing, treating, or preventing disease with this supplement (69a).

## Cesium

Cesium chloride has the highest alkaline level of any mineral. It is believed that it may kill cancer cells by preventing them from absorbing sugar, thus starving them to death, as well as raising the cells' alkalinity. Cesium goes right inside the cells, but beware, because taking large amounts of this mineral can lead to dangerous cardiac arrhythmias (71). Do not take cesium unless you are under the strict guidance of your physician.

## Chelation Therapy

Chelation therapy involves giving substances (usually intravenously) which are said to strip toxic metals from tissues and ream out the arteries. A synthetically-made amino acid by the name of EDTA *(ethylene diamine tetra-acetic acid)* is usually used for this form of detoxing the body (608). EDTA has been used to treat those with heavy-metal poisoning. The EDTA binds with the heavy metals and removes them from the body. There is now a form of EDTA that is referred to as *EDTA Liposome* which is supposed to do the same thing, but it is not given by I.V., which can take many hours to perform (608). PubMed details a study at *http://www.pubmedcentral.nih.gov/articlerender.Fcgi?artid=2111156* using this liposomal *EDTA* (608). You can find oral forms of liposomal EDTA with alpha lipoic acid at website: *http://organicpharmacy.org/products/EDTA/SKU:LF-EDTA2.* Also: *http://www.bio-genesis.com/pdf/EDTALiposomal.pdf.* Taking EDTA liposomal before you go to sleep is supposed to pull heavy metals out of your cells while you sleep (608). Be sure that you drink plenty of water to keep your body flushed, otherwise the heavy metals will reabsorb right back into the cells. This is why drinking water is so important when you are detoxing and juicing. Toxins are removed from your tissues and cells, but you must be well-hydrated to flush them out of the body.

## Chlorophyll & Chlorophyllin for Cancer Prevention

Scientists have discovered that eating green foods, which are high in natural chlorophyll, could protect from all cancers, but especially those of the colon and liver (76). Many animal studies have shown that natural chlorophyll and chlorophyllin (an extract made from chlorophyll) fight cancer. They discovered that this substance can also protect against a dangerous fungus that often affects nuts and cereals known as *aflatoxin,* a source of liver cancer, especially in nations that do not have adequate safety measures for storing their grains (76).

Chlorophyll and chlorophyllin also protect against the DNA damage from other cancer-causing substances, especially those found in *grilled meats* and *diesel exhaust.* Dr. George S. Bailey discussed the protective effects of this green substance in the LPI Research Newsletter "Chlorophylls and Cancer Prevention: passing the First Hurdle" (76). He describes a human study using chlorophyllin, which was conducted in Eastern China for a group of people who were at risk for liver cancer from the *aflatoxin* mold (76). They were given the chlorophyllin *thrice daily* in 100 mg pills for a total of 300 mg. The participants in the clinical trial experienced a 55% decrease in urinary output of the aflatoxin compounds, indicating that the chlorophyllin was destroying the toxins which are responsible for *DNA damage* (which causes liver cancer) (76). A new 20-year clinical trial is being done in China to test chlorophyllin. They explained that eating a *moderate-to-high* amount *of green vegetables* would be necessary to obtain the *300 mg per day of chlorophyllin* given in the clinical trial (76). High amounts of chlorophyll in the diet via green vegetables could also help prevent the type of colon cancer caused by an iron found in red meats (76). There is no toxicity in natural chlorophyll and chlorophyllin, however, do check with your physician or Naturopath before supplementing in large amounts.

## Cholesterol Drug Kills Deadly Cancer Cells Without Toxic Side Effects

As described by NeoPlas Innovation Director of Research, Dr. Stephen Cantrell, when they gave melanoma patients a "regimen of low-dose interferon with lovastatin," a common cholesterol-lowering drug, they saw tumors start to regress, often in a *few weeks* (76a). Not only that, but most participants complained only of *fatigue* (76a). They did not have the adverse effects usually found with chemo drugs and *radiation* (76a). Amazingly enough, they are also considering this new treatment for other lethal cancers, such as "pancreatic cancer, colon cancer, renal (kidney) cancer, mesothelioma, and a group of sarcomas, including osteosarcoma, chondrosarcoma and malignant fibrous histiocytoma" (76a). For more information on this exciting new development, see NeoPlas website *www.neoplas.org* (76a). This treatment has "arrested or eradicated tumors in more than 80% of initial patients" (76a). They first used the treatment in 2000 on a man with "stage 4 melanoma, he remains disease-free today" (76a). Just be aware that statin drugs strip CoQ10 out of your body. If you choose this treatment, let your doctor know this so they can advise you on CoQ10 supplementation. Some physicians are not aware of this.

## Cryo Treatment/CryoTherapy

Usually guided by doppler imagery, cryo treatment involves freezing cancerous growths with a controlled method that seeks to leave healthy tissue undamaged. It has been used effectively in many types of cancer. It usually causes less damage to the body than radiation or chemo, and is less invasive. It is more painless than using heat and is being mentioned here simply because it may be a more favorable choice than chemo or radiation, depending on the type cancer. It has been successfully used for abnormal cells of the cervix, retinoblastoma, skin cancers (before they become malignant), prostate cancer, and others and is sometimes used in combination with other therapies (see article below).

## Cryospray Ablation for Barrett's Esophagus & Throat Cancer

This is a new type of nearly painless, non-toxic treatment for throat cancers, as well as the abnormal *esophageal* cells found in *Barrett's esophagus* (usually caused by GERD or *acid reflux* disease). It uses *liquid nitrogen* to *freeze* the cells, and is being used at Loyola Medical Center in Chicago (480), and other facilities. It is planned for other cancers, such as those of the *colon,* in the not-so-distant-future. Though the treatment may need to be repeated, reports say that usually the first treatment takes out *70 to 90 percent* of the unwanted cells. Physicians were amazed that the response was so rapid. The treatment typically requires only *15 minutes to a couple of hours*, with patients going home the same day and resuming normal activities. Before now, the use of liquid nitrogen has been limited to *warts and skin cancer* (480).

## CyberKnife® for Killing Cancer

CyberKnife® is a sophisticated treatment being used, not only on brain tumors, but other cancers throughout the body. Unlike the Gamma Knife®, CyberKnife® is painless, bloodless, requires no anesthesia, *no recovery time*, no frame application, *no sedation,* a short duration of treatment, and it has fewer risks and side effects than traditional surgery (89a). This procedure, if used on parts of the body **outside** the brain, may require that *markers* or *fiducials* be put in place beforehand in order to assist the physician in precisely defining the targeted *area* (89b). This may require needles, which are not painless. These markers are not required for use in brain tumors.

The patient may be given a mesh-type mask to wear, then gets up and goes home immediately when the procedure is finished. It can even be used for soft tumors (e.g., those of the *lung, pancreas and liver lesions,* as well as growths in the *Kidney*), in a new treatment using CyberKnife®, known as *Synchrony*. Georgetown University in Washington, D.C., has been a pioneer in Synchrony (89a). This procedure "uses a miniature linear accelerator (LINAC) mounted on a robotic arm to deliver concentrated beams of radiation to the targeted tumor from multiple positions and angles" (89a). It has " lower risk" and "fewer complications than traditional open surgery," and while the Gamma Knife® is only used on brain lesions and tumors, the CyberKnife® is successfully being used on many other tumors located elsewhere in the body (89a). Another new accessory that the CyberKnife® will be using, which just came out, is what is known as "The AXUM automatic patient positioning system" (89a). Georgetown University's phone number is: (202) 342-2400. (CyberKnife® is discussed later in this chapter.) Just realize that the CyberKnife® does involve some radiation, and it can damage nearby healthy cells.

## Cytoluminescent Therapy®

Cytoluminescent Therapy ® (CLT) is a form of light therapy, also referred to as *photodynamic therapy*. Patients are given an injection of a light-sensitive chemical, then diodes and lasers are used against the sensitized cancer cells. Later, the patients themselves would take an oral form of the chemical and activate it (while back at home), using an infrared light. Though some people advocate this treatment, I have read some negative comments about it. Patients using the infrared lights had deteriorating health with complaints of pain, malaise, overall weakness, and weight loss. Now, when given, it is recommended that it is only done by professionals in an outpatient setting, rather than having the patients activate the treatment at home.

## Cytotron Therapy - QMR

A new cancer (and arthritis) treatment developed and available in India that you will not yet be able to get in the U.S., is being successfully used on humans and is known as *Cytotron Therapy*. This therapy uses a rapidly rotating nuclear magnetic field, which comes from more than 200 beams, so precise that they can renew and restore tissues that have degenerated, without harming healthy tissues (90). They can also destroy diseased tissue. It is available at Sibia Medical Center, Ludhiana, in Northern India, in use since 2006. It is completely painless, without harmful side effects, and considered non-invasive therapy (90). It is mostly for solid tumors, rather than systemic cancers. It is also being used to treat osteoarthritis, making total knee surgeries (and other degenerative joint surgeries) unnecessary (90). See their website at: *www.sssibia.com*, as well as *www.cytotrontreatment.com*. This treatment is also being used in Malaysia. Since it is non-invasive, painless, and has no toxic side effects, don't look for quick FDA approval in the U.S. You may hear this referred to as *QMR* or *Quantum Magnetic Resonance*—they are the same thing.

## DCA - Dichloroacetate

Touted as a cancer killer (in laboratory tests), this compound has not yet been subject to broad clinical trials for cancer, though it has been used for pulmonary hypertension and other disorders. It is only used in its sodium or potassium (salt) form and has been known to cause nerve problems.

## DaVinci® Surgical System

See below under *Robotic Technology*.

## Dendritic Cell Therapy

A type of vaccine that stimulates the body's own immune system to fight cancer (aka *Immunotherapy*), dendritic cell therapy is helpful even for those with stage IV disease, who have failed all other conventional treatments. It is also being used for HIV patients (6). Dendrite cells are actually immune cells occurring in the body, but not in sufficient amounts to fight cancer. The patient's own blood cells are taken, treated outside the body (so that dendritic cells are produced en masse) with UV light, then re-injected, thus triggering the immune response (6). Though not a painless process, it is being mentioned here since it does not involve chemo and radiation. More information can be found at website *dendritic.info* (6). Since the patient's own cells are used, there is no danger of rejection. Also, see the paragraph below under **Extracorporeal Photopheresis**, which is another name for this treatment.

## Epigenetic Therapy

Epigenetics is a study of DNA changes: some beneficial, some harmful. For example, the genes of identical twin girls are studied at six-years-old and found to be very similar. Again, when they are 15, they are studied, but found to have more dissimilarities. Scientists are shocked to find that when they again check the genetic profile of the identical twin girls at age 50, there are varied and dramatic changes in their genetic blueprint. They believe that these changes prove that our environment, the food we eat, the stresses we endure, the career path we choose, the toxins we are exposed to—all of these things can causes changes in our DNA—some beneficial, some potentially harmful. This is why one twin might be more prone to develop arthritis and cancer, while the other twin escapes arthritis and cancer, but may be more prone to mood swings and/or cardiac abnormalities—things that neither of them may have experienced at age six, yet the changes in their genes that they experienced at age 15 would have been passed on to their children (483a).

Epigenetics help scientists understand how genes are passed from parents to their children (483a). This means that "we are not only what we eat, but also what our parents and grandparents ate" (483a). Everything that we are exposed to affects us at the cellular level: cigarette smoking, food additives, mental disorders, traumatic stress, anti-oxidants, minerals, vitamins, antibiotics, perm chemicals, molds, bacteria, viruses, radiation; any of these things can affect our genes, thus the genes of our children (483a). It is hoped that epigenetics will eventually make chemo and radiation unnecessary. For example, Dr. Jean-Pierre Issa of M.D. Anderson Cancer Center did a study on a type of *incurable* leukemia, *Myelodysplastic Syndrome.* As a result of "epigenetics therapy," he was able to bring about half of his "clinical trial patients... into remission," and with fewer "side effects" (483a). Those involved in epigenetics hope to reverse negative genetic changes that occur in families and target (or mark) the good ones (483a).

## Essiac Tea

See chapter six of this book for greater detail on this amazing tea formula that a Canadian nurse used to cure hundreds (possibly thousands) of her cancer patients, even those given up by conventional medicine as terminal, hopeless, and inoperable.

## Extracorporeal Photopheresis with Autologous Dendritic Cell Vaccine (Ultraviolet Light Therapy)

Another treatment that is available at Issels, and also approved by the FDA for "cutaneous T-cell lymphoma," this ultraviolet light therapy eliminates cancer cells. A type of white blood cell is extracted, treated with UV light, allowed to multiply, then "injected into the patient in small doses over a certain period of time" (290). Issels website is *http://www.issels.com.* Ph# 888-447-7357 (290). Also, see in this chapter (above) under *Dendritic Cell Therapy*, which is the same thing.

## Far Infrared Hyperthermia Treatment

This detoxifying heat treatment is also available at Issels Medical Center Integrative and Complementary Medicine. They are located in Phoenix, Arizona, and Santa Barbara, California. This hyperthermia is considered safe. It uses infrared heat in treating the body (113). I am not associated with this center and cannot personally vouch for them. This information is included here because this treatment center provides alternative therapy as well as conventional therapies. You will be able to find alternative treatments at Issels that you may not find in your own area of the country.

For one of America's largest alternative health care centers, the Whitaker Wellness Center, which is in Newport Beach (4321 Birch Street), California, see this link: ***http://whitakerwellness.com/about_us/medical_team.*** Dr. Julian Whitaker, who runs this health care center, has written many books on alternative healing. He has an excellent website with a great deal of helpful information. They use many of the alternative health treatments that I have mentioned in my books, including chelation, hyperbaric oxygen, and intravenous therapies.

## Forskolin fights Cancer Spread

Derived from the roots of a plant, this is one blood thinner that has shown the ability, in animal testing, to fight the spread of cancer. It has shown an ability in **humans** to help fight glaucoma and asthma, and as an appetite suppressant. See website: *www.raysahelian.com/forskolin.html,* for standardized formulas for this and many other health supplements (544).

## Gamma Knife® & CyberKnife® for Inoperable Lesions & Tumors

The CyberKnife® is painless and non-invasive. The Gamma Knife uses a stereotactic head frame that is attached to the skull with four screws, which is painful, but it does not really involve the use of any sort of knife. Both of them use what is known as *radiosurgery,* or intense concentrated beams of radiation to target a tumor or lesion within the brain that would be difficult, if not impossible, to reach with surgery. They are often used on hard-to-reach tumors, such as pituitary tumors and acoustic neuromas (schwannomas). They do not require general anesthesia and usually just an overnight stay (GammaKnife®) or an outpatient hospital stay (CyberKnife®), with resumption of normal activities within hours. You may hear of this type treatment referred to as *stereotactic* surgery or *stereotactic* radiotherapy, though the CyberKnife® does not require the stereotactic frame attachment to the skull.

CyberKnife® is newer than the Gamma Knife®. An advantage of this type treatment is that there is usually less damage to nearby healthy cells, as found in standard radiation therapies, and patients are less likely to have the severity of side effects that standard radiation causes. Side effects depend on the size of the lesion or tumor, how long it is treated, and other factors that you would discuss with your physician. With the CyberKnife® there are few side effects and they are normally mild. Severe side effects are rare. Just realize that this is a form of radiation. Radiation treatments have the potential for some immune depression, and this treatment can cause some damage to nearby healthy cells.

Though not what I consider *natural*, I would not discourage anyone from having Gamma Knife® or CyberKnife®, though I have heard more positive things about CyberKnife® than Gamma Knife®. It has saved many lives and has also been used to treat trigeminal neuralgia and vascular malformities. It is often used on hard-to-reach tumors, such as pituitary tumors. It is being included here because sometimes the side effects associated with the procedure may be less severe than other types of radiation that are given over longer periods of time, depending on where in the brain the tumor is located and how long it is treated. It is also used to immediately shrink brain tumors that are causing life-threatening brain swelling, in order to provide time until other treatments can be considered. (Also, see later in this chapter for information on the new, non-toxic, painless NanoKnife™ technology.)

## Glandulars

These compounds are given to cancer patients with the intention of strengthening the thymus, liver, thyroid, and adrenals. You can find glandulars at most health food stores. They are often administered by alternative health physicians.

## Glyconutrition

There is a good deal of information on the internet on the benefits of glyconutrition, as well as some controversy. For more details on this nutritional energy source, see website: *http://www.gotglyconutrition.com/strengthen-the-imune-system.html*. There are also many other sites that promote this plant-based substance that uses plant sugars for boosting the immune system, including *www.mannatech.com* and *http://www.glycoscience.org/RDInsight_v3aboutambrotose121207.pdf*, as well as *glycoscience.org*, which sells the product under the name of *Ambrotose*®. *Mannatech* is another name for glyconutrient technology. Glyconutrients are not stated to cure or heal the body—but rather to improve the body's ability at self-healing. For some amazing testimonials of people who used glyconutrition to help boost their immunity and heal their cancers and other illnesses, contact Dr. Norman G. Marvin, M.D., at 913-681-9710 (fax#). *Mannatech* has been popularized on ABC's 20/20 program.

Also, see chapter seven in this book for the case of an 80-year-old grandmother cured of advanced ovarian cancer using a glyconutrition mushroom formula (RM-10) developed by her son, Jordan Rubin, which is now available through ***Garden of Life*** products. See website: *http://www.crohns.net/Miva/education/testimonial_rosemenlowe.shtml* (30).

## HGH—Human Growth Hormone

HGH is yet another hormone produced by our bodies in lesser amounts as we age. In their book, *What Your Doctor May Not Tell You About Immune Disorders*, Dr. Stephen Edelson and Lynn Sonberg tell us that by the time you hit 60, your body is only producing about one-fourth of the HGH found in younger counterparts, however, this growth hormone does not last long in the body (390). It is normally released from the pituitary while you are sleeping and after high activity. Almost immediately, the liver changes most of it to "insulin-like growth factor type 1 (IGF1)" (390). If your physician wants to see if you are deficient in HGH, he or she won't measure the HGH circulating in your body, since it doesn't last very long. They will measure the amount of IGF1 that you have, since it lasts about a day-and-a-half (390). As Edelson and Sonnberg explain, often those with *auto-immune disorders* or *chronic fatigue* have deficient levels of IGF1, and they will benefit from HGH supplements. Sub-normal levels can cause "fatigue, loss of muscle and bone strength, reduced healing capacity, diminished memory…weight gain, and loss of skin tone" (390). When taken in supplement form, both authors say that HGH fights osteoporosis, aging, sleep disorders, depression, and helps libido, stamina, *mood* and *memory* (390). HGH is available as an injectable form and "over the counter" supplements, however, you should check with your physician before taking this, or any other hormone (390).

## HMR Lignans From Spruce Knot Heartwood May Help Fight Hormonal Cancers

Not only is tree bark high in a cancer-fighting substance known as *stilbene,* but there are also some amounts of *resveratrol* in tree bark (276). You may find *HMR lignan* as a new food additive. Besides fighting hormonal cancers, it may also have positive effects against menopausal disorders and cardiac problems (276). Some findings suggest that resveratrol lowers LDH cholesterol and can be used with niacin to increase this effect. Exercise will also lower LDH and raise good cholesterol in the body.

## Hyperthermia for Cancer Treatment (Including Interstitial Radio Frequency)

Hyperthermia, discussed elsewhere in this book, can also be obtained at **Advanced Alternatives Cancer Center.** They have locations in Las Vegas, Nevada, and the Bahamas. It has been discovered that this non-toxic treatment can use heat in many areas of the body to quickly kill cancerous cells (303). For growths less than 3 cm deep, heating can safely be done through microwaves. Growths that are deeper in the body (e.g., 8 cm) are more likely to respond to *ultrasound hyperthermia units* (303). The positive effect of this treatment is that the heat can be targeted just to kill the cancer cells, leaving nearby healthy cells unharmed. In *Interstitial Radio Frequency*, needles that are placed into the tumor are heated, and the heat kills the tumor. There is also the use of hyperthermia to heat the entire body using a gradual process in a *sauna or whirlpool unit* (303). The patient must be monitored closely since reaching high body temperatures can create a dangerous strain on vital organs. (Another example of a treatment that deliberately causes a fever to the body is *Iscador, the mistletoe extract)* (303).

## Immunotherapy - Global First Of a Kind, Non-Toxic Miracle Cure for Acute Myeloid Leukemia - Breast & Ovarian Cancer Next?!

In a history-making event by physicians at the Royal Free Hospital in London, a woman suffering from *acute myeloid leukaemia*, who had already failed chemo and three routine transplants, was put into total remission with *natural killer* cells taken from her 21-year-old daughter (568a). The cells were removed, treated, then *injected* into her mother. Just *two days* after receiving *57 million* of the treated *natural killer cells*, they had multiplied into *137 million of the cells* (568a). Within one week the procedure was a success, making it a *world first!* A dozen more patients are lined up for the procedure, and it is hoped that the *same technique* will be successful against other cancers, such as those of the ovaries and breast. If the patient relapses, the procedure can be repeated (568a).

For many years, alternative health advocates have been promoting products and procedures that boost the body's immunity. They have been telling the public that it is the body's IMMUNITY that will heal disease. In this world record, it is ironic that a daughter's immune system was used to help heal her own mother's immunity. Also, see the other article in this chapter on the development of individualized vaccines for treating cancer, a similar treatment.

## Insulin-Induced Hypoglycemic Therapy—IHT

IHT treatment is based on the belief that, in order to survive, cancer cells must have sugar. At one time, insulin was given intravenously to deliberately induce a state of hypoglycemia for about an hour (starving the cells of sugar), during which time the patient was closely monitored; however, with today's new technology, this dangerous step no longer has to be done (165). One of the labs that uses IHT, BioPulse (in Mexico), reports that thus far, they have had success with everyone on which it has been used. Growths either shrank or disappeared entirely (165).

## Intracellular Hyperthermia (ICHT) & Magnetite Nanoparticles or Cationic Liposomes

In a laboratory study (reported in *Jpn J. Cancer Res.* 89, 463-470, April 1998), rats were treated for solid gliomas using ICHT with Magnetite Cationic Liposomes (501). As described at one website in particular, they were put directly into the cancerous growths, then irradiated through the use of an *alternating magnetic field* (501). Nearly 90% of the test animals in one of the groups went into total remission. Final results were very impressive. Most importantly, the procedure was safe. The animals had no serious adverse *effects*. The *magnetic nanoparticles* had worked against the *solid tumors* (501). Nanoparticles are being tested against breast cancer, melanoma, prostate cancer, and many other cancers.

Hyperthermia is very promising and is already being used on humans, however, the heated needles are painful. Quick-thinking researchers have devised needles which are not nearly as large. They are less painful and more efficient (501). They went on to develop *magnetite cationic liposomes* (MCLs), ten times more potent at attracting the cancer cells than the earlier nanoparticles (501).

## IPT (Insulin Potentiation Therapy) & Hyperthermia Cancer Treatments

IPT therapy uses insulin to treat cancer. This is because insulin makes cell membranes more efficient in transporting nutrients and compounds into cells, and helps get medications into the brain (167). First, the patient is given small doses of insulin IV, and a short while later, another medication of choice is given. Apparently, the insulin helps make the other medication given (whatever is chosen) work more effectively by getting it into the cells more rapidly and more efficiently (167). IPT also means that other drugs of choice can be given in smaller amounts, yet still be effective at killing cancer cells, while minimizing the adverse *side effects* that larger doses would cause, if they happen to be drugs that cause undesirable reactions (167). As noted by website: *http://iptq.com/fact_sheet.htm,* IPT has been used, not only in treating tumors, but "arthritis and related rheumatic syndromes…pancreatic cancer, multiple sclerosis, [and] paralysis after stroke" (167).

Realize that using toxic drugs damages the body's natural immunity, though they are sometimes used with IPT therapy. You need a strong immune system to help you get well. Hopefully, the information on the many non-toxic alternative cancer therapies in this book will give you the background that you need to assist you in choosing the therapy (or combination of therapies) that you feel most comfortable with. Either way, be sure to read this book in its entirety so that you are well-informed on making that important decision.

## IP-6 (Inositol Hexaphosphate) Fights Cancer

Cancer cells use a lot of iron and must have iron to survive. Drugs that remove iron from the body, thus fighting cancer cells, have adverse side effects, however, IP-6 is a natural substance which effectively strips cancer cells of iron without depleting the body's natural stores of iron (554). It is a safe, gentle, non-toxic ingredient and relatively inexpensive. Taken from nuts, rice bran, and other cereals, it is without the toxicity of chemo drugs. Extensive human trials have yet to be done on IP-6 (554). Most health food stores carry this supplement.

## Intensity Modulated Radiotherapy (IMRT)—Tomo Therapy

This radiation treatment is currently under testing in Europe and is being used in the U.S as well. It uses targeted radiotherapy to help minimize damage to nearby normal cells. It is used for lung tumors, thyroid, and breast cancers, as well as prostate, esophageal, nasal, head cancers, liver, brain, ovarian, cervical cancers, and uterine growths. You may also see this treatment referred to as ***TOMO Therapy*** or *TOMO Treatment*—they are the same thing.

IMRT was first used at Memorial Sloan-Kettering Hospital for treating cancer of the prostate (163a). Rather than using one large radiation beam to target the tumor, this type radiation uses many beams to target cancer tumors more precisely, thus hoping to prevent excess damage to nearby normal cells (163a), however, it is still considered radiation and will have some of the same side effects as any radiation would cause.

IMRT has been popular at treating tumors located around or near critical, vital organs (163a). It has been successfully used in treating children with many types of cancer, including those with *rhabdomyo-sarcomas*, who otherwise had little hope of survival (163a). One side effect of treating children with *medulloblastomas* with standard radiation has been not only severe radiation side effects, but possible hearing loss as well. With IMRT, medulloblastoma has been treated without the hearing loss (and other less severe side effects) due to the ability to more precisely direct the beams (163a). For more information on pediatric treatment of tumors using IMRT, see website: *http://www.mskcc.org/mskcc/html/8442.cfm* (163a).

## IOERT – Intraoperative Electron Radiation Therapy – The Mobetron

Though this is still considered a form of radiation treatment, and will have possible side effects (just as any radiation treatment does), it is being included here because it can be used right during surgery, while the tumor is open and exposed, thus minimizing damage to healthier nearby cells (165a). It is cost-efficient, portable, and *less risky* for the patient. It is already being extensively used on humans with fewer adverse effects than seen with traditional closed radiation. This treatment, also known as IOERT or "Intraoperative Electron Radiotherapy," has been used for cancers of the GI tract, throat, kidney, and many other sites (165a). The IOERT machine is also known as the *Mobetron* (165a).

## Kansius Machine

After going through many rounds of chemo for leukemia, John Kansius developed a radio wave machine (currently under testing) for killing cancer cells (563). The machine works on the premise that physicians first inject the patient's tumor with metallic nanoparticles, then use high-frequency radio waves, heating up the nanoparticles until the tumor is destroyed—and Mr. Kansius claims—with no side effects (563). The procedure is still in the testing stages (e.g., M.D. Anderson and others) and if it is pursued, it is not yet known how expensive the treatment could be (563). (I have discussed other forms of nanoparticle therapy elsewhere in this book.)

## Koch Cancer Cure

Dr. William Frederick Koch developed a cure for cancer by creating a substance known as *Glyoxylide*. It was such a success that he was ultimately closed down by the cancer establishment, and he eventually left the U.S. altogether. Though he fought many battles with organized medicine, Dr. Koch was not a fraud. He earned several degrees from prestigious American colleges and even taught at two of them. It was reported that

Glyoxylide had the ability to enable the elimination of toxins from the body. When Dr. Koch announced that he had successfully cured several of his cancer patients, it sounded the death bell for his career in the U.S. His peers quickly ostracized him. There is a great deal of information on Dr. Koch on the internet, and his cancer treatment has been written up in many books and journals in great detail.

## Laetrile (B17)

This vitamin is also discussed elsewhere in this book and in this chapter earlier, under B17. As described at website: *World Without Cancer.* "The Story of Vitamin B17," Dr. Manuel Navarro, M.D., who has a distinguished record in the medical field from Manila, wrote in 1971 that he had "treated over 500 patients with Laetrile…in various routes…including…oral and…I.V…The majority…have been in a terminal state…" and that this substance gave him "…comparable or superior results" as that "obtained with the use of the more toxic standard cytotoxic agents"(410).

## Low Dose Naltrexone for Cancer

In human testing, thus far, many people have benefited from using low doses of the drug, *Naltrexone*, for cancer treatment. Many cancers have responded, including carcinoid, leukemias, lymphomas, pancreatic, glioblastomas, and nearly all other cancers (179a). Patients with lymphomas, neuroblastoma, multiple myeloma, non-small cell lung cancer, and prostate cancers, have gone into remission using this treatment (179a). For individual case studies of people with various cancers using this treatment, see website: *http://starfishproject.wordpress.com/2008/11/29/low-dose-naltrexone-ldn-for-cancer-treatment.* Also, see website: *www.lowdosenaltrexone.org/ldn_and_cancer.htm* (179a).

## Malaria Cancer Therapy

The doctor responsible for the life-saving *Heimlich Maneuver* to save choking victims (that he also recommends to save drowning victims and to treat acute asthma attacks), Dr. Henry Heimlich, has been treating patients with a non-deadly form of malaria to cure their cancer. They first give the patient a healable type of malaria. The malaria invades the body, greatly boosting the immunity, which then fights the cancer. When the cancer is overcome, the patient is given a cure for the malaria (149b). You can read more at website: *http://www.scribd.com/doc/2057316/Heimlich-Uses-Malaria-to-Treat-Cancer-Philadelphia-Daily-News-22988*. He has also used this for HIV patients. See URL: *http://www.scribd.com/doc/2199011/11794-Heimlich-Using-Malaria-to-Treat-AIDS-Patients-Cincinnati-Post* (149b).

## Marine Phytoplankton & Carcinoid Tumors

Though carcinoid tumors are considered *incurable*, a mother of three, who was told she had invasive carcinoid tumor, was pleasantly surprised when she was told that diagnostic testing showed 8 of her 9 tumors had disappeared after she began drinking one ounce (in the morning and one at bedtime) of a marine phytoplankton drink. These one-celled entities are known as *dinoflagellates*. This woman's testimony can be found at *http://www.shirleys-wellness-café.com/cancer.htm* (187). For more information on marine phytoplankton, there are several websites, including this one: *http://planktonstar.com/order.htm* and *http://www.marinephytoplankton.net*. As with any supplement, be sure to check with your physician first.

## Max Gerson Treatment

As described at the Gerson® Institute website, *http://www.gerson.org/g_therapy/default.asp*, Gerson® therapy uses *natural* ingredients that enhance the *immune system*, enabling it to fight off chronic illnesses and diseases, like cancer. It uses 13 glasses a day (a glass hourly) of *fresh, organic juices* (149), as well as organic vegetarian meals and fresh fruits on a daily basis, and a colon detox program. This therapy has had a *60 year history of success*, with more than *200 articles* published in well-known prestigious journals describing its *effectiveness* at curing diseases in a safe, non-toxic manner (149). The therapy was introduced by Max Gerson, M.D. He used it successfully for many years, treating his own patients until he died at *78* years-of-age in 1959. He used it for *advanced* T.B, *heart disease, cancer,* and other ailments (149). The website says that he cured "his most famous patient…Dr. Albert Schweitzer, of advanced diabetes when Schweitzer was 75," and Schweitzer said of him: "I see in Dr. Gerson one of the most eminent geniuses in the history of medicine" (149). On May 14, 2005, Dr. Gerson "was inducted into the Orthomolecular Medicine Hall of Fame in Ottawa, Canada" (149). The Gerson Institute itself does not run clinics, but they will let you know "which clinics are licensed…to provide the Gerson Therapy" (149).

At first *JAMA* was so impressed with his work, that they published one of his articles, then later had a change of heart, and referred to him as a *quack*. An investigation spearheaded by Senator Claude Pepper (Fl.) asked him to present actual patient success cases with related dates, which he did. They were so impressed with the results, that Gerson was given a commendation (519).

Author of *Hydrogen Peroxide & Ozone*, Conrad LeBeau, met Gerson's daughter, Charlotte Gerson, in 1986 at the "National Health Federation Convention in Chicago" (463). He said that the thing that impressed him the most about the lecture she gave was when she described how they had successfully contacted scores of people her father "had treated for terminal cancer 30 years ago and found that many of them were still alive" (463)! There is an enormous amount of information on Gerson on the internet.

## MGN-3

MGN-3 is a *naturally-occurring* product that is derived from rice bran and mushrooms. Dr. Mamdooh Ghoneum, from the Department of Immunology at Charles Drew University of Medicine and Science in Los Angeles, has studied this supplement for many years and reports that MGN-3 stimulates the entire immune system (478). For personal testimonies of people who have used MGN-3 to fight numerous types of cancer (breast, multiple myeloma, leukemia, Non-Hodgkins lymphoma, prostate, colon cancer, melanoma, and cervical dysplasia), see website: *http://www.polymvasurvivors.com/what_you_know_mgn3_article2.html* (478). You can also find MGN-3 marketed under the name BioBran® at *wwwbuy-biobran.com/index.com.*

## MSM Plus Vitamin C & B12

*MSM (Methyl Sulfonyl Methane)* supplies sulfur to cells, apparently making the membranes more accessible. As described at *cancertutor.com,* it is popularly used in treating arthritis because of its positive effect on cells and pain control. It may help reverse malignancies (199). MSM also assists the body in balancing pH, detoxification, and helping maintain important levels of one of our most valuable anti-oxidants, *glutathione* (199). A study from 1986 revealed that glutathione could help the body fight the progression of breast tumors (199). MSM is best taken with vitamin C and

B12 if you are taking it for cancer prevention and treatment (199). (An excellent source of natural B12 is **spirulina and chlorella**. Be sure if using chlorella, to get the broken cell-wall chlorella for maximum absorption.)

Note that if you already have a diet rich in sulfur ("e.g., from eggs and onions"), MSM may do you little good (199). If you have allergies to sulfites, you may or may not have problems taking MSM. If so, try taking a mineral known as *molybdenum*, a lack of which may cause sulfur allergies (199). MSM is very important in bone joint health, and many supplements for joint health now include MSM in their formulas. Seek your doctor's advice about beginning any new supplement.

## MycoPhyto® Mushroom Formula

This is a six-mushroom blend of disease-fighting, immunity-boosting mushrooms. The producers grow Chinese herbs, then grow this formula on the herbs. According to website *http://www.advancedbionutritionals.com/immunity*, "Over a six-hour period, Mycophtyo® Complex increased NK cell activity by 45.2% more than the other formula" (211). This formula contains a blend of the ABM mushroom, coriolus, cordyceps, maitake, polyporus, and reishi, as well as Beta-glucan (211).

## Non-Toxic Immunotherapy—Including Individualized Vaccines

More and more health care researchers are studying the effectiveness of using immunotherapy for fighting cancer. This is taking on many new forms, such as removing white blood cells from patients and mixing them (in the laboratory) with the cancer cells. Once the immune cells multiply against the cancer, the new individualized vaccine that has been developed is re-injected into the patient. Since the patient's own cells were used, there is no danger of rejection. Sometimes, as described elsewhere in this book, the white blood cells are taken from a relative, allowed to multiply in the laboratory, then injected into the cancer patient. This individualized vaccine treatment is done at Issels. Their website is *http://www.issels.com.* Ph#888-447-7357.

## Noscapine – Cough Medicine Ingredient for Fighting Various Cancers Without Toxic Side Effects

A natural, common cough medicine ingredient, noscapine, is already being used off-label to kill some forms of cancer, including prostate cancer. It has also been studied for use in fighting leukemia, lymphomas, *breast, ovarian, colon, lung…brain* and skin cancers (323a).

## Olive Oil—Great Heart Benefits & Anti-Cancer Properties

Research continues to point to the heart-healthy benefits of extra virgin olive oil. Apparently, the extra virgin oil benefits exceed other types of olive oil for helping lower blood fats and for its anti-oxidant properties. For best results, the *unrefined*, organic EVOO is considered best (595).

## Oregano Oil

Oil of oregano, including wild oil of oregano, has been studied and written about extensively for its anti-oxidant properties and anti-bacterial benefits. Any ingredient that is high in anti-oxidant value is also an immune-booster. For those suffering from chronic sinus infections, you may want to try the oregano product, known as *Oregacyn,* which contains wild oil of oregano, cumin and sage. It is available at many health food stores and websites such as: *http://www.myhealthpro.com* (123).

## Oxalic Acid for Cancer

Some in the alternative medicine community believe that oxalic acid insufficiency in the body causes cancer, and that oxalic acid, though deadly to cancer cells, leaves healthy cells untouched. Foods that have high amounts of oxalic acid include wine, fish, teas, and chocolate (225). Isn't it interesting that these foods that are high in oxalic acid (and others, such as green drinks and leafy green vegetables), are also extraordinarily high in anti-oxidants (225)? Just realize that consuming high levels of oxalic acid, such as in the leaves of rhubarb, can be deadly. It is okay to eat the stalks of rhubarb, but **never the leaves.**

Other natural sources of oxalic acid include leafy greens, such as kale and spinach, asparagus, brussel sprouts, beet greens, chives, purslane, and parsley. (Do not consume large amounts of parsley.) Green drinks, such as wheat grass and barley, also contain some oxalic acid. Some people are not able to synthesize oxalic acid in their body and they develop bladder and kidney stones when they ingest too many foods containing oxalic acid. Gout is not usually caused from high oxalic acid consumption, but from the inability of the body to utilize purines, which form crystals in the joints, causing the pain of gout. Eating high amounts of oxalic acid foods, though not usually the cause of gout, can exacerbate gout episodes in individuals who are prone to this ailment. It would be next to impossible to poison oneself with natural food sources of oxalic acid (except for eating things like rhubarb leaves), but harm can be done to those who are prone to kidney or bladder stones.

## Polarizing Solutions

This is a treatment that was originally formulated by Dr. Demetrio Sodi-Pallares, and given intravenously. The solution contains *GKI (glucose, potassium, and insulin),* and works by increasing the acidity of tumors, thus helping to destroy them. It also helps in repairing cells that have been injured by tumors. This treatment is also available at Issels. Their website is *http://www.issels.com.* Ph#888-447-7357. (Note that this chapter also discusses how extreme alkalinity is used to destroy tumors.)

## Polyerga® Therapy

Polyerga® has something in common with Burzynski's antineoplastons (and Poly-MVA), in that it is a polypeptide. It is used extensively in Europe and Asia to enhance the body's immune system and was developed by Dr. Walter Kuhlmeg, M.D. A great deal of German research has been done on the compound. It is an extract from pig spleen. There is also a great deal of information on this substance on the internet.

## Pomegranate Juice for Cancer Prevention & Therapy

Pomegranate is one of the newest superstars among the anti-oxidants. A fruit that you rarely saw in stores ten years ago is appearing everywhere, and for good reason. This biblical fruit is packed with nutrients and anti-oxidants that fight free radicals in the body (376). It is now being touted as a deterrent for all types of cancer. Just 8 ounces a day is all that you may need to keep your immune system healthy (376). The seeds and juice from the seeds also promote heart health by fighting arterial plaque, lowering cholesterol, and preventing the type of inflammation in the colon that can lead to cancer (376). You can also find pomegranate extract capsules in health food stores.

## Proteolytic Enzyme Therapy

These are enzymes that work in the pancreas (trypsin and chymtrypsin), also known as *proteases.* Many alternative practitioners believe that these enzymes have cancer-healing properties, and human studies have borne this out. These type enzymes are also found in papaya (papain) and pineapple (bromelain), as well as in the silk worm (serrapeptase or serratia peptidase). Some of these enzymes, such as bromelain and papain, are discussed in other chapters of this book.

Complementary medicine sometimes combines chemo with these enzymes (514). In fact, a **human** study on advanced colon cancer patients treated with chemo, showed that adding proteolytic enzymes was able to prolong the lives of those taking them (514). You will find these enzymes sold in various compounds under the names: *Wobenzyme, Zymactive* and other names. When taking these enzymes, it is best to take them about 30 minutes before meals. Do not take proteolytic enzymes if you have allergies to pineapple, papaya or pork. Some researchers believe that cancer is caused by deficient levels of proteolytic enzymes in the body. Entire therapies have been developed on this premise.

## Proton Beam Therapy

Proton beam therapy, though not a natural treatment, may offer new choices to those who are fearful of conventional (photon) radiation treatments for cancer. Though it has been around for more than 50 years and is not really considered *new*, many people have never heard of it. Though I do not personally advocate radiation therapy, I am including proton beam therapy for informational purposes, and because this type therapy is touted as being safer than conventional radiation. Details are given in an article at OncoLink website, *www.oncolink.com,* from the Abramson Cancer Center of the University of Pennsylvania by James Metz, M.D (489). Apparently, proton beam therapy is aimed in such a way that more of the actual tumor is treated, with less damage to surrounding tissues, which means that the tumor can be treated with *higher doses* (489). Their website article has several graphs showing some very dramatic differences in side effects between conventional photon therapy and proton beam therapy, depending on the type cancer treated.

## Quercetin - Amazing Anti-Oxidant

Discussed in many chapters of this book, quercetin is an amazing anti-oxidant that helps in the prevention of disease. There is probably a good deal of truth in the old adage "an apple a day keeps the doctor away," because apples are packed with this anti-oxidant. Just remember that when you are eating apples—try to get organic—wash them thoroughly, and eat the skins too!

Other good sources of this nutrient are red and yellow onions (white onions have lesser amounts)(440), teas, beans (378), cayenne, green tea (551), grapes, ginkgo biloba, berries, broccoli, and some nuts and seeds, as discussed elsewhere in this book. Not only is quercetin a terrific anti-oxidant, but if you are having allergy problems or joint pain, it is also a natural anti-inflammatory and anti-histamine.

## R-A Therapy & Telomerase for Genetically Healing Cancer

As described at Advanced Alternatives Cancer Center website, R-A therapy targets the body's ability to heal itself. Provided certain stimuli, the cancer cells are prodded (via *natural substances)* to re-differentiate—in other words—completely change back into normal non-cancerous cells (246). Thus, the R represents *re-differentiation* and the A represents *apoptosis* (the cancer cells basically commit suicide). The human body is born with the ability, via its genetic makeup, to heal itself. R-A Therapy, and other therapies at Advanced Alternatives Cancer Center, is aimed at enhancing this self-healing process (246). They have treatment centers in Las Vegas, Nevada, as well as the Bahamas. Their main thrust in treating cancer is through detoxing the body, empowering the immune system to heal itself, and other natural alternative approaches to fighting cancer (246). See information on hyperthermia treatment (earlier in this chapter), which can also be obtained at Advanced Alternatives Cancer Center. Telomerase is produced by cancer cells, which unfortunately makes them stronger. They eventually take over a host, causing its demise and ultimately, theirs as well (246). Our own cells age and die, yet cancer yells stay healthy and young due to the presence of telomerase. New treatments are aimed at neutralizing this telomerase enzyme so that the cancer cells can then be destroyed (246). Advanced Alternatives Cancer Center website is: *http://www.aacancer.com/alternative_cancer_treatment.html.*

## Radio Wave Therapy from Australian Physician for Cancer Treatment

Dr. John Holt from Perth, Australia, is said to be having amazing results with an inexpensive radio wave treatment for his cancer patients. First, the patient is given a substance that inhibits glucose, then their body subjected to radio waves at a specified frequency (483). For more information on this alternative treatment, and the story of a bone cancer and brain cancer survivor who credit their lives to this treatment, see website: *www.cam. net/ uk/home/aaa315/healing/john-holt-cancer-treatment.htm,* and *www.the-institute. com.au* (483).

## Recancostat

This is a treatment that has been popular in Europe for several years for cancer, used minimally in the U.S., yet has no adverse side effects (382). As described by Dr. Joseph A. Debé, it can be combined with conventional therapy and is believed to help relieve side effects from chemo and radiation (382). It is taken *on an empty stomach,* and can be given through your health care practitioner. The substance was developed by scientists in Germany, and its advantages have been lauded in many health journals (382). It contains a form of *reduced glutathione,* which (once inside the cells) supplies extra electrons, thus destroying free radicals in the body (382). You can read more on this substance at *http://www .pwpgroup.com/rec ancostat%20description.htm* (382).

## Red Meat - Culprit in Causing Many Cancers

Curbing the ingestion of red meats could prevent you from all forms of cancer, especially those of the liver, lung, and esophagus. This according to a **human study** (for eight years) that involved half-a-million people, male and female. Processed meats are also unhealthy (481). Examples of red meats are: goose, lamb, goat, mutton, and beef. White meat is rabbit, chicken, pork, turkey, seafood, and fish, though you will find some disagreements when it comes to labeling meat *white* or *red.*

The controversy is ongoing about organic versus non-organic foods. Recently, studies have come out in favor of organic food being healthier for the body. This is no surprise for those who have been advocating the superiority of organic food for years. Organic foods are not grown with herbicides, pesticides, and other poisonous chemicals. Organic meats and dairy are not supposed to contain hormones, herbicides, and pesticides.

## Resveratrol - Potent Cancer-Fighter from Grapes

Resveratrol is discussed in many other chapters in this book, especially chapter three. It is not only found in grapes, but in red wine, fruits (cranberries, blueberries, pomegranates), and many types of nuts (328). An important study, conducted by Case Western Reserve University and University Hospitals of Cleveland, revealed that this anti-oxidant caused the death of cancer in *human epidermoid carcinoma A431 cells* (328). For intricate details of the study, see website NCBI PubMed from the U.S. National Library of Medicine and National Institutes of health. The PMID is 11350919 (328). When you get to PubMed's site, enter the PMID number and this research will pull up.

Resveratrol is also being touted as a way to fight obesity and high cholesterol, since it keeps the body from storing fat.

## Retinoblastoma Treatment that May Preserve Eyesight

Though I have mentioned alternative therapies (e.g., cryotherapy) for retinoblastoma, a cancer that invades the eye and occurs mostly in children, a new conventional therapy, which sometimes is able to preserve the eyes in these children is being discussed here, though it does involve some chemo. Usually, the cancer is removed by removing the child's eye.

Researchers have found that when the cancer is detected early in children, they may be able to preserve the eye and avoid giving the child radiation (102a). In a test involving 30 children with the disease, they were given the chemo drugs *etoposide* and *carboplatin,* along with *cryotherapy, photocoagulation* and *plaque therapy* (102a). In the children with low-grade cancer, nearly 70% had total remission with this treatment and did not require radiation and removal of their eye. Should you wish to enroll your child in clinical trials (like this one) contact the National Cancer Institute, as well as *eCancerTrials.com* (102a). Etoposide and carboplatin are not natural therapies, but the other treatments used are non-toxic. This is an example of combining chemo drugs with non-toxic therapies to get results. (More and more physicians are using a combination of CAM (complementary and alternative medicine) and conventional medicine. See earlier in this chapter for details on **CyberKnife®** therapy, which is also used on tumors involving the eye. It is painless, bloodless, requires no sedation, no hospital stay, no incision and is said to have low risk and mild side effects in comparison to conventional surgery, chemo and radiation. (Also, see later in this chapter for info on NanoKnife™ therapy.)

## Rexin-G™ —New Gene Therapy for Cancer

Rexin-G™ has been undergoing clinical trials at Mayo Clinic, M.D. Anderson, and a few other facilities. It is a drug for cancers that have spread, and those types of cancer that conventional medicine says do not respond to chemo drugs (256). Human clinical studies, thus far, have had good results. In the very first human trial, 83% of the patients experienced tumor shrinkage. The patients all had spreading pancreatic cancer (256). Good responses were also achieved in human studies involving several other types of metastatic cancer. Due to the reports, this drug is now used for treating all forms of *solid tumors* in the Philippines that are resistant to conventional therapy (256). The U.S. FDA has given the drug its *orphan drug status* (drugs approved for rare diseases) for use with pancreatic cancers in the US, as well as other types of cancer metastases (256). It is given intravenously, so isn't exactly natural or painless, but could be considered gentler than older chemo drugs because it is said to be a non-chemo drug, showing itself in **human** clinical trials, not to have the adverse side effects normally associated with standard chemo drugs (256). You can get more information on this drug at *epeiusbiotech.com/rexin_g-factsheet.asp*. Epeius Biotechnologies produce Rexin-G™ (257).

## Rife Machine

During the 1930s, a scientist by the name of Royal Raymond Rife invented a very powerful microscope which had the ability to magnify organisms, but it could do so without having to destroy the objects being studied, something that science had not done before. This enabled Mr. Rife to actually study and observe living specimens (261). Rife used an electronic treatment to destroy viruses, thus enabling the weakened immune system to recover and bring healing to the body. According to reports, doctors using this new treatment were successfully curing hundreds of cancer patients (261). They were also using the therapy for treating other ailments and diseases. His work was noted in multiple prestigious medical journals, and Rife was praised by many prominent physicians of his day; however, he met with great opposition from the

AMA until eventually his work was completely suppressed. He later died under mysterious circumstances (261).

## Robotic Technology

Many people facing surgery for cancer cannot withstand prolonged invasive surgeries. A type of surgery that is known as MIS or *minimally invasive surgery,* where very tiny incisions are made (especially useful in kidney and gynecological cancer procedures), is sparing patients from major invasive procedures by using robotic technology (92). One such place that provides this surgery is the *Karmanos Cancer Center* in Detroit, Michigan. It is known as the *DaVinci® Surgical System*. This type surgery is used when doing laparoscopies and endoscopies (92).

## Scorpion Venom

Radioactive scorpion venom from a yellow scorpion in Israel may be the next, newest and most powerful anti-cancer treatment. This according to World Science at: *http://www.world-science.net/othernews/060626_venom.htm*, which reports that the U.S. FDA has already (since 2003) given the drug produced from the venom (*TM-601*) expeditious review, especially for its use in treating gliomas. **No serious side effects** have been noted from the compound, which was developed by TransMolecular, Inc (247).

An article from Havana, Cuba, reports that the scientists at Guantanamo have developed a medication known as *Escoazul* from a blue scorpion Cubans have used for the past decade to treat cancer (326). Cases of complete cancer cures are documented at website: *http://www.lt ierramerica.net/2001/0819/iacentos.shtml* (326). Human studies involving thousands of patients have been performed in Guantanamo on *Escoazul.* These studies are still being conducted on the drug, which has also been used for kidney ailments, Parkinson's, and inflammation of the pelvic area. See website: *tierramerica.net/2001/0819/ia centos.shtml* (326), as well as *main.uab.edu/show.asp?durki=10990,* for more information on gliomas and scorpion venom.

University of Alabama researchers are also studying the effects of scorpion venom on **glioma** (brain) cancers (449). Physicians are looking at a giant Israeli scorpion which kills cockroaches with its venom, but does not harm humans. When they isolated a drug made from the venom and directly injected it into glioma cells, they discovered that only the cancer cells died. The surrounding cells were left untouched. They are still testing the substance (449). One of the drugs is known as TM-601.

## Stereotactic Surgery (aka Stereotactic Therapy) for Difficult Tumors

Look under Gamma Knife®, earlier in this chapter, and also in chapter 14 on brain cancers. It is sometimes referred to as *stereotactic surgery, stereotactic* therapy, or radiotherapy. It is often used on hard-to-reach tumors such as pituitary tumors and acoustic neuromas (schwannomas). Stereotactic Body Radiotherapy has recently been introduced at Northwest Indiana's Methodist Hospital for destroying lung tumors (220). An *Elekta Stereotactic Body Frame* is used in the procedure, which aims precisely-controlled *radiation beams* at cancer cells for lung tumor destruction. Many people diagnosed with lung tumors are not physically able to undergo surgery and this is another option available to those with lung cancer, especially as found in stage I. Considered painless with few complications, and requiring less than an hour and only three treatments, this procedure is normally done on an outpatient basis. See website: *insideindianabusiness.com/newsitem.asp?ID=27347* for more details (220). See the information in this chapter on CyberKnife®. When used for brain tumors, the CyberKnife® is painless, the Gamma Knife® is not painless. (Also, see later in this same chapter for information on the newer, non-toxic, gentle NanoKnife™ therapy.)

## TAP - Tumor-Activated Prodrug or TAP Technology for Cancer

Researcher, Dr. Anne Kellogg, a pathologist from East Carolina University, is the developer of a new type of monoclonal antibody that may pave the way for treating breast, ovarian, and *other cancers* more effectively and perhaps with fewer side effects as mainstream chemo (207). She called the new antibody *DS-6* and describes it as a *delivery vehicle* for a cancer-killing agent that was produced by a company known as *ImmunoGen.* The antibody works by sticking onto tumor cells and allowing itself (as well as the cancer-killing agent) to get inside the cell where it then destroys the cell (207). It is in an inactive state within the body and is only *activated* once it gets into the abnormal tumor cell (207). Dr. Kellogg says that even if the technology does not *cure cancer,* if it were able to"convert cancer to [merely] a chronic disease," then it could be treated as such, offering *oncologists* more choices for therapy (207).

## ThermoDox

This treatment, still in clinical trials, uses liposomes activated by heat to kill cancer cells, and may be especially useful for liver cancers.

## TOMO Therapy for Cancer - New, Safer Radiation Therapy

A new type of radiation, known as *TOMO* Therapy, which causes less harm to healthy tissue while killing cancer cells, was recently installed at the *Karmanos Cancer Center* in Detroit (294). It is known as the *Tomo Therapy HI-ART® System,* and it simply means that patients can be given concentrated, more precise doses of radiation (294). It is also known as *(Intensity Modulated Radiotherapy).* I have discussed IMRT in several other chapters of this book. More information about this type therapy can be found at the article from Barbara Ann Karmanos Cancer Institute: *http://www.karmanos.org/app.asp?id=1118* (294). See other areas in this book that discuss IMRT therapy. Just realize that although this therapy is said to be safer than some other conventional forms, it still involves radiation and will have some potential for side effects and immune depression.

## Transfer Factor - More Success with Immunotherapy

Transfer Factor is an immune factor that is extracted from white blood cells. Dr Sherwood Lawrence discovered this ability of transferring an immune response from one person to another nearly half a century ago, and millions of dollars have been spent on research, which has proven it safe and effective at fighting diseases, including cancer (295)(592). Transfer factors are actually molecules of protein made by cells of our immune system known as *T-cells.* We receive many of these transfer factors from our mothers colostrum, one of the many reasons that breast-feeding is recommended over bottle-feeding for babies. Transfer factors seem to train our immune system how to recognize certain bacteria, viruses, and fungi, and destroy them (295)(592). Many Transfer Factor supplement products on the market today are taken from bovine colostrum.

## Ukrain Fights Carcinoma in Clinical Trial

In a clinical trial involving 27 patients with carcinoma, there was an important overall stimulation in the body's own immune system after they received intravenous Ukrain at *10 mg every three days*, and the dosage was *well tolerated* (518). Details of the results can be seen at the U.S. National Library of Medicine (and National Institutes of Health) PubMed website. Go to the site and enter PMID 1713821 to pull up this clinical trial. (518). Also, see the animal study at PMID 15929607, on Lewis carcinoma and Ukrain. (Ukrain is discussed in several cancer-specific chapters in this book.)

## Ukrain May Help Overcome Cancers that are Cisplatin-Resistant

Cisplatin is a commonly known chemo drug used for various types of cancer. Many people who choose this conventional treatment go on to develop cancers that are resistant to this drug (458). Laboratory testing has shown that Ukrain, which is non-toxic, acts very much like the drug Cisplatin and for those who have Cisplatin-resistant cancers, it is believed that Ukrain may be helpful in overcoming this problem (458). For more information on this study, see the National Library of Medicine's PubMed NCBI website: *http://www.ncbi.nlm.nih.gov/sites/entrez?db=pubmed*, and enter the PMID #10190087 (458).

## Ukrain May Help Protect Cells Exposed to Radiation Treatment

Ukrain is described in nearly every chapter on cancer in this book, however, one item that is not discussed is the research that was done on Ukrain showing that this non-toxic substance may protect normal cells against radiation (377). Ukrain has been shown to promote health in the patients that receive it, fight allergies and inflammation, even stimulate the body's T-lymphocytes, and yet it is a completely non-toxic cancer treatment, without adverse side effects (381).

## Umbelliferae - Angelica Keiskei Root Fights Cancer

This plant root, *Angelica keiskei Koizumi*, also known as *umbelliferae*, has been used as an herbal and root healing remedy (448). Animal testing, conducted by the School of Medicine in Japan, has revealed that an extract of this root (*4-hydroxyderricin*) can be helpful in preventing tumors and their spread by preventing the growth of blood vessels that supply the tumors, and by assisting the immune system (448). For more information on this study, see PubMed NCBI website. The PMID is 15114497 (448). The root is commonly found in Asian countries as a health food. Be sure to consult with your physician before beginning any new herbal or extract remedy. Some extracts, such as this one, can interact with prescription meds and may also cause sensitivity to sunlight and other problems. (Note that shark cartilage also works at blocking blood vessel growth in tumors, a term known as *anti-angiogenesis*, without toxic side effects. It is discussed in greater detail in chapter seven. Also, see information on bindweed earlier in this chapter.)

## Vitamin C Shown to Destroy Cancer Cells

An article from the National Institutes of Health 08/04/2008, says that three decades ago, interest in vitamin C for fighting cancer and other diseases was at its height (307a). That is, until other researchers [who did not know what they were doing], stated that taking mega-doses of vitamin C by mouth did not produce *benefits* for cancer patients enrolled in their "two double-blind, placebo-controlled clinical trials" (307a).

There was just one gross problem with this study. Had it not been so flawed, multitudes of people possibly could have been saved from cancer and other diseases by the thousands before now. The reason I say it was "flawed" (which was not just my personal opinion, but the opinion of many others in the health industry), and the reason I say that the researchers did not know what they were doing, is because many years ago Dr. Irwin Stone, Dr. Virginia Livingston, Dr. William J. Saccoman, Dr. Paul Klenner, Dr. Abram Hoffer, Dr. Bernard Rimland, Linus Pauling, Dr. Robert Cathcart, and many others (who checked their research), tried to explain to the public (and to those doing research), that vitamin C taken orally can only be absorbed in limited amounts by the body, then excesses are excreted. However, if it is given in the form of Sodium Ascorbate INTRAVENOUSLY, which bypasses the GI tract, and is absorbed directly into the circulatory system, into the cellular level, patients can tolerate 100-300 GRAMS (that is not a typo—it is GRAMS, not milligrams) a day, sometimes more, depending on if doses are spread out over the day, and the condition of the patient. Some physicians will start out giving megadoses (known as Orthomolecular Medicine), the patient begins to improve, then they lower the dose. The patient then gets worse. This is typical, because the writings of Irwin Stone, Linus Pauling, and Robert Cathcart agree that you cannot suddenly reduce vitamin C megadosing, or the patient may regress. You MUST keep the megadoses going continuously until there is full recovery!

Researchers are just now [after 30 years of ignoring men smarter than them], figuring out that these early pioneers of Vitamin C intravenous mega-dosing knew exactly what they were doing (307a). Also, there are normally no toxic side-effects to intravenous vitamin C in the form of sodium ascorbate or calcium ascorbate (the ascorbic acid is too acidic to be given intravenously) (307a). Oral doses will eventually cause diarrhea. Chemo can cost thousands of dollars per dose. Vitamin C therapy usually runs about $125.00 per dose (149a), depending where you live. And even though Vitamin C doses are so much cheaper than chemo, insurance companies will pay for the chemo, but not the Vitamin C (149a). (Of course not—that would make too much sense—and our current health system in the U.S. operates with absolutely no common sense whatsoever!) More studies (using intravenous vitamin C) are planned in humans. These are studies that should have been done decades ago, had anyone taken Linus Pauling, Ewan Cameron, Irwin Stone, and Robert Cathcart seriously, instead of dragging their feet for decades, while people who could have been saved by megadoses of C died prematurely. Not only did researchers discover that high levels of ascorbate could kill cancer in lab studies, without harming normal cells, they found "that these high ascorbate concentrations could be achieved in people" (307a), something that Linus Pauling and Irwin Stone already knew (when the current researchers were mere babes), had anyone just listened to them and taken them seriously!

In chapter 12 of this book (on pancreatic cancer), I discuss the case of an email friend of mine who was totally cured of "terminal" pancreatic cancer with megadoses of **intravenous** vitamin C. This was more than THREE years ago. She worked the entire time she was receiving the treatment, had no adverse effects, felt healthy and well, and her cancer totally disappeared, in spite of the fact that her conventional physician told her she was dying. She obtained the megadose intravenous vitamin C from a Naturopathic physician. When she returned to her conventional doctor, he told her that this was impossible and he must have made an error in diagnosing her.

The sad fact is that Dean Burk of the NCI knew nearly 40 years ago that ascorbate (vitamin C) could destroy cancer cells, and leave normal cells unharmed, and he shared the information with his peers. They even published the results in the *Oncology* paper, revealing their *findings*:

> "In our view, the future of effective cancer chemotherapy will not rest on the use of host-toxic compounds now so widely employed, but upon virtually host non-toxic compounds that are lethal to cancer cells of which ascorbate…represents an excellent prototype." They also point out that ascorbate **was never tested for its anticancer effects by the Cancer Chemotherapy National Service Center, because it was too non-toxic to fit into their screening program. They don't want to test anything unless it helps kill the cancer patient**. [Emphasis mine] (571a).

If you scanned that very last paragraph briefly, you should read it again, because this is exactly what has happened in the last **40 years**! The Cancer Industry, historically, has NOT been interested in promoting non-toxic drugs. They are only interested in drugs (and treatments) that are so toxic, that they often kill the patient before the cancer does! You will find in this book, that just recently, some pharmaceutical companies (probably due to public outcry, competition with European drug makers, and perhaps all the new competition from alternative therapies), are beginning to develop drugs and treatments for fighting cancer that are less toxic to the body, many of which are described in this book.

Cameron and Campbell did, in fact, conduct a clinical trial in 1974, giving "50 advanced cancer patients…10,000 mg of ascorbate a day either intravenously or orally." They discovered that the "large doses of ascorbic acid" were able to "enhance natural resistance to cancer" (571a).

Scientists have proven that vitamin C, in laboratory testing, at "3 mgms per 100 mls" can effectively wipe out cancer and without any adverse side effects (166). This was discovered by scientists from the *Bio-Communications Research Institute in Wichita, USA*. The article is available at website: *http://www.alternative-doctor.com/cancer/ca_advanced.htm* (166). The blood level of vitamin C needed to achieve this amount would be available if 50 grams of vitamin C (50,000 mg) were given intravenously to a patient (166). This amount of sodium ascorbate, given intravenously, is usually well-tolerated by the patient, as stated earlier. As noted by Dr. Irwin Stone in *The Genetics of Scurvy and the Cancer Problem,* "Dr. Paul Klenner uses up to 300,000 mg of sodium ascorbate, intravenously, each day in his successful therapy of the viral diseases" (571a).

See page 544 in my book for information on the amazing new *liposome-encapsulated vitamin C,* taken by mouth, that is said to be clinically more effective than intravenous vitamin C (466b)!

## Vitamin D Prevents Nearly All Types of Cancer

Multiple human studies have proven that a lack of vitamin D will raise your risk for nearly all types of cancer, especially those of the colon, stomach, and breast. The best source of vitamin D is natural sunlight—about 20-30 minutes/day with no sunscreen, or at least 20-30 minutes a day for 3-4 days a week. Those who have a tendency toward (or history of) skin cancer will need to check with their physician first.

Being deficient in this vitamin may promote other chronic illnesses, such as MS and *Type I diabetes* (311). Nutritional experts are now concluding that most people need *1,000 to 2,000 IU* per *day* of vitamin D, a much higher amount than the RDA of *200 to 600 IU* for maintaining health and preventing disease (311). Adequate amounts of this vitamin are especially crucial to preventing colon, breast, and gastric cancers. The best natural source is sunshine. A nutritious diet and *supplements* can also provide vitamin D (311) for those unable to get out in the sun. (Mushrooms are the only vegetables that contain natural vitamin D.)

A research study that spanned eight years and involved more than 3000 people, showed that those people having the lowest vitamin D levels were twice as likely to die from all causes (575).

## White Blood Cell Transfusion - A Cure for All Cancers?

A scientific discovery from the late 90s that has been undergoing years of testing in animals, is set to begin in human trials, and hoped to be a cure for cancer—all cancers (523)! It was discovered that when mice were given deadly cancers, one mouse didn't develop cancer, even when all his counterparts were dying out. As a matter-of-fact, researchers at the Wake Forrest University Medical Center (N. Carolina), found that no amount of cancer affected the mouse. The mouse had a cancer-resistant immune system! Per Dr. Zheng Cui, who led the research, even giving the mouse increasingly larger amounts of the lethal cancer injections did not phase the rodent (523). For clinical trials, scientists will take white blood cells *(granulocytes)* from humans who are resistant to cancer, and transfuse them into those who have cancer. They succeeded in curing mice and hope that the same principle will work on humans (523). The treatment merely involves a blood-transfusion.

## 714X—Gaston Naessens

See chapter sixteen for information on Gaston Naessens and 714X, as well as the remarkable story of a young man who used 714X to cure **Hodgkins disease**. He also changed his diet and used Resperin Canada Essiac® tea and other nutrients described in that case. Note that there is some competition between the tea produced by Resperin Canada Essiac® and Flor-Essence® Essiac tea. Both companies claim that they have the original Essiac formula (the drinkable formula, not the injectable) that Rene Caisse used in treating her cancer patients. A website that has Resperin Canada Essiac® is also given in chapter sixteen. Also, see other chapters in this book.

## Zeolites (Megamin)

A supplement initially derived from volcanic rock (zeolites), Megamin has been successfully used for cancer treatment in over 100 **humans** in Austria. For example, a complete remission was reported in thirteen out of sixteen cancers which were treated over a three year time frame. This included patients with melanoma that had spread (4 cases) "3 liver cancers…2 bronchial carcinoma, 1 bladder cancer, and 1 hepato-cellular carcinoma." The rest had "partial remission and stabilization…(2 lung cancer and 1 breast cancer)" (324).

# IV. The Newer, Safer Conventional Therapies

See other cancer-specific chapters in this book for some of the newer, non-toxic, gentler drugs and therapies for treating cancer (besides the ones listed in this chapter). Examples are drugs like: Lodamin, Onconase, Avemar, Lapatinib (Tykerb®), Rexin-G®, and therapies like mammosite treatment, TAP Technology, and autohemotherapy; some gentler and safer than others. Some are totally non-toxic, but can be combined with chemo drugs that are toxic, so be sure to question your physician thoroughly about the side effects of prescribed treatments.

## V. Gentle & Painless – The IRE-NanoKnife™

A new procedure, still undergoing **human** trials, has been able to shrink solid tumours within fourteen days, painlessly and without toxic side effects. It is referred to simply as the *IRE-NanoKnife*™ or "irreversible electrocorporation" (354a). The procedure, using *needle electrodes* within and surrounding a tumor, creates holes through the *tumour cells* via *electric pulses* sent through the electrodes. It has been tested in the U.S. and Australia. Developed by Angio Dynamics®, Inc., it is gaining popularity (354a). This minimally-invasive procedure may become more popular than chemo for solid tumors, and with no harmful side effects (354a)! Human testing has been very positive, especially with pancreatic cancer.

## VI. Virastatin - Anti-Viral, Anti-Cancer & It's Natural

A natural substance made from chaparral (*Larrea tridentata*), known as Virastatin, is a known viral-killer. Some researchers believe that certain cancers could be caused by viruses. Is it logical then to believe that an extract that kills viruses may also help fight some forms of cancer? Virastatin has shown the ability at fighting the herpes virus, cold sores, shingles, Kaposi's sarcoma, HIV, Bell's Palsy, cytomegalovirus, and even helping against rheumatoid arthritis and candida yeast.

## VII. *Ecklonia Cava* - Super Antioxidant from the Deep

This brown seaweed (marketed under the name ***Seanol®***) is said to be much more potent in antioxidant power than green tea. It is a phlorotannin, shown (in **human testing)** to be important for brain health, treating fibromyalgia, asthma, killing parasites, improving circulation, immunity, fighting skin cancer, arthritis pain, inflammation, and high cholesterol, while actually raising HDL cholesterol in the body. It is possible that it is hundreds of times more powerful than any plant antioxidant found outside the oceans, and it has the ability to cross the *blood-brain barrier*. Go to website: *www.iherb®.com* and do a search for *Ecklonia cava* for more details and where to order.

# CHAPTER 35

# FASTING & DETOX

*"Is not this the fast that I have chosen? To loose the bands of wickedness, to undo the heavy burdens, and to let the oppressed go free, and that ye break every yoke?" (Isaiah 58:6)*

## Healing Through Fasting

Though fasting is controversial—it shouldn't be—because everyone fasts at some time or another in their life, and occasional fasting is a health boost. Fasting can be intentional or imposed by illness, pending surgery or other circumstances, sometimes those beyond our control. While most people are convinced that fasting several days will make them ill, what they don't realize is that it is usually too much food (even the right kind of food) that makes one ill, not fasting.

While I never recommend a total fast that even excludes water, I do believe that partial fasting (half day), juice-fasting, and complete food fasting (drinking water only), is very beneficial to the body if done in moderation. Not only that, but for Christians it is not merely a simple recommendation, but commanded and expected that they fast from time to time. Other religions also engage in occasional fasts as part of their belief system. Most people look at a juice-fast as drinking ONLY juice, and a water-fast as drinking ONLY water, however, the opposite is actually true. A water-fast means not drinking water and a juice-fast means no juice. For clarification purposes, when a water or juice-fast is discussed in this chapter, it will pertain to including ONLY water or ONLY juice in the diet. For those who want to maintain or recover optimal health, I believe the safest and healthiest fast is the juice-fast. This is a liquid fast, where no solid food is taken, but plenty of fresh raw vegetable and fruit juices (strained) are allowed.

This type of fast is very cleansing and detoxifying to the body (372). A juice-fast will also do something that may revitalize you beyond anything else you can possibly do; it will raise the pH of your body and alkalize the tissues (372). I have been on water-only fasts and juice-fasts. I've noticed that I actually get hungrier on a juice-fast. I believe it is because on a water-only fast, after a few days, the hunger went away. On the juice-fast it didn't, and I'm sure it's because carbs cause the body to release insulin and insulin makes you hungry; however, even juice-fasts will often begin with the first two or three days of water only, as suggested in the case of *The Grape Cure* diet by Johanna Brandt (discussed earlier in chapter three).

Water-only fasting is also very healthy for the body. It can help reverse plaque build-up in the arteries and halt painful inflammations. The same thing happens with a juice-fast, though it might take longer (372). It was after experiencing a 40-day fast that Moses, Elijah, and Jesus were greatly empowered (372). Remember, never go without water.

For Christians undertaking a fast, there are many promises from the Bible that they can claim. Several are found in the Old Testament from Isaiah Chapter 58 in regards to fasting:

> Then shall thy light break forth as the morning, and thine health shall spring forth speedily: and thy righteousness shall go before thee; the glory of the Lord shall be thy reward. Then shalt thou call, and the Lord shall answer; thou shalt cry, and he shall say, Here I *am*...then shall thy light rise in obscurity, and thy darkness be as the noonday: And the Lord shall guide thee continually, and satisfy thy soul in drought, and make fat thy bones: and thou shalt be like a watered garden, and like a spring of water, whose waters fail not. Isaiah 58: 8,9,11. *(AV 1611 KJV)*

Can you see that there are many blessings promised for those who undertake a scriptural fast? There are, however, reasons that God instructs people to fast. Not just for answers to prayer "[t]o make your voice to be heard on high" (Is 58:4 KJV), but God explains why he chooses fasts:

> Is not this the fast that I have chosen? To loose the bands of wickedness, to undo the heavy burdens, and to let the oppressed go free, and that ye break every yoke? Is it not to deal thy bread to the hungry, and that thou bring the poor that are cast out to thy house? When thou seest the naked, that thou cover him; and that thou hide not thyself from thine own flesh?" *(Is: 58:6-7 KJV)*

In other words, we are also to fast to loose the chains of those in bondage to sin, to help in feeding those who are hungry and clothing the poor.

Just a note here about the early church helping out the poor. We are told that they had everything in common. This is not socialism or communism where all the wealth of the upper and middle class is redistributed indiscriminately. They were sharing their wealth with those in the CHURCH, other BELIEVERS! It is one thing to help out a fellow believer, or a widow in the CHURCH, and another thing to just hand out donations to people who do not belong to the body of believers. We are to give alms wisely. This does not mean indiscriminately giving your hard-earned money out to just anyone that passes by. Who are you giving it to? Are you handing out donations to people who are part of the Body of Christ, to needy children, or to those who are worshipping Satan, Hare Krishna, Buddha, etc? And perhaps the reason they are begging in the streets could be because they are bowing down to idols, or dealing drugs, and bringing a curse upon their own head. Are you giving donations to people who hate Christians and despise Jesus? Are you blindly giving to "charities" that support organizations that have pledged themselves to destroy Israel and to kill Christians, and determined to destroy Democracy? How many people still remember the "food for oil" program? Don't be a gullible Christian, handing out donations to groups that are a front for terrorist organizations! Be WISE when you are asked to donate. One of the best ways to give your alms is to support your local church's missionaries. Inviting just anyone into your home who is not a believer, that you know nothing about, is asking for trouble. In the day and age in which we live, registered sex offenders, drug dealers, and murderers conceal themselves in every community. When you have small children, or even older children in your home, you have no business entertaining strangers. In the times in which we are living, you could be putting your family at risk. Don't set up meetings or dates with internet "friends" you know nothing about! Use discernment!

Recall that at one point, when Jesus' disciples were trying to cast out demons, they failed. When they asked him why, he told them: "Howbeit this kind goeth not out but by prayer and fasting." *(Matt: 17:21 KJV.)* This means that there will be times in your life that praying in itself will not get answers to prayer for you. You will have to combine it with fasting to get results. Thus, we see that not only is fasting great for cleansing and detoxification for the Christian, but it also has spiritual implications as well! There are many other instances in the Bible where great answers to prayer came as a result of fasting. Esther fasted three days and saved the Jewish people from total destruction at the hands of Haman, their adversary. Daniel fasted 21 days and received an angelic visitation in answer to his prayers. Cornelius fasted in Acts 10:30 and received an angelic visitation and answer to prayer. Many times the Jewish people fasted, not only in response to biblical commands, but in their prayers to God for assistance or deliverance in times of great distress.

In the Old Testament, fasting was even part of the law given to the Hebrews. There were special feast days in the Old Testament that required everyone to fast. Fasting was an important part of their lives, emphasized by God as an important way to come before Him in humility.

According to Tony Evans, author of *Tony Evans Speaks Out On Fasting,* fasting meets a need in the human soul and (as stated in Isaiah 58 of the Bible) causes "your voice to be heard on high." Mr. Evans also believes that fasting sharpens the spiritual senses (399).

When a Baptist youth pastor embarked on a 40 day fast, he did so for many reasons, including his desire for a family. He and his wife had been unable to have a child after several years of marriage. God answered his prayers, though in an unexpected way. He and his wife were not able to have a child that was biologically theirs, but they were able to adopt a beautiful baby girl!

When a dedicated Christian Bible school teacher went on a partial fast to break her daughter's drug and alcohol addiction (she could not do a total fast due to blood sugar problems), God answered her fasting and prayer by breaking her daughter's addictions and at the same time, bringing salvation to another family member.

When the pastor of a Baptist Church in New England embarked on a fast to pray for his wife who had been diagnosed with cancer, God heard his prayers and honored his fast; his wife was completely healed.

When a minister's wife was diagnosed with a very painful arterial blood vessel inflammation, she was told she would die without a steroid regimen. She refused the treatment much to the dismay of her friends, though her immediate family was supportive of her. She embarked on a 21 day fast and was completely healed.

As stated earlier in this book, perhaps we need to take a lesson from the animals when they are ill. When animals are sick, "they rest, drink water and fast" (372). There are many cases of chronic illnesses being cured after a period of fasting—I know of one in particular—a woman who was completely healed of lupus after she underwent a 21 day period of prayer and fasting. Just remember, you must clear a fast with your physician first, especially if you have any type of health condition.

## When You Should NOT Fast

There are certain situations where fasting is not recommended. As described by Dr. Don Colbert, author of *Toxic Relief*, women who are "pregnant or nursing" should not fast, nor should you fast if you are extremely ill, or fighting a chronic illness (372). Individuals with mental disorders may worsen with fasting. Those with heart problems should not fast (372). Children should not fast unless their physician has them on a fast (e.g., when a child develops severe diarrhea, the doctor may advise eating only certain foods or liquids until the diarrhea clears up). If you are on a water-restricted or salt-restricted diet, you should not be fasting without your physician's approval. If you've just had major surgery, you should not fast unless your physician has restricted your intake, nor should you fast if you are taking chemotherapy. You need adequate nutrients for healing. If you are awaiting a transplant, or just had one, you should not be fasting, unless ordered by your physician.

Never go on a fast without first consulting your physician. A water-only fast (drinking water only and avoiding all solid foods and juices) can cause low levels of potassium and other vital minerals, which can result in irregular heartbeat and even death. Many juices are mineral-rich (372).

Fasting requires large amounts of water. Realize that when you increase your water consumption, you should also **add salt**, or you may end up with a dangerous sodium deficiency, which can bring on severe weakness, arrhythmias, and death. You need "1/4 tsp. of salt for every **quart** of water you drink" (non-refined ocean or sea salt is best) (341). See chapter 23 of this book for more details on the importance of water.

## Juicing to Detoxify

Cherie Calhoun and Maureen Keane in their book, *Juicing For Life*, describe juices that are good for cleansing. "...[B]eet root" juice "(no more than three ounces should be consumed the first day, but this amount can be increased gradually up to six ounces), cabbage, wheat grass, sprouts, lemon, carrot, celery, and apple" (362). Always mix beet root juice with small amounts of another juice, such as celery or carrot.

## Ending the Fast

Whether you go on a water-only fast or a juice-fast, you need to end the fast gradually. You cannot go on an extended fast, and then begin eating a regular cooked diet the same day. Your body will protest violently. Doing so has landed many unfortunate individuals in the hospital. When you are fasting, your intestines and stomach contract. How you break the fast depends on how long the fast was and the type of fast. The longer the fast you have been on, the more time you need for ending the fast. A short fast of three days will not take nearly as long to break as a 21 day or 40 day fast. If you have been on an extended water-only fast, you can begin drinking decaffeinated teas and diluted fresh juices (not full strength), then begin introducing solids slowly into your diet over a period of days. Begin with raw fruits such as bananas, whole grain or gluten-free breads (especially if you are allergic to gluten) broth, soups, cooked cereals, like oatmeal, or cream of wheat and cream of rice, unless you are on a totally raw diet.

If you are breaking an extended juice-fast, you have already been taking juices, so you just need to slowly start introducing solid foods again (as above), though this fast is not as delicate to break as the water-only fast. You can begin with a breakfast of raw fruit such as bananas, and a slice of whole grain bread, a broth soup for lunch with whole grain bread, and a cooked cereal (such as cream of rice) for supper, with a sliced banana, or the Budwig diet. If you have been on a 21 day or longer fast, you will need to spend several days readjusting your body to eating solids. If you have been on a fast of seven days or more, you still have to begin slowly introducing solids into the body. (Note: if you are going to opt for a total raw foods diet, you will not be eating breads, cooked soups or cooked cereals.) Do not ruin the benefits of the fast by eating junk food and highly processed sugary foods.

# CHAPTER 36

# WHAT'S NEXT?

*"Death and life are in the power of the tongue:…" (Proverbs 18:21) "A merry heart doeth good like a medicine:…" (Proverbs 17:22) "For the joy of the Lord is your strength." (Nehemiah 8:10)*

## I. Purpose of Detox

Remember that detoxifying your body will make you feel worse initially. You are ridding your body of poisons that (unless you have detoxed before) have had many years to accumulate. The older you are, the more poisons have built up in your system. You may experience headaches and skin breakouts where poisons are being eliminated from your body. The type fast that you choose will be up to you, your own strength, and how you feel that the Lord is leading you. Pray and seek the Lord before ever beginning any fast. You should gradually begin to introduce more and more solids into the diet, even if you stay with raw foods only. If you begin adding cooked foods, do so slowly, beginning with one meal a day, such as cream of rice with fruit and toasted rye bread for breakfast, or a large baked potato for lunch, or items such as organic, poached eggs (unless you are going completely vegan), steamed broccoli, or stewed tomatoes for supper. If you are using cooked foods, you may want to begin eating organic rye breads (great for lowering high blood pressure), and whole wheat breads. Be sure to get gluten-free breads, especially if you already have gluten allergies. Many people who have been on raw food only diets report having a return of their old problems when they begin incorporating cooked meals back into their diet. Do not use gluten cereals if you have allergies to gluten. Don't eat organic eggs if you are allergic to eggs. Regardless of which you choose, you should stay with the prayer and praise program (see chapter one).

Make a covenant with God to spend time every day praising Him, not just at the worship service you attend. Search out the many healing verses in the Bible. Memorize them—claim them—and remember that God has also promised that: *"If ye abide in me, and my words abide in you, ye shall ask what ye will, and it shall be done unto you."* (John 15:7) God operates on faith. Your own words can determine your destiny. If you get up in the morning declaring verbally that everything will go wrong, it probably will! If you start declaring positive outcomes for each day (and for your health), God will honor your faith and move mountains for you. Take healing verses from the Bible, write them down and recite them OUT LOUD every morning when you arise. One of the best books I have ever read on how to put your faith into action is by Darlene Bishop, *Your Life Follows Your Words.* You can find Darlene's book at her website *www.darlenebishop.org.* She was miraculously healed of breast cancer and has a tremendous testimony. Just be aware that I do not advocate avoiding medical care for yourself or your children, as I have discussed earlier in this book. I have heard horror stories of so-called "believers," who have newly-diagnosed children with diabetes, refusing to get help for them and letting their children die. This is totally absurd, it is murder!

See the first chapter of my book for more information on the importance of prayer and worship, and the words that come out of your mouth. Realize too that prayer and worship are alkalizing to the body!

## II. Where To Start—Healthy Tips

There are no *quick-fixes* for optimal health, but the very first thing that you need to do is to purchase a good quality **juicer**! By the time you've gotten this far in this book, you should have a pretty good idea which juicer you are going to use (if you don't already have one). Once you've done that, you are ready to begin. You can also begin by taking green powdered drinks before you even get a juicer. See further in this chapter for a sample detox program you may wish to choose. Just be sure to check with your physician or Naturopath first, since it does involve fasting. It is not set in stone. You can try it for 3 days, 7 days, or longer, as you feel led. Always pray first, seeking God's will for you.

## III. Wholesome Recipes

Below is a recipe for a tea mix that you may wish to try. This tea mix is a recipe that I combined several years ago because I liked the variety of herbs used. You will end up with several cups of DRY ingredients, once blended. If you want a smaller amount, use half the ingredients given for ½ the recipe. As noted earlier, be sure to discuss any new herbal tea, such as this one, with your physician before beginning. You want to be sure you will not be ingesting anything that could be incompatible with prescription medications you are taking. You also want to be sure that you do not have a chronic disease or condition that may negate the use of herbal preparations. Some items, for example, can cause uterine contractions, so pregnant women should avoid them.

## Alphabet Tea Blend

Combine the following DRY herbal ingredients in a large glass or polycarbonate jar with a reclosable, sealing lid. You will need a large jar to be able to mix and combine the contents of this tea unless you cut the amount in half for fewer total cups. You will end up with several cups of dry ingredients, depending on whether or not you choose to use them all. Obtain these certified organic ingredients from your local herbal supplier or natural health food store. This tea should last you several weeks, depending on how many times a day you drink it. Be sure to consult with your physician about using this or any other herbal blend if you have a blood disorder, are on prescription medications, are pregnant or nursing, a transplant patient, or have any type of chronic health problems. Do not give to children without first consulting with their physician. Do not use if you have allergies to any of the ingredients. I use a large glass jar, put the ingredients inside, close the lid, and shake them all together for several minutes to mix them well (Store in a cool, dry area as with any dry tea) away from moisture and the sun. Do not refrigerate.

- ½ cup dried **alfalfa leaf** (omit this ingredient if you have lupus!)
- ¼ cup dried **astragalus tea** (decaffeinated)*
- ¼ cup dried **cat's claw** tea or purchase the herb in bulk (decaffeinated) (I buy the certified organic tea bags and cut them open until I have ½ cup total)* (see note below)
- ¼ cup dried **dandelion leaf**
- ¼ cup dried **dandelion root**
- ½ cup dried **Enchinacea purpura**
- ¼ cup dried **ginkgo leaf**
- ¼ cup dried **golden ginger**
- 1 cup dried **green tea** (decaffeinated)
- ¼ cup dried **hyssop**
- ¼ cup **kelp granules** (check with your Dr. first if you have thyroid problems before using kelp)
- ¼ cup dried **indian sage**

- 1 cup dried **milk thistle seeds**
- 1 cup dried **mixed mushrooms** - e.g., shiitake, maitake (don't use maitake if you have multiple sclerosis) (184), ABM (agaricus blazeill) kawaratake (coriolus versicolor), reishi, morels, and cordyceps sinesis. You may not be able to find all of these in the dried bags, but some you will. Break them into smaller pieces (you can break them up before you ever remove them from the bags you purchase them in). The water in the tea will reconstitute them. Sometimes you will find bags of dried mushrooms in health food stores with seven or eight varieties that will make one cup. Be sure to choose certified organic. You can also chop them into very small pieces. You can find mushroom variety teas that can be substituted for the dried mushrooms and use one cup total of the teas.
- ½ cup dried **orange peel**
- ¼ cup dried **Pau d'arco bark**
- ¼ cup dried **peppermint**
- ½ cup dried **red clover blossom**
- 1 cup dried **rose hips**
- ½ cup dried **sheep sorrel**
- ¼ cup **slippery elm bark**
- ¼ cup dried **spearmint**
- ½ cup **Turkish rhubarb** root
- ¼ cup dried **yellow dock root**

This sounds like a lot of ingredients, but most are easy to find. You can break it up into 6 separate lists, hand them out to friends and go to the health food store on a scavenger hunt. It is fun to mix all the ingredients. I have been able to find all of them in ONE local health food supplier. It takes a while to get them all combined, and mixed up, but it is well worth the effort. The tea will last you several weeks, depending on how often you drink it. Use a reliable supplier. You don't want moldy mushrooms!

*Do not use cat's claw herb if you have an "auto-immune illness, multiple sclerosis, and/or tuberculosis. European practitioners avoid combining this herb with hormonal drugs, insulin or vaccines" (67). Do not take cat's claw if you are *pregnant* or breast-feeding (67). Check with your physician about using this herb, especially if you have an infection or are running a temperature (36). (Do not use caffeinated teas. They act as diuretics in the body.) When you make the tea, you can also add herbs such as celery seed or dill to taste, if desired. When you make an 8 oz. cup of tea, you will be using two teaspoons (one if you want a milder strength) of the *Alphabet Tea* blend. Use a stainless steel tea ball and put two teaspoons of the dried tea mixture inside the tea ball and put the tea ball into a large cup. If you have a kit where you can make your own tea bags, go for it. Then pour

8—10 oz. of boiling water over the tea ball (or bags) and let it steep until it gets cool. (Or drink when still warm if you prefer warm tea.) Add fresh lemon to taste if you like, and ¼ tsp of royal jelly or honey (use LifeMel Honey if you are ill) to sweeten. Add powdered cinnamon to taste, if desired. Put the royal jelly in the tea while it is still **hot** so that it will dissolve. (Remember, do not give honey and other bee products to children under two. Also, some individuals are allergic to bee products.) This tea is very detoxifying and rich in anti-oxidants. For those who love iced tea, you can let the tea cool, and add ice cubes, rather than drinking it warm. You can also make a fruit smoothie or slushie of choice, and add the cooled tea to the slushie. If you like the taste of cloves, you can add 2 or 3 whole or chopped cloves to your tea ball. Cloves are great anti-oxidants, plus they kill parasites. Cloves are so popular, that even candy makers use them, but they are more potent against parasites when chopped.

## Liver Flush

The following is a liver tonic recipe of mine that I use occasionally for its detoxification and nutritional value. Juice the following organic items in your juicer after they have been thoroughly cleaned:

- 2 medium carrots
- 3 medium tomatoes
- Small bunch of parsley
- ¼ sweet green or red pepper (seeds and all)
- 1 medium beet
- 2 kale or collard leaves
- 6-12 spinach leaves
- 1 large celery stalk
- 1/2 small red or yellow onion
- Small bunch of cilantro

¼ peeled raw potato

- ¼ tsp. grated ginger (optional)
- ¼ tsp. grated lemon peel

To the finished juice, add 1 tblspn lemon juice, ½ tsp. of turmeric,* one tblspn flax oil, ¼ tsp. cayenne pepper (optional, as tolerated), the juice of 1 crushed garlic clove, and one serving of a green powder such as chlorella, barley, or kamut (or 1 oz. fresh wheat grass juice if available). Add three ounces of distilled water to further dilute, if desired. Mix well with the juice and drink. Drink six to eight ounces. This drink is very nutritious, and detoxifying. (Be aware that some of the ingredients in this flush have blood-thinning properties.) You will find more curcumin in turmeric than you will in curry powder. Use organic turmeric rather than curry. (*Do not use turmeric if you have gallbladder problems, if you are pregnant, on blood-thinners, contemplating or just recovering from surgery or transplant, nor if you are breast-feeding (571). Do not use the fresh ginger unless you really LIKE the taste of ginger. I love ginger in some vegetable dishes and in capsule form, but I do not care for the taste of raw ginger mixed in vegetable drinks. (With this recipe, you may end up with two or three servings depending on the size of your vegetables and the output of your juicer. If so, use in the detox regimen, refrigerate one or two servings for later in the day, or for tomorrow (or share with a family member). Do not save in refrigerator for longer than 24 hours. Not for small children. If you have added fresh wheat grass juice to your mixture, do not let it sit overnight. If you are going to save some of this mixture overnight, do not put the fresh wheat grass juice (or the powdered green juice) into the drink until right before consumption.

## Power Seed Mix

This power seed mix can be used once you have advanced off your juice-fast for several days and you are already back on solids, but not before. Use organic products. Do not use salted nuts or products that have sulfur preservatives in them. Mix all the fiber-rich ingredients thoroughly, **refrigerate,** and use ½ to ¾ cups once or twice per day. (If you want a smaller mix, use half the amounts given.) Not only is this mix packed with fiber and nutrients, it is high in ORAC units. Combine the following in a large bowl:

½ cup raisins
½ cup sunflower seeds
½ cup sesame seeds
1 cup almonds
½ cup walnuts
¼ cup macadamias
½ cup pecans
½ cup pine nuts
¼ cup pistachios
1 cup Brazil nuts

1 cup unsalted pumpkin seeds
½ cup red-skinned peanuts

## IV. Nutrient Supplements—Why Do We Need Them?

Most people do not get the amount of vitamins and minerals they need in their daily diet, especially in this fast-paced society in which we live. You should consider taking a potent multiple vitamin/mineral supplement daily, such as the *OLA LOA*™ varieties, found in health food stores, or a mineral drink, such as *Mineral Rich*®, marketed by Maureen Kennedy Salaman. You can find *Mineral Rich*® at her website *www.mksalaman.com.* It is a form of minerals in a good tasting, easily absorbable liquid. Some natural health food stores also carry *Mineral Rich*® and *OLA LOA*™. Do not take grape-seed extracts at the same time that you take Vitamin C. Research suggests that taking them at the same time may raise blood pressure in some individuals.

## Recent Studies on Vitamins & Cancer

There has been a lot of publicity in the news in the latter part of 2008 that vitamins such as C, E, and selenium, in human studies, were not shown to prevent cancer. When you read about these studies, many factors need to be taken into consideration:

- In the study on vitamin C, only 500 mg a day was given. You will read throughout this entire book that not a single advocate of vitamin C therapy ever proposed such a ridiculously LOW amount of vitamin C for fighting cancer! You can probably burn that much vitamin C in 5 minutes waiting in a traffic jam! It has also been proven that vitamin C given in huge doses intravenously is much more effective at fighting cancer than C taken orally! Also, some forms of vitamin C are better than others (e.g., vitamin C from rose hips and vitamin C with other bioflavonoids). See p. 544 for a new potent form of vitamin C!
- In the study using vitamin E, only 400 IU were given every OTHER day, not every day. Why was it not given daily? Also, what KIND of vitamin E was given? The synthetic dl-alpha? The natural d-alpha, mixed tocotrieols? This would make a HUGE difference. Even synthetic beta-carotene is so far inferior to natural beta-carotene, prior human studies showed that the SYNTHETIC variety can actually increase the risk for lung cancer in smokers – not so with the natural!

- There are numerous other human studies that have been done using vitamin therapy that contradict the findings of these studies. What about the control group? How healthy were they? Did they eat normally? If so, how do they know that the group not receiving the vitamin or mineral supplements did not get the SAME amounts in their daily diets, via food intake, as those given the supplements, making the entire study flawed. In other words, is it possible that BOTH groups received the exact same amount of nutrition in their daily intake? Did anyone bother to monitor food intake of the same nutrients during this time period, or keep track of the type of diets both groups were consuming?
- Anytime I have read research studies on the importance of minerals like selenium and vitamin C antioxidants for cancer prevention, then along comes another study that tries to contradict 30 that were done before it, a red flag goes up. WHO sponsored these studies? How many drug companies were involved in these studies? Pharmaceutical companies are ALWAYS trying to discredit natural substances like vitamins and minerals. They would like to see every man, woman, and child in the country taking their prescription medications for things like high-cholesterol, rather than natural foods and nutrients that lower cholesterol levels without drugs. Most of them test 200 mg of vitamin C against a disorder, then pitch it as useless when it does not work. (What they need to be testing is 100-500 GRAMS of vitamin C intravenously at a time! Or using the new *liposome-encapsulated Vitamin C* that is taken orally (466b). They should try using 50 mg of an antibiotic (rather than 2 grams and see where it gets them in fighting disease!)
- Two new studies by German scientists showed that selenium boosts the body's natural immunity. Of significance was the fact that all the men in the study with prostate cancer already had low levels of selenium in their body. What about the other recent study that claimed that selenium did nothing to prevent prostate cancer? Were blood levels of selenium taken BEFORE the study began to determine if some of the men were already deficient in selenium before even beginning the study?
- While it was shown that those men taking selenium alone (rather than with vitamin E) had increased incidence for diabetes, this should come as no surprise, because minerals and vitamins need each other for best performance. Our bodies were meant to function at optimal level when adequate amounts of all nutrients and vitamins are supplied, not just one or two.
- While one large study said that selenium did not affect melanoma, the same study revealed that it decreases the risk for all other cancers.
- Those giving the results of the study said that natural foods are a better source of vitamins and minerals than supplements. Of course, this has always been true, however, there are some nutrients that you just can not

get sufficient amounts of without supplementing (e.g., alpha lipoic acid, vitamin C, and CoQ10), and there are many areas of the country, for example, where you can eat foods that SHOULD be rich in selenium, but they are not because the soil has been stripped of selenium, so you need to supplement.

- Individual situations will also determine vitamin and nutrient needs. If you have just had a devastating illness or blow (e.g., death of a loved one in your family), you are going to require more vitamin C to offset the stress in your life than someone dealing with no stress.
- Be VERY suspicious of people who tell you that you don't need vitamin and mineral supplements, but it's fine to take multiple prescription drugs and that your only CHOICE for cancer is chemo or radiation!

## Vitamin-Mineral-Herbal Supplement Choices

There are many available choices on the market for vitamin-mineral-herbs and other health ingredients. Many mushroom (and other nutrient) supplements can be found at *www.newchapter.info*. Their supplements are marketed under the brand name Mycomedicinals® or New Chapter®. Life Extension (for example at *www.lef.org)* advertises pharmaceutical grade supplements. So does *Usana*® Health at website: *http://www.usana.com*, and Dee Simmons at *www.ultimateliving.com*. (Some of these brands may cost more, but you will be getting a pharmaceutical grade product, higher in quality, and often lower in additives, than other brands.) There are also mushroom supplements available at *http://www.advancedbionutritionals.com/immunity* and from *http://www.medicinalmushrooms.net/index.html*. Also, see *http://www.Agaricusfarm.com/index.html* and *http://www.herbal remedies.com*, as well as health supplements at *www.swansonvitamins.com*, and other websites mentioned in several chapters of this book. (See *Appendix II* at the back of this book.)

Some other vitamin, mineral, herbal and natural brands that you will see are: Green Foods™, Kyolic® (garlic supplements), Spring Valley®, Carlson®, Country Life®, Enzymatic Therapy®, Jarrow Formulas®, Nutramax Laboratories®, Inc., New Chapter®, Garden of Life®, TWINLAB®, Alacer®, All One®, American Health®, Bach® Flower Remedies, Boiron® Homeopathics, Body Rescue®, Chromalux®, Dessert Essence® Organics, EarthRise®, Essiac® International, Flora®, FoodScience® of Vermont, Green Foods®, Halo® Purely for Pets, Hylands® Homeopathic Remedies, Irwin Naturals®, Jason® Cosmetics, Life-Flo®, Maximum Living®, NaturalCare®, Nature's Secret®, Natural Vitality®, Nature's Way®, NOW® Foods, NutriCology®, ReNew life,

Shen Min®, Spectrum Essentials®, Trace Minerals®, Udo's Choice®, Weil™ Supplements, Weleda®, Willard Water®, Xenna®, Xlear®, Inc., Natrol®, Now® Foods, Schiff®, Nature's Life®, Sundown®, Solaray®, Nature Made™, Nature's Bounty®, and many others. Website *http://www.discount-vitamins-herbs.net,* has discount prices, great nutritional information, and a large variety of supplements. You can even buy your own home mushroom growing kits at some websites such as: *http://www.fungi.com/kits/index.html.* There are many other internet sites that have nutritional supplements at reasonable prices, such as *www.swansonvitamins.com* and *www.puritan.com.* There are also places where you can buy vitamins and mineral supplements in bulk, free of additives. Try to avoid supplements which contain additives like magnesium stearate and titanium dioxide.

## V. Detoxification

Each day you should be drinking (depending on your size) about six to eight (eight ounce) glasses of water per day, unless your physician has you on a special water-restricted or salt-restricted diet. There are many ways to detox. You can try drinking only fresh juices for several days, but the key is to remember that you also need plenty of water, whichever detox means you choose. If you have diabetes or other chronic diseases, blood disorders, are pregnant or breast-feeding, or are taking prescription medications, do not attempt to detox (or any type of fasting program) without first consulting with your physician. You should also be praying about it; seeking spiritual guidance.

Of course, anyone who is severely ill needs to consult with their physician before beginning a new health regimen or detox program. Many times, those who are severely ill cannot tolerate fasting, juicing, and strict detox regimens. You are flushing out your system, so you will need extra water every day during detox. (You will not be doing strenuous exercise during a detox program. Mild exercise is fine.) Don't take alkalizers on a stomach full of food. Your food will just sit there and not digest!

## Tips on the Detox

Do not mix Essiac tea with anything else. Take it on an empty stomach. Always wait one hour before ingesting anything else after taking Essiac. Always wait one hour AFTER you have eaten anything else, before taking

Essiac. Day 4 through 7, you are drinking (or eating) fresh grapes or juice. You can choose purple, red, green, or black grapes, or mix them to your taste. Remember to also be drinking water during any detox program. Don't forget to get ten to twenty minutes of fresh air and sunshine in your routine (at least 3 days per week) during this time. (See earlier precautions if you or a family member have a history of melanoma.) Do not get sunshine during the hottest time of the day. Use a mineral drink such as *Ola Loa*® or *Mineral Rich*® daily with these detox programs to be sure you are getting other essential minerals during the day.

## 3 Day Apple Cider Vinegar Detox – Rapid Alkalizer

Mix one teaspoon of apple cider vinegar in 8 ounces of fresh water and drink this mixture 3 or 4 times each day for three days, adding additional glasses of water during the day as desired. If you already have cancer, drink 2 oz of Essiac tea (as instructed and prepared on the brand you choose) when you first arise in the morning, and 2 oz of the tea on retiring. Do not drink the apple cider vinegar at least one hour before or one hour after you have ingested the Essiac tea. Use a mineral drink such as *Ola Loa*® or *Mineral Rich*® daily with these detox programs to be sure you are getting other essential minerals during the day. Be sure to spend time praising God and in Bible study.

## 3 Day Soda Bicarb Detox – Very Rapid Alkalizer

You will find this alkalizer on the *Arm & Hammer*® soda bicarb that you find in your grocers. It is used for "sour stomach," for example. They instruct that you check with your physician first. Use ½ teaspoon of the bicarb in ½ glass of water (4 ounces) every two hours, not to exceed 7 doses within a 24 hour period, and no more than 3 doses in 24 hours if you are over 60 years of age. Do not use the maximum dose for more than 2 weeks. (This is a 3 day program only.) You should always seek your physician's advice with a detox, or any alkalizer, especially this one, since soda bicarb has a high salt content. Use a mineral drink such as *Ola Loa*® or *Mineral Rich*® daily with these detox programs to be sure you are getting other essential minerals during the day. Do not take soda bicarb on a stomach full of food. It alkalizes stomach acidity, so your food will just sit there and not digest!

# 7 Day Detox Programs – Rapid Alkalizers

- **Day 1 through Day 3:**
Water, at least 8 glasses per day (8 ounce glasses), if you are not on a water-restricted diet. Do not use water that has chlorine or fluoride. If you already have cancer, drink 2 oz of Essiac tea (as instructed and prepared on the brand you choose) when you first arise in the morning, and 2 oz of the tea on retiring. Be sure to spend time praising God, and in Bible study (e.g., 15-30 minutes in the am and 15-30 minutes in the pm) or longer, every day. Always praise him FIRST, then present your requests before him.

- **Day 4 through Day 7:**
  1. Essiac tea, 2 oz on arising
  2. An hour later, drink 6 oz of fresh grape juice from your juicer, or you can eat a handful of fresh organic grapes, whichever you prefer (when using seeded grapes chew them into tiny bits.) Choose mostly the purple, red, and black grapes. The green grapes are okay, but only occasionally. Try to avoid bitterly sour grapes, and stick to sweeter varieties. (Purple concord grapes are great if you can get them organic and in season!) Remember when you juice grapes, you will juice seeds and all. When you eat grapes, eat the seeds and skin.
  3. Two hours later, you will again drink the grape juice or eat the grapes. You will do this every two hours on day four through day seven, until one hour before bedtime.
  4. At bedtime, again take 2 oz of the Essiac tea preparation. (Your hours may vary from day to day, depending on when you go to bed at night, and when you rise in the morning.) You may find yourself taking Essiac at 6 or 7 one morning, then at 8 the next. Just be sure that you eat or drink nothing within one hour of taking the Essiac. Remember that ALL your juices should be organic and fresh-squeezed that you juice yourself, or a family member juices for you. By the end of day 7, you should be well on your way to detox and alkalinity.

Be certain that you are taking sufficient salt each day (e.g., for every eight to ten glasses (8 oz) of water (or liquids) you will need about ½ tsp of salt total (341). If you are diabetic, pregnant, or have any health disorders, you will need to consult with your doctor before beginning a detox program.

Use a mineral drink such as *Ola Loa®* or *Mineral Rich®* daily with these detox programs to be sure you are getting other essential minerals during the day.

## 7 Day Lemonade Detox

Use fresh-squeezed lemon juice (and/or lime juice) diluted in water to concentration of your taste. Drink as often as you like with extra water as desired for seven days. This is a rapid alkalizer and detox. Use a mineral supplement such as *Ola Loa®* or *Mineral Rich®* once or twice daily on this fast as with any fast you embark on. Also, drink water as desired. Remember to discontinue any fast such as this one GRADUALLY.

## 10 Day Lemonade Detox

*Lemonade Diet* by Stanley Burroughs. Mix 2 tablespoons of fresh-squeezed lemon juice, 2 tablespoons of maple syrup and 1/8 tspn cayenne pepper into 8 oz of water. Drink as often as needed to maintain energy. Follow for a ten day period, but eat and drink nothing else (340).

## 7 Day/21 Day/40 Day Detox

This is a juice fast and can be followed for anywhere from 24 hours to 40 days. You will be taking juices only. Just realize that when you come off this fast, you must do so **very gradually**.

Take 2 oz of Essiac tea each day upon rising and at bedtime. Do not drink or eat anything within one hour of the time you take Essiac. One hour after taking the Essiac in the morning, drink 6 – 8 oz of a vegetable juice of choice. You can mix carrot juice with celery, sprout and/or greens, whatever you choose. Then two hours later and every two hours for the rest of the day until one hour before you take the last dose of Essiac for the day, you will drink 6 – 8 oz. of a vegetable juice of choice. This should be a fresh blend that you juice from a juicer, not a store-bought juice. The only exception would be if you would like two or three glasses a day of LOW SODIUM V8® juice. You can also use citrus juice (oranges or grapefruit, lemon or lime) once or twice a day during this fast. When you are juicing vegetables, use celery, carrots, tomato, cucumbers, greens, broccoli, onion, radish, cabbage, lettuce, beets, squash, potato, asparagus, sprouts, etc. It is also permissible to add the juice of an apple occasionally to the vegetable juices or the juice of berries or grapes. You can also add cinnamon to any of the drinks or other herbs or spices (e.g., ginger, garlic, cayenne, cilantro, parsley, paprika, etc.) to your preference. Use a mineral supplement such as *Ola Loa®* or *Mineral Rich®* once or twice daily on this fast as with any fast you embark on. Also, drink water as desired.

## Cancer-Fighting Soda-Bicarb Recipe

**(See Chapter 34)**

> Add one part baking soda with three parts maple syrup in a small saucepan. Stir briskly. Heat for five minutes. Take one teaspoon daily, as needed. Be sure you use ALUMINUM-FREE baking soda and 100% maple syrup (no synthetics). Use organic (obtain from your health food store) (377a). [Do not use an aluminum pan.]

Note that this formula can be varied. It can be heated just until it foams. You can substitute organic blackstrap molasses or honey for the maple syrup, and if so, you do not need to heat them. This per Dr. Mark Sircus in his book *Sodium Bicarbonate Rich Man's Poor Man's Cancer Treatment* (566c). This recipe is not part of a daily fast, but added to your daily diet.

## Soda-Bicarb Used to Cure Spreading Prostate Cancer

Dr. Sircus also discusses a man who was diagnosed with prostate cancer that had gone into his bones, and he was basically sent home to die. Before this patient began using the soda bicarb, he had been treated with *Finasteride*, a drug given for prostate enlargement, and *Casodex*, a drug that treats prostate cancer by reducing levels of testosterone (566c). [The drugs did nothing to stop his cancer.] He cured himself within just **11 days** using the oral soda bicarb, which he mixed with blackstrap molasses. On day 1 through day 4, he added one teaspoon of soda bicarb and one teaspoon of blackstrap molasses to 8 ounces of water and drank the solution (at room temperature) once a day (566c). [On day 5, I could not tell from the notes if he was taking one teaspoon of the bicarb and one teaspoon of the blackstrap molasses twice a day or TWO teaspoons of each twice a day.] By day 6 and 7, he definitely is using 2 teaspoons each of soda bicarb and the blackstrap molasses in 8 ounces of water twice a day and using pH testing paper to check his urine and saliva. On day 8 and 9, he drank the same mixture 3 times a day. [This is a lot of salt!] On day 10, he used the same mixture, but took it only twice a day. On the 11th day, he used one-and-a-half teaspoons each of the soda bicarb and the blackstrap molasses in 8 ounces of water twice a day. On day 12, a bone scan was done. Results were mailed to him and showed that he had no trace of cancer anywhere. He did experience night sweats, some loose stools, and headaches during the process and said afterwards that he probably should have added some potassium to his diet (566c). I would not recommend this protocol unless you were also taking potassium and magnesium supplements each day; and, as stated earlier, this mixture (especially on days 6 through 10) is very high in sodium! If you are already fighting illness and on a salt-restricted or water-restricted diet, you should be using great caution and checking with your physician. I am sure individual results would vary depending on your body weight, the rest of your diet, and your overall health to begin with, including the health of your kidneys! The patient did not say what else he was consuming during the day, if anything. Eating a lot of cooked foods, meat, or dairy would skew the results. Some people could probably get their urine pH up to 8 and keep it there for 2 or 3 days with a much lower amount of the soda bicarb, or by using lemon juice and/or apple cider vinegar (without all that salt). Also, realize that most conventional doctors won't agree to this regimen. You would need the guidance and second opinion of a Naturopathic physician. This regimen kept the patient's alkalinity at 8 for about 3.5 to 4 days. I would hope that he was also drinking lots of water to keep his body flushed from all the salt intake.

Remember, you MUST go off any fast gradually, as described earlier in **chapter 35**. You cannot immediately begin eating solid and cooked foods in large amounts. It must be gradual, or you can end up in severe distress. You cannot break a detox program like this in ONE day, then go back to eating cooked foods and a regular diet!

If you already have cancer, you may wish to keep taking the Essiac every day until you have healed your immune system.

Read the cancer-specific chapter in this book for the type cancer you have, to see what other supplements you may find helpful (e.g., if you have breast cancer, you will want to check the breast cancer chapter in this book, and discuss with your physician about working up to at least 390 mg/day of CoQ10, milk thistle, and many other nutrients that can help you recover. You will need a good multi-vitamin and multi-mineral. You will need sufficient calcium, selenium, zinc, B vitamins, iodine, magnesium, lycopene, omega-3s, and you may wish to take AHCC, B17, resveratrol, or PBs (which the liver converts into antineoplastons). You may wish to consider intravenous vitamin C injections, PSK injections, mushroom supplements, LifeMel Honey, liposome-encapsulated vitamin

C, and any number of items to help boost your immunity, as described in this book.

## Johanna Budwig Program Next - for Those with Cancer

Once you finish a detox program (if you already have cancer), you may wish to begin the Johanna Budwig flax oil program. Use it after the detox is finished or any time before or after a detox. The mix is as follows:

> Blend 2 Tbsp. organic flaxseed oil with 4 Tbsp. organic low-fat cottage cheese or *quark (100) [obtain the cottage cheese or quark from a dairy farmer who makes this fresh in your area, if possible)]. Blend until you can no longer see the oil (100). [ONCE mixed thoroughly (a blender works fine), you can add cinnamon to taste, or fruit of choice, such as organic raisins. *Quark is a pasty type of white cheese. Some farmers make their own.]
>
> See chapter 18 for the rest of the items that go along with the Budwig diet (e.g., no processed oils, animal fats, sugars, no meat, no diet drinks, no margarines) (100).

# VI. Other Helpful Steps

## Comedy, Color, Aroma, Touch

There is a great deal of research going on in the field of relaxation, comedy, balance, and the things you think about (your thought life), for healing the body. Studies are showing that what we put into our mind, influences us nearly as much as the food we put into our body. Having patients lie down and quiet their thoughts in a relaxing atmosphere, surrounded with things that they love (ocean waves, bubbling aquariums, children, music, or pets), greatly reduces stress and has beneficial effects on blood pressure and immunity. Even watching beautifully-colored marine life swimming about in a fish tank can reduce stress level and blood pressure. Stroking your pet cat or dog lowers your stress level (and theirs), and has a positive effect on your immunity, though scientists haven't figured out exactly why this occurs, except that it strengthens the immune cells.

Many health clinics and hospitals are taking advantage of this new-found data to keep their patients in more relaxed atmospheres, even putting attractive colors on the walls and piping in classical music to relax the body. Some are also using aroma-therapy, plants, bringing pets in to interact with patients, and comedy movies to stimulate the body's own immunity for self-healing. Vigorous belly-laughing is healthy for the immune system!

Jesus touched people, laying his hands upon many of them to heal them. Be sure if you have someone laying hands on you and praying over you, that they are praying in the name of Jesus. There are many Eastern cults that are practicing touch for healing, and it has nothing to do with the God of the Bible. Do not open yourself up to negative spiritual influences and gods of Eastern philosophy! (You may find yourself in a worse situation than when you began!

## Music for the Muted Soul

Music has often been called the universal language. Many people do not realize that music affects not only the body, but the mind, the soul, and the spirit as well. Scientific experiments have been done showing that flowers and animals flourish when they are exposed to long hours of classical music, but shrivel up and die when exposed to long hours of heavy-metal rock music. Why would humans think that they are any different? Why would anyone think that they can subject their body to hours of incessant, deafening cadence and loud rhythmic beats and believe it is good for them? Many teens who thought boom-boxes were *totally rad* twenty years ago, are now having psychological, emotional, and hearing problems!

# VII. Most Important Items for Fighting Cancer

(Also, see the cancer-specific chapters in this book for other important minerals, nutrients & other items, depending on the type cancer you have)

| | | |
|---|---|---|
| Almonds | Brewer's Yeast | Flaxseed |
| Alpha lipoic acid | Calcium | Folic acid |
| Apple cider vinegar | Cherries | Fruits (all) |
| Artichoke | Chlorella | Garlic |
| Avocados | Cinnamon | Ginger |
| B vitamins | Citrus fruits | Glutathione |
| Barley grass juice | CoQ10 | Grapes |
| Bee Pollen | Cruciferous foods | Haelan |
| Berries | Dark leafy greens | Honey (LifeMel) |
| Beta-carotene | Essiac Tea | Iodine |

Magnesium
Melatonin
Mushrooms
Natural progesterone
Niacin
Olive oil
Omega 3
Onions
Papaya
Pecans
Pomegranates
Potassium
Prunes
Raisins
Resveratrol
Royal Jelly
Selenium
Soda Bicarb
Spirulina
Sprouts
Squash
Sunflower Seeds
Sunshine (Vitamin D)
Tea
Turmeric
Vitamin B17
Vitamin C
Vitamin E
Walnuts
Water
Wheat germ
Wheatgrass juice
Yellow vegetables
Zinc

## VIII. LAST—But Not Least

What you choose to do with the information in this book you have just read is up to you! If you are fighting a terminal illness, pray *Psalm 119:17 every day! "Deal bountifully with thy servant, that I may live, and keep thy word,"* and declare *Psalm 118:17* BOLDLY every day: *"I shall not die, but live, and declare the works of the Lord."* Take these verses, type and print them off on your PC, and tape them on your mirror so that you can memorize them and repeat them when you get up in the morning, and declare them throughout the day all day long! Verbally declare Jesus as your HEALER! If you have a young child who is fighting a terminal illness, obtain some CD and/or DVD praise songs and play them at your child's bedside 24 hours a day! During sleep time, turn the volume down if the music keeps your child awake. The WORD of God is powerful. You may wish to get a CD of the Bible that is being read aloud and play it at your child's bedside! Remember to proclaim these same verses over your child throughout the day. You can also claim *Psalm 118:17* for them. Get several family members and friends together. Go to your child's (or friend's) hospital room. Form a circle around the perimeter of the bed and join hands. Pray for your child or friend. Lay hands on them. Then raise both arms and begin to praise God over the one who is ill. Praise music will clear evil spirits out of your home. Evil spirits do NOT like worship music, especially songs elevating the Blood of Jesus. Sing to God and praise him at your child's bedside, and most importantly—if they are old enough to learn and well enough that they can participate— (e.g., tapping a smalltambourine) teach your children to **PRAISE THE LORD!**

# APPENDIX I

Below is a sample prayer that you can pray asking Jesus to come into your life. As you pray this prayer, God knows your heart and he can tell how sincere you are. As you say the words—mean them. When you finish, sign your name at the bottom and put the date. (You will always REMEMBER this date as the most important of your life—because it is the day that you were BORN AGAIN!)

**Prayer:**

Dear Jesus: I am a sinner. I realize that I can do nothing to save myself and that you have done everything necessary for me to be saved. I am willing to put my trust for eternal life in you alone. I have broken your holy commandments. I am guilty and deserving of your wrath, but I am trusting your holy WORD where you have said in Romans 10:9 "*That if thou shalt confess with thy mouth the Lord Jesus, and shalt believe in thine heart that God hath raised him from the dead, thou shalt be saved.*" I am confessing you now as my Savior and willing to tell others that I have done so. I forsake my own righteousness and take yours. I repent and turn from my sinful life. I ask you to let your Holy blood cleanse me now of all my sins. Come into my life and change me and be the Lord of my life. Show me your will for my life. Guide me and direct me. Fill me with your Holy Spirit right now and make me a new creature forever. Amen.

______________________________ ________________

Your Name Date

Be willing to follow Jesus in the commandment of being baptized and most importantly, find a Bible-believing church where you can fellowship with other Christians and GROW as a Christian! It is God's will that you fellowship with other believers, and always keep your EYES on Jesus, not on the performance or failures of others. Remember, other Christians will always come up short and disappoint you because no Christian is perfect. Only Jesus was and IS perfect. Keep your eyes on other Christians, and if they fail, you will become discouraged and disheartened. Keep your eyes on JESUS, and he will NEVER forsake you, fail you, or disappoint you!

# APPENDIX II

__Valuable Links:__ Note that these links are given for informational purposes only. The author and publisher are not affiliated with any of these websites except the author's own site at *gentlecures.org*.

- Aloe vera website: ***aloeverahealthbenefits.info.***

- Alternative health doctor list is at this link: ***http://heartspring.net/naturopathic_directory.html*** and here: ***http://www.altmedangel.com.*** For the American Holistic Medical Association's link to finding a physician in your area, see website: ***http://www.holisticmedicine.org/displaycom mon.cfm?an=1&subarticlenbr=49.***

- Alternative health websites: for more information about Johanna Budwig, and many other alternative health websites, see this link: ***http://www.heal ingcancernaturally.com/budwig_protocol.html,*** and for a link which has dozens of testimonials of people who cured their cancers using natural non-toxic therapies, most of which are discussed in this book, see: ***http://www.healingcancernaturally.com/naturalcancer-curetestimonials.ht ml#herbal%20healing%20of%20cancer.***

- Bob's Red Mill Products: ***www.bobsredmill.com***. They have soda bicarb that is guaranteed to be free of aluminum. (*Arm & Hammer*® also says that their soda bicarb is aluminum-free.)

- Burzynski Patient Group: ***http://www.burzynskipatientgroup.org/stori es.htm*** and also see link: ***http://www.burzynski patientgroup.org.*** At these two links you can read the amazing true case histories of many of Dr. Burzynski's patients who were cured of all forms of cancer using his non-toxic antineoplastons and PBs (oral form).

- Burzynski's website: ***http://www.burzynskiclinic.com/ph/index.html*** - here you can get all the details about his amazing non-toxic cancer cure known as antineoplastons and PBs (oral form). Also see website: ***http://w ww.cancure.org/burzynski_institute.htm.***

- Cancell testimonial - here is a link for a testimonial on a person who used Cancell for curing a bone tumor and a brain tumor: ***http://cancerfighter. wordpress.com/2008/06/19/cancell-testimony.***

- Cansema-like skin formula, see website: ***http://www.mnwelldir.org/doc s/cancer1/altthrpy.htm#formula.***

- Encyclopedia for health: ***http://www.polymvahealthclub.com/hd.*** This website by Poly-MVA has an encyclopedia of more than 75,000 health-related items that you can search.

- eXcella™ sweetener – for a sweetener that does not affect blood sugar, see website: ***livonlabs.com.*** This sweetener is a natural sucrose substitute.

- Gentle cures website: ***gentlecures.org***

- Herbs in bulk can be purchased here: ***http://www.sunbreezeherbsho p.com, http://www.herbalhealer.com/bulk-herbs.html,*** and ***http://e sutras.com/index.Ph p?cPath=1.***

- Hodgkin's Lymphoma cure testimonial - To read the interview with Sue Best whose son, Billy, was healed of Hodgkin's lymphoma several years ago, and also a resource for dozens of other links, see this site: ***http://curezon e.com/forums/fm.asp?i=67143.***

- I.P.T. (insulin potentiation therapy) - see the LifeWorks Wellness Center at 301 Turner Street in Clearwater, Florida; their link is here: ***http://www.life workswellnesscenter.com/succan.asp.*** You can also email them here: ***lifeworksinfo@bodyhealth.com***., and another link to some of their success stories at: ***http://www.lifeworkswellnesscenter.com/success. asp.***

- Liposome-encapsulated vitamin C (**Lypo-Spheric™**) - see website: ***livon labs.com***. Also, see Dr. Thomas Levy's website for info on this product as well: ***peakenergy.com*** and ***http://tomlevy.com.***

- Magnascent Iodine, also known as Nascent Iodine, ***www.magnascent.com*** and ***www.magneticclay.com.***

- **Magnesium Chloride Transdermal Oil - Sources:** *http://www.magnetic clay.com*, as well as website: *www.ancient-minerals.com* and *http://www.swan sonvitamins.com.*

- Mercury-free dentists closest to your area: see this link: ***http://library.alt medangel.com/2a.htm.***

- Morgellon's Disease cure: see website: ***http://www.loveforlife.com.au/node/4578.***

- Non-Hodgkin's lymphoma testimonial - to read the amazing testimonial from Maryjo Siegel who was healed of non-Hodgkin's lymphoma using non-toxic antineoplastons, see this link: ***http://burzynskipatientgroup. org/maryjo.htm.***

- Poly-MVA info and amazing case histories of cancer survivors who used Poly-MVA to completely heal their cancers, see this link: ***http://www.polymvasurvivors.com.***

- Probiotic specialists – NATREN® - see their website at ***www.natren.com.***

- Testimonials of people who used natural methods to cure deadly cancers - see this link: ***http://www.cancure.org/cancer_victors.htm.***

- **Ultimate Living** - see Dee Simmons website: ***www.ultimateliving.com,*** for pharmaceutical-grade products.

- **USANA** has pharmaceutical-grade products: ***http://www.usana.com.***

- Vitamin site with nutrient information: ***http://www.mcvitamins.com/default.htm.***

- Whitaker Wellness Center is in Newport Beach (4321 Birch Street), California, see this link: ***http://whitakerwellness.com/about_us/medical_team.*** Dr. Julian Whitaker who runs this health care center, has written many books on alternative healing. He has an excellent website with a great deal of helpful information. They use many of the alternative health treatments that I have mentioned in my books, including chelation, hyperbaric oxygen, and IV therapies. (Also, for those suffering from depression, obsessive-compulsive disorders, and anxiety, Dr. Whitaker says that he has had excellent results treating his patients with low-dose **Dilantin** for these problems. Contact them for more info.) He also has a great newsletter.

- Zeolites websites: ***http://liquidzeolite.zoxic.com,*** or ***http://www.ghchealth.com/zeotrex.php?gclid=CKnb0c25iZcCFQFqxwodh1p6dA*** and ***http://www.zeoliteshealth.com.*** There are many others that either carry the product or discuss it in detail.

# REFERENCES


1. "100% Science. Pure Juice." POM Wonderful Health. Online posting. Accessed 3 Nov. 2007 <http://www.pomwonderful.com/pdf/Clinical_Cancer_Research>. See this site for the Phase II study of the benefits of pomegranate juice for men with prostate cancer.

2. "3F8 Monoclonal Antibody Therapy Q & A." Online posting. Accessed 12 Dec. 2007. <http://www.mskcc.org/mskcc/html/3215.cfm>. © Memorial Sloan-Kettering Cancer Center: ph# 212-639-2000. 1275 York Avenue, New York, N.Y. 10065.

3. "1999 Independent Study by Institute of Longevity Medicine." Online posting. Accessed 8 Nov. 2007 <http://www.realsuccess4life.com/cgi-bin/home.cgi?6038864. Professional Net-workers, Hutchinson, K.S.

4. "A Unique Sugar May be Key to Energizing the Failing Heart." "Bioenergy Life Science's D-ribose offers promising options for energy-deprived hearts." From Minn., MN, 3-22-2007, online posting. Accessed 02 Jan. 2008. <http://bioenergy.com/Papers/FailingHeart.JEJMO32207 .pdf>. Also, see NutraBio.com website © 2007 NutraBio.com., Inc.

5. "A summary of the 20 successful case histories of long-term survivors using Binzel Nutritional Program." Online posting from *Brave-Souls.com Fighting Cancer Around the World.* Accessed 28 Nov. 2007. <http://www.brave-souls.com/learnfromothers/Binzel. html>. Stanley Cua. © 2001-2002 Brave-Souls.com.

6. "About Dendritic Therapy." Online posting. Accessed 13 Jan. 2008. <http://www. Dendritic.info>. © 2004 by The Dendritic Cell Therapy for Cancer.

7. "Abstracts of Published Studies indicating Aloe's Potential Efficacy Against Cancer." Online posting Life Extension Magazine, April 2002. Accessed 8 Nov. 2007. (Also see LEF Protocol Book) <http://www.lef.org/magazine/mag2002_report_clinic_04.ht ml>. When you reach this website, do a search and the article will come up. © 1995-2007 Life Extension Foundation.

8. "Acai Fights Leukemia Cells." Online posting. Accessed 3 Nov. 2007. <http://www. discount-vitamins-herbs.net/n-309-cancer_acai.htm>. From Health News Archive 309 - Leukemia.

9. "Advanced Cancer Alternative Remedies." "Alternative Testing For Cancer." "ORTHO-IMMUNE." Online posting from Cancer Alternatives website. Accessed 20 Jan. 2008. <http://www.alternative-doctor.com/cancer/ca_advanced.htm>. Copyright © 2003 Keith Scott-Mumby.

9a. "Advances in Breast Cancer Treatment." 01/25/08. "A Report from the 2007 Annual San Antonio Breast Cancer Symposium." Online posting accessed or retrieved 26 Aug. 2008. <http://patient.cancerconsultants.com/CancerNews_Breast_Cancer.aspx?DocumentID=41236> © 1998-2008 CancerConsultants.com.

10. "Agaricus Blazei Murill." Newsletter August 2001, from the Wellness Directory of Minnesota™'. Updated 05/05/07. Online posting. Accessed 8 Nov. 2007. <http://www.mnwell dir.org/docs/Cancer1/altthrpy.htm#Agaricus.htm>. Copyright © 1995-2004 International Wellness Directory.

11. "Agaricus." Wellness Directory of Minnesota™, Alternative Cancer Therapies, updated 05/05/07. Online posting. Accessed 8 Nov 8, 2007. <http://www.mnwelldir.org/docs/Cancer1/altthrpyhtm>. Copyright © 1995-2004 International Wellness Directory.

12. "Amargo." Online posting. From Raintree's Tropical Plant Database. Updated 1-14-2007. © 1996 to present - Raintree Nutrition, Inc., Carson City, NV 89701. This information is also found in Leslie Taylor's book, *The Healing Power of Rainforest Herbs*, Square One Publishers, Jan. 2005.

13. "Amazing fruits, when an apple a day just is not enough." "ARONIA BERRIES." From the Amazing journey weblog online posting. Accessed 30 Dec. 2007. <http://scottsports.wordpress.com/2007/11/03/when-an-apple-a-day-is-not-enough/>.

14. "Amla Fruit," from oneearthherbs.com, "Chrysalis Natural Medicine Clinic: Amla Fruit," which they say is a selection from Alan Tillotson's *One Earth Herbal Sourcebook*. Online posting. <http://www.oneearthherbs.com/AmlaFruit.htm>. Also, see The Tillotson Institute of Natural Health: http://oneearthherbs.squarespace.com.

15. "An overview of medicinal mushrooms, mushroom preparations and their medicinal properties." From Mushroom Harvest website online posting "Medicinal Mushrooms." Accessed 31 Dec. 2007. <http://www.mushroomharvest.com/extra_ pages/med_mush rooms.htm>.

16. "Anamu." Online posting. Raintree Nutrition's Tropical Plant Database. "Biological/anamu.htm>. © 1996 to present. Raintree Nutrition, Inc., Carson City, NV. 89701. Updated 1-15-2007. This information is also found in Leslie Taylor's book, *The Healing Power of Rainforest Herbs*, Square One Publishers, Jan 2005.

17. "Anticarcinogenic effect of refined Amorphophallus Konjac on MNNG-induced lung cancer in LACA mice," by Luo Deyuan and Li Yugiong. Institute of Cancer Research, West China University of Medical Sciences, Chengdu. Online posting. Accessed 30 Oct. 2007 <http://www.springerlinkcom/content/g513862nw2551641. Copyright © Springer. Part of Springer Science+Business Media.

18. "Anti-cancer Activities of Pomegranate Extracts." From the Health News Archive 204-Breast Cancer at website www.discount-vitamins-herbs.net online posting. Accessed 8 Dec. 2007. <http://www.discount-vitamins-herbs.net/n-204-breast-cancer-pomegranate.htm>. © 2001-2007 Discount Herbs & Vitamins, Inc. Source given was "Anti-cancer activities of pomegranate extracts and genistein in human breast cancer cells." Jeune, M.A., Kumi-Diaka J.,Brown, J., *Journal of Medicinal Food* 2005 Winter;8(4);469-475.

19. "Andiroba." Online posting. Raintree Nutrition's Tropical Plant Database. Updated 1-14-2007. Accessed 8 Nov. 2007. <http://www.rain-tree.com/andiroba.htm>. This information is also found in Leslie Taylor's book, *The Healing Power of Rainforest Herbs*, Square One Publishers, Jan 2005.

20. "Andrographis." Online posting from herbs2000.com. Accessed 8 Nov. 2007. <http://www.herbs2000.com/herbs/herbs_andrographis.htm>.

21. "Antineoplastons." Online posting. Alternatives in Cancer Therapy, from their excerpt of the book *Alternatives in Cancer Therapy*, by Ross, R., Ph., Pelton, Lee Overholser. Accessed 8 Nov. 2007. <http://www.curezone.com/diseases/cancer/anti-neoplastons.asp>.

22. "Anti-Tumor Effect of Cranberry." Online posting. "Health News Archive 105 - Cancer." Accessed 4 Nov 2007. <http://www.discount-vitamins-herbs.net/n-105-cancer-cranberry.htm. © 2001-2007, Discount Herbs & Vitamins, Inc.

23. "Apple Juice May Help Keep Colon Cancer At Bay." By ANI. From OneIndia™ website, online posting. Accessed 29 Jun. 2008. <http://living.oneindia.in/health/wellbeing/2008/apple-juice-colon-cancer-treatment-280308.html>. © Greynium Information Technologies Pvt. Ltd.

24. "Artemisinin." Alternative Cancer Therapies. Online posting. Updated 5/5/07. Wellness Directory of Minnesota. Accessed 8 Nov. 2007. <http://www.mnwelldir.org/docs/cancer/alt thrpy.Htm#Artemisinin>. from Dr. Lam, M.D. at website <http://www.drlam.com/A3R _brief_ in_doc_ format/Artemisinin.cfm>.

25. "Aspartame (Nutra-Sweet or Equal) Causes Cancer—Lymphoma, Leukemia." Health News Archive 263 - Cancer - Online Posting. Accessed 4 Nov. 2007. From Discount Vitamins & Herbs website <http://www.discount-vitamins-herbs.net/n-263-cancer-aspartame.htm>. © 2001 - 2007, Discount Herbs & Vitamins, Inc.

26. "Ashwagandha." From herbs2000.com. Online posting. Accessed 27 Dec. 2007. <http://herbs2000.com/herbs/herbs_ashwagandha.htm>. © 2002-2008 herbs2000.com.

27. "Aspilia." Online posting. Accessed 8 Nov. 2007. <http://www.herbs2000.com/herb/herbs _aspilia.htm> © 2004-2007 herbs2000.com.

28. "Autumn Crocus." Online posting. Accessed 8 Nov. 2007. <http://www.herbs2000.com/herbs/herbs_autumn_crocus.htm> © 2002-2007 herbs2000.com.

29. "Avanex 7-1037 Demonstrates Chemotherapeutic Potential Without Toxic Side Effects for the Treatment of Colorectal Cancer, Other Types of Solid Tumors." Online posting. Press release from Geneva, Switzerland 01/16/08 (PR.com) from Avanex Life Sciences Corp. See their website at www.avanex.com. Accessed 16 Jan. 2008. <http://www.pr.com/press-release/678 28>.

30. "Beating Ovarian Cancer at 80 with RM-10." Interview with Rose Menlowe. "Jordan Rubin's Grandmother from Garden of Life." "Rose Menlowe cured of ovarian cancer with Jordan Rubin RM 10." Online posting. Accessed 23 Jun. 2008. <http://www.crohns.net/Miva/education /testimonial_rosemenlowe.shtml>.

31. "Beres Drops." Online posting. Accessed 8 Nov. 2007. Cancer Tutor website. Alternative Cancer Treatment Information Center™ - Over 200 Alternative Cancer Treatments Plus Other Information. Accessed 23 Jul 2008. <http://www.cancer tutor.com/Other/Big_List. htm>.

32. "Berry Young Juice Advantages." Online posting. Accessed 8 Nov. 2007 <http://www.aroma-essence.com/catalog/berry-young-juice.htm. © 1996-2006 World Direct™ and its licensors.

33. "Beta-Sitosterol." Online posting. Accessed 8 Nov. 2007. <http://www.drlam.com/opinion/beta_sitosterol.cfm>. © Copyright 2001-2004 by Michael Lam, M.D.

34. "Billion Dollar Drug Company Nearly Squashes Astounding Research On Natural Cancer Killer," "Natural Cancer Killer." Online posting. (H.S.I.) Health Sciences Institute, Members Alert for January. 2001, Vol. 5, No. 7. Accessed 8 Nov. 2007. <http://www.hisbaltimore.com/articles/his_2001ds/his_200101_awb9.html. Copyright © 1997-2007 by Institute of Health Sciences, L.L.C.

34a. "BioCancell. Cancer Therapy Breakthrough." Online posting from BioCancell Therapeutics, Inc. Accessed 03 Aug. 2008. <http://www.biocancell.com>. © BioCancell Therapeutics, Inc.

35. "Bioenergy RIBOSE™ and Your Blood Sugar." Online posting from Nutra Bio.com® website. Accessed 01 Jan. 2008. <http://www.nutrabio.com/Products/ribose_blood_sugar.htm>. © 2007 NutraBio.com., Inc. Also see their article "Research: Benefit of Ribose in a Patient With Fibromyalgia," from 01-31-2005 Journal Pharmacotherapy. Benjamin Gebhart, Pharm.D., James A. Jorgenson, M.S., FASHP. <http://www.nutrabio.com/Products/ribose_fibromyalgia_research.htm>. Copyright © 2007 NutraBio.com, Inc. as well as the article: "Unique Sugar Improves Energy, Pain and Quality of Life in Fibromyalgia and Chronic Fatigue Patients!" "New Study on D-ribose published *in Journal of Alternative and Complementary Medicine.*" Minneapolis, MN. From Nov. 13, 2006. See website: <http://bioenergy.com/Papers/Expo%20WestPress%20release%20JACM.pdf>, from NutraBio.com website © 2007 NutraBio.com, Inc.

36. "Bladder Cancer." Online posting. Accessed 8 Nov. 2007. <http://www.herbs2000.com/disorders/cancer_bladder.htm>. © 2002-2007 herbs2000.com.

37. "Blueberries Contain Chemical That May Help Prevent Colon Cancer." From American Chemical Society (2007, March 26). *ScienceDaily*. Retrieved July 8, 2008, from <http://www.sciencedaily.com/releases/2007/03/070325111552.htm>. Online posting from Science Daily website. Also related article: "Blueberry Compound Shows Promise of Lowering Cholesterol as Effective as Drug" (from Aug. 31, 2004) © 1995-2008 ScienceDaily LLC.

38. "Blueberries Stop Liver Cancer Growth." Wed Jun. 7, 2006. Online posting. Accessed 8 Nov. 2007. <http://www.discount-vitamins-herbs.net/n-311-liver-cancer-blueberry.htm>. © 2001 - 2007 Discount Herbs & Vitamins, Inc.

39. "Blue Light Used To Harden Tooth Fillings Stunts Tumor Growth." Medical College of Georgia (2008, June 28). *ScienceDaily*. Retrieved July 8, 2008, from http://www.sciencedaily.com/releases/2008/06/080624110831.htm. © 1995-2008 ScienceDaily, LLC.

40. "Bone Cancer - Another Flax Cure." Online posting. Accessed 8 Nov. 2007. <http:// www.curezone.com/diseases/cancer/testimonials/Bone-cancer_another_flax_cure.asp>. Copyright © 1996 - 2005 Curezone.com.

41. "Bone Cancer." Online posting. Accessed 8 Nov 2007. <http://www.herbs2000.com/disorders/cancer_bone.htm>. © 2002-2007 herbs2000.com.

42. "Bone Marrow and Stem Cell Transplants." Online posting. Accessed 8 Nov 2007. <http://www.cancerindex.org/ccw/guide2bm.htm>. Page last updated 11 Jan. 2003.

43. "Borage Oil – Borage Oil, Essential Fatty Acids And Gamma Linolenic Acid, GLA." Online posting from Dr. Vikrama's friendly holistic herbalist website. Accessed 24 Jul 2008. <http://www.holistic-herbalist.com/borage-oil-1.html>. Dr. Vikrama © www.holistic-herbalist.com2005.

44. "Brain Stem Gliomas." Online posting. Accessed 8 Nov. 2007. <http://www.braintumor.org/PediatricFAQ/#q3565>. Also see website <http://www.braintumor.org/GlobalSearch>. © 2007 National Brain Tumor Foundation.

45. "Brazilian Peppertree." Raintree Nutrition's Tropical Plant Database. Online posting. Accessed 8 Nov. 2007. Their page updated 15 Jan. 2007. <http://www.rain-tree.com/pepper tree.htm>. This information is also found in Leslie Taylor's book, *The Healing Power of Rainforest Herbs*, Square One Publishers, Jan 2005. © Copyrighted 1996 to present by Raintree Nutrition, Inc., Carson City, NV 89701.

46. "Breast Cancer – healing with herbs, vitamins and minerals." Online posting. Accessed 8 Nov. 2007. <http://www.herbs2000.com/disorders/cancer_breast.htm>. © 2002-2007 herbs2000.com.

47. "Breuss Total Cancer Treatment." Online posting. Accessed 8 Nov, 2007. Alternative Cancer Treatment Information Center™. <http://www.cancertutor.com/Cancer/Breuss.html>.

48. "Broccoli and tomatoes prevent prostate cancer better than leading prescription drugs, research shows." Online posting. Accessed 8 Nov. 2007. <http://www.newstargetcom/ 001391.html>. News Target Network – Information That Empowers™. News Target Network © 2004, 2005, 2006, 2007.

49. "Broccoli sprouts cut bladder cancer risk by half. From CHINESE MEDICINE NEWS online posting. A "CM NEWS, American Association for Cancer Research release," 02/28/2008. Accessed 24 Jul. 2008. <http://chinesemedicinenews.com/2008/02/28/broccoli-sprouts-cut-bladder-cancer-risk-by-half>. © 2007-2008 CHINESE MEDICINE NEWS.

50. "Bupleurum." Online posting. Accessed 8 Nov. 2007. <http://www.herbs2000.com/herbs/herbs_bupleurum.htm>. © 2002-2007 herbs2000.com.

51. "Burzynski Patient Group." "Crystin S." Online posting. Accessed 8 Nov 2007. <http://burzynskipatientgroup.org/cyrstins.htm>.

52. "Burzynski Patient Group." "Dustin K." Online posting. Accessed 8 Nov. 2007. <http://www.burzynskipatientgroup.org/dustink.htm>.

53. "Burzynski Patient Group." "Jodi G." Online posting. Accessed 8 Nov. 2007. <http://www.burzynskipatientgroup.org/jodig.htm>.

53a. "Burzynski Patient Group." "Roy H." Online posting. Accessed 8 Nov. 2007. <http://www.burzynskipatientgroup.org/roy_hash.htm>.

53b. "Burzynski Patient Group." "Sophia G." Online posting. Accessed 8 Nov. 2007. <http://burzynskipatientgroup.org/sophiag.htm>.

54. "Butcher's Broom." Online posting. Accessed 8 Nov. 2007. <http://www.herbs2000.com/herbs/herbs_butchers_broom.htm>. © 2002-2007 herbs2000.com.

55. "Cancer: Can food prevent cancer?" Reported by Fiona Macdonald-Smith from telegraph.co.uk, updated Jun 16, 2008. Online posting. Accessed 22 Jun. 2008. <http://www.telegraph.co.uk/health/main.jhtml?xml=/health/2008/06/16/hcancer116.xml>. © Telegraph Media Group Limited 2008.

56. "Cancer-fighting herbs." "Schisandra." Online posting. Accessed 23 Oct 2007. <http://www.namastestu.addr.com/page2.html>. As seen on The Golden Almond Natural Food Store website. Wholesome Directions, Inc.

57. "Cancer-fighting Foods/Spices." "Rosemary." Online posting. Accessed 20 Oct. 2007. <http://thecancerfreekitchen.tripod.com/id6.html.

58. "Cancer Adjuvant Therapy." "Health Concerns." Online posting. Accessed 9 Nov. 2007. <http://www.lef.org/protocols/prtcl-027b.html>. (Also see the LEF Protocol Book) p. 3. Life Extension Foundation.

59. "Cancer Adjuvant Therapy." Cancer Adjuvant Treatment. Online Reference for Health Concerns. Online posting. Accessed 9 Nov. 2007. (Also see the LEF Protocol Book) <http://www.lef.org/protocols/prtcl-027b.shtml>. Life Extension Foundation.

60. "Cancer and Immunity." Online posting. "Immune Building Agents." "Olive Leaf." An Insider's Guide to Natural Medicine. Accessed 9 Nov. 2007. <http:/www.drlam.com/A3R_brief_in_doc_format/cancer_and_immunity.cfm#2-2>. © 2001-2004 by Michael Lam, M.D.

61. "Cancer-Fighter Perillyl Alcohol Found in Tart Cherries." Online posting. Accessed 9 Nov. 2007. <http://www.fruitinstitute.org/cherry_health3.htm>. Copyright © 2005 Fruitinstitute.org, Inc.

62. "Cancer-fighting Foods and Spices." The Cancer Cure Foundation. Online posting. Accessed 27 Dec. 2007. <http://cancure.org/cancer_fighting_foods.htm>.

63. "Cancer Issues: New Non-Invasive Cancer Treatments." Online posting. Accessed 21 Oct. 2007. See article at HealthNewsDigest.com from 3/27/06. <http://www.hifu. ca/news/cancer-issues.php>.

64. "Cancer Killer Found In The Ocean." "Marine Biotechnologists Treat Cancer With Mud-loving Ocean Bacteria." Note that this story and the video were made for the American Institute of Physics series by Ivanhoe Broadcast News. Online posting Nov. 1, 2007 from ScienceDaily website. Accessed 01 July 2008. <http://www.sciencedaily.com/videos/2007/1107-cancer_killer_found_in_the_ocean.htm>. Copyright © 1995-2008 ScienceDaily LLC.

65. "Canelim Capsule." "Product Direction." Online posting. Accessed 16 Jan. 2008. TraditionalChineseMedicine.HongKong. FuQiZheng–Alternative Cancer TCM. <http://www.tcm.hk/index.cfm?fuseaction=browse&id=158407&pageid=98.

66. "Carigent Awarded NSF Phase I SBIR to Develop Targeted Nanoparticle Ovarian Cancer Therapeutic." Article Preview is from the "PharmaLive.com News Archive" 01-22-2008. Online posting at "TherapeuticsDaily©. Accessed 22 Jan. 2008. <http://www.therapeuticsdaily.com/news/article.cfm?contenttype=newsarchive&contentValue=507714&contentType=newsarchive&channelID-28>. © 2005 PharmaLive.com.

67. "Cat's Claw." Online posting. Accessed 10 Nov. 2007 <http://www.herbs2000.com/herbs/herbs_cats_claw.htm>. © 2002-2007 herbs2000.com.

68. "Caveats: Conflicting Reports on Vitamins and Minerals." Jane Russell's Health Facts. "Vitamins – Anti-oxidants: Beta-carotene and Vitamins A and E." Online posting. Accessed 10 Nov. 2007. <http://www.jrussellshealth.org/caveats_vit_min.html>.

69. "Cayenne Pepper." Alternative Cancer Therapies. Online posting. Wellness Directory of Minnesota™. Accessed 10 Nov. 2007. <http://mnwelldir.org/docs/cancer1/alt thrpy.htm>. Site updated 05/05/07. Copyright © 1995, 1998-2004 International Wellness Directory.

69a. CellQuest™ Dietary Supplement. Online information. Accessed 5 Sept. 2008. See website: <http://www.mypracticemarketer.com/ProductsCellQuest.pdf>.

70. "Cervical Cancer." Online posting. Accessed 10 Nov. 2007. <http://www.herbs2000.com/disorders/cancer_cervical.htm>. © 2002-2007 herbs2000.

71. "Cesium Chloride Alternative Cancer Treatment Comparison." Online posting. Accessed 13 Jan. 2008. http://www.alternativecancer.us/cesiumchloride.htm

72. “Chaparral.” www.curezone.com’s excerpt from the book: Alternatives in Cancer Therapy by Ross, Pelton, R. Ph., Lee Overholser. AlternativesInCancerTherapy3.htm. Online posting. Accessed 10 Nov. 2007. <http://www.curezone.com/diseases/cancer/chaparral.asp>.

72a. “Chemo Pill Shows Promise for Advanced Lymphoma, Leukemia.” 8 Dec. 2008 by Insciences. Online posting, accessed 30 Dec. 2008. <http://insciences.org/article.php?article_id=570> from the University of Rochester Medical Center.

73. “Chemotherapy: A Dull Weapon! Kyle Slavik A Success Story,” Jun. 1995 from website article “Cancer & Biopsy—OPTIONS—Revolutionary Ideas on the War on Cancer.” Online posting. Accessed 10 Nov. 2007. <http://www.karlloren.com/biopsy/p60.htm>.

74. “Chicory Root.” Over 200 Alternative Cancer Treatments Information Center™ Cancer Tutor website. Online posting. Accessed 10 Nov. 2007. <http://www.cancertutor.com/Other/Big_List.htm>.

75. “Chinese asparagus.” Earthnotes Herb Library. Online posting. Accessed 10 Nov. 2007 <http://earthnotes.tripod.com/asparagus.htm>. © 2000 by Ernestina Parziale CH.

75a. “Chinese salad may harbor cancer cure.” Online posting Oct. 22, 2008. Accessed 14 Dec. 2008. <http://www.entertainmentandshowiz.com/chinese-salad-may-harbour-cancer-cure-200810223789>. © 2008-09 entertainmentandshowbiz.com.

76. “Chlorophyll and Cancer Prevention.” From an online posting 06/28/2008 at cancer solutions.org website. Accessed 29 Jun. 2008. <http://www.cancersolutions.org/2008/06/chlorophyll-and-cancer-prevention.html>.

76a. “Cholesterol Drug Plays Role in Melanoma Remission.” From www.medilexicon.com. See NeoPlas Innovation site at http://www.neoplas.org. Accessed 04 Sept 2008. <http://www.medilexicon.com/medicalnews.php?newsid–11 8059>.

77. “Chronic Fatigue Immune Dysfunction Syndrome CFIDS”: “Original Trusted Molo Cure Formulation Since 1996.” Online posting. Accessed 10 Nov. 2007. This website by the “Founder, former Officer and Stock Holder of AMP MoloCure.” Name of new company is AMPFLORACEL™. See website: <http://ampfloracel.com/CFIDS_chronic_fatigue_immune_dysfunction_syndrome.html>. Copyright © AmpFloracel, 2007. Not affiliated with Digestinol®, Doctors Aloe®, AMP Molo®, SeroVera® or BuyAmpNow® - See website FDA disclaimer.

78. “Cilantro: A Common Spice/Herb That Can Save Your Life.” Online posting. Wellness Directory of Minnesota™. Accessed 10 Nov. 2007. <http://www.mnwell.dirorg/docs/detox/cilantro.htm> © 2004, 2005 International Wellness Directory.

79. “Clodronate.” Online posting. Cancer Tutor™, Alternative Cancer Treatment Information Center™. Accessed 23 Oct. 2007. <http://www.cancertutor.com/Other/Big_List.htm>.

80. “Coffee Intake Linked To Lower Diabetes Risk.” *JAMA* and Archives Journals (2006, June 28). *ScienceDaily*. Retrieved July 8, 2008, from http://www.sciencedaily.com/releases/2006/06/060628091738.htm. © 1995-2008 ScienceDaily, LLC.

81. “Coffee May Be Linked To Rheumatoid Arthritis.” Center For The Advancement Of Health (2000, July 27). *ScienceDaily*. Retrieved July 8, 2008 from http://www.sciencedaily.com/releases/2000/07/000727080902.htm © 1995-2008 ScienceDaily, LLC.

82. "Coffee May Protect Against Breast Cancer, Study Shows." Lund University (2008, April 25). *ScienceDaily.* Retrieved July 8, 2008 from http://www.sciencedaily.com/releases/2008/04/080424115324.htm. © 1995-2008 ScienceDaily, LLC.

82a. "Colon cancer: Now, a simple blood test to detect colon cancer." Online posting of Nov. 28, 2008. Accessed 14 Dec. 2008. <http://www.entertainmentandshowbiz.com/colon-cancer-now-a-simple-blood-test-to-detect-colon-cancer/200811286098>. © 2008-09 entertainmentandshowbiz .com.

83. "Colorectal Cancer." Online posting. Herbs2000.com. Accessed 7 Nov. 2007. <http://www.herbs2000.com/disorders/cancer_colorectal.htm>. © 2002–2007 herbs 2000.com.

84. "Colorectal Cancer." Online posting from 4uherb.com. Accessed 16 Jan. 2008. <http//www.4uherb.com/cancer/colorectal/treat.htm>. © 2002 FOYO Herb.

84a. "Combo Therapy Helps Multiple Myeloma Patients." "Three-quarters of those who had relapsed saw disease stabilize or improve, study shows." Online posting – report from study at the Mayo Clinic, news release, Dec. 9, 2008. Accessed or retrieved 14 Dec. 2008. Article at *HealthDay News* Friday Dec. 12. <http://www.healthfinder.gov/news/newsstory.aspx?docID= 622118>.

85. "Comparison of Glutathione in Fresh vs. Cooked Foods (in milligrams per 3 ½ oz. (100 gm serving)." Online posting. Accessed 10 Nov. 2007. <http://www.nutritionadvisor.com/glutathione_foods.php>. © Nutritionadvisor, Inc.

85a. "Compound from olive-skin pomace protects against colon cancer." Online posting Dec. 18, 2008. Accessed 25 Dec. 2008 at <http://www.news-medical.net/?id=44397>. © 2008 News-Medical.Net.

86. "Compound Identified In Grapes May Fight Cancer And Diabetes." American Chemical Society (2002, May 22). *ScienceDaily.* Retrieved July 8, 2008 from http://www.sciencedaily.com/releases/2002/05/020522073916.htm. © 1995-2008 ScienceDaily LLC.

87. "Congestive Heart Failure." "Co-enzyme Q10. This is Very Important." Online posting. Accessed 10 Nov. 2007. <http://www.doctoryourself.com/congestive.html>. © 2003 and prior years by Andrew W. Saul. From the book *Doctor Yourself*, available from Andrew Saul, 23 Greenridge Crescent, Hamlin, NY 14464 USA.

88. "Could Milk Be Causing Your Acne?" Online posting from CareFair.com. Accessed 06 Jun. 2008 <http://www.carefair.com/print_article.asp?id=4740&url=http%3A%2Fwww>. Copyright © 2006 - 2008 CareFair.com.

88a. "Cup of Black Tea Could Defend Against Anthrax Threat, Research Suggests." From an article at *ScienceDaily* 16 March 2008. Their information from Cardiff University. Online posting. Accessed 25 Dec. 2008. <http://www.sciencedaily.com/releases/2008/03/080312100045.ht m>. © 1995-2008 *ScienceDaily LLC.*

89. "Curcumin/Turmeric." Online posting. Cancer Tutor. Accessed 10 Nov. 2007. Alternative Cancer Treatments Information Center™. <http://www.cancertutor.com/Other/Big_List.htm>.

89a. "CyberKnife® Stereotactic Radiosurgery System – New Treatment Option for Patients with Tumors and Lesions of the Brain and Spine." Online posting. Accessed 8 Oct. 2008. <http://www.georgetownuniversityhospital.org/body.cfm?id=451>. © Georgetown University Hospital.89b. "Cyberknife – The non invasive radio surgery using robotic arm CybeKnive Center, Miami." "Miami cancer treatment center." 2008-04-01 from Caymanmama.com – Health News, online posting. Accessed 8 Oct. 2008. <http://www.caymanmama.com/2008/03/31/cancer-treatment-plan_200803311213.html>. Copyright © 2007 Caymanmamma.com.

90. "Cytotron the New No Side Effect Cancer Treatment." MEDINDIA. Online posting. Accessed 25 Oct. 2007. <http://digitalvillages.org/blogs/announcements/archive/2007/07/30/2758.aspx> at Digital Village Global Healthcare Perspectives website.

91. "Dairy Products Danger." "Study Links Dairy Products to Prostate Cancer." Online posting. Accessed 10 Nov. 2007 <http://jparisi.com/dairy_products.htm>.

91a. Daily Mail Reporter. "Red Grapes 'are wonder cure for high blood pressure and cholesterol'" Mail Online health. Last updated 20th Aug 2008. Online posting. Accessed 21 Aug 2008 <http://www.dailymail.co.uk/health/article-1047217/Red-grapes-wonder-cure-high-blood-pressure-cholesterol.html#>. © 2008 Associated Newspapers Ltd.

92. "DaVinci Robot Surgery for Gynecological and Urologic Cancers - Karmanos Leads the Way in Robotic Technology." Online posting. Accessed 19 Jan. 2008. <http://www.karmanos.org/app.asp?id=1116> © 2008 Karmanos Cancer Institute, Member of the Michigan Cancer Consortium. Their ph#1-800-527-6266.

93. "Dandelion Plant (herb–NOT just the root)." Online posting. Cancer Tutor. Accessed 10 Nov. 2007. <http://www.cancertutor.com/OtherBig_List.htm>. Alternative Cancer Treatments Information Center™.

94. "Detecting Breast Cancer Early." "Doctors Catch Cancer Earlier With Special MRI." This story and accompanying video were originally produced for the American Institute of Physics series by Ivanhoe Broadcast News. Online posting from an article at ScienceDaily Science Video website 01/01/2006. Accessed 02 Jul. 2008. Http://www.sciencedaily.com/videos/2006/0102-detecting_breast_cancer_early.htm>. © 1995-2008 ScienceDaily, LLC.

95. "DHEA protects against prostate cancer." Online posting. Accessed 31 Oct. 2007. <www.yourhealthbase.com/prostate_cancer.htm> © 1998-2007 Hans R. Larsen. ISSN 1203-1933.

96. "DIM (diindolylmethane)." Online posting. Cancer Tutor. Accessed 10 Nov. 2007. <http://www.cancertutor.com/OtherBig_List.htm>. From Alternative Cancer Treatments Information Center™.

97. "D-limonene," and "Perillyl Alcohol." Online posting. Cancer Tutor website. Accessed 10 November 2007. <http://www.cancertutor.com/Other/Big_List.htm>. Alternative Cancer Treatments Information Center™.

98. "Doctors Discover Lapacho." Online posting. Red-Purple Lapacho (also known as Pau D' Arco or Taheebo). Accessed 10 Nov. 2007. <http://www.oralchelation.com/taheebo/lapacho2.htm>. © December 21, 2006 6:42 PM by Karl Loren on behalf of Vibrant Life.

99. "Dr. Budwig's Diet & Cancer Healing Protocol," at website *Healing Cancer Naturally*. "Dr. Budwig's Protocol." The quote is from Dr. Johanna Budwig in *Flax Oil as a True Aid*. Online posting. Accessed 7 Nov. 2007. <http://www.healingcancernaturally.com/budwig_protocol.html>. © 2004, 2005, 2006 & 2007 www.healingcancernaturally.com.

100. "Dr. Budwig's Diet & Cancer Healing Protocol." at website Healing Cancer Naturally. Online posting 17 Jan. 2005. <http://www.healingcancernaturally.com/budwig_protocol.html> from Dr. Budwig in "Der Toddes Tumors, Band II." (The Death of the Tumor, Vol. II) transcribing an

interview broadcast by the Siddeutscher Rundfunk Stuttgart (South German Radio Station) on 11 Sept. 1967. © 2004, 2005, 2006 & 2007 www.healingcancernaturally.com.

101. "Dyer's Woad (Isatis Indigotica Fortune)." Online posting from Nutrition2000. Accessed 10 Nov. 2007. "Prostate Gland – Prostate Health – Prostate Problems – PC Hope Testimonies – Free Prostate Assessment." <http://www.nutrition2000.com/prostate_and_health/prostate-health-facts.asp>.

102. "Eat Cranberries—Reduce Ulcer Risk." 06/24/2008. Online posting. Accessed 27 Jun. 2008. <http://www.reddressdiary.blogspot.com">. Colette Bouchez On Health, Beauty, Style & Attitude for Fabulous Women Over 40!

102a. "Effective New Treatment Strategy for Retinoblastoma Avoids Removal of Eye and Radiation Therapy in Selected Patients." Also see *Journal of Clinical Oncology,* Vol 18, No 15 pp 2990-2995. Online posting from CancerConsultants.com. Retrieved 26 Aug 2008. <http://patient.cancerconsultants.com/CancerNews_Retinoblastoma.aspx?DocumentId=18692>. Copyright © 1998-2008 CancerConsultants.com.

103. "Effects of Estrogen Dominance." Diagnose-Me: Condition: Progesterone Low or Estrogen Dominance. Online posting. Accessed 10 Nov. 2007. Site last updated Oct. 26, 2007. <http://www.diagnose-me.com/cond/C8779.html>.

104. "Ellagic Acid." Online posting. Accessed 10 Nov. 2007. <http://www.cancerprevention.net>.

105. "Ellagic Acid." Online Posting. Wellness Directory of Minnesota™, Alternative Cancer Therapies. Site updated 05/05/07. The Information on H. Pylori is from Dr. Glen Halvorson's book, *Chemo-preventive Properties of Phytochemicals.* Accessed 10 Nov. 2007. <http://www.mnwelldir.org/docs/cancer1/altthrpy.htm.> © 1995, 1998 - 2004 International Wellness Directory.

106. "Emmanuel Revici." Online posting. Accessed 10 Nov. 2007. <http://www.cancertutor.com/Other/Big_List.htm>. Alternative Cancer Treatments Information Center™.

107. "Endometrial Cancer." Online posting. Accessed 10 Nov. 2007. <http://www.herbs2000.com/disorders/cancer_endometrial.htm>. © 2002-2007 herbs2000.com.

108. "Erlotinib (Tarceva®)." From the cancerbackup.org.uk website online posting. Accessed 30 Jan. 2008. <http://www.cancerbackup.org.uk/Treatments/Biologicaltherapies/Cancergrowthinhibitors/Erlotinib>.

109. "Espinheira Santa." Online posting. Accessed 10 Nov. 2007. <http://www.herbs2000.com/herbs/herbs_espinheirasanta.htm.> © 2002-2007 herbs2000.com.

110. "Essential Fatty Acids." "Well Being Abounds Volume Three Number One," by Birgette Necessary. Online posting. Accessed 10 Nov. 2007. <http://www.absolutelythepurest.com/other%20parts/essentialfattyacids.html>. © 2006 Thymely Solutions, Inc.

111. "Estrogen Information Summary." National Institute of Neurological Disorders and Stroke, "Estrogen." Online posting. Accessed 10 Nov. 2007. <http://www.nindsnih.gov/funding/research/parkinsonsweb/drug_summaries/estrogen.htm.>. Last updated Feb. 9, 2005.

112. "Ewing's sarcoma in children." CANCERBACUP Helping people live with cancer. Online posting. Accessed 10 Nov. 2007. <http://www.cancerbacup.org.nk/Cancertype/Childrenscan

cers/Typesofchildrenscancers/Ewingssarcoma>. © Cancer BACUP 2003. Page last modified Oct. 18, 2007.

112a. "Extracts From Reishi Mushroom And Green Tea Shows Synergestic Effect To Slow Sarcoma." Federation of American Societies for Experimental Biology. Online posting from *ScienceDaily*, 14 April 2008, who adapted their article from the information provided by Federation of America Societies for Experimental Biology, via *EurekaAlert*, a service of AAS. Accessed or retrieved 25 Dec. 2008. <http://www.sciencedaily.com/releases/2008/04/08040 8175308.htm>. © 1995-2008 *ScienceDaily LLC*

113. "Far Infrared Hyperthermia Treatment." From the Issels Medical Center website. Online posting. Accessed 26 Dec. 2007. <http://www.isselsmedicalcenter.com/therapies/firthermal .aspx>. © 2005-2007 Issels Treatment.

114. "First Human Use Study Of Third Eye Retroscope ™ Underway – Suggests That New Device May Improve Detection of Colon Cancer." 11 Oct. 2006. Online posting from Medicalnewstoday.com. Accessed 21 Jul. 2008. <http://www.medicalnewstoday.com/articles /53780.php>. © 2008 MediLexicon Int'l., Ltd.

115. "FIT Testing Detects Colorectal Cancer Earlier." Online posting from emax health.com. Accessed 22 Jun. 2008. <http://www.emaxhealth.com/100/22493.html>. © 2004-2008 eMax Health.com. Hareyan Publishing LLC does not provide medical advice.

116. "Flax seed Protects Against Breast Cancer." Online posting. Accessed 2 Nov. 2007. <http:/ /www.Discount-Vitamins-herbs.net/health-news21.htm." Copyright © 2001—2007 Discount Herbs & Vitamins, Inc.

117. "Food as Medicine: Protective Foods Other Phytochemicals. How Other Phytochemicals Help Protect Against Cancer." Online posting. The Cancer Project. 12 Nov. 2007. <http:// www.cancerproject.org/protective foods/phytochemicals.php>.

117a. FOODNEWS from ENVIRONMENTAL WORKING GROUP - foodnews.org. Online posting - shows ranking of 43 fruits and vegetables in order of those having highest pesticide load (non-organic foods). Accessed 16 Aug 2008. <http://www.food news.org>.

118. "Food sources of Lysine." From the "Lysine Amino Acid Information page." Zest for Life® Specialized Vitamin Supplements webpage. Online posting. Accessed 12 Nov. 2007. <http://www.anyvitamins.com/lysine-info.htm>. © Salamander Concepts 1998–2007. Site last updated November 11, 2007.

119. "Foods that Harm, Foods That Heal – Tasty Ways to Keep the Doctor Away." Reader's Digest, from the book, April 2004. The book itself was published (1st edition) in Mar. 2004.

120. "Fruits, Vegetables, Teas May Protect Smokers From Lung Cancer." Online posting from UCLA Healthcare Jun 09, 2008. Website: emaxhealth.com. Accessed 21 Jul. 2008. <http://www. emaxhealth.com/58/22898.htm>.

121. "Gamma-Linolenic Acid Cuts Levels of Breast Cancer-Causing Gene." From the Health News Archive 138 – Breast Cancer online posting at website http://www.discount-vitamins-herbs.net. Accessed 8 Dec. 2007. © 2001-2007 Discount Herbs & Vitamins, Inc. Source given as Javier A. Menendez, Luciano Vellon, Ramon Colomer, Ruth Lupu. "Effect of Gamma-Linolenic Acid on the Transcriptional Activity of the Her-2/neu (erbB-2) Oncogene." *Journal of the National Cancer Institute*, Vol 97, No. 21, 1611-1615, Nov. 2, 2005.

121a. "Gene therapy ups survival in end-stage head & neck cancer." Boston. Online posting from consultantlive.com. Accessed 26 Aug 2008. <http://www.consultantlive.com/otorhinolaryngologic-diseases/article/10165/1165449#>. © 1996–2008 CMP Medica LLC, a United Business Media Company.

122. "Geraniol." Online posting. "Health conditions starting with C and herbal remedies used to treat them." Accessed 12 Nov. 2007. <http://www.earthnotes.tripod.com/ckbk_c.htm>. Site updated 16 Oct. 2007. © 1998-2007 by Ernestina Parziale, CH.

123. "Ginger Compound Prevents Growth of Colorectal Cancer Cells." Online posting. Accessed 2 Nov. 2007. <http://www.discount-vitamins-herbs.net/health-news17.htm>. © 2001-2007 Discount Vitamins, Inc.

124. "Ginger root can treat ovarian cancer." 26 Jan. 2008 article from Press TV. Accessed 26 Jan. 2008. <http://www.presstv.ir/detail.aspx?id=40449&sectionid=3510210>. © Press TV 2007.

125. "Ginkgo Slows Breast Cancer Growth 80%." Online posting. Accessed 4 Nov. 2007. Their source is given as: Anti-cancer Research, Jan – Feb. 2006. <http://www.discount-vitamins-herbs.net/n-242-breast-cancer-ginkgo.htm. © 2001-2007 Discount Vitamins, Inc.

126. "Ginseng and Cancer: A follow-up." Perspectives Research and Creative Activities, Spring 2004, Southern Illinois University Carbondale. Online posting. Accessed 12 Nov. 2007. <http://www.siu.edu/~perspect/04_sp/ginseng.html>. Copyright © 2004, Board of Trustees, Southern Illinois University.

127. "Glandulars." Cancer Tutor, Alternative Cancer Treatment Information Center™. Accessed 12 Nov. 2007. <http://www.cancertutor.com?Other/Big_List.htm>.

128. "Good Vibrations." From website Israel21c.org 06/29/03 HEALTH article, published by the American Assoc. for Cancer Research. Based on the research by Prof. Yona Keisari & assoc. Online posting. Accessed 13 Jun. 2008. <http://www.israel21c.org/bin/en.jsp?enPage=BlankPage&enDisplay=view&enDispWhat=object&enDispWho=Articles%5E1441&enZone=Health>.

129. "Grape Juice Inhibits Breast Cancer Cell Growth in Animal Study." From Health News Archive 21 – Breast Cancer. Online posting. Accessed 2 Nov 2007. <http://www.discount-vitamins-herbs.net/health-news21.htm#127>. © 2001–2007 Discount Herbs & Vitamins, Inc.

130. "Grape Vitis Vinifera." Online posting. Accessed 12 Nov. 2007. <http://www.herbs2000.com/herbs/_grape.htm>. © 2002-2007 herbs2000.com.

131. "Grape." Online posting. Accessed 12 Nov. 2007. <http://www.herbs2000.comherbs/herbs_grape.htm>. © 2002-2007 herbs2000.com.

132. "Grapes Inhibit Cancer Growth." Online posting from CNN interactive, Jan 10, 1997. Accessed 12 Nov. 2007. <http://www.cnn.com/HEALTH/9701/10/grapes.Cancer/index.html>. © 1997 Cable News Network, Inc.

133. "Graviola." Online posting. Alternative Cancer Therapies. Accessed 7 Nov. 2007. <http://www.mnwelldir.org/docs/cancer1/altthrpy2.htm#Graviola>. From the International Wellness Directory. © Copyright 2006 Minnesota Wellness Publications, Inc.

134. "Green Tea Compound Blocks Bladder Tumors in Rats." Online posting. Accessed 2 Nov. 2007. <http://www.discount-vitamins-herbs.net/health-news5.htm>. © 2001 – 2007 Discount Herbs & Vitamins, Inc.

135. "Green Tea Found to Fight More Kinds of Cancer." Online posting from an article "cancer treatment" 12-31-2007. Accessed 19 Jan. 2008. <http://health-cancertreatment.blogspot.com /search?q=green+tea>.

136. "Green tea may cut the risk of gastric cancer in women." Research Update article #2 online posting at *swansonvitamins.com* website. From Cancer Epidemiology, Biomarkers & Prevention 17(2):343-351, 2008. Accessed 29 Mar. 2008. <http://video.swansonvitamins.com/c_files/ResearchUpdate/080327_Rua2.html>.

137. "Green Tea." "Saving Your Skin with Green Tea." Golden Moon Tea Nov. 9, 2006. Online posting. Accessed 12 Nov. 2007. <http://www.goldenmoontea.com/Articles/Articleage.aspx?pageId=369>. © 2001-2006 Papugai, Inn.

138. "Green Tea Fights Killer Disease." Online posting. FoodNavigator.com, News Headlines—Science & Nutrition, 2/4/2004. Accessed 12 Nov. 2007. <http://www.foodnavigator.com/news/news-NG.asp?id=51104>. © 2000/2007 - Decision News Media SAS.

139. "Green Tea Supports Ovarian Health." Online posting. Accessed 4 Oct. 2007. From Larsson SC, Wolk A. "Tea consumption and ovarian cancer risk in a population-based cohort." Arch Intern. Med 2005 Dec. 12-26;165(22)2683-6. <http://www.Discount-vitamins-herbs.net/n-143-ovarian-cancer_green-tea.htm>.

140. "Grocery warning: curry sauces contain dangerous levels of food coloring chemicals." News Target Network, News and Commentary on Today's Top Stories. Monday, Jan. 23, 2005 commentary. Online posting. Accessed 12 Nov. 2007. <http://www.newstarget.com/001027.html>. Information That Empowers™. News Target Network © 2004, 2005, 2006, 2007.

141. "Guacatonga." Raintree Nutrition's Tropical Plant Database. Online posting. Accessed 12 Nov. 2007. <http://www.rain-tree.com/guacatonga.htm>. Site updated 1-17-2007. Copyright © 1996 to present by Raintree Nutrition, Inc., Carson City, NV 89701. This information is also found in Leslie Taylor's book, *The Healing Power of Rainforest Herbs*, Square One Publishers, Jan. 2005.

142. "Gymnema Sylvestre for Diabetes." Brain Wave Entrainment Technology. Online posting. Accessed 27 Dec. 2007. <http://www.intelegen.com/nutrients/gymnema_sylvestre_for_diabetes.htm>. © Vitamin Research Products, Inc. 2001.

143. Haelan Products, Inc. See their website at: http://www.haelan951.com, and haelanresearch foundation.com. They make no medical claims on their products. © 2008 Haelan Products, Inc.

144. "Harkach Kanta to fight liver cancer?" Jan. 17, 2008. Online posting at oneindia™. Accessed 24 Jul. 2008. <http://news.oneindia.in/2008/01/17/medicinal-plant-acanthus-harbou r-liver-cancer-cure-1200553320.html>. © Greynium Information Technologies, Pvt. Ltd.

145. "Harvard Researchers Link Vitamin D Levels to Colon Cancer Survival." GEN News Highlights online posting Jun 19, 2008. Accessed 21 Jun. 2008. <http://www.genengnews.com/news/bnitem.aspx?name=37488385>. © 2008 GeneticEngineering & Biotechnology News.

145a. "Has a cancer killer been discovered?" From NatusVita website online posting. Accessed 03 Apr. 2008. <http://www.raax11.net/products.htm>. Copyright © A.D. Ser. Prov. Int. Ltda.

146. "Headway on Natural Chemotherapy for Prostate Cancer." News Headlines Research, 20/04/2004, "Natural Treatments for Prostate Cancer are Fast Gaining Scientific Evidence for

their efficacy in human patients." Online posting. Accessed 12 Nov 2007. <http://www.nutraingredients.com/news/news-NG.asp?id=51500>. © 2001/2007 – Decision News Media SAS

147. "Healing Colon Cancer with RAW Food: A personal account." Online Posting. Holistic Health: Testimonials of Amazing Health Recovery. Accessed 04 Nov. 2007. <http://www.shirleys-wellness-café.com/cancer.htm>. © 1996 – 2007.

148. *Healing With Vitamins,* by the Editors of Prevention Health Books (City, State, not given), Rodale, Inc. 1996.

149. "Healing Your Body with the Gerson Therapy." Online posting from GERSON Institute "Alternative Cancer Treatment" website. Accessed 28 Jul 2008. <http://www.gerson.org/g_therapy/default.asp>. © 1992-2003 Gerson Institute. Location: Gerson Institute/Cancer Curing Society – 1572 Second Avenue, San Diego, CA 92101. (619) 685-5363. Fax (619) 685-5363. U.S. only #888-443-7766. U.S. and Canada #800-838-2256.

149a. "Health Alert: Cancer treatment with Vitamin C." Posted & Updated Aug 29, 2008. Online posting. Accessed 04 Sep 2008. Wistv.com. <http://www.wistv.com/Global/story.asp?S=8922907&nav=menu36_8>. Copyright © 2000-2008 WorldNow and WISTV, a Raycom Media Station.

149b. "Heimlich Uses Malaria to Treat Cancer, Philadelphia Daily News 2-29-88," online posting. Accessed 19 Sept 2008. <http://www.scribd.com/doc/2057316/Heimlich-Uses-Malaria-to-Treat-Cancer-Philadelphia-Daily-News-22988> © 1988, Philadelphia Daily News. Also, see website: <http://www.scribd.com/doc/2199011/11794-Heimlich-Using-Malaria-to-Treat-AIDS-Patients-Cincinnati-Post>. © 1994, The Cincinnati Post.

150. "Herbal Extract Inhibits Angiogenesis." Online posting at springboard4health.com/Notebook/health_bindweed.html. Accessed 13 Jan. 2008. Also see "Letter From A Patient" Nov. 24, 2000. <http://www.springboard4health.com/store/more_arg_bindweed.htmlandwww.springboard4health.com/Notebook/health_bindweed.html>. Copyright © 1998-2007 Springboard. (Also, see bibliography #301a.)

151. "Herbal Remedies for Immunity." CancerHolisticonline.com. Online posting. Accessed 20 Oct. 2007. <http://www.holisticonline.com/cancer_lapacho_herb-rem.htm>. Copyright © 2007 – 2008 ICBS, Inc.

152. "Herbs & Supplements." "Milk Thistle." See under "Dosage and Administration." Online posting from Express Scrips website (updated 16 Oct. 2007). Accessed 03 Jul. 2008. <http://www.drugdigest.org/DD/DVH/HerbsTake/0,3927,551935%7CMilk%2BThistle,00.html>. © 2008 Express Scripts, Inc.

153. "High dietary boron linked to reduced risk for prostate cancer." From Reuters Health Information. Available: <http://www.oncolinkcom/resources/article.cfm?c=3&s=8&ss=23&id=1188&month=04&year=2001>. Oncolink Cancer News Accessed 12 Nov. 2007. Copyright © 2007 Reuters Limited. Reuters shall not be liable for any errors or delays in the content, or for any actions taken in reliance thereon.

154. "Highly Active Compound Found In Coffee May Prevent Colon Cancer." American Chemical Society (2003, October 15). *ScienceDaily.* Retrieved July 8, 2008, from http://www.sciencedaily.com/releases/2003/10/031015031251.htm>. Copyright © 1995-2008 ScienceDaily, LLC.

155. “Hodgkin Lymphoma and Non-Hodgkin Lymphoma.” Cancer Types, Classification. Online posting. Accessed 28 Dec. 2004. <http://www.cancer-healing.com/cancer_type.php>. Copyright 2004-2007 © Life Enthusiast Co-op.

156. “Hoelen.” Online posting. Accessed 12 Nov. 2007. <http://www.herbs2000.com/herbs/herbs_ hoelen.htm>. © 2002-2007 herbs2000.com.

157. “Horseradish.” Online posting. Herbs2000.com. Accessed 12 Nov. 2007. <http://www.herbs2000.com/herbs/herbs_horseradish.htm>. © 2002-2007 Herbs2000. com.

158. “How Shark Cartilage Works…” see new article “Shark Cartilage Report.” Online posting. Accessed 23 Oct. 2007. <http://www.nutritionfarm.com/GLOSSARY/REPORTS/sharkrept.php>. © 1996-2006, The Nutrition Farm®.

159. “How The Brain Can Protect Against Cancer.” Rutgers University (2008, June 10). *ScienceDaily*. Retrieved July 8, 2008, from <http://www.sciencedaily.com/releases/2008/06/080609171202.htm>. © 1995-2008 ScienceDaily, LLC.

160. “Hoxsey Formula.” Wellness Directory of Minnesota™. Alternative Cancer Therapies. Online posting. Accessed 12 Nov. 2007. <http://www.mnwelldir.org/docs/cancer1/altthrpy 2.htm>. Copyright © 1995, 1998, 1999, 2000, 2001, 2002, 2003, 2004, 2005, 2006 International Wellness Directory.

161. “HRT Comes With Serious Risks and Side Effects.” Online posting. Accessed 12 Nov. 2007. <http://www.safemenopausesolutions.com/hrt.html>. © Personal Wellness Network, Inc. FDA disclaimer.

162. “HSI Members Battle Prostate Cancer with Herbal Complex From the Amazon.” Health Archives. The Health Sciences Institute. 2/1/2002. Online posting. Accessed 13 Nov. 2007. <http://www.hsibaltiore.com/articles/his_2002wh/his_200202_cv4j.html>. Copyright © 1997 2007 by Institute of Health Sciences, L.L.C.

163. "Improved prognosis of postoperative liver cancer patients when treated with AHCC." From Health News Archive 62 – Cancer and AHCC Research at website http://www.discount-vitamins-herbs.net online posting. Accessed 8 Dec. 2007. Reported in the *Journal of Hepatology*, vol 37/1, pp 78-86, July 2002. Also, see website: <http://www.discount-vitamins-herbs.net/health-news62.htm>. © 2001-2007 Discount Herbs & Vitamins, Inc.

163a. “IMRT Reduces Side Effects in Pediatric Patients.” Online posting from Sloan-Kettering website. Accessed 12 Dec. 2007. <http://www.mskcc.org/mskcc/html/8442.cfm>. © 2007 Memorial Sloan-Kettering Cancer Center. (ph# 212-639-2000) located at 1275 York Avenue, New York, N.Y. 10065.

164. “Intravesical Immunotherapy.” “Information Resources > Cancers > Intravesical Immunotherapy. Online posting. Accessed 30 Nov. 2007. <http://www.nuhospitals.com/inimmunotherapy.php>. © 2007 NU Hospitals.

165. “Insulin-induced Hypoglycemic Therapy (IHT).” Online posting. Accessed 13 Nov. “Over 200 Alternative Cancer Treatments Plus Other Information.” <http://www.cancertutor.com/Other/Big_List.htm>.

165a. “IntraOp Mobetron.” Online posting from intraopmedical.com. Accessed 04 Sept 2008. <http://www.intraopmedical.com/?q=node/4>. © Copyright 2000-2007 Intraop Medical Corp.

166. "Intravenous Therapy" "ORTHO-IMMUNE." Online posting, accessed 20 Jan. 2008. <htt p:www.alternative-doctor.com/cancer/ca_advanced.htm>. © 2003 Keith Scott-Mumby.

167. "IPT Fact sheet." Online posting. Accessed 13 Nov. 2007. <http://iptq.com/fact _sheet.htm>. Entire IPTQ website Copyright © 1999-2002 by Chris Duffield, Ph.D.

168. "Israeli clinical trials help new breast cancer drug Tykerb win FDA approval." By ISRAEL 2 1c staff March 11, 2007. Online posting. From ISRAEL21c–A Focus Beyond website. Accessed 13 June 2008. <http://www.israel21c.org/bin/en.jsp?enDispWho=Articles%5El1584&enPage= BlankPage&enDisplay=view&enDispWhat=object&enVersion=0&enZone=Health>. © 2001 — 2007 ISRAEL21c.

169. "Israeli Science – Green Tea Is Good For the Brain?" Oct 16, 2007. From an online posting accessed 13 Nov. 2007. "Kosher News About Israeli Jews." <http://www.isragood.com /2007 /110/israeli-science-geen-tea-is-good-for.html>. IsraGood © 2006-2007.

170. "Is the Budwig Protocol 'just flax seed oil and cottage cheese'"? Online posting. Accessed 13 Nov. 2007. <http://www.healingcancernaturally.com/budwig_protocol. html>. © 2004, 2005, 2006 & 2007 www.healingcancernaturally.com.

171. "Johanna Budwig Revisited," "or How to Heal Cancer." Online posting. Wellness Directory of Minnesota™. Accessed 13 Nov. 2007. <http://www.mnwelldir.org/docs/cancer1budwig. htm>. Copyright © 2001 International Wellness Directory.

171a. "Just one chemo jab can cure testicle cancer." Online posting of Oct. 13, 2008. Accessed 14 Dec. 2008. <http://www.entertainmentandshowbiz.com/just-one-chemo-jab-can-cure-testicle - cancer-200810133102>. © 2008-09 entertainmentandshowbiz.com.

172. "Kidney Cancer (Renal Cell Carcinoma)." Online posting. Accessed 13 Nov. 2007. <http ://www.herbs2000.com/disorders/cancer_kidney.htm>. © 2002-2007 herbs2000.com.

173. "Kiwifruit." The World's Healthiest Foods: Eating-Healthy Cooking-Healthy Feeling-Great, George Mateljan Foundation. "Protection Against Asthma. Online posting. Accessed 13 Nov. <http://www.whfoods.com/genpagephp?tname=foodspice&dbid=41>. Copyright © 2001-2007 The George Mateljan Foundation.

174. "Krill Oil Shows Promise Against Skin Cancer." Online posting. Health News 42 –Skin Cancer at Discount Vitamins & Herbs. Accessed 2 Nov. 2007. <http://www.discount-vitamins-herbs.net/health-news42.htm#162>. © 2001–2007 Discount Herbs & Vitamins, Inc.

175. "LabCorp announces new colon cancer test." From TheTimesNews.com online posting Jul. 14, 2008. Accessed 14 Jul. 2008. <http:www.thetimesnews.com/news/labcorp_15590_article .html/new_test.html>. © 2008 Freedom Communications, Inc.

176. "Lactose Intake May Increase Ovarian Cancer Risk in Postmenopausal Women." HSI, Health Sciences Institute. Online posting. Accessed 30 Dec. 2004 and 13 Nov. 2006 <http:// www.hsialert.com/ealerts/ea200412/ea20041214.html>. Also rec'd this as an email alert on 12/14/04 from HSI/Research@healthiernews.com. Copyright © 1997–2007 by Institute of Health Sciences, L.L.C.

176a. "Light Sciences Oncology Completes Patient Enrollment In Phase 3 Clinical Trial of Litx As A Treatment For Hepatocellular Carcinoma." By Allsoch. Online posting Nov. 29, 2008. Accessed 25 Dec. 2008. <http://www.canceraids.org/2008/11/29/light-sciences-oncology-completes-patient-enrollment-in-phase-3-clinical-trial-of-litx-as-a-treatment-for-hepatocellular-car cinoma>.

(Also see website <http://www.lsoncology.com/litx_therapy>. © 2009 Light Sciences Oncology, Inc.)

177. “Light Therapy Tackles Cancer.” BBC News Health. Online posting. Thursday 14 March, 2002, 01:14 GMT. Accessed 13 Nov. 2007. <http://news.bbc.co.uk/1/hi/health/1871474.stm >. © BBC News.

178. “Liver Cancer.” Online posting. Liver Cancer – Healing with Herbs, Vitamins and Minerals. Accessed 13 Nov. 2007. <http://www.herbs2000.com/disorders//cancer_liver.htm>. © 2002-2007 herbs 2000.com.

179. “Lorenzo’s oil for adrenoleukodystrophy and adrenomyeloneuropathy.” “Evidence based thinking about health care.” Online posting. “Lorenzo’s oil for AMN and ALD.” Accessed 13 Nov. 2007. <http://www.jr2.ox.ac.uk/bandolier/booth/neurol/lorenz.html>. © 1994–2007.

179a. “Low Dose Naltrexone (LDN) for Cancer Treatment.” Online posting of The Starfish Project. Accessed 25 Dec. 2008. <http://starfishproject.wordpress.com/2008/11/29/low-dose-naltrexone-ldn-for-cancer-treatment>.

180. “Lung Cancer.” Online posting. Accessed 13 Nov. 2007. <http://www.herbs2000.com/ disorders/cancer_lung.htm>. ©2002-2007 herbs 2000.com.

181. “Lung Cancer Reduced 90% with Omega-3 Fatty Acids.” From Health News Archive 119 – Lung Cancer at website http://www.discount-vitamins-herbs.netonline posting. Accessed 8 Dec. 2007. <http://www.discount-vitamns-herbs.net/n-119-lung-cancer_omega-3.htm>. Their source given was: Pardini RS, Wilson D, Schiff S, Bajo SA, Pierce R. “Nutritional Intervention With Omega-3 Fatty Acids in a Case of Malignant Fibrous Histiocytoma of the Lungs.” Nutrition and Cancer, 52(2), 121-129.

182. “Lyprinol.” Online posting. Accessed 13 Nov. 2007. <http://www.primohealth.com/PILy prinol.a.html>.

183. Macela.” Raintree Nutrition’s Tropical Plant Database. Online posting. “Biological Activities and Clinical Research.” Site updated 1-18-2007. Accessed 13 Nov. 2007. <http://www.rain-tree. com/macela.htm>. This information is also found in Leslie Taylor’s book, *The Healing Power of Rainforest Herbs*. Square One Publishers, Jan. 2005 - © Copyrighted 1996 to present by Raintree Nutrition, Inc., Carson City, NV. 89701.

184. “Maitake.” Herbs 2000.com. Online posting. Accessed 13 Nov. 2007. <http://www.herbs 2000.com/herbs/herbs_maitake.htm>. ©2002–2007 herbs2000.com.

185. “Mangosteen Treatment for Cancer.” Online posting. Alternative Cancer Treatments Information Center™. Accessed 13 Nov. 2007. <http://www.cancertutor.com/Cancer/Mango steen.html>. Their given source for this article: research: “‘Antiproliferation, antioxidation and induction of apoptosis by Garcinia mangostana (mangosteen) on SKBR3 human breast cancer cell line,’ by Moongkarndi P, Kosem N, Kaslungka S, Luanratana O, Pongpan N, Neungton N.”

186. “Marijuana Compound Shows Promise In Fighting Breast Cancer.” California Pacific Medical Center (2007, November 26). *ScienceDaily*. Retrieved July 8, 2008, from <http://www. sciencedaily.com-/releases/2007/11/071123211703.htm>. © 1995-2008 ScienceDaily LLC.

187. “Marine Phytoplankton Tumor and Cancer.” Online posting. Accessed 25 Oct. 2007. <http://www.shirleys-wellness-café.com/acancer.htm#plankton>. From Shirleys Wellness Café - “Holistic Health Care for People and Animals.

188. "Mayo Clinic Researchers Develop A New Imaging Test For Diagnosing Breast Cancer." Mayo Clinic (2002, June 26). *ScienceDaily*. Retrieved July 8, 2008, from <http://www.sciencedaily.com-/releases/2002/06/020626071110.htm>. © 1995-2008 ScienceDaily, LLC.

189. "Medical Conditions." "Botanicals." Online posting. Accessed 13 Nov. 2007. <http://www.naturalopinion.com/nmp/Sample.html>. Natural Medical Protocols. A reference program for doctors on natural medicine.

190. "Melanoma, Cancer, Metastasis." Online posting. Accessed 4 Nov. 2007. Vitasearch website. <http://search.vitasearch.com/get-clp-summary35010>. Also, see reference: "Low plasma coenzyme Q10 levels as an independent prognostic factor for melanoma progression," Rusciani L, Proietti I., et al, Jam Acad Dermatol, 2006;54(2):234-41. From *Vitasearch Clinical Pearls* website.

191. "Melatonin." "Melatonin for Sleep Disorders and anti-oxidant protection." Online posting. Accessed 13 Nov. 2007. <http://www.health-n-energy.com/melatonin.htm>. Health-n-Energy website. FDA disclaimer.

192. "Melatonin: Supplements, What Works." Online posting. Accessed 13 Nov. 2007. <http://www.healthyroads.com/mylibrary/data/pelletier/chapter3/p_melatonin.asp>. Last reviewed 12/06. From *The Best Alternative Medicine* by Kenneth Pelletier. Copyright © 2000 by Dr. Kenneth Pelletier, Inc.

193. "Mercury fillings post health risks, FDA warns." From CBC News article online posting (updated Thurs. June 5, 2008.) Accessed 03 July 2008. <http://www.cbc.ca/consumer/story/2008/06/05/dental-amalgam.html>. © CBC 2008.

194. "Microvascular Ultrasonographic Imaging for the Detection of Early Stage Epithelial Ovarian Carcinoma." Online posting from ClinicalTrials.gov website, a service of the U.S. National Institutes of Health. New York University School of Medicine, Aug 2007, was recruiting participants for the study under the ClinicalTrials.gov Identifier NCT00531570. Site accessed 29 Jan. 2008. Also see the U.S. National Library of Medicine and U.S. Department of Health & Human Services and USA.gov. <http://www.clinicaltrials.gov/ct2/show/NCT005315 70?term=NCT00531570&rank=1>.

195. "Migraine." Online posting. Accessed 13 Nov. 2007. <http://www.mcvitamins.com/migraine.htm>. FDA disclaimer.

196. "Milk Thistle Protects Against Lung Cancer." Health News Archive 341 – Lung Cancer from website www.discount-vitamins-herbs.net online posting. Accessed 12 Dec. 2007. <http://www.discount-vitamins-herbs.net/n-341-lung-cancer_milk-thistle.htm>. Source given was: Singh, R.P., G. Deep, et al. (2006) "Effect of Silibinin on the growth and progression of primary lung tumors in mice." J Natl Cancer Inst 98(12): 846-55.

197. "Milk Thistle." Side Effects and Cautions. Online posting. Herbs 2000. Accessed 13 Nov. 2007. <http://www.herbs2000.com/herbs/herbs_thistle_milk.htm>. Copyright © 2002-2007 herbs2000.com.

197a. "Mistletoe 'may prolong' lives of cancer patients." Dec. 25, 2008, London. Online posting from expressindia.com website. Accessed 30 Dec. 2008. <http://www.expressindia.com/story_print.php?storyId=402861>. © 2008 Indian Express Newspapers (Mumbai) Ltd.

198. "Modified Citrus Pectin Holds Promise for Prostate Cancer." Online posting from *Medical News Today* website. 14 Sept. 2007. Accessed 28 Nov. 2007. <http://www.Medicalnewstoday.com/articles/82455.php>. © 2007 MediLexicon International Ltd.

199. "MSM Plus Vitamin C and B12 Cancer Treatment." Online posting. Accessed 13 Nov. 2007. <http://www.cancertutor.com/Cancer/MSM.html>. This study was done by "Dr. McCabe, Dr. P. O'Dwyer, Dr. B. Sickle-Antanello, Dr. E. Woltering, Dr. H. Abou-Issa and Dr. A. James, published in the Archives of Surgery, 12/1986." Article from Alternative Cancer Treatments Information Center™.

200. "Mullaca." Online posting. "Plant Chemicals." Tropical Plant Database of Raintree Nutrition. Accessed 14 Nov. 2007. <http://www.rain-tree.com/mullaca.htm>. Updated 1/20/07>. This information is also found in Leslie Taylor's book, *The Healing Power of Rainforest Herbs.* Square One Publishers, Jan. 2005. © Copyrighted 1996 to present by Raintree Nutrition, Inc., Carson City, NV. 89701.

201. "Muscular Dystrophy." Online posting from Alternative Health & Herbs website. Accessed 24 Jul. 2008. <http://www.healthherbs.com/conditionitem.php?id=192>. Copyright © 2008 ALTERNATIVE Health & Herbs REMEDIES.

202. "Mushrooms." Online posting. Accessed 28 Dec. 2007. <http://www.iconocast..com/News_Files/Hnews9XE_X_05/Health6.htm>. © 2002-2006.

203. "Myeloma Cancer." Online posting. Discount Vitamins & 4 Herbs Health News. Accessed 14 Nov. 2007. <http://www.discount-vitamins-herbs.net/healthnews30.htm#121> p. 4. Their reference is given as: "Bharti AC, Donato N, Singh S, Aggarwal B. 'Curcumin (diferuloylmethane) down-regulates the constitutive activation of nuclear factor-kappa B and I kappa Balpha Kinase in human multiple myeloma cells, leading to suppression of proliferation and induction of apoptosis.' From *Blood.* 2003 Feb 1;101(3):1053-62.'"

204. "Nanoparticle Implant Measures Tumor Growth, Treatment." Massachusetts Institute of Technology (2006, December 29). *ScienceDaily.* Retrieved July 8, 2008, from <http://www.sciencedaily.com/releases/2006/12/061219095316.htm>. © 1995–2007 Science Daily LLC.

205. "Neuroblastoma: Innovative Treatments." "High-risk Neuroblastoma." Online posting. Accessed 12 Dec. 2007. <http://www.mskcc.org/mskcc/html/32107.cfm> and <http://www.mskcc.org/mskcc/html/62106.cfm>. Copyright © Memorial Sloan Kettering Cancer Center ph# 212-639-2000. 1275 York Avenue, New York, N.Y. 10065.

206. "NK-Immunomodulation by AHCC in 17 Cancer Patients." From Health News Archive 62 – Cancer and AHCC Research at the www.discount-vitamins-herbs.net website online posting. Accessed 8 Dec. 2007. <http://www.discount-vitamins-herbs.net/health-news62.htm>. © 2001-2007, Discount Herbs & Vitamins, Inc.

207. "New Antibody Offers Hope for Treating Ovarian, Breast Cancer." Online posting from ne Wswise.com 22 May 2008. Accessed 22 June 2008. <http://www.newswise.com/p/articles/view/541074>. © 2008 Newswise.

208. "New Broccoli Compound Appears Promising Against Breast Cancer." American Chemical Society (2002, August 19). *ScienceDaily.* Retrieved July 8, 2008, from <http://www.sciencedaily.com/releases/2002/08/020819064835.htm>. © 1995–2008 Science Daily, LLC.

209. "New Cancer Treatment Targets Both Tumor Cells And Blood Vessels." University of Missouri-Columbia (2008, June 19). *ScienceDaily.* Retrieved July 8, 2008 <http://www.sciencedaily.com/releases/2008/06/080618133718.htm>. © 1995-2008 ScienceDaily, LLC.

210. “New Colon Cancer Screening Being Tested Out.” “Picture Your Future.” Online posting 06/26/08. Accessed 27 Jun. 2008. <http://www.scandirectory.com/blog/2008/06/new_colon_cancer_screening_bei.html>.

211. “New breakthrough boosts immune cell activity 45.2% more than ordinary mushrooms.” “MycoPhyto® Complex.” Online posting. Accessed 28 Dec. 2007. <http://www.advancedbio nutritionals.com/immunity>.

212. “New Research on Cancer-fighting Foods, Supplements.” (Also see: “Drinking cloudy apple juice daily may help prevent colon cancer.”) American Chemical Society (2007, March 26). *ScienceDaily*. Retrieved July 8, 2008, from http://www.sciencedaily.com/releases/2007/03/0703 25111619.htm. © 1995-2008 ScienceDaily LLC.

213. “New Research on Cancer-fighting Foods, Supplements.” (Also see: “Black raspberries show promise for preventing cancer of the esophagus, colon.”) American Chemical Society (200 7, March 26). *ScienceDaily*. Retrieved July 8, 2008, from <http://www.sciencedaily.com/releases/2007/03/070325111619.htm>. © 1995–2008 ScienceDaily LLC.

214. “New Research on Cancer-fighting Foods, Supplements.” (Also see: Grape seed compounds may prevent skin cancer by boosting immune system.”) American Chemical Society (2007, March 26). *ScienceDaily*. Retrieved July 8, 2008, from <http://www.sciencedaily.com/releases/2007/03/070325111619.htm>. © 1995-2008 ScienceDaily LLC.

215. “New Research on Cancer-fighting Foods, Supplements.” (Also see: “Compound found in high-fiber foods shows promise against prostate cancer.”) American Chemical Society (2007, March 26). *ScienceDaily*. Retrieved July 8, 2008, from http://www.sciencedaily.com/releases /2007/03/070325111619.htm. © 1995-2008 ScienceDaily LLC.

215a. “New Tests That Could Make Mammograms Obsolete - But first the bad news: neither of these tests has been approved by our FDA.” Online posting from Wellness Directory of Minnesota. “Newsletter: Wellness Update.” Accessed 26 Aug 2008. <http://www.mnwelldir.org/nw_current.htm>. © 2008 Minnesota Wellness Publication, Inc.

215b. “New Test Appears Promising At Detecting Breast Cancer.” Online posting from NBC-10.com HEALTH article 09/25/2008, accessed 26 Sept. 2008. <http://www.nbc10.com/health /17556752/detail.html>. © 2008 NBC Universal, Inc.

216. “NIH Awards. Grant to Study the Dietary Supplement Nexrutine for Prevention of Prostate Cancer.” Online posting. Accessed 2 Nov. 2007. <http://www.discount-vitamins-herbs.net /health-news5.htm>. © 2001–2007 Discount Herbs & Vitamins, Inc.

217. “NINDS Adrenoleukodystrophy Information Page,” from the National Institute of Neurological Disorders and Stroke. Online posting. Accessed 14 Nov. 2007. <http://www.ninds.nih.gov/disorders/adenoleukodystrophy/adrenoeukodystrophy.htm>. Last updated October 02, 2007.

218. “Non-Hodgkin’s Lymphoma – oncology channel.” From the Oncology Channel®, online posting, accessed 14 Nov. 2007. <http://www.oncology/channel.com/non hodgkins>. © 1998–2007 by Healchcommunities.com, Inc.

218a. “Noninvasive test accurately identifies advanced liver disease without biopsy.” “Transient elastography evaluates liver stiffness to diagnose cirrhosis.” Bethesda, MD. Sept 1, 2008. From the *Clinical Gastroenterology and Hepatology*, “official journal of the American Gastroenterological

Association (AGA) Institute." Online posting. Accessed 02 Sept. 2008. <http://www.eurekalert.org/pub_releases/2008-09/aga-nta082708.php>. For more information, see www.gastro.org.

219. "Non-Small Cell Lung Cancer Treatment (PDQ®)," from an online posting at the National Cancer Institutes, U.S. Institutes of Health website www.cancer.gov, last updated Jun 12, 2008. Accessed 15 Jul 2008. <http://www.cancer.gov/CANCERTOPICS/PDQ/TREATMENT/NON-SMALL-CELL-LUNG/PATIENT#Keypoint2>.

220. "Northwest Indiana Hospital Offering New Lung Cancer Treatment." Online Posting from website "Inside Indiana with Berry Dicks," Press Release. Accessed 16 Jan. 2008. <http://www.insideindianabusiness.com/newsitem.asp?ID=27347. © Grow Indiana Media Ventures, LLC (Grow Indiana).

220a. "Novel Vaccine May Improve Survival in Brain Cancer." Online posting at "Brain Cancer News – CancerConsultants.com" Jun 5, 2008. Accessed 26 Aug 2008. <http://patient.cancer consultants.com/CancerNews_Brain_Cancer.apx?DocumentId=42104>. © Brain Cancer Information Center on CancerConsultants.com.

221. "Oat Beta-glucan." Effective Natural Cancer Treatments. Online posting. Natural Cancer Support. Accessed 14 Nov. 2007. <http://www.cancer-treatments.net/cancer.html>.

222. "Onconase Mesothelioma Treatment." Online posting from Mesothelioma Cancer Treatment Center website. Accessed 8 Jul. 2008. <http://www.mesothelioma-cancer-treatment.com/pages/onconase.html>. Also, see: http://www.mesothelioma-cancer-treatment.com/index.html. © 2008.

223. "North American Herb & Spice – Oregacyn Respiratory," online posting. Accessed 08 Jan. 2008. <http://myhealthpro.com/shop/detail.cfm?sku=D0861&rfr=ggl&kid=16905&gclid=CL> "North American Herb & Spice — Oregacyn Respiratory P-73-90 veg cap."

224. "Oil of Oregano." Online posting. Accessed 14 Nov. 2007. <http://www.cancertutor.com/OtherBig_List.htm>. "Over 200 Alternative Cancer Treatments Plus Other Information."

225. "Oxalic Acid The Cure For Cancer." Online posting 1-7-2008 "Cancer Treatment." Accessed 19 Jan. 2008. <http://health-cancertreatment.blogspot.com/2008/01/oxalic-Acid-cur e-for-cancer.html>.

226. "PET/CT Scan Could be Valuable Non-invasive Tool For Determining Stages Of Ovarian Cancer." From Photonics Online website. Online posting. Accessed 24 Jun. 2008. <http://www.photonicsonline.com/article.mvc/PETCT-Scan-Could-Be-Valuable-Noninvasive-Tool-0001>. So urce: Society of Nuclear Medicine. Copyright © 1996-2008 VertMarkets, Inc.

227. "Pancreatic Cancer: Story of Maribel C. Lim." Cancer Central (Aug. 2003), Manila, Philippines. Online posting. Accessed 14 Nov. 2007. <http://www.cancer-central.com/pancreas-cancer/pancreas-cancer-3.htm>. Copyright 2003 Green & Gold International Exports.

228. "Parsley." Online posting. Accessed 14 Nov. 2007. <http://www.herbs2000.com/herbs/herbs_parsley.htm>. ©2002-2007 herbs 2000.com.

229. "Pau d' arco and Cancer." Herbal Remedies for Immunity, Cancer, Lapacho, Natural Herbal Remedies for Cancer. Online posting. Accessed 14 Nov. 2007. <http://www.holistic-online.com/cancer/Cancer_lapacho_herbrem.htm>. Holisticonline.com is developed and maintained by ICBS, Inc.

230. "PawPaw Alternative Cancer Treatment Comparison." Online posting. Accessed 14 Nov. 2007. <http://alternativecancer.us/pawpaw.htm>.

231. "Pharmaceutical Advances—Ancient Medicinal Offers New Hope to Young Adults." Online posting from Innovation.org. "Advances in the Treatment of LEUKEMIA," Accessed 08 January 2008. <http://www.innovation.org/index.cfm/InnovationToday/InnovationinRareDiseases/Rare_Diseases_-_Leukemia>.

232. Philippine Information Agency. "Research boosts 'kamunggay' as effective anti-cancer cure." Online posting from *Tagbilaran City (28 September)*, at *PIA Daily News Reader.* Accessed 3 February 2008. PIA Press Release 2007/09/28. <http://www.pia.gov.ph/?m=12&fi=p070928.htm&no=77>. © 2005 Philippine Information Agency.

233. "Phyllanthus." Online posting. Accessed 14 Nov. 2007. <http://www.herbs2000.com/herbs/herbs_phyllanthus.htm>. © 2002-2007 herbs2000.com.

233a. "Pituitary Tumor (pituitary adenoma, nervous system tumor)." "Minimally Invasive endoNeurosurgery Center." Online posting. Accessed 8 Oct. 2008. <http://www.upmc.com/Services/minc/conditionstreatments/Pages/Pituitary-Tumor.aspx?> © Copyright 2008 UPMC /Affiliated with the University of Pittsburg Schools of the Health Sciences.

234. "Pituitary Tumors." National Institute of Neurological Disorders and Stroke. Online posting. Accessed 14 Nov. 2007. <http://www.ninds.nih.gov/disorders/pituitary_tumors/pituitary_tumors.htm>. "NINDS Pituitary Tumors Information Page." Last updated, September 06, 2007.

235. "Poly-MVA New hope for cancer patients. New hope for brain cancer patients." Online posting. Accessed 14 Nov. 2007. <http://www.mnwelldir.org/docs/cancer1/poly.htm>. Wellness Directory of Minnesota™. Copyright © 2001, 2002 International Wellness Directory.

236. "Polysaccharide Kureha (PSK)." Online posting. Herbs2000.com. Accessed 14 Nov. 2007. < http://www.herbs2000.com/h_menu/psk.htm>. © 2002-2006 herbs2000.com.

237. "Pomegranate extract blocks skin tumors in mice." New York, Reuters Health from OncoLink Cancer News, *Reuters Health Information.* Accessed 14 Nov 2007. <http://www.oncolink.com/resources/article.cfm?c=3&s=8&ss=23&id=11481&month=01&year=2005>. Online posting January 20, 2005. © 1994-2005 © Trustees of the University of Pennsylvania. Reuters shall not be liable for any errors or delays in the content, or for any actions taken in reliance thereon.

238. "Pomegranate Inhibits Lung and Prostate Cancer." Online posting. Accessed 3 Nov. 2007. <http://www.discount-vitamins-herbs.net/blog/2006_06_01discountsupplements_archive>.

239. "Preserving the living and the dead." New Agriculturist on-line—Reporting Agriculture for the 21st Century. "Spice Preservatives." Online posting. Accessed 14 Nov. 2007. <http://www.new-agri.co.uk/02-1/focuson/focuson8.html>. Wren Media.

240. "Probiotics Reduce Risk of Liver Cancer." Online posting. Accessed 3 Nov. 2007. "Anti-aging Research: June 2006." <http://www.discount-vitamins-herbs.Net/blog/2006_06_01_discount-supplements_archive. © 2001-2007 Discount Herbs & Vitamins, Inc.

241. "Promising Results with Epratuzumab and Chemotherapy in Children with Acute Lymphoblastic Leukemia." Online posting from Bio-Medicine.org website. Accessed 11 Jul. 2008. <http://www.bio-medicine.org/medicine-technology/Promising-Results-with-Epratuzumab-and-

Chemotherapy-in-Children-0Awith-Acute-LymphoblasticLeukemia-491-1/>. © 2003-2008 Bio-Medicine.

242. "Prostate cancer drug 'breakthrough.'" From The Press Association 22 Jul. 2008 online posting. Accessed 24 Jul. 2008. <http://uk.news.yahoo.com/pressass/20080722/tuk-prostate-cancer-drug-breakthrough-6323e80.html>. © 2008 The Press Association. © 2008 Yahoo!

243. "Prostate Cancer." Herbs 2000. Online posting. Accessed 15 Nov. 2007. <http://www. herbs 2000.com/disorders/cancer_prostate.htm>. © 2002-2007 herbs2000.com.

244. "Provera Side Effects, and Drug Interactions—Medroxyprogesterone Acetate – RxList Mon…" Side Effects. Online posting. Accessed 15 Nov. 2007. <http://www. rxlist.com/cgi/generic/medrox_ad.htm>. The Internet Drug Index. Copyright © 2007 by RxList Inc.

245. "Psoralea." Online posting. Accessed 15 Nov. 2007. <http://www.herbs2000.com/herbs/herbs_psoralea.htm>. © 2002-2007 herbs2000.com.

246. R-A Therapy. "Introducing R-A Therapy," from Advanced Alternatives Cancer Center online posting. Accessed 26 Dec. 2007. <http://www.aacancer.com/alternative_cancer_treat ment.html>. © 2005-2007 Advanced Alternatives Cancer Center.

247. "Radioactive scorpion venom deemed safe cancer treatment." Online posting Jun. 26, 2006. "Special to World Science." <http://www.world-science.net/othernews/06/06 26_venom.htm>.

247a. "Radiofrequency Ablation Effective for Primary Lung Tumors and Lung Metastases from Other Cancers." Online posting from Daily Cancer News—Cancer Consultants.com 7/30/2008. Accessed 03 Jul. 2008. <http://patient.Cancerconsultants.com/CancerNews.aspx?DocumentId= 42404&Keywords=ca>. © 1998–2008 Cancer Consultants.com.

248. "Raw Dairy Sales Illegal in Manhattan." HSI Health Sciences Institute. "The Milkman Cometh." Online posting. Accessed 15 Nov. 2007. <http://www.hsialert.com/ealerts/ea2004 12/ea20041222.html>. Also received this as an email on 12-22-04 from HSIResearch@health iernews.com. Copyright © 1997–2007 by Institute of Health Sciences, LLC

248a. "Raw Milk is Catching on in the UK." From *Belfast Telegraph* Nov. 6, 2007. Also see Dr. Mercola'a website <http://articles.mercola.com/sites/articles/archive/2007/11/29/raw-milk-is-catching-on-in-the-UK>. Online posting. Accessed 8 Dec. 2007.

249. "Recent Scientific Advances in Rare Diseases Research," Report on the Rare Diseases Research Activities at the National Institutes of Health FY 2003," "Beta-Sitosterolemia," Online posting. Accessed 15 Nov. 2007. <http://rarediseases.info.nih.gov/html/reports/fy2003/nhlbi. html>. Last reviewed November 4, 2005.

250. "Red Beet." "Leukemia," from website: Herbal Formulas for Leukemia. Online posting. Accessed 15 Nov. 2007. <http://www.herballegacy.org/Leukemia.html>. From "Dr. Christopher's Herbal Legacy" "Natural Healing with Herbs for a Healthier You." Also see website: <http://www.herballegacy.org/Incurables.html>.

251. "Red Clover (Trifolium praetense)." Online Posting. Cancer Tutor. Alternative Cancer Treatment Information Center™. Accessed 15 Nov. 2007. http://www.cancertutor.com /Other/Big_List.htm.

251a. "Reduce Your Brain's Exposure to Cell Phone Radiation." From Mercola.com Take Control of Your Health" website. Online posting. Accessed 16 Aug 2008. <http://www.mercola.com/forms/ferrite_beads.htm>. © 2008 Dr. Joseph Mercola.

252. "Red Wine Anti-oxidant May Help Destroy Pancreatic Cancer." From living.One india.in/health/wellbeing website – by ANI from the March edition of *Advances in Experimental Medicine and Biology* journal. Online posting article accessed 29 Jun. 2008. © Greynium Information Technologies Pvt. Ltd.

252a. "Regular Vegetables Discovered to Work against Colon Cancer." Posted by Maggie at cancer-prevent.com 23 Dec. 2008. Accessed 31 Dec. 2008. <http://www.cancer-prevent-com/colon-rectal-cancer/regular-vegetables-discovered-to-work-against-colon-cancer-679.html>. © 2007-2008 Prevent Cancer.

253. "Renowned Cardiothoracic Surgeon Calls Ribose Results 'Astounding,' Pioneering Beating Heart CABG Doc Presenting ATS Paper on Using Ribose to Rebuild the Energy Supply of the Heart Prior to Bypass Surgery." From Bioenergy, Inc., press release. Online posting, accessed 02 Jan. 2008. <http://bioenergy.com/Papers/BioenergyPerkowski:Release.pdf>.

254. "Repeated-Radioimmunotherapy-With-131I-Labetuzumab Appears Safe and-Effective-in Colorectal Cancer with Liver Metastases." Bio-Medicine website online posting Jun 04, 2007. Washington PR Newswire. Accessed 24 Jun 2008. <http://www.bio-medicine.org/medicine-technology/Repeated-Radioimmunotherapy-With-131I-Labetuzumab-Appears-Safe-and-OAEffective-in-Colorectal-Cancer-with-Liver-Metastases-483-2/>. © 2003–2008 Bio Medicine.

255. "Researchers Discover That A Protein In Grape Skins Can Kill Cancer Cells." University Of Virginia Health System (2004, May 28). *ScienceDaily*. Retrieved July 8, 2008, from <http://www.sciencedaily.com-/releases/2004/05/040526065457.htm>. © 1995–2008 ScienceDaily LLC.

255a. "Resveratrol—Another Look Some call it the Fountain of Youth," Newsletter Update from Minnesota Wellness Publications, Inc. Online posting, accessed 26 Aug 2008. <http://www.mnwelldir.org/nw_current.htm>. Copyright © 2008 Minnesota Wellness Publications, Inc. Also see their reference: Gunnlaugsdoitter, E., et al., "Prevalance and causes of visual impairment and blindness in Icelanders aged 50 years and older: the Reykjavik Eye Study," Acta Opthamol, 2008 May 3, in regards to the info on resveratrol and cataracts.

256. "Rexin-G™, The World's First Tumor-Targeted Gene Therapy Vector, Stymies Metastatic Cancer." Online posting from 11-7-2006 online article posted at medicalNewstoday.com. Accessed 13 Jan. 2008. <http://www.medicalnewstoday.com/Articles/56021/php>. © 2008 MediLexicon International Ltd.

257. "Rexin-G™ Fact Sheet." Online posting from Epeius Biotechnologies. Accessed 16 Jan. 2008. <http://www.epeiusbiotech.com/rexin_g-factsheet.asp>.

258. "Rhodiola Rosea." New Page 5. Online posting. Planet Herbs. Accessed 15 Nov. 2007. < http://www.planetherbs.com/showcase/>. © 2005 Planet Herbs. Site is now referred to as: *Michael Tierra's East West Coast Herb Course & Planetary Herbs & Formulas.*

259. "Rhodiola Rosea." Online posting. Planet Herbs. Now site is referred to as: *Michael Tierra's East West Coast Herb Course & Planetary Herbs & Formulas.* Accessed 15 Nov. 2007. <http://www .planetherbs.com/showcase/>. © 2005 Planet Herbs. See their reference from: *Arctic Root (Rhodiola Rosea): The Powerful New Ginseng Alternative* by Carl Germano, R.D., C.N.S. L.D.N., and Zakir Ramazanov, Ph.D., published by Kensington Health Books.

260. "Royal Jelly (a bee product)." Online posting. Alternative Cancer Treatment Information Center™. Accessed 15 Nov. 2007. <http://www.cancertutor.com/OtherBig_List.htm>.

261. "Royal Rife Machine." Online posting. Accessed 15 Nov. 2007. <http://www.cancertutor.com/Other/Big_List.htm>.

262. "Saliva vs. Serum or Plasma Testing For Progesterone." Special Report from the John R. Lee, M.D. Medical Letter, Saliva Hormone Testing. Online posting. Accessed 15 Nov. 2007. <http://www.johnleemd.com/store/saliva_serum.html>. Copyright © Hormones Etc.

263. "Sarcoma." Online posting. Accessed 15 Nov. 2007. Cancer-healing.com website. "Cancer Types." Accessed 15 Nov. 2007. <http://www.cancer-healing.com/cancer_type.php>. copyright 2004-07 © Life Enthusiast Co-op.

264. "Schisandra Berries More Than a Liver Aid," From the January 2001 issue of Nutrition Science News, NewHope.com. Online posting. Accessed 15 Nov. 2007. "Protects the Liver." <http://www.newhope.com/nutritionsciencenews/NSN_backs/Jan_01/schisandra.cfm>. Copyright © Penton Media Inc.

265. "Seaweed extract blocks HPV cervical cancer virus, scientists discover." Online posting Jul 14, 2006 from naturalnews.com website. Accessed 17 Feb. 2008. <http://www.naturalnews.com/019649.html>. Truth Publishing, Ltd. Natural News Network © 2008.

265a. "Selective Internal Radiation Therapy (SIRT): SIR-Spheres – About Selective Internal Radiation Therapy (SIRT)." Online posting. Page last updated 04/22/2008. Retrieved 14 Aug 2008. Greenbaum Cancer Center – UMGCC. <http://www.umgcc.org/sir-spheres/about_sirt.htm>. © 2008 University of Maryland Greenbaum Cancer Center (UMGCC).

266. "Selenium Reduces Cancer Risk." From the British Journal of Urology 81(5):730-4, 1998 May. Online posting at website alkalizeforhealth.net. Title: "Decreased incidence of prostate cancer with selenium supplementation: results of a double-blind cancer prevention trial." Accessed 25 June 2008. <http://www.alkalizeforhealth.net/Lselenium.htm>. © 2000–2008 AlkalizeForHealth.

266a. "Selenium to prevent recurrence of colorectal polyps." "Phase III Randomised Study of Selenium in Patients with Adenomatous Colorectal Polyps." Online posting, published 28/05/2008. Accessed 22 Jun. 2008 from Insider News – "Cancer Journal: Latest cancer research Selenium to prevent recurrence of colorectal polyps" at ecancermedicalscience.com. <http://www.ecancermedicalscience.com/news-insidernews.asp?itemId=189>. *e*cancermedicalscience is published by Cancer Intelligence Limited, a private limited company, incorporated in the United Kingdom, company registration number 4595666. The registered office is situated at 53 High St, Keynsham, BS311DS, Avon.

267. "Seven Essentials." Healthy-Living.org. Online posting. Accessed 15 Nov. 2007. <http://www.healthy-living.org/html/essential_seven.html>. Copyright © Healthy-Living.Org 2002 – 2006.

268. "Shark Cartilage." Online posting. Accessed 15 Nov. 2007. <http://www.enerex.ca/articles/shark_cartilage.htm>. From www.Enerex.ca.

269. Sharma, Nidhi. "Cancer Immunotherapy Saves Life of Advanced Melanoma Patient." 06/18/2008. Online posting from allheadlinenews.com. Article was also published in the *New England Journal of Medicine.* Website accessed 03 Jul. 2008. <http://www.allheadlinenews.com/articles/7011316473>. © 2003 – 2008 AHN.

270. "Sheep Sorrel." Online posting. Cancer and Immunity, Immune Building Agents, Dr.Lam.com. Accessed 15 Nov. 2007. <http://www.drlam.com/A3R_brief_in_doc_format/cancer_and_immunity.htm.> ©2002 Michael Lam, M.D.

271. "Silymarin (Milk Thistle): how effective and safe is it? Milk Thistle Extract, an herbal remedy." Online posting. Accessed 13 Dec. 2007. <http://www.ndri.com/news/silymarin_milk_thistle_how_effective_and_safe_is_it-384.html>.

272. "Simarouba." Online posting. "Simarouba glauca, amara Simaruba—Simarouba glauca," Tropical Plant Database of Raintree Nutrition. "Biological Activities & Clinical Research." Accessed 15 Nov. 2007. <http://www.rain-tree.com/simaruba.htm>. Updated 1-22-2007. This information is also found in Leslie Taylor's book, *The Healing Power of Rainforest Herbs.* Square One Publishers, Jan. 2005.

273. "Snow Fungus." Online posting. Accessed 15 Nov. 2007. <http://www.herbs2000.com/herbs/herbs_snow_fungus.htm>. © 2002-2007 herbs2000.

274. See website – gentlecures.org

275. Solco Biomedical – World class products enterprise club. Online posting – World-class products from Korea. Accessed 25 Feb. 2008. <http://wopeclub.kotef.or.kr/eng/next_generation/electronics/solcobio.shtml>. © Electrochemical Cancer Therapy.

276. "Spruce HMR lignan may slow development of hormonal cancers: Health effects from bioactive substances in free knots." Online posting 02/06/2006 from Innovations–Report website. Accessed 23 Jun. 2008. <http://www.innovationsreport.de/html/berichte/agrar_forstwissenschaften/bericht-60615>. © 2000–2008 by innovations-report.

277. "St. John's Wort Extract Fights Cancer." From Health News Archive 41-Canceronline posting at website www.discount-vitamins-herbs.net. Accessed 8 Dec. 2007. © 2001–2007 Discount Herbs & Vitamins, Inc. From researchers at the University of Freiburg's Department of Dermatology. <http://www.discount-vitamins-herbs.net/health-news41.htm>.

278. "Stomach Cancer." Online posting. Accessed 15 Nov. 2007. <http://www.herbs2000.com/disorders/cancer_stomach.htm>. © 2002-2007 herbs2000.

279. "Suma." Raintree Nutrition Tropical Plant Database. Online posting. Accessed 15 Nov. 2007. <http://www.rain-tree.com/suma.htm>. Updated 1-22-2007. This information is also found in Leslie Taylor's book, *The Healing Power of Rainforest Herbs.* Square One Publishers, Jan. 2005.

280. "Sun exposure prevents prostate cancer." Yourhealthbase.com. Online posting. Accessed 15 November 2007. <http://www.yourhealthbase.com/cancer_prostate.htm>. ISSN 12031933 Copyright © 1998-2007 by Hans R. Larsen.

280a. "Susan Hale." Article from Burzynski Patient Group. Online posting. Accessed 28 Aug 2008. <http://www.burzynskipatientgroup.org/susanhale.htm> on Glioblastoma multiforme.

281. "Sushi May Protect Against Rare Type of Lung Cancer." From Health News Archive 6 - Cancer online posting of website www.discount-vitamins-herbs.net. Accessed 8 Dec. 2007. © Discount Herbs & Vitamins, Inc. Source given as *British Journal of Cancer* 2001;84. <http://www.discount-vitamins-herbs.net/health-news6.htm>.

282. "Sweet Wormwood (herb)." Online posting. The Cancer Tutor, Alternative Cancer Treatment Information Center™. Accessed 15 November 2007. <http://www.cancertutor.com/Other/Big_List.htm>.

283. *Taber's Cyclopedic Medical Dictionary.* 20th Edition, Philadelphia, PA: F.A. Davis Co., © 2005.

284. "Tea for Cancer-Free Cells." Online posting from uncommoncures.org website. Accessed 28 Mar. 2008. <http://www.uncommoncures.org/diseases/cancer.htm>.

284a. "Ten-minute test for cancer." Online posting. Accessed 20 Dec 2008. <http://www.daily mail.co.uk/health/article-1095091/A-round-latest-health-news-Vitamin-B-battle-depression-min ute-test-detect-cancer.html?ITO=1490>.

285. "Tetrahydrocannabinol (THC–medical marijuana)." Cancer Tutor, Alternative Cancer Treatment Information Center™. Online posting. Accessed 16 Nov. 2007. <http://www.cancertutor.com/Other/Big_List.htm>.

286. "The Benefits of Beta-glucan and MSM Supplements from a Terminal Cancer Survivor's perspective." Why Beta-glucan for Immune System Response? Online posting. Accessed 16 Nov. 2007. <http://www.aboutbetaglucan.com>. Copyright © 2002–2004, AboutBetaGlucan.com.

286a. "The CyberKnife Advantage." From the CyberKnife® Center – St. Catherine Hospital in East Chicago, Indiana. Online posting. Accessed 8 Oct. 2008. <http://www.comhs.org/cyber knife/advantage_pr.asp>.

287. "The Effect of Ukrain on Cancer." Online posting. Accessed 13 Oct. 2004 and 16 Nov. 2007. <http://www.ukrin.com>. This website is now titled "Nowicky Pharma." © 2006 Nowicky Pharma.

288. "The Healing Power of Vitamins, Minerals, and Herbs." *Reader's Digest*, Pleasantville, N.Y. Reader's Digest Assoc., Inc. 1009, 1999, 2000.

289. The website – see gentlecures.org.

290. "The Issels Treatment: Comprehensive Immunotherapy for Cancer." Online posting. "Co-Enzyme Co-Q10." Accessed 30 Nov. 2007. <http://www.issels.com/TreatmentSummary.as px>. © 2005–2007 Issels Treatment.

291. The website – see gentlecures.org.

292. The website – see gentlecures.org

293. "Tian Xian." Cancer Alternative Treatments. Online posting. Tian Xian liquid. Accessed 16 Nov. 2007. <http://www.tianxian.com>. © 2004 Green & Gold Int'l.

294. "Tomo Therapy. More Healthy Tissue Spared with New Radiation Procedure." Online posting from the Barbara Ann Karmanos Cancer Institute. Accessed 19 Jan. 2008. <http://www.karmanos.org/app.asp?id=1118>.

295. "Transfer Factor." *Over 200 Alternative Cancer Treatments Plus Other Information.* Online posting. Accessed 16 Nov. 2007. <http://www.cancertutor.com/Other/Big_List.htm>.

296. "Treatment: Hydrazine Sulfate." Online posting. Accessed 16 Nov. 2007. <http://www.diagnoseme.com/treat/T396383.html>. Last Updated May 10, 2007.

297. "Tumor Types: Non Gliomas." Online posting. Accessed 17 Nov. 2007. <http://www.braintumor.org/SurvivorshipTopics/?bPrintStyle=1>. © Copyright 2007 National Brain Tumor Foundation.

298. "Tumor Types: Other Brain-Related Conditions." Online posting. Accessed 17 Nov. 2007. <http://www.braintumor.org/OtherConditions.html>. Copyright © 2007 National Brain Tumor Foundation.

299. "Turmeric May Be Effective Adjunct Cancer Therapy." Discount Vitamins & Herbs Health News. Online posting. Accessed 16 Nov. 2007. <http://www.discount-vitamins-net/health-news30.htm#123>. © 2001–2007 Discount Herbs & Vitamins, Inc.

299a. "Two Endometrial Cancer Treatments May Not Work." Online posting Dec. 14, 2008. Accessed 21 Dec. 2008. <http://dreddyclinic-project.blogspot.com>. From dreddyclinic.com.

299b. "UCSB scientists show how certain vegetables combat cancer." Dec 23, 2008 online posting. Accessed 25 Dec. 2008. <http://www.bio-medicine.org/biology-news-1/UCSB-scientists-show-how-certain-vegetables-combat-cancer-6457-1/>. © 2003-2008 Bio-Medicine.

300. "Using Nanotechnolody to Kill Cancer." From an Ivanhoe.com medical alert — online posting 06/23/2008. Accessed 23 Jun. 2008. <http://www.ivanhoe.com/channels/p_channel story.cfm?storyid=19059>. Their source given was *Proceedings of the National Academy of Sciences, 2008.* © 2008 Ivanhoe Broadcast News, Inc.

301. "Uncovering Mushroom's Magic." "BREAST CANCER." From "Shiitake–Enoki–Lenti nan," Online posting. Accessed 31 Dec. 2007. <http://www.a-zbreastcancer.com/articles/amus hroom.htm>. © a-zbreastcancer.com © 1999-2008.

301a. "VascuStatin" - by Allergy Research Group®. "A Breakthrough in Angiogenesis Inhibition - 100 times Stronger than Shark Cartilage Powder." Online posting. The VascuStatin is available at this website in capsules. Accessed 09/04/2008. <http://organicpharmacy.org/products /VascuStatin>. © 1994-2008 Organic Pharmacy. (Also see biblio# 150).

302. "Vassourinha." Online posting. Raintree Nutrition's Tropical Plant Database. "Plant Chemicals." Accessed 16 Nov. 2007. <http://www.rain-tree.com/vassourinha.htm>. Updated 1-22-2007. © 1996 to present by Raintree Nutrition, Inc., Carson City, NV 89701. This information is also found in Leslie Taylor's book, *The Healing Power of Rainforest Herbs.* Square One Publishers, Jan. 2005.

303. "Victory Over Cancer: Hyperthermia for Cancer." Article at Advanced Alternatives Cancer Center website, online posting. Accessed 26 Dec. 2007. <http://www.aacancer.com/article4.html>. All content © 2005–2007 Advanced Alternatives Cancer Center.

304. "Vitamin A may prevent prostate cancer." Yourhealthbase.com. Online posting. Accessed 16 Nov. 2007. <http://www.yourhealthbase.com/cancer_prostate.htm>. © 2002–2007 by Hans R.Larsen. *International Health News* website.

305. "Vitamin A and Carotenoids." "Dietary Supplement Fact Sheet," National Institutes of Health Office of Dietary Supplements. Online posting. Accessed 16 Nov. 2007. <http://ods.od.nih.gov/factsheets/vitamina.asp>.

306. "Vitamin B12 and Folate Deficiency, Presenting as Leukemia." Online posting. Donkal, I.S., et al British Medical Journal May 12, 1990;300:1263-1264. From Vitasearch. Accessed 4 November

2007. Summary #8666 <http://www.vitasearch.com/get/C/summaries/get.php?id= 5021>. © Vitasearch.

307. "Vitamin B6 Stops Pancreatic Cancer Growth." From online posting at website www.discount-vitamins-herbs.net. Accessed 8 Dec. 2007. © 2001-2007 Discount Herbs & Vitamins, Inc. <http://www.discount-vitamins-herbs.net/health-news41.htm>. Source given as *Nutrition Research*, May 2003.

307a. "Vitamin C Injections Slow Tumor Growth in Mice," from the U.S. Department of Health and Human Services - NIH - National Institutes of Health. From an article "Embargoed for Release Monday Aug 4, 2008 5:00 pm EDT. Contact given is J. Chamberlain, NIDDK. Online posting. Accessed 29 Aug 2008. <http://www.nih.gov/news/health/aug2008/niddk-04.htm>. For more information about NIH and its programs, visit www.nih.gov.

308. "Vitamin D Cuts Pancreatic Cancer Risk by 43%." Online posting. Accessed 2 Nov. 2007. <http://www.discount-vitamins-herbs.net/n-417-pancreatic-cancer_vitamin-D.htm>. © 2001 - 2007 Discount Herbs & Vitamins, Inc.

309. "Vitamin D Deficiency Found in Patients with Lupus." From article: "Vitamin D deficiency in patients with active systemic lupus erythematosus," Borba VZ, Vieira JG, et al, Osteoporosis Int, 2008 July 4; [Epub ahead of print]. (Address: Division of Endocrinology, Universidade Federal de São Paulo, São Paulo, Brazil. E-mail: familiabborba@terra.com.br). Online posting. Accessed 10 Jul. 2008. <http://www.vitasearch.com/get/PC/summaries/get.php?id=37506>. Copyright © Vitasearch.

310. "Vitamin D supplements to protect against MS." 03/01/2005. NUTRAingredients com/Europe. Online posting. Accessed 16 Nov. 2007. <http://www.nutraingredients.com/news/news-ng.asp?n=56996-vitamin-d-supplements>. Industry & Science News © 2001/2007—Decision News Media SAS.

311. "Vitamin D: How Much is Enough?" "Many Americans are deficient, studies show." Online posting from Harvard Public Health Review website, Harvard School of Public Health. Spring/Summer 2007. Nutrition. Accessed 09 Feb. 2008 <http://www.hsph.harvard.edu/review/spring07/spr07vitaminD.html>. Copyright © 2007, President and Fellows of Harvard College.

312. "What are Clinical Trials? – Patient's Library." Online posting from cellgenesys.com. Accessed 19 Jan. 2008. <http://www.cellgenesys.com/what-are-clinical-trials.shtml>. © 2007 Cell Genesys, Inc.

313. "What are the reasons to have a hysterectomy?" "When is a hysterectomy necessary?" Online posting. Accessed 16 Nov. 2007. <http://www.safemenopausesolutions.com/hysterectomy.html>. © Personal Wellness Directory, Inc.

314. "What Is Graft-versus-host disease?" Online posting. CANCERBACUP Helping people live with cancer. Accessed 16 Nov. 2007. <http://www.cancerbackup.org.uk/QAs/TreatmentsQAs/StemcellbonemarrowtransplantsQAs/related_faqs/QAs/688. © Cancerbacup 2003.

315. "What is Leukodystrophy?" National Institute of Neurological Disorders and Stroke. NINDS Leukodystrophy Information Page. Online posting. Accessed 16 Nov. 2007. See <http://www.ninds.nih.gov/disorders/leukodystrophy/leukodystrophy.html>.

316. "What is the health risk of too many carotenoids?" Facts About Dietary Supplements "Vitamin A and Carotenoids," National Institutes of Health Office of Dietary Supplements. Online posting. Accessed 16 Nov. 2007. <http://ods.od. nih.gov/factsheets/vitamina.asp#h8>.

317. "What's in Garden of Life's RM 10 Formulated by Jordan Rubin?" Online posting. Accessed 23 Jun. 2008 <http://www.crohns.net/Miva/productinfo/whatsinR10.shtml>. For the story of Jordan's grandmother, who was cured of advanced ovarian cancer using RM 10, see website: <http://www.crohns.net/Miva/education/testimonial_rosemenlowe.shtml>.

318. "Wheat Germ Extract Inhibits Breast Cancer." Online posting from New Hope Cancer Centers online article of Jun. 7, 2007. Accessed 13 Jan. 2008. "http://www.newhopeblog.com/archives/2007/06/wheat_germ_ext.php>.

319. "Wheat Grass Treatment For Cancer." Cancer Tutor website. Online posting. Alternative Cancer Treatments Information Center™. Accessed 19 Nov. 2007. <http://www.cancertutor.com/Cancer/Wheat grass.html>.

320. "Whole World Botanicals' Product: Royal Camu® (Camu-Camu)." "Camu-Camu." Online listing. Accessed 30 Dec. 2007. <http://www.wholeworldbotanicals.com/info_ royalcamu.html>.

321. "Wobenzyme: what your body has been aching for!" From online posting at website International Antiaging Systems. Accessed 08 Jan 2008. <http:///www.antiaging-systems.com /a2z/wobenzym.htm>.

322. "Wormwood." Alternative Cancer Therapies. Dr. Lam, M.D. at http://www.drlam.com/A3R_brief_in_doc_format/Artemisinin.cfm; info from the Wellness Directory of Minnesota™ website, online posting. Accessed 19 Nov. 2007. <http://www.mnwelldir.org/docs/cancer1 /altthrpy.htm>. Copyright © 1995, 1998, 1999, 2000, 2001, 2002, 2003, 2004 International Wellness Directory.

323. "Xi Shu." Online posting. Accessed 19 Nov. 2007. <http://www.herbs2000.com/herbs/herbs_xi_shu.htm>. © 2002–2007 herbs2000.com.

323a. "Your Cough Medicine May Treat Prostate Cancer." Online posting Dec. 19, 2008. Accessed 20 Dec. 2008. <http://www.scientificblogging.com/news_releases/your_cough_medicine_may _treat_prostate_cancer>. © 2008 ION Publications LLC.

324. "Zeolite: Powerful New Supplement from Volcanic Rock." Online posting. Accessed 25 Oct. 2007. "HUMAN CANCER CASE RESULTS." <http://www.Net/~drbrewer/zeolite.htm >. © 1998-2006 Brewer Science Library.

325. Abernathy, Michael. TIMES-News. "LabCorp develops ovarian cancer screening process." From the TimesNews.com June 24, 2008. "Burlington company works with Yale to create 100 percent effective product, officials say." Online posting. Accessed 24 Jun 2008. <http://www.thetimesnews.com/news/cancer_14926_article.html/ovarian_women.html>. © 2008 Freedom Communication, Inc.

326. Acosta, Dalia. "Scorpion Venom a New Weapon in Fighting Cancer." Online Posting. Accessed 13 Jan. 2008. <http://www.tierramerica.net/2001/0819/iacentos.shtml>.

326a. Adams, Mike. "Grapeseed Extract Kills 76% of Leukemia Cancer Cells in 24 Hours." From an online posting at Natural News website Jan 6, 2009 by Mike Adams, Natural News Editor. Accessed 08, Jan. 2009. <http://www.naturalnews.com/025249.html>. Natural News Network © 2008.

327. Adams, Mike. "Merck Caught in Massive Scientific Fraud as In-House Authors were Disguised as Independent Scientists (opinion)." Online posting from naturalnews.com. 04/18/2008. Accessed 18 Apr. 2008. <http://naturalnews.com/z023052.html>. Natural News Network © 2008.

327a. Adams, Mike. "Why Moxxor makes fish oil, krill oil and many painkiller medications obsolete." From an article at Natural News website. "The safe, natural way to ease inflammation." Online posting. Accessed 8 Jan. 2009. <http://www.naturalnews.com/moxxor_health_benefits.asp>. Natural News Network © 2008. Moxxor can be purchased at website http://www.mymoxxor.com/productListPage.aspx?ID=consumerwellness.

328. Ahmad N, Adhami VM, Afaq F, et al. "Resveratrol causes WAF-1/p21-mediated G(1)-phase arrest of cell cycle and induction of apoptosis in human epidermoid carcinoma A431 cells." Online posting. Clin Cancer Res. 2001 May;7(5):1466-73. From the U.S. National Library of Medicine and National Institutes of Health PubMed NCBI website. Accessed 20 Jan. 2008. <http://www.ncbi.nlm.nih.gov/pubmed/11350919?ordinalpos=1&itool=EntrezSystem2.PEntrez.Pubmed.Pubmed_ResultsPanel.Pubmed_RVAbstractPlus>.

329. Aldersberg, Dr. Jay. "Early Detection of Ovarian Cancer" from "Seven's On Call with Dr. Jay Aldersberg," by Dr. Jay Aldersberg, New York (WABC-TV) from Monday June 23, 2008. Online posting. Accessed 24 June, 2008. <http://abclocal.go.com/wabc/story?section=news/health&id=6222990>. © 2008 WABC-TV/DT.

329a. Aldhous, Peter. "Vitamin C jabs may combat cancer." From an online posting at newscientist.com 08/04/08. Accessed 04 Aug. 2008. <http://www.newscientist.com/article/dn14460-vitamin-c-jabs-may-combat-cancer.html>. © Reed Business Information, Ltd.

330. Anandasabapathy, Sharmila, M.D. "Endoscopic Imaging: Emerging Optical Techniques for the Detection of Colorectal Neoplasia." Posted on 1/8/2008 at medscape.com. "Mortality Rates." Online posting. Accessed 22 Jan. 2008. <http://www.medscape.com/viewarticle/568371>. Copyright © 1994-2008 by Medscape.

331. Andersen, Ella. "Middle-Eastern Herb Effective Against Pancreatic Cancer." From naturalnews.com website 06/04/2008. Online posting. Accessed 3 Jun. 2008. <http://www.naturalnews.com/023348.html>. Natural News Network © 2008.

332. Anderson, Nina. "120 and Healthy! It's Common in the Republic of Georgia." Online posting. Many Hands Feature Articles at the *Alternative Medical Journal of New England.* Accessed 19 Nov. 2007. <http://www.manyhands.com/articles/georgia.html>. © 1995-2000 Many Hands. Per their website, "This information provided by Professor Dr. Zakir Ramazanov, Ph.D., and excerpted from the book *The Secrets of Staying Young* (Safe Goods: 1-800-903-3837)."

333. Antol, Marie N. *Healing Teas: How to Prepare and Use Teas to Maximize Your Health,* (City, State, n.g.) Avery Publishing, Penguin Group (USA), Inc., 1996.

334. Aschhoff B. "Retrospective study of Ukrain treatment in 203 patients with advanced-stage tumors." Online posting. Drugs Exp Clin Res 2000;26(5-6):249-52 from the Villa Medica Clinic of Edenkoben, Germany. At National Health Library's PubMed NCBI site PMID: 11345032. <http://www.ncbi.nlm.nih.gov/pubmed/11345032?Ordinalpos=39&itool=EntrezSystem2.PEntrez.PubMed.PubMed_ResultsPanel.Pubmed_RVDocSum>.

335. Aschoff B. "Ukrain and hyperthermia treatment in a patient with Ewing's sarcoma (case report)." Online posting. Drugs Exp Clin Res. 1998;24(5-6):241-2. Accessed 20 Jan. 2008. From the National Institutes of Health and U.S. National Library of Medicine website PubMed, NCBI –

the PMID is 10190081. <http://www.ncbi.nlm.nih.gov/pubmed/10190081?ordinalpos=1&ito ol=EntrezSystem2.PEntrez.PubMed.PubMed_ResultsPanel.Pubmed_RVAbstractPlus>.

336. Aschoff B. "Ukrain treatment in a patient with stage IV neuroblastoma. A case report." Online posting. Drugs Exp Clin Res. 1998;24(5-6):243-5. From the National Institutes of Health and U.S. National Library of Medicine website PubMed, NCBI. The PMID is 10190082. Access ed 20 Jan. 2008. <http://www.ncbi.nlm.nih.gov/pubmed/10190082?ordinalpos=1&itool=Entre zSystem2.PEntrez.PubMed.PubMed_ResultsPanel.Pubmed_RVAbstractPlug>.

336a. Attiyeh E, London W, Mosse Y, et al. "Chromosome 1p and 11q Deletions and Outcomes in Neuroblastoma." *New England Journal of Medicine.* 2005; 353:2243-2253. Taken from website CancerConsultants.com article: "Chromosome Abnormalities Affect Outcomes of Neuro-blastoma." Online posting 11-29-2005. Accessed 26 Aug 2008. <http://patient.cancerconsul tants.com/CancerNews_Neuroblastoma.aspx?DocumentId=35491>. Copyright © 1998-2008 CancerConsultants.Com.

337. Balch, James F., M.D. *The Super Anti-Oxidants–Why They Will Change the Face of Healthcare in the 21st Century.* New York: M. Evans and Co., Inc., 1998.

338. Balch, Phyllis A., C.N.C and J.F. Balch, M.D. *Prescription for Nutritional Healing.* New York: Avery Publishing, 2000.

339. Baron JA, Cole BF, Mott L, Haile R, et al. Oxford University Press. Ingenta-*connect* website online posting. "Neoplastic and Antineoplastic Effects of Beta-Carotene on Colorectal Adenoma Recurrence: Results of a Randomized Trial." Accessed 26 Dec. 2007. <http://www.ingentacon nect.com/content/oup/jnci/2003/00000095/00000010/art00717>. *Journal of the National Cancer Institute.* Website © 2007 Ingenta.

339a. Barrett, John, M.D. Director, Bone Marrow Transplant Program, National Institutes of Health. "Allogeneic Blood Stem Cell Transplants Using Less Toxic Treatment Regimens (Minitransplants) are a Promising New Cancer Treatment Approach." Online posting from "Cancer Tips" at CancerConsultants.com. Accessed 26 Aug 2008. <http://patient.cancerconsul tants.com/CancerTips.aspx?DocumentId=217 © 1998-2008 CancerConsultants.com.

340. Baroody, Theodore A., N.D., D.C., Ph.D. Nutrition, C.N.C. *Alkalize or Die* – Superior Health Through Proper Alkaline-Acid Balance. Waynesville, N.C: Holographic Health Press, 1991.

341. Batmanghelidj, F., M.D. *Your Body's Many Cries For Water.* Vienna, VA: Global Health Solutions, Inc. 1992, 1995, 1997.

342. Becker, Sue. "Bulk Up On Fiber." Online posting. Accessed 19 Nov. 2007. <http:// www.breadbeckers.com/bulkuponfiber.html>.

343. Beetstra, Sasja, Carolyn Salisbury, Julie Turner, Meryl Altree, Ross McKinnon, Graeme Suthers, and Michael Fenech. "Lymphocytes of BRCA1 and BRCA2 germ-line mutation carriers, with or without breast cancer, are not abnormally sensitive to the chromosome damaging effect of moderate folate deficiency." Molecular Epidemiology and Cancer Prevention. Online publication by Carcinogenesis on 14 Sept. 2005. Online posting. Accessed 25 Jun. 2008. © Their Author 2005. Published by Oxford University Press. <http://carcin.oxfordjournals.org/cgi/cont ent/short/bgi226v1>.

344. Berkson, Bert, M.D., Ph.D. *The Alpha Lipoic Acid Breakthrough.* New York: Prima Publishing, Division of Random House, Inc., 1998.

344a. Berkson, B.M. "A conservative triple antioxidant approach to the treatment of hepatitis C. Combination of alpha lipoic acid (thioctic acid), silymarin, and selenium: three case histories. Online posting from the National Library of Medicine. Accessed 15 May, 2009. <http://www .ncbi.nlb.gov/pubmed/10554539?dopt-abstract.> PubMed ID is 10554539.

344b. Berkson, B.M, Rubin, D.M., Berkson, A.C. "The long term survival of a patient with pancreatic cancer with metastases to the liver after treatment with the intravenous alpha-lipoic acid/low dose Naltrexone protocol." Accessed 16 May, 2009. <http://www.ncbi.nlm.nih.gov/pubmed/16484716?ordinalpos=2&itool=EntrezSystem2.PEntrez.Pubmed.Pubmed_ResultsPanel.Pubmed_DefaultReportPanel.Pubmed.RVDocSum.> PubMed ID is 16484716.

344c. Berkson, B.M., Rubin, D.M., Berkson, A.J. "Reversal of signs and symptoms of B-cell lymphoma in a patient using only low-dose Naltrexone." Accessed 20 May, 2009. <http://www.ncbi.nlm.nih.gov/sites/entrez.> PM ID is 17761642.

345. Best, Billy and Sue Best. "The Boy Who Ran Away From Chemotherapy, Billy's Story." Online posting. Accessed 7 Jan. 2005 and 19 Nov. 2007. <http://wwwgrandstrand.com /suebest/boywho.htm>. © 2004 Grand Strand Information Technologies.

346. Bharat B, Aggarwal, Anjana Bhardwaj, et al. "Role of Resveratrol in Prevention and Therapy of Cancer: Preclinical and Clinical Studies." Anti-cancer Research 2004 online posting. Accessed 25 Jan. 2008. <http://www.agrawal.org/PDF/ACR-Resveratrol1.pdf>. Study from M.D. Anderson Cancer Center and the UCLA Center for Human Nutrition.

347. Bharti, A.C., et al. "Turmeric May Be Effective Adjunct Cancer Therapy." Discount Vitamins and Herbs Health News (from "The Annual Meeting of the American Assoc. for Cancer Research," San Francisco, CA. April 9, 2002. Online posting. Accessed 19 Nov. 2007. <http://www.discount-vitamins-herbs.net/health-news30.htm#123>. Copyright © 2001-2007 Discount Herbs & Vitamins, Inc.

348. Bhatia N, Agarwal C, Agarwal R. "Differential responses of skin cancer chemopreventive agents silibinin, quercetin, and epigallocatechin 3-gallate on mitogenic signaling and cell cycle regulators in human epidermoid carcinoma A431 cells." Online posting from the U.S. National Library of Medicine and National Institutes of Health, PubMed NCBI. NutrCancer 2001;39(2):292-9. Accessed 20 Jan. 2008. <http://www.ncbi.nln.nih.gov/pubmed/.11759294?ordinalpos=1&itool=EntrezSystem2.PEntrez.PubMed.PubMed_ResultsPanel.Pubmed_RVAbstracPlus>.

348a. Birnbauer, William. "Drug Gives New Hope in Breast Cancer Fight." Aug 17, 2008. Online posting. Accessed or retrieved on 19 Aug. 2008. <http://www.theage.com.au/action/printArticle?id=182417>. © 2008 Fairfax Digital.

349. Blackburn, Nicky. "Israeli honey offers hope to cancer patients." From website: Israel21c A Focus Beyond, online posting Jan 21, 2008. Accessed 25 Jun. 2008. <http://www.israel21c.org/bin/en.jsp?enDispWho=Articles%5El1933&enPage=BlankPage&enDisplay=view&enDispWhat=object&enVersion=0&enZone=Health&>. Copyright © 2001–2007 ISRAEL21c.

350. Blauer, Stephen. *The Juicing Book: A Complete Guide to the Juicing of Fruits and Vegetables for Maximum Health.* (City, State, n.g.) Avery Publishing, 1989.

351. Blaylock, Russell. L., M.D. *Natural Strategies For Cancer Patients.* New York: Twin Streams, Kensington Publishing Corp. © 2003.

352. Block, Betsy. "Barley Green: On the Medicinal Benefits of Barley Grass Powder." From an article at healingcancernaturally.com, "Barley Green as Medicine in Cancer And Other Diseases." Online posting. Accessed 16 Jan. 2008. <http://www.healingCancernaturally.com/barley-green-powder-medicine.html>. © 2004, 2005 & 2006 www.healingcancernaturally.com.

353. Bondar GV, Borota AV, Yakovets YL and Zolotukhin SE. "Comparative evaluation of the complex treatment of rectal cancer patients (chemotherapy and X-ray therapy, Ukrain monotherapy)." Online posting. Drugs Exp Clin Res, 1998;24(5-6):221-6. NCBI, National Library of Medicine PubMed website PMID: 10190078. Accessed 20 Jan. 2008. <http://www.ncbi.nlm.nih.gov/pubmed/10190078?ordinalpos=10&itool=EntrezSystem2PEntrez.PubMed.PubMed_ResultsPanel.Pubmed_RVDocSum>.

354. Borek, C., Ph.D. "Beta-glucan Boosts Immunity," by Carmia Borek, Ph.D. Online posting. New Hope Online. Accessed 19 Nov. 2007. <http://www.newhope.com/nutritionsciencenews/NSN_backs/Jan_01/betaglucan.cfm>. From The January 2001 Issue of *Nutrition Science News.* © 2007 Penton Media, Inc.

354a. Bradford, Katie. "Painless zap gives hope in battle against cancer." From *The Canberra Times.* Online posting Nov. 25, 2008. Accessed 27 Nov. 2008. <http://www.canberratimes.com.au/news/local/news/general/painless-zap-gives-hope-in-the-battle-against-cancer/1369152.aspx>. © 2008 Fairfax Media.

355. Brandt, Johanna. *The Grape Cure.* Yonkers, New York: Ehret Literature Publishing Co., Inc., P.O. Box 24, Dobbs Ferry, N.Y., 10522, 1971. Their website is at www.arnoldehret.org.

356. Brandt, Johanna., N.D. *How to Conquer Cancer Naturally.* Joshua Tree, Ca: Tree of Life Publications, 1989.

357. Bridwell, Brenda. "Skin Cancer Cure Using Curaderm BEC5." Online posting at BellaOnline(SM). The Voice of Women Body Care Site. Accessed 07 Jun. 2008. <http://www.bellaonline.com/articles/art56016.asp>.

358. Broadhurst, C. Leigh, Ph.D. *Health and Healing with Bee Products.* Vancouver, Canada: Alive Books, Burnaby BC, 2000.

359. Brown, Anthony J., M.D. Reuters Health. New York, posting date May 23, 2005. "Pomegranate juice shows promise as treatment for recurrent prostate cancer." Accessed 19 November 2007. <http://www.oncolink.com/esources/article.cfm?c=3&s=8&ss=23&id=11913&month=058&year=2005>. Oncolink Cancer News. Last Updated: 2005-05-23 14:00:01-0400 (Reuters Health). © 1994-2007 Trustees of the University of Pennsylvania. Reuters shall not be liable for any errors or delays in the content, or for any actions taken in reliance thereon. © 2007 Reuters Limited.

360. Brown, Arlin J. "Comprehensive Cancer Therapy." Online posting. The Cancer Homepage. Accessed 19 Nov. 2007. <http://www.curezone.com/diseases/cancer/cancer_arlin_therapy.asp>.

361. Browning, Leslie Dru. "A Little Rosemary Can Go a Long Way in Reducing Acrylamides in food." From Natural News website online posting 04/18/08. Accessed 18 April 2008. <http://www.naturalnews.com/z023043.html>. Also see website: http://www.alphagalileo.org and website: http://www.dtu.dk/english.aspx. Truth Publishing, LLC.

361a. Butler S, Oliver D, Youker S. Proceedings from the 2008 annual meeting of the American Academy of Dermatology. February 2008. P2205. Retrieved from an online posting article:

"Patients Undergoing Organ Transplant at Increased Risk for Skin Cancer," 04/28/08 by "Skin Cancer News" CancerConsultants.com website. Accessed 26 Aug 2008. <http://patient.cancer consultants.com/CancerNews_Skin_Cancer.aspx?DocumentId=41917>. © Skin Cancer Information Center on CancerConsultants.com, © Melanoma Cancer Information Center on CancerConsultants.com, © 1998-2008 CancerConsultants.com.

362. Calhoun, Cheri and Maureen Keane. *Juicing For Life.* (City, State, n.g.) Avery, member of Penguin Putnam, Inc., 1992, Trillium Health Products.

363. Carper, Jean. *The Food Pharmacy – Dramatic New Evidence That Food Is our Best Medicine.* New York: Bantam Books, 1988.

364. Carper, Jean. *Miracle Cures: Dramatic New Scientific Discoveries Revealing the Healing Power of Herbs, Vitamins and Other Natural Remedies.* New York: Harper Perennial, 1998 (Harper Collins, 1997).

365. Cathcart, Robert F., M.D. "Vitamin C – Orthomed.com," "Polio (Klenner's Cure 1949)." Online posting. Accessed 26 Nov. 2007. <http://www.orthomed.com>. © 2005 & prior years, Robert F. Cathcart, M.D.

366. Challem, Jack. *All About Carotenoids Beta-Carotene, Lutein & Lycopene.* Garden City Park, N.Y: Avery Publishing, 1999.

367. Cheraskin, E., M.D., D.M.D. *Vitamin C Who Needs It?* Birmingham, AL: Arlington Press & Co., 1993.

368. Chinkwo, KA. "Sutherlands frutescens extracts can induce apoptosis in cultured carcinoma cells." Biochemistry lab at the Department of Biotechnology, University of the Western Cape, Cape Town, South Africa. Online posting. 3 Ethnopharmacol. 2005 (Apr 8;98(1-2):163-70. Accessed 03, April 2008. <http://www.sutherlandia.org/cancer.html>. © 2001–2005 Sutherlandia.org.

369. Clark, Hulda Regehr, Ph.D., N.D. *The Cure For All Cancers: Including Over 100 Case Histories Of Persons Cured*, Chula Vista, CA: New Century Press, 1993.

370. Clark SS, Zhong L, Filiault D, Perman S, Ren Z, Gould M, Yang X. "Anti-leukemic Activity of Perillyl Alcohol in Bcr/Abl-transformed Cells Indirectly Inhibits Signaling Through Mek in a Ras–and Raf-independent Fashion." Online posting. Accessed 26 Nov. 2007. University of Wisconsin Comprehensive Cancer, Madison, WI 53792, PubMed website. Entrez, PubMed, Clin Cancer Res. 2003. <http://www.ncbi.nln.nih.gov/sites/entrez>. PMID 14555523. PubMed - indexed for MEDLINE.

371. Colbert, Don, M.D. *Walking in Divine Healing.* Lake Mary, FL: Siloam, A Strang Co., 1999.

372. Colbert, Don, M.D. *Toxic Relief.* Lake Mary, FL: Siloam, A Strang Co., 2001, 2003.

373. Colbert, Don, M.D. *What You Don't Know May Be Killing You.* Lake Mary, FL: Siloam, A Strang Co., 2000.

374. Condor, Bob. "Researcher: Flax meal beats flax oil to prevent colon cancer." June 4, 2008. Online posting from bartonpublishing.com. Accessed 22 Jun. 2008. <http://www.barton publishing.com/blog/2008/06/04/flax-meal-beats-flax-oil-to-prevent-coloncancer>. © 2008.

375. Connor, John G. "Cancer Prevention and Diet." Online posting. Accessed 26 Nov. 2007. <http://www.compassionateacupuncture.com/cancer.htm>. Copyright © 2005 John G.Connor. Updated Oct. 2004.

376. Coolridge, James. "Pomegranate linked to reducing prostate cancer risk." Online posting May 28, 2008 from arxmanhealth.com website. Accessed 22 Jun. 2008. <http://www.arxman health.com/pomegranate-linked-to-reducing-prostate-cancer-risk/print>. © 2008 Arxman Health Blog.

377. Cordes N, Plasswilm L, Bamberg M, Rodemann HP. "Ukrain, an alkaloid thiophosphoric acid derivative of Chelidonium majus L. protects human fibroblasts but not human tumour cells in vitro against ionizing radiation." Online posting from PubMed website—Int J Radiat Biol. 2002 Jan;78(1):17-27. Accessed 20 Jan. 2008. <http://www.ncbi.nlm.nih.gov/pubmed/1174755 0?ordinalpos=64&itool=EntrezSystem2.PEntrez.PubMed.PubMed_ResultsPanel.Pubmet_RVDo cSum. See the study by Boyko VN, and Zholus RR. "A comparative evaluation of the influence of the complex drug Ukrain and its components on the effects of radiation." Online posting also found at PubMed NCBI website. From the U.S. National Library of Medicine and National Institutes of Health. Accessed 20 Jan. 2008. Drugs Exp Clin Res 1998;24(5-6)331-33. <http:/ /www.ncbi.nlm.nih.gov/pubmed/10190098?ordinalpos=85&Itool=EntrezSystem2.Pentrez.Pub Med.PubMed_ResultsPanel.Pubmed_RVDocSum>.

377a. "Country Doctor Cures Cancer With Baking Soda & Maple Syrup." "Cancer, Cure, Cure for, Alternative Method." Online posting Ashville, N.C. Website "Clayton's Canine Closet." "Country Doctor" is actually a truck driver with no medical degree, but 185 of the patients he has used his simple remedy on (out of 200) with "terminal cancer," lived "at least 15 more years." Accessed 31 Aug 2008. <http://www.claytonscaninecloset.com/cureforcancer>. © Ann Clayton Photographic Imaging Fernley, NV.

378. Daniels, Stephen. 06-17-2008 "Flavonols may slash colorectal cancer risk: study." "An increased intake of anti-oxidant flavonols from tea, onions, beans, and apples may slash the risk of colorectal cancer by a whopping 76 percent, suggests a new US study." Online posting. From Beveragedaily.com website. Accessed 27 Jun. 2008. <http://beveragedaily.com/news/ng.asp?id =85959>. Also see: http://www.beveragedaily.com/Industry-Markets/Flavonols-may-slash-colo rectal-cancer-risk-study. Decisionnewsmedia copyright © 2002/2008 — Decision News Media SAS.

379. Daniels, Stephen. 13-11-2007 "Black Cohosh Stops Breast Cancer Growth in the Lab." From Foodanddrinkeurope.com website. Provided by NutraIngredients.com.Europe.NewsHead lines. Online posting. Accessed 8 Dec. 2007. <http://www.foodanddrinkeurope.com/news/ng.a sp?n=81302&m=1FDEN13&c=eepddtxhp>Decisionnewsmedia © 2002-2007—Decision News Media SAS. The in vitro study was published in *Phytomedicine.* Information was also from *Anti-cancer Research* (Vol. 2, pp. 697-712) and the *International Journal of Cancer* (Vol. 121, pp. 2072-2983).

380. Daniels, Stephen. 6-29-2007 "Low intake of vitamin B6 may increase a man's risk of colorectal cancer by 31 per cent, suggests a study from Japan." Online posting from nutraingredients-usa.com. Accessed 16 Jan. 2008. <http://www.nutraingredients-usa.com/ne ws/ng.asp?n=77795-vitamin-b-folate-colorectal-cancer. © 2002/2008—Decision News Media SAS.

381. Danilos J, Zbroja-Sontag W, Baran E, et al. "Preliminary studies on the effect of Ukrain: (Tris(2-[5bS-(5ba,6b,12ba)]-5b,6,7,12b,13,14-hexahydro-13-methyl[1,3]benzodioxolo[5,6-v[1-3-dio xolo]4,5-I]phenanthridinium-6-ol]-Ethaneaminyl)Phosphinesulfide,6HC l) on the immunological response in patients with malignant tumors." Drugs Exp Clin Res 1992;18 Suppl:55-62. Online posting from the U.S. National Library of Medicine and National Institutes of Health PubMed

NCBI website. PMID 1305046. Accessed 20 Jan. 2008. <http://www.ncbi.nlm.nih.gov/pubmed/1305046?ordinalpos=119&itool=EntrezSystem2.PEntrez.PubMed.PubMed_ResultsPanel.Pubmed_RVDocSum>.

382. Debé, Joseph A., D.C. D.A.C.B.N., C.C.S.P., C.C.N. "Recancostat – Premier Supplement For The 21[st] Century." Online posting. Accessed 23 Jun. 2008. <http://www.pwpgroup.com/recancostat%20description.htm>. © Mar. 19, 1998 by Joseph A. Debé, D.C., D.A.C.B.N., C.C.S.P., C.C.N.

382a. DeNoon, Daniel J. "Food-Poisoning Bug Trained to Attack Tumors." From an online posting Jul. 29, 2008 at WebMD Health News. Accessed 03 Aug. 2008. <http://www.webmed.com/cancer/news/20080729/salmonella-vs-cancer>. Copyright © 2008 WebMD, LLC.

383. DeNoon, Daniel J. "Prostate Cancer Health Center." "New Form of Fiber Fights Cancer - Human Trials Under Way for Citrus-Skin Derivative." WebMD Medical News. Jan 28, 2003. Online posting. Accessed 28 Nov. 2007. <http://www.webmd.com/prostate-cancer/news/20030128/new-form-of-fiber-fights-cancer>.

384. Derbyshire, David. "Three cups of coffee a day 'can cut the risk of ovarian cancer.'" From Dailymail.co.uk – Health article website online posting From Associated Newspapers Ltd. <http://www.dailymail.co.uk/pages/live/articles/health/healthmain.html?in_article_id=509596&in_pageid=1774>. © 2007 Associated Newspapers Ltd.

385. Deoul, Kathleen. "Cancer Cover-Up The Neal Deoul Story." Frequently Asked Questions from cancer-coverup.com. Online posting. Accessed 26 Nov. 2007. <http://www.cancer-coverup.com/faqs/is-this-treatment-safe.htm>. © 2001 Cancer-CoverUp.com.

385a. Doheny, Kathleen, HealthDay Reporter. "Magnesium Sulfate Reduces Threat of Cerebral Palsy." 08/27/2008. Online posting. HealthDay News. Accessed 01 Sept. 2008. <http://www.washingtonpost.com/wp-dyn/content/article/2008/08/27/AR2008082702634.html>. © 1996 - 2008 The Washington Post Company. Their sources for this article: Dwight J. Rouse, M.D., professor of obstetrics and gynecology, University of Alabama at Birmingham; William Zinser, M.D., pediatric neurologist, Children's Medical Center, Dallas, and associate professor of pediatric neonatology, University of Texas Southwestern Medical Center at Dallas; Aug 28, 2008, *New England Journal of Medicine.*

386. Dubin, Reese. From *Miracle Food Cures From The Bible* by Reese Dubin. © 1999 by Prentice-Hall.

387. Duke, James A., Ph.D. *The Green Pharmacy, The Ultimate Compendium of Natural Remedies from the World's Foremost Authority on Healing Herbs.* New York: St. Martin's Paperbacks, 1998, published in arrangement with Rodale Press, Inc.

388. Duke, James A., Ph.D., with Michael Castleman. *The Green Pharmacy-Anti-Aging Prescriptions Herbs, Foods, and Natural Formulas to Keep You Young.* (City, State, n.g.) Rodale Press, Inc., 2001.

389. Dummert, Erin, R.D., C.D. "Flax seeds Reduce Breast Cancer Risk." Jan. 11, 2007. Online posting the Diet Channel. Accessed 9 Jul. 2008. <http://www.thedietchannel.com/flax seed-and-health-flaxseeds-reduce-breast-cancer-risk.htm>.

390. Edelson, Stephen.B., M.D., and Deborah Mitchell. *What Your Doctor May Not Tell You About Immune Disorders: The Revolutionary Drug-free Treatments for Thyroid Disease, Lupus, MS, IBD, Chronic Fatigue, Rheumatoid Arthritis, and Other Diseases.* New York: Warner Books, A Lynn Sonberg Book,

2003. From What Your Doctor May Not Tell You About™ Auto-immune Disorders by Stephen Edelson, M.D. © 2003 by Stephen Edelson and Lynn Sonberg.

391. Eftekhar, J.L. *Heal Yourself.* Globe Digests. Boca Raton, FL and New York: Globe Communications Corp., 1995.

392. Elkins, Rita, M.H. *Healing From the Hive Bee Pollen Royal Jelly Propolis and Honey.* Pleasant Grove, UT: Woodland Publishing, 1996.

393. Elkins, Rita, M.H. Cat's Claw *(Una de Gato),* Pleasant Grove, UT: Woodland Publishing, Inc., 1995.

394. Elkins, Rita, M.H. *D-Glucarate™, Powerful Protector Against Breast and Prostate Cancers.* Pleasant Grove, UT: Woodland Publishing, Inc., 1999.

395. Elkins, Rita, M.H. *Natural Alternatives to HRT.* Orem, UT: Woodland Publishing, 2003.

396. Elkins, Rita, M.H. *Noni (Morinda citrifolia) Prize Herb of Tahiti and the South Pacific.* Pleasant Grove, UT: Woodland Publishing, 1997.

397. Elkins, Rita. *Chinese Red Yeast Rice.* Pleasant Grove, UT: Woodland Publishing, 1998.

398. Evans, Marcus C. "Acai Found to Kill Cancer Cells." Online posting from health-and-diseases.blogspot.com. Accessed 17 Jul. 2008. <http://health-and-diseases.blogspot.com/2008/07/acai-found-to-kill-cancer-cells.html>. Also see article: "Brazilian berry destroys cancer cells in lab, UF study shows," from Jan. 12, 2006 article at University of Florida News http://news.ufl.edu/2006/01/12/berries © University of Florida. Accessed 29 Jul. 2008. Writer, Tom Nordlie; Source: Stephen Talcott and Joshua Bomser.

399. Evans, Tony. *Tony Evans Speaks Out on Fasting.* Chicago: Moody Press, 2000.

400. Forgionne, Guisseppi. A., Ph.D. "Nutritional Therapy for Primary Peritoneal Cancer: A Case Study." From the CancerLynx website. Jul. 8, 2002. Online posting. Accessed 26 Nov. 2007. <http://www.cancerlynx.com/peritonealcase.html>.

401. Fox, Maggie. "Accidental fungus leads to promising cancer drug." Jun 29, 2008, from Reuters.com online posting. Accessed 29 Jun. 2008. <http://www.reuters.com/article/marketsNews/idUSN2936154720080629?pageNumber=3&>. Copyright © Thomson Reuters 2008.

402. Fox, Marilyn. "Multiple Sclerosis Testimonials." Online posting. Accessed 26 Nov. 2007. <http://www.watercure2.org/multiple_sclerosis.htm>.

402a. Frassoni F, Gualandi F, Podesta M, et al. "Direct intrabone transplant of unrelated cord-blood cells in acute leukemia: a Phase I/II study." Lancet Oncology, online publication. Aug 9 2008. DOI:10. 1016/S1470-2045(08)70180-3. Also, see Daily Cancer News website article: "Injection of Umbilical Cord Stem Cells into Bone Appears Promising for Leukemia." Online posting 08-12-2008. Accessed 26 Aug 2008. <http://patient.cancerconsultants.com/CancerNews.aspx?DocumentId=42450&Keywords=cancer,news,information,treatment,umbilical%20cord,stem%20cells,leukemia,acute,allogeneic,transplant>. © 1998-2008 CancerConsultants.com.

403. Freya Walter, Antje Clausnitzer, Bora Akoglu, et al. "Piceatannol, a Natural Analog of Resveratrol, Inhibits Progression through the S Phase of the Cell Cycle in Colorectal Cancer Cell Lines." From Journal *Nutrition* online posting. Accessed 24 Jan. 2008. <http://wwjn.nutrition.org/cgi/content/abstract/132/2/298>. Also see Mar Larrosa, Franciso A, Tomas-Barberan, et al.

"The grape and wine polyphenol piceatannol is a potent inducer of apoptosis in human SK-mel-28 melanoma cells." From the *European Journal of Nutrition* Vol 43, Number 5, Oct 2004 pp. 275-284. Publisher is given as *Steinkopff* – and publication date online 2-19-2004. Accessed 24 Jan. 2008. <http://www.springerlink.com/content/patxrdbrgml9yacg/>. Copyright © Springer, Part of Springer Science+Business Media.

404. Gale, K. Reuters Health. "Herbal COX-2 Inhibitor Induces Prostate Cancer Cell Apoptosis." 29 Jul. 2003, Online Posting. Oncolink – Abramson Cancer Center of the Univ. of Pennsylvania. "Prostate Cancer." Copyright 1994-2007 © Trustees of the University of PA. Acce ssed 26 Nov. 2007.<http://www.oncolink.com/resources/article.cfm?c=3&s=8&ss=23&id=9953&month=07 &year=2003>. © 2005 Reuters Limited. Reuters shall not be liable for any errors or delays in the content, or for any actions taken in reliance thereon.

405. Gardiner, Eric. *How I conquered Cancer – A Naturopathic Alternative.* Houston, TX: Emerald Ink Publishing, 1997.

406. Gittleman, Ann Louise, M.S. *Natural Healing For Parasites.* New York: Healing Wisdom Publications, 1995.

407. Getsinger, Annie. H & R Staff Writer. Herald Review online posting. Accessed 16 Jan. 2008. "TheraSphere vial packs a big punch against cancer." Herald&Review.com. "Central Illinois #1 News Source!" From Decatur, Illinois. <http://www.herald-review.com/articles/2008/01/16/lifefeatures/1029341.txt>. © 1996-2007 Herald & Review, Decatur, Il, a division of Lee Enterprises.

407a. Goh Yl, Bollano E, Einarson TR, et al. "Prenatal multivitamin supplementation and rates of pediatric cancers: A meta-analysis." *Clinical Pharmacology and Therapeutics*, online posting, Feb 21, 2007. DOI: 10:1038/sj.clpt.6100100. From "Neuroblastoma News" CancerConsultants.com website 02/23/07. Accessed 26 Aug 2008. <http://patient.cancerconsultants.com/CancerNews _Neuroblastoma.aspx?DocumentId=39373>. Copyright © Brain Cancer Information Center on CancerConsultants.com. © Leukemia Information Center on CancerConsultants.com. © 1998 - 2008 CancerConsultants.Com.

408. Gordon, Serena. HealthDay Reporter. "Vitamin K Might Prevent Liver Cancer." Online posting. Accessed 26 Nov. 2007. <http://news.healingwell.com/?p=news1&id=520187. From Healingwell.com website. © 1999-2007 Healingwell.com. © 1999-2007 e-Healthcare Solutions.

409. Gottlieb, Bill. *Alternative Cures – The Most Effective Natural Home Remedies for 160 Health Problems.* (City, State, n.g.) Rodale, Inc., 2000.

410. Griffin, G. Edward. "The Laetrile 'Quacks.'" From the book *World Without Cancer* Ch. 8. Online posting from WWC England, World Without Cancer website. "The Story of Vitamin B17." Accessed 30 Nov. 2007. <http://www.worldwithoutcancer.org.uk/quacks.html>. © 2000 and 2001 Worldwithoutcancer.org.uk.

411. Griffith, H. Winter, M.D. *Vitamins, Herbs, Minerals & Supplements, The Complete Guide.* Rev. Edition. (City, State, n.g.) Fisher Books, Member of Perseus Books Group, 1988, 1998.

412. Groth, Robert. "6 Risk Factors for Multiple Sclerosis." Ezine Articles®. Online posting. Accessed 27 Mar 2008. <http://ezinearticles.com/?6-Risk-Factors-for-Multiple-Sclerosis&id=782577> © 2008 EzineArticles.com.

413. Gupta, C. "The FDA versus Folic Acid." Share the Wealth, July 14, 2003. Online posting. Accessed 26 Nov. 2007. <http://www.newmediaexplorer.org/chris/2003/07/14/the_fda_versus_folic_acid.htm>.

414. Gupta, Chris. "The FDA Versus Folic Acid – Share The Wealth." "It's time to revolt." Online posting. Accessed 26 Nov. 2007. <http://www.newmediaexplorer.org/chris/2003/07/14/the_fda_versus_folic_acid.htm>.

415. Gursche, Siegfried. *Fantastic Flax, A Powerful Defense Against Cancer, Heart Disease and Digestive Disorders.* Burnaby BC V5J 5B9: Vancouver, Canada: Alive Books, 2003.

416. Gursche, Siegfried. *Good Fats and Oils, Why We Need Them and How to Use Them in the Kitchen.* Vancouver, Canada: Alive Books, 2000.

417. Gutierrez, David. "Acrylamides From Fried, Grilled Foods Linked to Ovarian Cancer." From NaturalNews.com online posting. Accessed 24 Jun. 2008. <http://www.naturalnews.com/z023500.html>. © 2003, 2004, 2005, 2006 by Truth Publishing, Inc. ("Natural News.")

418. Gutierrez, David. "Berries and Onions Slash Pancreatic Cancer Risk By Up To 59 Percent." Online posting from naturalnews.com 12/11/2007. Accessed 27 Jun. 2008. Truth Publishing, LLC. © 2003-2006 by Truth Publishing, Inc. ("Natural News.")

419. Gutierrez, David. "French Volcanic Clay Kills Antibiotic-Resistant MRSA Superbug." Online posting from naturalnews.com website. Accessed 18 Apr. 2008. <http://www.naturalnews.com/z023022.html>. © 2003, 2004, 2005, 2006 by Truth Publishing, Inc. ("Natural News.")

420. Gutierrez, David. "How Drug Companies Covertly Influence the Content of Medical Literature," 04/16/08. Online posting. Accessed 18 Apr. 2008. <http://www.naturalnews.com/z023033.html>. Natural News Network © 2008.

421. Gutierrez, David. "Painkiller Patch Fentanyl May Have Killed 3,500 People, Warns FDA." Jul. 17, 2008 online posting from natural news.com. Accessed 17 Jul. 2008. <http://www.naturalnews.com/023649.html>. Natural News Network © 2008.

422. Guzman, Monica L, Rossi, Randall M, et al. "The sesquiterpene lactone parthenolide induces apoptosis of human acute myelogenous leukemia stem and progenitor cells." Online posting from *Blood Journal* 1 Jun 2005, Vol. 105, No. 11, pp. 4163-4169. Accessed 01 Jan. 2008. <http://bloodjournal.hematologylibrary.org/cgi/content/full/105/11/4163>. See the article: *Parthenolide* by Ray Sahelian, M.D. "Parthenolide benefits Parthenolide Research Update," online posting. Accessed 01 Jan. 2008. <http://www.ray sahelian.com/parthenolide.html>, which gives source as *Blood* online Feb. 1, 2005.

423. Hall, Celia, Medical Editor. "I've seen herbal remedy make tumours disappear, says Respected cancer doctor." Telegraph.co.uk website online posting – last updated 20/09/2004. Accessed 13 Jan. 2008. <http://www.telegraph.co.uk/news/main.Jhtml?xml=/news/2004/09/20/ncarc20.xml>. © Copyright of Telegraph Media Group Ltd 2008.

423a. Halliday, Jess. "Bilberry and pine bark combo wards off glaucoma: study." From website NUTRAUSA ingredients.com 24 Jul 2008. Accessed 20 Aug 2008. <http://www.nutraingredients-usa.com/Research/Bilberry-and-pine-bark-combo-wards-off-glaucoma-study>. Decision News Media. © 2000/2008-Decision News Media SAS.

424. Hamler F., Hiesmayr W., Korsh O., Melnyk A. "Ukrain monotherapy in malignant melanoma (case report)." Online posting from www.pubmed.gov. Accessed 21 Dec. 2007. <http ://www.ncbi.nlm.gov/sites/entrez>. PMID 8899338.

425. See website gentlecures.org

426. Hawken, C.M. *Green Foods, "Phyto Foods" for Super Health*. Pleasant Grove, UT: Woodland Publishing, 1998.

427. Hayes, Norvel. *Worship Your Foundation For The Victorious Life.* Tulsa, OK: Harrison House, 1997.

428 Heinerman, John. *Healing Power of Herbs.* Boca Raton, FL: Globe Digests, Globe Communications Corp., 1995.

429. Heinerman, John. *Heinerman's Encyclopedia of Healing Juices,* New York: Reward Books by Penguin Putnam, Inc., 1994.

430. Heinerman, John. *Heinerman's New Encyclopedia of Fruits & Vegetables,* Reward Books 1995, p. 75 by Penguin Putnam, Inc., New York, 1995.

431. Hoffer, Abram, M.D., Ph.D., "Clinical Procedures in Treating Terminally Ill Cancer Patients with Vitamin C." Supportive Vitamin C Therapy for Cancer Patients. Online posting. Accessed 27 Nov. 2007. <http://www.doctoryourself.com/hoffer_cancer_ 2.html>.

432. Hoffer, Abram, M.D., Ph.D., "Hoffer's Home Page - Orthomolecular Treatment of Cancer." Online posting. Accessed 27 Nov. 2007. <http://www.islandnet.com/~hoffer>.

433. Hoffer, Abram, M.D., Ph.D., with Linus Pauling, Ph.D. *Healing Cancer—Complementary Vitamin & Drug Treatments*, Toronto, Ontario Canada: CCNM Press, Inc. 2004.

434. Hong, S.A., Kim M.K., et al., in J Cancer 2007 Oct. 17. "Breast Cancer, Postmenopausal - Eating More Mushrooms May Reduce the Risk of Breast Cancer in Post-menopausal Women." From Vitasearch-Clinical Pearls. Online posting. Accessed 4 Nov. 2007. <http://search. vitasearch.com/search?q=mushrooms&restrict=Summaries&btnG=Search&>. Also, see website: www.vitasearch.com/get-clp-summary/36794.

435. Howenstine, James, M.D. 12/23/03. "USE OF CoQ10 TO TREAT MALIGNANCIES." NewsWithViews.com website online posting. Accessed 20 Mar. 2008. <http://www.newswithvi ews.com/Howenstine/james2.htm>. Copyright © 2003 Dr. James Howenstine.

436. Hunsberger, Mae Eydie with C. Loeffler. *How I Conquered Cancer Naturally*, Garden City Park, N.Y.: Avery Publishing Group, Inc., 1992.

437. Isaacs, Tony. "Father of the 'Oleander Soup' Cancer Remedy." Online posting. Accessed 03, Apr. 2008. <http://www.buzzle.com/articles/father-of-the-oleander-soup-cancer-remedy.html>. © 2000-2007, 2008 Buzzle.com®.

438. Isaacs, Tony. "Mushrooms for Health Immune System and Cancer." "Yun Zhi Mushroom." 10/29/2007online posting from disabled-world.com website. Accessed 09 Apr. 2008. <http:// disabled-world.com/artman/publish/printer/printer_mushrooms.shtml>. Copyright © www. disabled-world.com.

439. Jaehnig, K.C. "Ginseng Root May Help Slow Growth of Cancer Cells." Jan. 11, "Promising Research From SIUC." Online posting. Accessed 27 Nov. 2007. <http://news.siu.edu/news/January05/011105kj4109.htm>. Copyright © 2003. Board of Trustees, Southern Illinois University. Last updated Apr. 12, 2005. From Board of Trustees, Southern Illinois University, Carbondale.

440. Jegtvig, Shareen. "Quercetin." "What is Quercetin and What are the Health Benefits." Online posting. Updated Jun. 1, 2007. From website About.com: Nutrition. Accessed 28 Nov. 2007. <http://nutrition.about.com/od/phytochemicals/p/quercetin profil.htm>.

441. Kadan P., Korsh OB., Hiesmayr W. "Ukrain in the treatment of urethral recurrent carcinoma (case report)." From www.pubmed.gov. Online posting. Accessed 21 Dec. 2007. <htt p://www.ncbi.nlm.nih.gov/sites/entrez>. PMID 8899346.

442. Kadan P., Korsh OB., Melnyk A. "Ukrain therapy of recurrent breast cancer with lung metastases (case report)." From www.pubmed.gov. Online posting. Accessed 21 Dec. 2007. <http://www.ncbi.nlm.nih.gov/sites/entrez>. PMID 8899340.

442a. Kahaleh M, Mishra R, Shami VM, et al. "Unresectable cholangiocarcinoma: comparison of survival in biliary stenting alone versus stenting with photodynamic therapy." *Clinical Gastroenterol ogy and Hepatology* online posting 2008 Mar; 6(3):290-7. Feb 6, 2008. Retrieved from "Liver Cancer News–CancerConsultants.com" online posting 05/05/08. "New Treatment Combination for Bile Duct Cancer May Improve Survival." <http://patient.cancerconsultants.com/CancerNews_Live r_Cancer.aspx?DocumentId=41944>. © Liver Cancer Information Center on CancerConsultants. com, © 1998-2008 CancerConsultants.com.

443. Keegan, Lynn, Ph.D., R.N. *Healing Nutrition.* Albany, N.Y: Delmar – A Division of Thomas Learning, www.thomsonrights.com. Fax 800-730-2215. From *Healing Nutrition* 2nd Edition by KEEGAN. © 2002.

444. Keenan, Sophia. "Breakthrough in Ovarian Cancer Fight." Online posting from eNews2.0. Accessed 15 Dec. 2007. <http://www.enews20.com/news_Breakthrough_in_Ovarian_Cancer_ Fight_04416.html>. © 2007 - eNews 2.0.

444a. Kerfoot, Jessica. From the Burzynski Patient Group website online posting at: <http://burzynskipatientgroup.org/jessicak.htm>. Accessed 12 Dec. 2008.

445. Kiefer, Dale. "A New Weapon to Fight Prostate Cancer." Online posting. Accessed 23 Oct. 2007.<http://search.lef.org/cgi-src-bin/MsmGo.exe?grab_id=0&page_id=972&query=milk%>. Also, see LE Magazine Nov. 2005.

446. Kimura Y, Okuda H. "Resveratrol isolated from Polygonum cuspidatum root prevents tumor growth and metastasis to lung and tumor-induced neovascularization in Lewis lung carcinoma-bearing mice." Online posting from NCBI, PubMed. J. Nutr 2001 Jun;131(6):1844-9. PMID 11385077. Accessed 20 Jan. 2008. <http://www.ncbi.nlm.nih.gov/pubmed/11385077?ordinalpos=1&itool=EntrezSystem2.PEntrez.PubMed.Pubmed_ResultsPanel.Pubmed_RVAbstrac tPlus>.

447. Kimura Y. Kido T, Takaku T, Sumiyoshi M, Baba K. "Isolation of an anti-angiogenic substance from Agaricus blazei Murrill: its antitumor and antimetastatic actions." Online posting. Cancer Sci 2004 Sep;95(9):758-64, from U.S. National Library of Medicine and the National Institutes of Health PubMed NCBI website. Accessed 20 Jan 2008 PMID 15471563. <http://www.ncbi.nlm.nih.gov/pubmed/15471563?ordinalpos=1&itool=EntrezSystem2.PEntrez.Pubmed.Pubmed_ResultsPanel_RVAbstractPlus.

448. Kimura Y. Taniguchi M, Baba K. "Antitumor and antimetastatic activities of 4-hydroxyderricin isolated from Angelica keiskei roots." Plants Med 2004 Mar;70(3):211-9. From PubMed NCBI website online posting - The U.S. National Library of Medicine and Institutes of Health. Accessed 20 Jan. 2008. <http://www.ncbi.nlm.nih.gov/pub med/15114497?ordinalpos= 1&itool=EntrezSystem2.PEntrez.PubMed.PubMed_ResultsPanel.Pubmed_RVAbstractPlus>.PMID 15114497.

449. Koerth-Baker, Maggie and Laurel Mills. "Deadly critters that might save your life," "mental_floss." "2. Scorpions: Leading the battle against brain cancer." Online posting updated Apr. 8, 2008. Accessed 9 Apr. 2008. From CNN.com/living. <http://www.cnn.com/2008/ LIVING/wayoflife/04/08/deadly.animals/>. Copyright © MENTAL FLOSS LLC.

450. Kolata, Gina and Andrew Pollack. Health article "Costly Cancer Drug Offers Hope, but Also a Dilemma." From an online posting of the New York Times July 6, 2008. Accessed 8 Jul. 2008. <http://www.nytimes.com/2008/07/06/health/06avastin.html?_r=1&em&em=12154032 00&en=61fb&oref=slogin. Copyright © 2008 The New York Times Company.

451. Kowalska, Elzbieta, Steven A. Narod, Tomaz Huzarski, Stanislaw Zajaczek, Jowita Huzarska, Bohdan Gorski and Jan Lubinski. "Increased Rates of Chromosome Breakage in BRCA1 Carriers Are Normalized by Oral Selenium Supplementation." Online posting at Cancer Epidemiology, Biomarkers & Prevention website Vol. 14, 1302-1306, May 2005. © American Association for Cancer Research. Accessed 25 June 2008. <http://cebp.aacrjournals.org/cgi/content/full/14/5 /1302>.

452. Kradjian, R.M., M.D. "The Milk Letter: A Message To My Patients," from Dr. Robert M. Kradjian, M.D. *Breast Surgery,* Chief Div. of General Surgery, Seton Medical Centre #302 – 1800 Sullivan Ave., Daly City, CA 94015 USA. Online posting. Accessed 27 Nov. 2007. <http://www .notmilk.com/Kradjian.html>. Article courtesy of Dr. Kradjian and <http://www.apafitness .com/articles/MILKDOC.HTM>.

453. Kramer, T.A., M.D. "Understanding Clinical Trials in Context." Posted 10/02/03, from Medscape General Medicine™, Medscape from WebMD. Online posting. Accessed 27 Nov. 2007. "Medscape Psychopharmacology Today." <http://www.medscape.com/viewarticle/462 046_3>. "Support and Sponsorship." From *Medscape General Medicine* 5(4), 2003 <http://www. medscape.com/viewarticle/462046>. © 2003 Medscape and © 1994-2007 by Medscape.

454. Kroeger, Hanna, Ms.D. *Free Your Body of Tumors and Cysts.* (City, State, n.g.) Hanna Kroeger Publications, 1997.

455. Kroeger, Hanna. *Parasites The Enemy Within.* (City, State, n.g.) Hanna Kroeger Publications, 1991.

456. Kroiss T, Melnyk A, Korsh OB. "Ukrain treatment in carcinoma of the cervix (case report)." Online posting from National Library of Medicine NCBI PubMed. Drugs Exp Clin Res 1996;22(3-5):255-7. Accessed 20 Jan. 2008. <http://www.ncbi.nlm.nih.gov/pubmed/8899342?Ordinal pos=4&itool=EntrezSystem2.P.Entrez.PubMed.PubMed_ResultsPanel.Pubmed_RVDocSum>. PMID 8899342.

457. Krystosik, James, D. C. *Nature's Prescription for Over 60 Diseases - Grape Seed and Pine Bark Extract* (The prior title of this book was: *Pycnogenols Pine Bark (OPC's) Grape Seed (OPC's) "Superstar Anti-oxidants."* Garrettsville, OH: Good News Press, 1995.

458. Kulik GI. "Comparative in vitro study of the effects of the new antitumor drug Ukrain and several cytostatic agents on the thiol groups in the tissue of Guerin carcinoma and its resistance to

cisplatin variant." Drugs Exp Clin Res 1998;24(5-6):277-80. Online posting from the U.S. National Library of Medicine and Institutes of Health PubMed NCBI website. Accessed 20 Jan. 2008. <http://www.ncbi.nlm.nih.gov/pubmed/10190087?ordinalpos=56&itool=EntrezSystem2.entrez.PubMed.PubMed_ResultsPanel.Pubmed_RVDocSum>. PMID 10190087.

459. Kumagai, Takashi, Claudia Muller, Julian C. Desmond, Yasufumi Imai, David Heber, H. Phillip Koeffler. "Scutellaria baicalensis, a herbal medicine: Anti-proliferative and apoptotic activity against acute lymphocytic leukemia, lymphoma and myeloma cell lines." Online posting. Accessed 24 Dec. 2007. Leukemia Research website <http://www.lrjournal.com/article/PIIS0145212606003365/abstract>. Volume 31, Issue 4. Apr. 2007 pp. 523-530. © 2007 Elsevier, Inc.

460. Laino, Charlene. MSNBC, "Chinese Folk Remedy Fights Cancer - Plant Compound Sparks Chain Reaction That Kills Tumor Cells." Dec. 4 (year n.g.) Online posting. Accessed 27 Nov. 2007. Dr. Eliaz News Article <http://www.DrEliaz.com>. "News Room." © 2007 by Dr. Eliaz.

461. Lam, Michael, M.D. "Medicinal Mushrooms." "Cancer and Immunity." Online posting. "An Insider's Guide to Natural Medicine." Accessed 27 Nov. 2007. <http://www.drlam.com/A3R_brief_in_doc_format/cancer_and_immunity.cfm>. © 2001–2004 by Dr. Michael Lam, M.D.

462. Lanvers-Kaminsky C, Nolting DM, Koster J, et al. "In vitro toxicity of Ukrain Against human Ewing tumor cells lines." Online posting. Anti-cancer Drugs, 2006 Oct;17(9):1025-30. Accessed 20 Jan. 2008. From the National Institutes of Health and U.S. National Library of Med icine website PubMed NCBI – PMID 17001175. <http://www.ncbi.nlm.nih.gov/pubmed/1700 1175?ordinalpos=1&itool=EntrezSystem2.PEntrez.PubMed.PubMed_ResultsPanel.Pubmed_RVAbstractPlus>. PMID 17001175

463. LeBeau, Conrad. *Hydrogen Peroxide & Ozone.* 13th Edition. West Allis, WI: Vital Health Publications, 2001.

464. Lee, Deborah. *JUICING Your Liquid Nutritional Supplement.* Pleasant Grove, UT: Woodland Publishing, 1998.

465. Lee, John R., M.D., et al. *What Your Doctor May Not Tell You About Breast Cancer How Hormone Balance Can Help Save Your Life* - New York: from What Your Doctor May Not Tell You About Breast Cancer by Dr. John Lee, M.D., Virginia Hopkins, M.A. and David T. Zava, Ph.D., Warner Books, Inc., 2002. © 2002 by John R. Lee, M.D., Virginia Hopkins, M.A. and David T. Zava, Ph.D

466. Lee, John R., M.D. with Virginia Hopkins. *What Your Doctor May Not Tell You About™ Menopause – The Breakthrough Book on Natural Progesterone.* New York: Warner Books, Inc., 1996. From What Your Doctor May Not Tell You About Menopause, by Dr. John Lee, M.D. © 1996 by John R. Lee, M.D. and Virginia Hopkins.

466a. LeMasters GK, Genaidy AM, Succop P, et al. "Cancer Risk Among Firefighters: A Review and Meta-Analysis of 32 Studies." *Journal of Occupational and Environmental Medicine.* 2006;48:1189-1202. Retrieved from an online article posted 11/15/06 by "Testicular Cancer News - CancerConsultants.com" website. Retrieved or accessed on 26 Aug 2008. Article: "Firefighters Face Increased Risk of Cancer." <http://patient.cancerconsultants.com/CancerNews_Testicular_Cancer.aspx?DocumentId=38563>. © 1998-2008 Cancer Consultants.com.

466b. Levy, Thomas, M.D. "Vitamin C For Heart, Cancer & Infectious Diseases." From a speech given by Dr. Levy at the 35th Annual Cancer Convention – Sept. 1-4, 2007, the Cancer Control Society.

467. Ley, Beth M., Ph.D. *Bilberry & Lutein: the Vision Enhancers Protect Against Cataracts, Macular Degeneration, Glaucoma, Retinopathy & Other Health Problems,* B. L. Publications, 2001.

468. Liau, Dr. Ming C. "CDA II - a type of urine therapy & nutrition." Article "Chapter 2: the history of my struggle and CDA II." "Determination to find a CURE FOR CANCER." From the book: *CDA II, The Smart Cancer Drug* by Dr. Ming C. Liau, 1999. Online posting. Accessed 28 Nov. 2007. <http://www.brave-souls.com/learn-from-others>.

469. Lieberman, Shari. Ph.D. and K. Balbal, C.N. *Maitake Mushroom AND D-Fraction.* Pleasant Grove, UT: Woodland Publishing, 2001.

470. Lin, P. F. "Antitumor effect of actinidia chinensis polysaccharide on murine tumor." Institute of Molecular Medicine, Zhejiang College of Traditional Chinese Medicine, Pangzbou, PubMed website, NCBI, National Library of Medicine. Online posting. Entrez PubMed, 1: Zhonghua Zhong Liu Za Zhi. 1988 Nov;10(6):441-4, PMID: 2855056. Accessed 27 Nov. 2007. <http://www.ncbi.nlm.nih.gov/entrez/query.fcgi?cmd=Retrieve&db=PubMed&dopt=Abstract&list_uids=2855056&query_hl=33>.

471. Liu, R.H. *Cornell News,* "Onions anti-cancer effects." Article name: "Onion a day keeps doctor away? Cornell researchers find some onions do indeed have anti-cancer benefits." Online posting. Accessed 25 December 2007. <http://www.news.cornell.edu/releases/Oct04/onions/cancer.ssl.html>.

472. Lockwood, K, S. Moesgaard and K. Folkers. "Partial and complete regression of breast cancer in patients in relation to dosage of coenzyme Q10." PubMed, NCBI, Biochem Biophys Res Commun. 1994 Mar 30;199(3):1504-8, p 1. Online posting. Accessed 27 Nov. 2007. <http://www.ncbi.nlm.nih.gov/sites/entrez>. PMID: 7908519.

473. Lockwood, K., S. Moesgaard, T. Yamamoto and K. Folkers. . "Progress on therapy of breast cancer with vitamin Q10 and the regression of metastases." PubMed, NCBI Online posting. Entrez PubMed, Biochem Biophys Res Commun 1995 Jul. 6;212(1)72-7. Accessed 27 Nov. 2007. <http://www.ncbi.nlm.nih.gov/entrez/query.fcgi?cmd=Retrieve&db=pubmed&dopt=Abstract&list_uids=7612003>.

474. Maintz D, R. Fischbach, et al. "Results of electrochemical therapy of colorectal liver metastases in rats followed up by MRI." From the Department of Diagnostic Radiology, University of Cologne Medical School in Germany. Online posting from PubMed website May 2000. Accessed 25 Feb. 2008. Invest Radiol. 2000 May;35(5):289-94. Indexed for MEDLINE. PMID 10803669. <http://www.ncbi.nlm.nih.gov/pubmed/10803669>.

475. Malkmus, Rev. George. "From Death to Life - A Miraculous Recovery." Rita Myers. Back to the Garden – Teaching Health From a Biblical Perspective. Hallelujah Acres - Publisher: Rev. George H. Malkmus, Fall 2004, Issue #29.

476. Malkmus, Rev. George. "How to Eliminate Sickness Seminar." "Hallelujah Acres Brings You Back to the Garden: the biblical natural diet." Online posting. Accessed 27 Nov. 2007. <http://hallelujahacres.org/publications/showtip.asp?tipid=387>.

477. Martarelli D., Martarelli B., Pediconi D., Nabissi M., Erfumi M., Pompeii P. "Hypericum perforatum methanolic extract inhibits growth of human prostatic carcinoma cell line orthotopically implanted in nude mice." *Cancer Letters* 210(1):27-33, Jul. 8, 2004, from Positive Health Magazine. "Integrated Medicine for the 21st Century." Online posting. Accessed 27 Nov. 2007. <http://www.positivehealth.com/research-view.php?researchid=3318>. © Positive Health Publications Ltd., 1994-2007.

478. McAllister, Emmalyn. "What You Must Know." "MGN-3: Personal Stories of Healing." Online posting. Accessed 28 Dec. 2007. <http://www.polymvasurvivors.com/what_you_know_mgn3_article2.html>. © 2000.

479. McArthur, Grant. "Australian cancer breakthrough will save women's lives." Jun. 04, 2008 from an online posting of the Herald Sun – website www.news.com.au. Accessed 22 Jun. 2008. <http://news.com.au/heraldsun/story/0,21985,23806750-661,00.html>. © Herald and Weekly Times.

480. McCoppin, Robert. "New Loyola treatment freezes cancer in its (gastro intestinal) tracts." Online posting from the dailyherald.com. 8 Jul. 2008. Accessed 10 Jul. 2008. <http://www.daily herald.com/story/?id=216347&src=1>. © 2008 Daily Herald, Inc.

481. McKenzie Jr., Donald. "Red Meat Connected to More Kinds of Cancer." 1-19-2008. "Updated Health News." Online posting. Accessed 19 Jan. 2008. <http:/Ezinearticles.com /?Red-Meat-Connected-to-More-Kinds-of-Cancer&id=878171>. © 2008 E-zineArticles.com.

482. Martin, Daniel. "The prostate cancer 'wonder pill' set to save thousands every year." Online posting from "Mail Online" health - 29 Jul. 2008. Accessed 29 Jul. 2008. <http: //www.mailons unday.co.uk/textbased/health/article-1037074/The-prostatecancer-wonder-pill-set-save-thousan ds-year.html>. © 2008 Associated Newspapers Ltd.

483. Martin, Ray. "The doctor many believe can cure cancer - 9 August 2004 - Reporter: Ray Martin." Online posting. Accessed 13 Jan. 2008. <http://www.cam.net.uk/home/aaa315/heal ing/john-holt-cancer-treatment.htm>.

483a. Medieros, Angela. "Epigenetics: A New Search Begins." Online posting Aug 21, 2008. Accessed 21 Aug 2008. From *Today's CAREGIVER. Magazine,* Jan-Feb 2008, <http: //www.caregiver.com/magazine/2008/jan-feb/epigenetics.htm>. © Caregiver.com, Inc. 1995-2008.

483b. Mercola, Dr. Joseph. "Alpha Lipoic Acid – One Powerful Antioxidant." Online posting. Accessed 20 May, 2009. <http://blogs.mercola.com/sites/vitalvotes/archive/2009/04/27/Alp ha-Lipoic-Acid--One-Powerful-Antioxidant.aspx.> © 2009 Dr. Joseph Mercola.

483c. Mercola, Dr. Joseph. "Drug Company Had Hit List for Doctors Who Criticized them." Online posting 04--23-2009. Accessed 13 June, 2009 <http://articles.mercola.com /sites/articles/archive/2009/04/23/Drug-Company-Had-Hit-List-for-Doctors-Who-Criticized-Them.aspx>. Copyright © by Joseph Mercola.

484. Mercola, Dr. Joseph. "Sunlight Actually Prevents Cancer." 04-03-02. Online Posting. Accessed 27 Nov. 2007. <http://www.mercola.com/2002/apr/3/sun_prevents_cancer.htm>. *Cancer* March 2002;94:1867-75.

485. Mercola, Dr. Joseph. "High Quality Chlorella." Online posting. Accessed 27 Nov. 2007. <http://www.mercola.com/chlorella>. © 2007 Dr. Joseph Mercola.

486. Mercola, Dr. J. "The Benefits of Probiotics 9/29/04." Issue 573. Online posting. Accessed 28 Nov. 2007. <http://www.mercola.com/2004/sept/29/probiotics_benefits.htm. © 2007 Dr. Joseph Mercola.

487. Merkle, Jason, Jay and Patty Merkle. "Jason Merkle," from Burzynski Patient Group stories website. Online posting. Accessed Nov. 2005, Mar, Apr. 2008 and Jun. 2008. <http://www. Burzynskipatientgroup.org/jasonm.html>.

488. Meschino, James, D.C., M.S. "Chinese Skullcap: A Viable Adjunct to Cancer Treatment." Online posting. Accessed 25 Dec. 2007. Dynamic Chiropractic 2007. Date website says this was last modified was 01-Oct-2007. <http://www.Chiro web.com/archives/21/22/10.html>.

489. Metz, James, M.D. "Reduced Normal Tissue Toxicity With Proton Therapy." Last modified June 29, 2006. Online posting. OncoLink website, The Abramson Cancer Center of the University of Pennsylvania. Accessed 28 Nov. 2007. <http://www.oncolink.com/treatment/article.cfm?c=9&s=70&id=211. Copyright 1994-2007 © Trustees of the University of Pennsylvania.

490. Michael, Nancy. From "Newsletter #46 Feb./Mar. 1998." "Rocket Fuel Ingredient Panacea or Placebo." Online posting. Accessed 9 Nov. 2007. <http://bcaction.org/index.php?page=newsletter-46f>. © 2000-2007 Breast Cancer Action. Also, see: http://www.hydrazinesulfate.org.

491. Miller EG, Peacock JJ, Bourland TC, Taylor SE, Wright JM, Patil BS, Miller EG. "Inhibition of oral carcinogenesis by citrus flavonoids." Online posting. Nutr Cancer 2008 Jan-Feb;60(1):69-74. PMID 18444138. PubMed - indexed for MEDLINE. Accessed 23 Jun. 2008. <http://www.ncbi.nlm.nih.gov/pubmed/18444138>.

492. Mindell, Earl L., R.Ph., Ph.D. with V.L. Hopkins. *Dr. Earl Mindell's What You Should Know About The Super Anti-oxidant Miracle.* New Canaan, CT: Keats Publishing, Inc., 1996.

493. Mindell, Earl, R.Ph., Ph.D. *Earl Mindell's Food As Medicine: What You Can Eat To Help Prevent Everything From Colds To Heart Disease To Cancer*, New York: Simon & Schuster Adult Publishing Group, 1994. © by Earl Mindell, R.Ph., Ph.D., and Carol Colman.

494. Mindell, Earl, R.Ph., Ph.D. *Earl Mindell's Herb Bible*, New York: Simon & Schuster Adult Publishing Group. © 1992 by Earl Mindell, R.Ph., Ph.D., and Carol Colman.

495. Mindell, Earl, R.Ph., Ph.D. *Earl Mindell's Soy Miracle.* New York: A fireside book, Simon & Schuster Adult Publishing Group. © 1995 by Earl Mindell, R.Ph., Ph.D.

496. Miners, Scott E. "Hope For Cancer Sufferers." Online posting. "An 'Official Miracle.'" Accessed 28 Nov. 2007. <http://www.1001herbs.com/webarticles/Essiac/Essiac-extras.html>. © 1993 The Herb Quarterly.

497. Minton, Barbara. "Study Reveals Benefits of Red Clover for Prostate and Liver Health." From naturalnews.com website online posting 4/15/2008. Accessed 18 April 2008. <http://www.naturalnews.com/z023019.html>. Natural News Network © 2008.

498. Mirkin, G., M.D. "Breast Milk Prevents Childhood Diabetes?" Online posting. Accessed 28 Nov. 2007. <http://www.drmirkin.com/diabetes/D216.htm>. © 2007 www.Dr.Mirkin.com.

499. Mitchell, Terri. "Prostate Cancer and Cruciferous Vegetables." From LE Magazine, Report July 2000. Online posting. Accessed 23 Oct. 2007. <http://search.lef.org/cgi-src-bin/MsmGo.exe?grab_id=0&page_id=4107&query=milk%20>.

500. Mitchell. T. "Resveratrol Powerful Protection Against Prostate Cancer." Online Posting. From Life Extension Magazine Report. Accessed 28 Nov. 2007. <http://www.lef.org/magazine/mag2004/apr2004_report_resver_01.html>. Also see the LEF Protocol Book. LE Magazine 2004. When the website comes up, do a search for resveratrol, and it will bring up this article. © 1995-2007 Life Extension Foundation.

501. Mitsugu Yanase, Masashige Shinkai, Hiroyuki Honda, Toshihiko Wakabayaski, Jun Yoshida and Takeshi Kobayashi. "Intracellular Hyperthermia for Cancer Using Magnetite Cationic Liposomes: An *in vivo* Study." *Jpn. J. Cancer Res.* 89, 463-470, April 1998. Online posting. Accessed 26 Dec. 2007. <http://www.blackwellsynergy.com/doi/pdf/10.1111/j.13497006.1998.tb600586 .x?cookieSet=1>.

502. Monchik JM, Donatini G, Iannuccilli J, Dupuy DE. "Radiofrequency ablation and percutaneous ethanol injection treatment for recurrent local and distant well-differentiated thyroid carcinoma." Online posting at PubMed website. Ann Surg 2006, Aug;244(2)296-304. From the Div of Endocrine Surgery, Brown Medical School, Rhode Island Hospital, PMID: 168 58194. Accessed 20 Jan. 2008. <http://www.ncbi.nlm.nih.gov/pubmed/16858194?ordinalpos=66&itool=Entrez System2.PEntrez.PubMed.PubMed_ResultsPanel.Pubmed_RVDocSum>.

503. Morse, Robert, N.D. *The Detox Miracle Sourcebook*, Prescott, AZ: Hohm Press, 2004.

504. Moss. Ralph W., Ph.D. *Cancer Therapy: The Independent Consumer's Guide to Non-Toxic Treatment & Prevention.* New York: Equinox Press, 1992.

505. Moss, Ralph W., Ph.D. *The Cancer Industry.* Brooklyn: Equinox Press, 2002.

506. Moss, Ralph W., Ph.D. "Intriguing New Anti-cancer Compound From East Europe." Online posting. From The Cancer Chronicles #27, © June 1995 by Ralph W. Moss, Ph.D. Accessed 28 Nov. 2007. <http://www.ralphmoss.com/ukrain.html>. Cancer Decisions® © 2007.

507. Moss, Ralph W., Ph.D. *Anti-oxidants Against Can*cer. State College PA: Equinox Press, Inc., 2000.

508. Moss, Ralph,W., Ph.D. "A Reply to Dr. Klausner: Natural Products Should be Tested First Against Cancer," from The Cancer Chronicles #29 © Sept. 1995 by Ralph W. Moss, Ph.D. *Landmark Study.* "Ralph Moss on Cancer – Expert Guidance for Crucial Decisions." Online posting. Accessed 28 Nov. 2007. <http://www.ralphmoss.com/html/try.shtml>. Cancer Decisions® © 2007.

509. Mowrey, D., Ph.D. "Rainforest Remedies," "Undiscovered Riches," Important Herbs from South American Rainforests. Online posting. "Lapacho." Accessed 28 Nov. 2007. <http://www.rain-tree.com/article4.htm>. © 1996-2005 Raintree Nutrition, Inc., Carson City, NV. 89701. This information is also found in Leslie Taylor's book, The Healing Power of Rainforest Herbs, Square One Publishers, Jan. 2005.

510. Mowrey, Daniel B., Ph.D. *The Scientific Validation of Herbal Medicine. How to Remedy and Prevent Disease With Herbs, Vitamins, Minerals, and Other Nutrients,* New York: McGraw-Hill Companies, 1986.

511. Mueller, Sue. "Coffee drinkers at lower risk of liver cancer." *DIET & HEALTH: CANCER* Online posting - updated Jun 28, 2008 from foodconsumer.org. Accessed 29 Jun. 2008. <http://foodconsumer.org/7777/8888/C_ancer_31/062809032008_Coffee_drinkers_at_lower_risk_of_liver_cancer.shtml.> © 2004-2008 by foodconsumer.org.

512. Murnal, Sarah. "Cancer Treatments on the Horizon." "Alternative Treatments." Oral Cancer Foundation website. Online posting. Accessed 30 Nov. 2007. <http://www.oralcancerfoundation.org/facts/cancer_treatments_horizon.htm. © 2001-2007 OFC, Inc.

513. Murray, Frank. *Remifemin: Herbal Relief for Menopausal Symptoms.* New York: McGraw-Hill Companies, 1996.

514. Murray, Michael T. ASK DR. MURRAY website. "What are proteolytic enzymes? Proteolytic enzymes in cancer therapy." Online posting. Accessed 23 June 2008. <http://www.doctormurray.com/articles/pdfs/ProteolyticsInCancer.pdf>. © 2001 Published by Mind Publishing Natural Factors Nutritional Products Ltd., www.naturalfactors.com.

515. Nefyodo LI, Uglyanica KN, Smirnov VY, et al. "Amino acids and their derivatives In blood plasma of patients with breast cancer treated with Ukrain. Part V." Online Posting at PubMed website. Drugs Exp Clin Res, 1996;(22)3-5):155-7. Accessed 20 Jan. 2008. Institute of Biochemistry, Belarus. PMID 8899320. <http://www.ncbi.nlm.Nih.gov/pubmed/8899320?ordinalpos=1&itool=EntrezSystem2.PEntrez.PubMed.PubMed_ResultsPanel.Pubmed_RVAbstractPlus>.

516. Nitha, B, Meers, CR, Janardhanan, K.K. "Anti-inflammatory and anti-tumour activities of cultured mycelium of morel mushroom, *Morchella exculenta.*" Online posting. Accessed 29 Dec. 2007. <http://www.ias.ac.in/currsi/jan252007/235.pdf>. "Research Communications" from *CURRENT SCIENCE*, Vol 92, No. 2, 25 Jan. 2007 pp.235-239.

517. Norton, Amy. "Bee Products Fight Tumors in Mice Study Shows." "News," from Reuters Health Information, New York. Reuters shall not be liable for any errors or delays in content, or for any actions taken in reliance thereon. Matria® Healthcare. Source: *Journal of the Science of Food and Agriculture*, Dec. 2004. Online posting. Accessed 28 Nov. 2007. <http://www.cancerpage.com/news/article.asp?id=7827>. Cancerpage.com 2000-2007.

518. Nowicky JW, Staniszewski A, Zbroja-Sontag, et al. "Evaluation of thiophosphoric acid alkaloid derivatives from Chelidonium majus L. ('Ukrain') as an immunostimulant in patients with various carcinomas." Online posting from the U.S. National Library of Medicine and Institutes of Health PubMed NCBI website. Drugs Exp Clin Res 1991; 17(2):139-43. Accessed 20 Jan. 2008. http://www.ncbi.nlm.nih.gov/pubmed/1713821?ordinalpos=1&itool=EntrezSystem2.PEntrez.PubMed.PubMed_ResultsPanel.Pubmed_RVAbstractPlus. Also, see the animal study that was done on Lewis carcinoma and Ukrain by Grinevich Y, Shalimov S, Bendyuh G, et al. "Effect of Ukrain on the growth and metastasizing of Lewis carcinoma on C57BL/6 mice." PMID 15929607. Online posting. Accessed 20 Jan. 2008. <http://www.ncbi.nlm.nih.gov/pubmed/1592960?Ordinalpo=104&itool=EntrezSystem2.Pentrez.PubMed.Pubmed_ResultsPanel.Pub_RVDocSum>.

519. Null, Gary. *The Complete Encyclopedia of Natural Healing: A Comprehensive A-Z listing of common and chronic illnesses and their proven natural treatments.* New York, N.Y. © 2000, 2001, 2002, Kensington Publishing Corporation: www. kensingtonbooks.com.

520. O'Brien, James E. *The Miracle of Garlic & Vinegar and other Exciting Natural Wonders.* Globe Mini Mags®. Boca Raton, FL: Globe Communications Corp., 1991.

521. Olsen, Cynthia with contributions by Jim Chan and Christopher Gussa. *Essiac A Native Herbal Cancer Remedy* by Cynthia Olsen, Lotus Press, P. O. Box 325, Twin Lakes, WI. 53181. ©1996.

522. Oski, Frank A., M.D. *Don't Drink Your Milk! New Frightening Medical Facts About The World's Most Overrated Nutrient.* Brushton, N.Y: Teach Services, Inc., 1996. Translated from the book, *Don't Drink Your Milk!* Copyright © 1996 by TEACH Services, Inc., 254 Donovan Road, Brushton, N.Y. 12916 518/358-3494.

523. Pal, Jyoti. "Cancer 'Cure' Approved For Human Trials." Online posting from themedguru.com. Accessed 30 Jun. 2008. <http://www.themedguru.com/articles/cancer_cure_approved_for_human_trials-7325303.html>. Copyright © 2006-2008 the medguru.com.

524. Patton, D. "Vitamin E has protective role in bladder cancer." Online posting. News & Analysis Science and Nutrition 30/03/2004. Accessed 3 Nov. 2007. <http://<http://www.foodnavigator.com/news/news-NG.asp?id=51009>. DECISIONNEWSMEDIA SAS © 2000-2007.

525. Peters, J.M., Preston-Martin S, London SJ, Bowman JD, Buckley JD, Thomas DC. "Processed meats and risk of childhood leukemias" (California, USA). From human research conducted by the University of Southern California School of Medicine - Los Angeles 90033. Online posting at NCBI, PUBMED website, PMID 8167267. Accessed 03 Jul. 2008. <http://www.ncbi.nlm.nih.gov/pubmed/8167267>.

525a. Pettersson A, Richiardi L, Nordenskjold A, et al. "Age at surgery for undescended testis and risk of testicular cancer." *New England Journal of Medicine.* 2007;356:1835-1841. Retrieved from an article posted online by CancerConsultants.com website - "Testicular Cancer News." 05/04/07. Article: "Surgery Earlier in Life Reduces Risk of Testicular Cancer Among Males with Undescended Testis." Accessed 26 Aug 2008. <http://patient.cancerconsultants.com/Cancer News_Testicular_Cancer.aspx?DocumentId=39769>. © Testicular Cancer Information Center on CancerConsultants.com, © 1998-2008 CancerConsultants.Com.

526. Phillips, Gavin. "The Cancer Racket." "The Hoxsey Remedies." Online posting. Accessed 28 Nov. 2007. <http://www.getipm.com/personal/cancer-racket.htm>.

527. Preidt, Robert. *Breast Cancer News,* "Hormone Could Ease Painful Lymphedema," Online posting from *Cancer Connections.* Accessed 22 Dec 2007. <http://body.aol.com/condition-center /breast-cancer/news/article/_a/hormone-could-ease-painfullymphedema/n2007122017060999 0062>. From *HealthDay News.* © 2007 Scout News, LLC.

528. Pressinger, R., M.Ed., and Wayne Sinclair. Allergy, Asthma & Immunology. "About Neuroblastoma." "Causes of Neuroblastoma Research." "Neuroblastoma and Chlordane." (CANCER, 59:1853-1859, 1987.) Online posting. Accessed 28 Nov. 2008. <http://www.chem-tox.com/neuroblastoma/default.htm>.

529. Prokopchuk OI, Zemskov SV, Susak YM. "Ukrain treatment in a patient with Metastatic renal cell carcinoma extending to the vena cava inferior. Case Report." From the U.S. National Library of Medicine, NCBI, PubMed online posting. PMID 11345035. Accessed 20 Jan. 2008. <http://www.ncbi.nlm.nih.gov/pubmed/11345035?ordinalpos=1&itool=EntrezSystem2.PEntre z.PubMed.PubMed_ResultsPanel.PubMed_RVAbstractPlus>.

530. Prokopchuk OI, Zemskov SV, Susak YM. "Ukrain treatment of a patient with Retro-Peritoneal synovial sarcoma. Case report." From the National Library of Medicine, NCBI, PubMed online posting. PMID 11345034. Accessed 20 Jan 2008. <http://www.ncbi.nlm.nih.gov/pubmed/11345034?ordinalpos=1&itool=EntrezSystem2.PEntrez.PubMed.PubMed_Resu ltsPanel.Pubmed_RVAbstractPlus>.

531. Rajkapoor, B., et al. "Antitumor Activity of Elephantopus scaber Linn Against Dalton's Ascitic Lymphoma." Online posting. IJPS – *The Indian Journal of Pharmaceutical Sciences.* The Indian Pharmaceutical Assoc (IPA). Accessed 28 Nov. 2007. <http://www.ijpsonline.com/article.asp?issn=0250;volume=64;issue=1;spage=71;epage=73;aulast=Rajkapoor;type=0>. © 2006 *Indian Journal of Pharmaceutical Sciences.* Published by MedKnow.

532. Raloff, Janet. "Selenium's Value to Prostate Health." Online posting. Was accessed 3 November 2007. <http://www.sciencenews.org/articles/20030510/food.asp>. © 2003 Science Service from Science News Online website.

532a. Reedy J, Mitrou P, Krebs-Smith S, et al. "Index-based dietary patterns and risk of colorectal cancer." From the *American Journal of Epidemiology.* 208; 168:38-48. Online posting. 08-04-2008. Accessed 27 Aug 2008. Daily Cancer News – "More Fruits and Veggies, Less Meat Reduces Colorectal Cancer." <http://patient.cancerconsultants.com/CancerNews.aspx?DocumentId=42458&Keywords=cancer,news,information,treatment,Fruits,Vegetables,red%20meat,colorectal.colon%20cancer,rectal%20cancer,whole%20grains,diet,prevention>. Copyright © 1998-2008 Cancer Consultants.com.

532b. Reid, Melanie. "MS link to Vitamin D deficiency hailed by politicians as giant leap forward." Online posting from The Times Online website. Accessed 8 Jun 2009. <http://www.timesonline.co.uk/tol/news/uk/scotland/article5672308.ece>. Copyright © 2009 Times Newspapers Ltd.

533. Ritter, Jim. *Chicago Sun Times*, Jan. 25, 2007. Article: "Picking the right poison: Tiny doses of arsenic help fight leukemia." Online posting. Accessed 08 Jan. 2008. <http://findarticles.com/p/articles/mi_qn4155/is_20070125/ai_n17165683>.

534. Rivers, Charmaine. *Manna from Heaven–Healing Foods From The Bible.* Boca Raton, FL and New York: Globe Digests™. American Media Mini Mags., Inc., 2002.

535. Roberts, John. "Citric Fruits - A Healthy Food." From foodconsumer.com by John Roberts. Online posting from letdiet.blogspot.com website. Accessed 8 Jul. 2008. <http://letdiet.blogspot.com/2008/07/citric-fruits-healthy-food.html>.

536. Rollins, Catherine P. "Auto-immune Disorders (Multiple Sclerosis, Lupus, Hashimoto's & Grave's Disease) and Natural Progesterone." Online posting. Accessed 28 Nov. 2007. <http://www.natural-progesterone-advisory-network.com/auto-immune-disorders-and-natural-progesterone.php>. © 2007 Making Plans Pty Ltd.

537. Rollins, Catherine P. "Estrogen Dominance and Natural Progesterone." Online posting. "Synthetic HRT and Cancer." Accessed 28 Nov. 2007. <http://www.natural-progesterone-advisory-network.com/estrogen-dominance-and-natural-progesterone.php>. © 2007 Making Plans Pty Ltd.

538. Rollins, Catherine P. "Natural Progesterone - A Safer Alternative." Online posting. Accessed 28 Nov. 2007. <http://www.natural-progesterone-advisory-network.com/is-natural-progesterone-safe.php>. © 2007 Making Plans Pty Ltd.

538a. Rossi M, Negi E, Lagiou P, et al. "Flavonoids and ovarian cancer risk: a case-control study in Italy." *International Journal of Cancer.* 2008;123:895-898. Online posting from article retrieved from CancerConsultants.com 08/26/08 - "Dietary Flavonoids Reduce Risk of Ovarian Cancer." Daily Cancer News - Cancerconsultants.com. Accessed 26 Aug 2008. <http://patient.cancerconsultants.com/CancerNews-Ovarian_Cancer.aspx?DocumentId=42517>. © Ovarian Cancer Information Center on Cancerconsultants.com, © 1998-2008 CancerConsultants.com.

539. Rubin, Jordan S., N.M.D., Ph.D. *The Maker's Diet.* Lake Mary FL: Siloam Publishing, 2004.

540. Ryan, Caroline. BBC News. "Sunshine 'Prevents Cancer.'" Feb. 15, 2002. From website The Greatest Herbs on Earth™. Online posting. Accessed 28 Nov. 2007. <http://www.greatestherbsonearth.com/articles/sunshine_prevents_cancer.htm>. Copyright © 2000-2007 Greatest Herbs on Earth.

541. Sage, Donna., M.S.S.A. "Healing Breast Cancer With Haelen." Online Posting. From "The Light Party" website. Accessed 28 Nov. 2007. <http://www.lightparty.com/Health/Haelen BreastCancer.html>.

542. Sahelian, Ray, M.D. "Ashwagandha: by Ray Sahelian, M.D., Ashwagandha Benefits." Online posting. Accessed 28 Nov. 2007. <http://www.raysahelian.com/ashwagandha.html>.

543. Sahelian, Ray, M.D. "Benefits of Rosemary." "Carnosol-induced apoptosis and downregulation of Bcl-2 in B-lineage leukemia cells." Online posting. Accessed 01 Jan. 2008. <http://www.raysahelian.com/rosemary.html>. Their resource: Cancer Lett. 2001 Sep 10;170(1) :33-9.

544. Sahelian, Ray, M.D. "Forskolin and cancer - Forskolin: a potential antimetastatic agent." From *Int. J. Cancer.* 1983 Dec 15;32(6):801-4. Online posting. Accessed 01 Jan. 2008. Site says page was last updated Jan. 2008. <http://www.raysahelian.com/forskolin .html>.

545. Sahelian, Ray, M.D. "Gymnema." "Gymnema and diabetes – gymnema and blood sugar." Online posting. Accessed 28 Nov. 2007. <http://www.raysahelian.com/ gymnema.html>.

546. Sahelian, Ray, M.D. "Neuroblastoma." Online posting. Accessed 02 Jan. 2008. <http:// www.raysahelian.com/neuroblastoma.html>. See under "Zeaxanthin and neuroblastoma," "The photoreceptor protector zeaxanthin induces cell death in neuroblastoma cells." Anti-cancer Res. 2005 Nov-Dec;25(6B):3871-6, and under "Resveratrol and neuroblastoma" - "Resveratrol-induced cellular apoptosis and cell cycle arrest in neuroblastoma cells and antitumor effects on neuroblastoma in mice," from Surgery 2004 Jul;136(1):57-66. Also see under "Curcumin, resveratrol and neuroblastoma" - "Curcumin and resveratrol induce apoptosis and nuclear translocation and activation of p53 in human neuroblastoma." From Anti-cancer Res. 2004 Mar-Apr;24(2B):987-98, http://www.raysahelian.com/neuroblastoma.html.

547. Sahelian, Ray. *Saw Palmetto Nature's Prostate Healer.* New York: Kensington Publishing, 1998.

548. Sakalo VS, Korsh OB, Melnyk A. "Ukrain treatment in a patient with non-seminomatous germ-cell tumour of testis" (case report). Online posting from National Library of Medicine website PubMed ID: 8899344. Accessed 20 Jan. 2008. Drugs Exp Clin Res, 1996;22(3-5):263-5. <http://www.ncbi.nlm.nih.gov/pubmed/8899344?ordinalpos=7&itool=EntrezSystem2.PEntrez. PubMed.PubMed_ResultsPanel.Pubmed_RVDoc Sum>.

549. Salaman, Maureen Kennedy, et al. *FOODS That Heal.* Menlo Park, CA: Statford Publishing, 1989.

550. Salaman, Maureen Kennedy. *Nutrition: The Cancer Answer II.* Menlo Park, Ca: Statford Publishing, 1995, 2002.

551. Salaman, Maureen Kennedy. *All Your Health Questions Answered Naturally.* MKS, Inc., 1998.

552. Salaman, Maureen Kennedy. *How to RENEW YOU.* Menlo Park, CA: MKS, Inc., 2003.

553. Sampalis, Tina, M.D., Ph.D. *The Healing Power of Neptune Krill Oil,* New York, N.Y. Rebus LLC, 2005.

553a. Sanjay Ramakumar, Jalaluddin Bhuiyan, Jennifer A. Besse, Steven G. Roberts, Peter C. Wollan, Michael L. Blute, Dennis J. O'Kane. "Comparison of Screening Methods In The Detection of Bladder Cancer. *The Journal of Urology* - Vol. 161, Issue 2, Pages 388-394 (February

1999). Accepted Aug 28 1998. Online posting. Accessed 02 Sept. 2008. <http://www.jurology.com/article/S0022-5347(01)61899-8/abstract>. © 2008 Elsevier, Inc.

554. Sardi, Bill. "The Overlooked Cancer Cure From Japan." Online posting. Accessed 28 Nov. 2007. <http://www.lewrockwell.com/sardi/sardi39.html>. © 2005 Bill Sardi Word of Knowledge Agency, San Dimas, Calif.

555. Saxion, Valerie. *How To Feel Great All The Time A Lifelong Plan for Unlimited Energy and Radiant Good Health,* Little Rock, Arkansas: Lions Head Publishing, 2002.

556. Schramm E, Nowicky JW, Godysh Y. "Biophysiological effects of Ukrain therapy in a patient with breast cancer (case report)." From the Ukranian Anti-Cancer Institute of Vienna, Austria. PubMed online posting accessed 20 Jan. 2008. PMID 8899341. <http://www.ncbi.nlm.nih.gov/pubmed/8899341?ordinalpos=13&itool=EntrezSystem2.PEntrez.PubMed.PubMed_ResultsPanel.Pubmed_RVDocSum>. PubMed NCBI website.

557. Schulick, Paul. *Ginger Common Spice & Wonder Drug.* Revised Edition. Brattleboro, VT: Herbal Free Press, Ltd., 1994.

558. Schwartz, J., Shklar, G., Reid, S., Trickler, D. "Prevention of experimental oral cancer by extracts of Spirulina-Dunaliella algae." PubMed, NCBI, National Library of Medicine, Nutr Canc er. 1998; 11(2):127-34. Online posting. Accessed 28 Nov. 2007. <http://www.ncbi.nlm.nih.gov/sites/entrez?db=pubmed&uid=3129701&cmd=showdetailview&indexed=google>. PMID 3129 701.

559. Scott, C., and Lust, John, Naturopath. *Crude Black Molasses, The Natural "WonderFood."* (City, State, n.g.) Benedict Lust Publications, 1980, 1992.

560. Shealy, C. Norman, M.D., Ph.D. *Natural Progesterone Cream:* Safe and Natural Hormone Replacement, New York. McGraw Hill Companies, 1999.

560a. Sheng-Hong Tseng, Swei-Ming Lin, Jin-Cherng Chen, Yen-Huo Su, Hsin-Yi Huang, Chia-Kang Chen, Po-Yin Lin and Yun Chen. "Resveratrol Suppresses the Angiogenesis and Tumor Growth of Gliomas in Rats." From *Clinical Cancer Research* Vol 10, 2190-2202, March 2004 © 2004 American Association for Cancer Research. Experimental Therapeutics, Preclinical Pharma-cology. Online posting. Accessed 25 Dec. 2008. <http://clincancerres.ascrjournals.org/cgi/content/abstract/10/6/2190?maxtoshow=&HITS=10&hits=10&RESULTSFORMAT=&fulltext=resveratrol&searchid=1137718106863_2349&FIRSTINDEX=O>.

561. Shogren, Elizabeth. "FDA kept suicide findings secret." Los Angeles Times, published on 4/6/4, Psyche Drug Truth. Online posting. Accessed 28 Nov. 2007. <http://www.prozactruth.com/article_fda_secret_findings.htm>.

561a. Sibley, Lisa. "BiPar Sciences developing cancer-killer." Online posting Dec. 5, 2008. Accessed 6 Dec. 2008. <http://sanjose.bizjournals.com/sanjose/stories/2008/12/08/focus32.html>. © 2008 American City Business Journals, Inc.

562. Siegel, Maryjo. See website Burzynski Patient Group at http://burzynskipatientgroup.org/maryjo.htm. Accessed 5-18-2008. Site updated 2-19-2008 <http://burzynskipatientgroup.org/maryjo.htm>.

563. Simon, Tanya. "Kanzius Machine: A Cancer Cure?" Reported by Lesley Stahl on CBS News 60 Minutes 4-13-08. Article 6-26-08, online. Accessed 27 June, 2008. <http://www.cbsnews.

com/stories/2008/04/10/60minutes/main4006951.shtml>. Copyright © MMVIII CBS Interactive, Inc.

564. Sinatra, Stephen, M.D., F.A.C.C. *The Coenzyme Q10 Phenomenon: The breakthrough nutrient that helps combat heart disease, cancer, aging and more*, New York: the McGraw-Hill Companies, 1998.

565. Sinatra, Stephen.T., M.D., F.A.C.C. *Coenzyme Q10 and the Heart*, New York: The McGraw-Hill Companies, 1999.

566. Sircus, Mark, Ac., OMD. "A Magnesium Deficiency Increases Cancer Risk Significantly." Online posting from naturalnews.com. Accessed 18 April 2008. <http://www.naturalnews.com/z023046.html>. Natural News Network © 2008.

566a. Sircus, Mark, Ac., OMD. *Iodine – Bringing Back the Universal Medicine;* e-book. See website: http://www.winningcancer.com.

566b. Sircus, Mark, Ac., OMD. *Magnesium The Ultimate Heart Medicine* (also see his book: *Magnesium Medicine Magnesium The Lamp of Life*; e-book. Available at website: http://www.magnesium forlife.com.

566c. Sircus, Mark, Ac., OMD, *Sodium Bicarbonate Rich Man's Poor Man's Cancer Treatment* (from IMVA Books) Dec. 2008. Available as e-book at: http://publications.imva.info.

567. Skousen, Max B. *Aloe Vera Handbook: The Ancient Egyptian Medicine Plant.* (City, State, n.g.) Aloe Vera Research Institute, 1992.

568. Smith, E.D. "Veterinarian: Effects of Homogenization and Pasteurization of Milk." Online posting. Accessed 28 Nov. 2007. <http://www.karloren.com/aajonus/p.17.htm>. From Karl Loren's website.

568a. Smith, Rebecca, Medical Editor. "Cancer victim treated with daughter's cells in world first - A British cancer victim has been given a transplant of cells from her daughter in a potentially life-saving world first that could revolutionise (sic) the treatment of advanced cancer." From an online posting by telegraph.co.uk/news website last updated 09 Aug 2008. Article retrieved 09 Aug 2008. <http://www.telegraph.co.uk/news/uknews/2524101/Cancer-victim-treated-with-daughters-cells-in-world-first.html> © Copyright of Telegraph Media Group Limited 2008.

568b. So FV, Guthrie N, Chambers AF, Moussa M, Carroll KK. "Inhibition of human breast cancer cell proliferation and delay of mammary tumorigenesis by flavonoids and citrus juices." Online posting from National Library of Medicine's PubMed website. NutrCancer1996;26(2):16 7-81. Accessed 03 Jul. 2008. PM ID 8875554. <http://www.ncbi.nlm.nih.gov/pubmed/8875554 ?ordinalpos=1&itool=EntrezSystem2.PEntrez.Pubmed.Pubmed_ResultsPanel.Pubmed_Discovey Panel.Pubmed_Discovery_RA&linkpos=1&log$=relatedarticles&logdbfrom=pubmed>.

569. Srinivas, G., Anto, R.J., Srinivas, Vidhyalakshmi, S., Senan, V.P. Karunagaran, D. "Emodin induces apoptosis of human cervical cancer cells through poly (ADP-ribose) polymerase cleavage and activation of caspase-9." Div. of Cancer Biology. Rajiv Ghandi Centre for Biotechnology, Poojapura, Thiruvananthapuram 695014, Kerala, India. Online posting. Accessed 1 Dec 2007 PubMed. <http://www.ncbi.nlm.nih.gov/entrez/query.fcgi?cmd=Retrieve&db=PubMed&list_uids=12892828>. Eur J. Pharmacol. 2003 JVL 25;473(2-3):117-25 p.1. PMID 12892828 Indexed for MedLine.

570. Steinacker J., Kroise T., Korsh, O.B., Melnyk A. "Ukrain therapy in a frontal anaplastic grade III astrocytoma (case report)." From www.pubmed.gov website. Online posting. Accessed 21 Dec. 2007. <http://www.ncbi.nlm.nih.gov/sites/entrez>. PMID 8899347.

571. Stengler, Mark, N.D. *The Natural Physician's Healing Therapies – Proven Remedies that Medical Doctors Don't Know About.* Stamford, CT: Bottom Line Books – Prentice-Hall Press, 2001. Avery Publishing, Penguin Group USA, Inc.

571a. Stone, Irwin. "The Genetics of Scurvy and the Cancer Problem." "I 1331 Charmwood Square, San Jose, California 95117. This is a Transcript of a talk presented at the meeting of The California Orthomolecular Medical Society, San Francisco, 14 Feb., 1976." Online posting. Accessed 14 Aug 2008. <http://www.seanet.com/~alexs/ascorbate/197x/stone-i-orthomol_psych-1976-v5-n3-p183.html>. From Orthomolecular Psychiatry, 1976, Vol 5, Number 3, PP. 183-190. HTML Revised 22 Feb, 2003. Formatting © 2001-2003 AscorbateWeb.

572. Strand, Ray D., M.D. with Donna K. Wallace. *Death by Prescription: The Shocking Truth Behind An Overmedicated Nation.* Nashville, TN: Thomas Nelson Publishers®, 2003.

573. Strand, Ray., M.D. *What Your Doctor Doesn't Know About Nutritional Medicine May Be Killing You.* Nashville: Thomas Nelson Publishers®, 2002.

573a. Sullivan, Jeff. "URI undergraduate finds Jamun berry could treat breast cancer." 12/04/2008. Online posting. Accessed 25 Dec 2008 <http://media.www.ramcigar.com/media/storage/paper366/news/2008/12/04/News/Uri-Undergraduate.Finds.Jamun.Berry.Could.Treat.Breast.Cancer3569498.shtml.

574. Susak YM, Zemskov VS, Yaremchuk OY, et al. "Comparison of chemotherapy and x-ray therapy with Ukrain monotherapy for colorectal cancer." Drugs Exp Clin Res, 1996;22(3-5):115-22. Online posting at National Library of Medicine NCBI PubMed site. Accessed 19 Jan. 2008. <http://www.ncbi.nlm.nih.gov/pubmed/8899313?Ordinalpos=1&tool=EntrezSystem2.PEntrez.Pubmed.Pubmed_ResultsPanel.Pubmed_RVAbstractPlus>. PMID 8899313.

575. Tanner, Lindsey. "Lack of Vitamin D Raises Risk of Death." Online posting of 06/24/Accessed 23 Jun. 2008. <http://news.aol.com/story/_a/lack-of-vitamin-d-raises-risk of death/20080624101309990001>. © 2007 AOL, LLC.

576. Tenney, D. *Medicinal Mushrooms: Cancer-fighters and Immunity Enhancers.* Pleasant Grove, UT: Woodland Publishing, 1997.

577. Tenney, L., M.H. *Health Handbook.* Pleasant Grove, UT: Woodland Publishing, 1996.

578. Thalmann GS, Markwalder R, Walter B, Studer UE. "Long-term experience with bacillus Calmette-Guerin therapy of upper urinary tract transitional cell carcinoma in patients not eligible for surgery." J Urol. 2002 Oct;168(4 Pt 1):1381-5, Dept of Urology, University of Bern, Switzerland. From the U.S. National Library of Medicine NCBI, PubMed website PMID 12352398. Online posting. Accessed 20 Jan. 2008. <http://www.ncbi.nlm.nih.gov/pubmed/12352398?ordinalpos=1&itool=EntrezSystem2.PEntrez.PubMed.PubMed_ResultsPanel.Pubmed_RVAbstractPlub>. PMID 12352398.

579. The Editors of Bottom Line Publications. *The World's Greatest Treasury of Health Secrets.* Greenwich, CT: Boardroom, Inc., 2000.

580. Thomas, Richard. *The Essiac Report - Canada's Remarkable Unknown Cancer Remedy.* Los Angeles, CA. The Alternative Treatment Information Network, 1993.

581. Tietze, Harald W. *Papaya The Healing Fruit.* Vancouver, Canada: Alive Books, Alive Natural Health Guides, 2000 (from Andrea Ehring, author of Das Krebsheilmittel Der Aborigines: Papaya: The Cancer Healing Remedy of the Aborigines.) <http://www.alive.com>. Alive Group, Inc., Canada.

582. Tullio, Simoncini, M.D. *Cancer Is A Fungus.* From the online posting article at cancerisafungus.com, accessed 06 Mar. 2008 <http://www.cancerisafungus.com/cancer-fungus-content.html>. Also see article "Cancer therapy with sodiumbicarbonate by Dr. Simoncini," at http://www.curenaturalicancro.com/2-treatment-sodiumbicarbonate.html Accessed 12 Jan. 2009. Also see website: <http://www.cancerfungus.com> and website: <http://www.curenaturali cancro.com, as well as http://www.curenaturalicancro.com/treatment-simoncini-protocol.html. And see website: http://www.curenaturalicancro.com/2-side-effects-sodiumbicarbonate.html and website: http://www.curenaturalicancro.com/2-treatment-sodiumbicarbonate.html.

583. Udall, K. Gilbert. *Immune and Stamina Booster Cordyceps Sinensis.* Pleasant Grove, UT: Woodland Publishing, 2000.

584. Uglyanica KN, Fomin KA, Nefyodov LI, et al. "Influence of Ukrain on patients with surgically treated breast cancer. Part II. Hormonal profile." Drugs Exp Clin Res. 1996;22(3-5): 139-41. From the Medical Institute of Grodno, Belarus. NCBI PubMed website online posting. Accessed 20 Jan. 2008. <http://www.ncbi.nlm.nih.gov/pubmed/8899317?ordinalpos=1&tool =EntrezSystem2.PEntrez.PubMed.PubMed_ResultsPanel.Pubmed_RVAbstractPlus>. PMID 88 99317.

585. Uglyanica KN, Maciuk JR, Fomin KA, Nefyodov LI, et al. "Influence of Ukrain on patients with surgically treated breast cancer. Part IV. Electronmicroscopic and cytochemical evaluation." Online posting. Drugs Exp Clin Res 1996;22(3-5);147-53. From NCBI PubMed online posting. Accessed 20 Jan. 2008. <http://www.ncbi.nlm.nih.gov/pubmed/8899319?ordinalpos=1&itool= EntrezSystem?PEntrez.PubMed.PubMed_ResultsPanel.Pubmed_RVAbstractPlus>. PMID 8899 319.

586. Uglyanitsa KN, Nefyodov LI, Doroshenko YM, Brzosko WJ. "Comparison of the efficacy of different doses of Ukrain in the combined treatment of breast cancer." Drugs Exp Clin Res 2000;26(5-6):201-21, online posting at the National Library of Medicine, NCBI, PubMed. Accessed 20 Jan. 2008. <http://www.ncbi.nlm.nih.gov/pubmed/11345028?ordinalpos=1&itool=EntrezSys tem2.PEntrez.Pub.PubMed_ResultsPanel.Pubmed_RVAbstractPlus>. PMID 113450 28.

587. Uglyanitsa KN, Nechiporenko NA, Nefyodov LI, et al. "Results of Ukrain monotherapy of prostate cancer." Drugs Exp Clin Res, 2000;26(5-6):191-3. Online posting. Accessed 20 Jan 2008. <http://www.ncbi.nlm.nih.gov/pubmed/11345026?Ordinalpos=1&Itool=EntrezSystem2. PEntrez.PubMed.PubMed_ResultsPanel.Pubmed_RVAbstractPlus>. PMID 11345026.

588. Uglyanitsa KN, Nechiporenko NA, Nefyodov LI, Brzosko WJ. "Ukrain therapy of Stage TINOMO bladder cancer patients." Drugs Exp Clin Res. 1998;24(5-6):227-30. Online posting. Accessed 20 Jan. 2008. U.S. National Library of Medicine website, NCBI, PubMed. <http: //www.ncbi.nlm.nih.gov/pubmed/10190079?ordinalpos=1&itool=EntrezSystem2.PEntrez.PubM ed.PubMed_ResultsPanel.Pubmed_RVAbstractPlus>. PMID 10190079.

588a. Van Seters, M, Van Beurden, M, Fiebo J., et al. "Treatment of intraepithelial neoplasia with topical imiqimod." *New England Journal of Medicine.* 2008;358:1465-1473. Article retrieved on "Vaginal Cancer News" – CancerConsultants.com. 04/11/08. "Aldara™ Effective Alternative to Surgery for Precancerous Changes to Vulva," online posting. Accessed 26 Aug 2008. http://patient.cancerconsultants.com/CancerNews_Vaginal_Cancer.aspx?DocumentId=41797 ©

Vaginal Cancer Information Center on CancerConsultants.com, Copyright © 1998-2008 Cancer Consultants.com.

588b. Von Hoff D, et al. "Efficacy data of GDC-0449, a systemic hedgehog pathway antagonist, in a first-in-human, first-in-class Phase I study with locally advanced, multifocal or metastatic basal cell carcinoma patients. Proceedings from the 2008 Annual Meeting of the American Association for Cancer Research (AACR). Abstract LB-138." Retrieved from a website article at CancerConsultants.com entitled: "GDC-0449 is Promising New Drug for Advanced Basal Cell Skin Cancer." 04/15/08. Accessed 26 Aug 2008. <http://patient.cancerconsultants.com/Cancer News_Skin_Cancer.aspx?DocumentId=41830>. © Skin Cancer Information Center on Cancer Consultants.com, © 1998-2008 CancerConsultants.Com.

589. Vyas J.J, Jain V.K, "Ukrain treatment in carcinoma of the oesophagus - (case report)." Tata Memorial Hospital. Bombay, India. Online posting. Accessed 21 Dec. 2007. <http://www.ncbi.nlm.nih.gov/sites/entrez>. "PMID 8899345 PubMed;Indexed for MedLine."

590. Wade, Carlson. *Carlson Wade's New FACT BOOK On Bee Pollen and Your Health.* New Canaan, CT: Pivot Original Health Books, Keats Publishing, Inc., 1978, 1992.

591. Ward, Bernard. "Garlic." Optimal Diet Healthy Eating Website, "Letters to Friends," "Glorious Garlic" 04 Oct. 2003. Taken from "Healing Foods of the Bible," by Bernard Ward. Online Posting. Accessed 1 Dec. 2007. <http://homodiet.Netfirms.com/otherssay/letters/garlic.htm>.

592. Warner, Jennifer, M.D. "Esophageal Cancer on the Rise—Fastest Rising Form of Cancer in the U.S," by Jennifer Warner WebMD Medical News Reviewed by Michael Smith, M.D. Online posting. Accessed 6 Nov. 2007. From website article at <http://www.shirleys-wellness-café.com /tf/s/cancer-testimonials.htm>.

593. Warner, Jennifer. "Substance in Peppers Kills Cancer Cells." Online posting. WebMD Medical News 9/3/02. Retrieved from the Annie Appleseed Project website. Accessed 1 Dec. 2007. <http://www.annieappleseedproject.org/caphotpepsub.html>.

594. Waters, Ed Jr. "New cancer drug being developed locally–Scientist returns to Frederick to establish company, originally published Jan. 22, 2008." From FrederickNewsPost.com online posting. Accessed 22 Jan. 2008. <http://www.fredericknewspost.com/sections/news/display.htm?StoryID=70291>. Copyright 1997-08 Randall Family, LLC.

595. Weatherby, Craig and Hartnell, Randy. "Extra Virgin Olive Oil Seen Superior for Reducing Cardiac and Cancer Risks: Anti-oxidants Get Credit. FDA OK's heart-health claim for 'mono' fats; Anti-oxidants abundant only in EVOO offer added health benefits." "Anti-oxidants in Extra Virgin Olive Oil Add Extra Cardiac Benefits. Phenols in extra virgin grade add cardiac benefits to those imparted by its 'mono' fats." Also see section 3 on "Olive Oil's 'Mono' Fats Seen Cutting Risk of Breast Cancer. New results support and explain hypothesized anti-cancer effect of the 'Mediterranean Diet.'" From Vital Choices website online posting. Jan 2, 2006. Accessed 01 January 2008. Vol. 3, Issue 55. <http://newsletter.vitalchoice.com/e_article000507623.cfm?x=b6qDMGw,blkJpvRw>. See section 4 - "Anti-oxidants in Extra Virgin Olive Oil May Curb Colon Cancer" - "Findings apply only to unrefined oils; standard 'pure' oils fall short in protective polyphenols." From Vital Choices website online posting. Jan 2, 2006 Accessed 01 Jan. 2008. Vol. 3, Issue 55. <http://newsletter.vitalchoice.com/e_article000507623.cfm?x=b6qDMGw.blkJpvRw>. Source given as: Gill CI, Boyd A, et al. "Potential anti-cancer effects of virgin olive oil phenols on colorectal carcinogenesis models in vitro. Int. J. Cancer. 2005 Oct 20;117 (1):1-7.

596. Whitaker, Julian, M.D. *Dear Dr. Whitaker.* From *Dr. Julian Whitaker's Health & Healing® Your Definitive Guide to Wellness Medicine.* Jul. 2007. Vol. 17. No. 7.

597. White, Linda B., M.D., Steven Foster and the staff of Herbs for Health. *The Herbal Drugstore—The Best Natural Alternatives to Over-the-Counter and Prescription Medicines!* (City, State, n.g.) Rodale, Inc., 2000.

598. Wigmore, Ann. *The Hippocrates Diet and Health Program.* (City, State, n.g.) Avery Publishing, 1984.

599. Wigmore, Ann. *The Sprouting Book: How to Grow and Use Sprouts to Maximize Your Health and Vitality.* Wayne, N.J: Avery Publishing Group, Inc., 1986.

600. Wigmore, Ann. *The Wheat grass Book: How to Grow and Use Wheat Grass To Maximize Your Health and Vitality* Nov. 1984 (City, State, n.g.) Avery Publishing, member of Penguin Putnam, Inc., and The Hippocrates Health Institute, Inc., 1985.

601. Willner, Robert, M.D., Ph.D. "Dr. Johanna Budwig Diet Cancer, Arthritis, Multiple Sclerosis, Psoriasis, Eczema, Acne…Flax seed oil and cottage cheese." Accessed 1 Dec. 2007. <http://www.alternativehealth.co/nz/cancer/budwig.htm>.

601a. Wilson, Anthony. "Diets High In Fat, Low In Fruit & Vegetables Linked To Bladder Cancer." From Cancer News, Articles & Information, Online posting Aug 23, 2008. Accessed 26 August 2008. <http://healthhubs.net/cancer/diets-high-in-fat-low-in-fruit-vegetables-linked-to-bladder-cancer/>. © Cancer News Articles & Information.

601b. Wilson, Anthony. "Folate May Reduce Pancreatic Cancer Risk," from Cancer News, Articles & Information. Online posting May 7, 2008. Accessed 28 Aug 2008. <http://health hubs.net/cancer/folate-or-vitamin-b9-may-reduce-pancreatic-cancer-risk/>. Copyright © *Cancer News, Articles & Information.*

602. Winters, Jason. "Sir Jason Winters Story – About Sir Jason Winters." Online posting. Accessed 1 Dec. 2007. <http://www.sirjasonwinters.com/story.htm>. © 1997-2007 Tri-Sun International.

603. Wright, Lloyd. "Milk Thistle Ancient Blessing." "Triumph Over Hepatitis C" website. Online posting. Accessed 1 Dec. 2007. <http://www.hepatitisCfree.com/milk_thistle_book. htm>.

604. Yeager, Selene, et al. *The Doctors Book of Food Remedies: The Newest Discoveries in the Power of Food to Cure and Prevent Health Problems - From Aging and Diabetes to Ulcers and Yeast Infections.* (City, State, n.g.): Rodale, Inc., 1998.

605. Yiamouyiannis, John. "Fluoride Toxicity, Immune System and Aging." Online posting. Accessed 1 Dec. 2007. <http://www.healthscience.com/fluoride_toxicity.html>. © 1995-2007 Health & Science Research, New York, N.Y. USA.

606. Young, Gary D. "New Discovery on the Chinese Wolfberry." Special Health Advisory on Immunity and Anti-Aging. Online posting. Accessed 1 Dec. 2007. <http://www.aroma-essence.com/research-reports/chinese-wolfberry.html>. © 1996-2004 aroma-essence.com and its licensors.

607. Young, Robert O., Ph.D., and Shelley Redford Young. *The pH MIRACLE Balance Your Diet, Reclaim Your Health.* New York: Warner Books, Inc. 2002. From *The pH Miracle* © 2002 by Robert Young, Ph.D.

608. YUEH-ERH, Rahman and Betty Jean Wright. From the Division of Biological and Medical Research, Argonne National Laboratory. Argonne, Illinois 60439 "Liposomes containing chelat-ing agents. Cellular penetration and a possible mechanism of metal removal." Online posting of JCB, the *Journal of Cell Biology,* PubMed Central, Cell Biol. 1975 April 1; 65(1): 112–122. Courtesy of The Rockefeller University Press. Accessed 26 Jul 2008. <http://www.pubmedcentral.nih.gov/articlerender.fcgi?artid=2111156>.

609. Zemskov VS, Procopchuk O.L., Susak Y.M., Zemskov, S.V., Hodysh, Y.Y., Zemskova, M.V. "Ukrain (NSC-631570) In the Treatment of Pancreas Cancer." "Kyiv Centre for Hepato-Pancreato-Biliary Surgery, Kiev, Ukraine and Ukrainian Anti-Cancer Institute, Vienna, Austria." Online posting. Accessed 1 Dec 2007 <http://www.ukrain-drug.net/papers/153.htm>. Also, see website: <http://www.ncbi.nlm.nih.gov/pubmed/11345025?ordinalpos=1&itool=EntrezSystem2.PEntrez.PubMed.PubMed_ResultsPanel.Pubmed_RVAbstractPlus>. PMID 11345025.

610. Zemskov SV, Prokopchuk OL, Susak YM. "Ukrain treatment in a patient with breast carcinoma. Case report." Online posting from NCBI PubMed website. Accessed 20 Jan. 2008. Ukrainian State Medical University, Kiev, Ukraine. Drugs Exp Clin Res.20 00;226(5-6):253-4. <http:///www.ncbi.nlm.nih.gov/pubmed/11345033?ordinalpos=1&tool=EntrezSystem2.PEnt rez.PubMed.PubMed_ResultsPanel.Pubmed_RVAbstractPlus>. PMID 11345033.

611. Zentaro, Nishimura. "With Tian Xian Liquid, I shall Never Surrender to Liver Cancer." Tian Xian. Online Posting. Accessed 1 Dec. 2007. <http://www.tianxian.com/testimonials /liver_cancer.asp>. © 2004 Green & Gold International Exports.

612. Zhang M., Binns CW, Lee AH. "Tea consumption and ovarian cancer risk: a case-control study in China." From website *Healthy Living with Nature's Garden.* Their article, "'New News' on cancer treatment?'" Dec. 13, 2005. Online posting. Accessed 28 Nov. 2007. <http://www.ncbi.nlm.nih.gov/sites/entrez>. "PMID 12163323 PubMed article; indexed for MEDLINE."

613. Ziff, S., Ziff, M.F., D.D.S. *Dentistry Without Mercury.* Orlando, FL: Bio=Probe, Inc., 1985.

614. Zidan, Jamal, Shetver, Likta, et al. "Prevention of chemotherapy-induced neutropenia by special honey intake." Online posting from SpringerLink Journal Article. Accessed 13 Jan. 2008. © Springer, Part of Springer Science+Business Media.

# INDEX


131-I Labetuzumab, 37, 135
2aG4, 73
2ME2, 36
3F8, 37, 380-381
3F8, monoclonal antibody, 380-381
3TP System – Cadscience MRI, 52
4-hydroxyderricin, 625
*7 Essentials* drink, 475-476
714X, 416-417, 629

## A

A10 (antineoplaston), 589-590
Abajeru, 71, 317
Abdominal cancer, 130-168
  & Budwig diet, 131-132
  & Canelim, 594
  & celery, 485
  & fenugreek, 150
  & garlic, 150-151
  & resveratrol, 144-145
  & shark cartilage, 163-164
  & suma, 153-154
  & tea, 152
  & zinc, 159
Abdominal cancer cure, 428
Abdominal liposarcoma, 132
Abiraterone, 103
Ablatherm (HIFU), 103-104
Ablation (liver), 264
ABM mushroom, 254-255, 524-525
  & cancer, 524-525
ABMT, 363
Abnormal clotting & ginkgo biloba, 456
Abscisic acid (ABA) 432
Acai berries, 462
*Acanthopanax senticosis*, 453
Acanthus (Harkach kanta), 240
Acemannan, 36
Acerola, 479
Acetyl cysteine, 295
Acetylenics, 485
Acid reflux disease, 598
Acid-free diet & Carctol, 594-595
Acidic-forming foods, 559-560
Acidity & cancer, 427, 557
Acidity in the body, 558-559
Acne:
  & kombucha, 570
  & milk, 533
  & propolis, 556
  & vitamin A, 479
Acoustic neuromas, 622
Acral melanoma, 37
Acrylamides, 221
  & rosemary, 566
ACSL3 gene, 36
Actinidia, 260
Active hexose correlated Compound (AHCC), 136
Acupuncture, 582
Acute myeloid leukemia cure, 205-206, 606
ADCs, 36
ADD, 487-488
Adenosine monophosphate injections, 474
ADH-1 trials, 36
Adrenal health & glandulars, 604
Adrenal Leukodystrophy, 162
Adrenal tumor, 397
Adriamycin, 151
Advanced Alternatives Cancer Center, 605, 617
Advexin, 304
Aflatoxin, 238, 596
  & chlorophyllin, 146
AFP, 170-171
*Agaricus Blazei Murrill*, 179, 524-525
Agarikon mushroom, 529
Agent Orange, 503
Agricur & MRSA, 204
AHCC, 62, 213-214, 269
  & rhabdomyosarcoma, 401-402
AIDS & lentinan, 339
Akashiba (red reishi), 527
Akee, 479
ALA, 284, 583-584
  & glutathione, 462-463
  & liver transplants, 246-247
ALA sources, 284, 463
ALD (Adrenal Leukodystrophy), 472, 473
Aldara, 197
Alkaline cancer cure, 561
Alkaline-forming foods, 559-560
Alkalinity, 427
  & wheat grass, 435
  & bladder cancer, 340
  & cancer, 594-595
  & fasting, 631-632
  & grapes, 45-46
  & health, 557-561
  & MSM, 612-613
*Alka-Seltzer Gold*, 129
ALL & scutellaria, 422
*Aller-Bee-Gone*, 553
Allergies:
  & bee pollen, 552-553
  & krill oil, 446-447
  & quercetin, 617
Allogeneic, 201-202
Aloe & intestinal problems, 542
*Aloe Mucilaginous Polysaccharide*, 542
Alpha lipoic acid, 243-245, 462-463
Alphabet Tea recipe, 639-641
Alpha-carotene, 483
*Aphanizomenon flos-aquae*, 71
Alsihum, 36
Aluminum & Alzheimers, 511
Alzheimer drugs for cancer 37
Alzheimers & HRT, 495
Amalgam fillings, 547
Amargo, 232-233
AMAS test, 30, 170-171, 582-583
Ambrotose (glyconutrition), 604
AML miracle cure, 73, 172
Amla fruit, 260
*Amorphophallus konjac*, 279
*AMP Molo-Cure*, 542
Amplichip, 170-171
Amygdalin (Laetrile), 585-587
Anamu, 232-233
Anaplastic astrocytoma:
  & antineoplastons, 354
  Inoperable, cured, 354
  (Stage III) cured, 354
Ancient Minerals, 129
Andiroba, 385, 415-416
Andrographis, 85, 233-234
  & lymphoma, 405
  side effects of, 405

Anemia & spirulina, 434
*Angelica keiskei* root (umbelliferae), 625
Angiosarcoma, 401
Annexin A3, 36
Anodyne therapy, 36
Anthrax & black tea, 567
Anti-angiogenesis, 587, 625
Antibiotics vs. honey, 554-555
Anti-Cancer Herbs & Foods, 448-461
Antigenics vaccine, 37
Anti-histamines (natural).
  jiaogulan, 458
  quercetin, 617
  grape seed, 469
  reishi, 527-528
Anti-inflammatories:
  (natural), 188, 212
  cherries, 161
  dandelion tea, 568
  echinacea, 455
  ginger, 563
  licorice, 458-459
  Lyprinol, 447
  morels, 527
  propolis, 556
  quercetin, 617
  skullcap, 185
Antineoplastics, 589
Antineoplastons (& see cancer specific)
Antineoplastons, 56-57, 106, 162-163, 354-355, 589-590
Anti-oxidants, 462-476
  acai berries, 462
  ALA, 462
  cat's claw, 463-464
  for the skin, 384
  rose hips, 460
  the wolfberry, 461
Anti-parasites, Mullaca, 232
Antiseptic, oregano, 459
Anthrax & vitamin C, 541
Anxiety & low-dose Dilantin, 658
Aoshiba (blue reishi), 527
Apis, 552
APL & vitamin A
APM, warning against, 455
Apoptosis, 617
Appetite suppressant, Forskolin, 602
Apples & lung cancer, 274
Arame, 433
Araza, 479
Arginine, 258
*Armoracia rusticana* (horseradish), 564
Aroma & healing, Ch 36
Aromasin, 72
Aronia berries, 136
ARQ-197, 36
Arrhythmias & ciwujia, 453
Artemisinin, 91, 549-550
Arterial plaque:
  & fasting, 632
  & pomegranate, 615-616
Arthritis:
  & aloe vera, 450
  & bromelain, 452
  & cytotron therapy, 365
  & dehydration, 512
  & ginger, 563, 569
  & gymnema sylvestre, 457
  & IPT, 607-608
  & kombucha, 570
  & Krill oil, 446-447
  & Lodamin, 395
  & Lyprinol, 447
  & Moxxor, 447
  & pomegranates, 471
  & propolis, 556
Artichokes, 258
  & cancer, 484
AS2-1 (antineoplaston), 589-590
Ascended Masters, 12
Ashwagandha, 405-406, 451
  & lymphoma, 405
Asian pears, 179
Asparagus:
  & cancer, 484
  & neural tube defects, 484
*Asparagus cochinchinensis*, 453
Aspartame:
  & leukemia, 406
  & lymphoma, 406
  & urinary tumors, 406
  warnings against, 455
Aspartic acid, warnings against, 455
*Aspartyl-L-phenylalanine*, 455
Aspilia, 85, 288
Astaxanthin, 483
  sources of, 363-364
Asthma:
  & aloe vera, 450
  & beta-carotene, 478
  & cordyceps mushroom, 517, 525
  & *Ecklonia cava*, 630
  & Forskolin, 602
  & Lyprinol, 447
  & propolis, 556
  & selenium, 397
  & sodium needs, 513
  & water hydration, 512-513
Astragalus, 146, 224, 331
Astrocytoma, 349-382, 401
  & antineoplastons, 350
  advanced – proof of cures, 355
  fast growing, 355
  & Ukrain, 378
Astrocytoma III, 358
Attitude & healing, 9, 10-11
A-type Lamins, 36
Atypical teratoid/rhabdoid tumor & antineoplastons, 351
Aubergines (eggplant), 468
Autism, 41
Autofluorescence, 133
Autohemotherapy, 584
Auto-immune disorders, 505-506
  & HGH, 604-605
  & IGF1, 605
Auto-immunity:
  & milk, 504
  & hydration, 514
Autologous dendritic cell vaccine, 403, 602
Autologous, 201
Autumn Crocus, 224
Avanex- 7-1037, 137, 584-585
Avastin, 34-35
Aveloz, 36
Avemar, 72
Avicine, 36
Avocados, 469
AXUM, 599
Ayurvedic therapy, 36

## B

B12 & B17, 585
B12, 57
  in spirulina, 433-434
  in vegans, 61
  nasal delivery form, 585
  patches for, 585
  sources, 218, 613
  sublingual, 585
B-17, Laetrile, 585-587
B6 & cancer, 465
B6, sources of, 154
Babies with tumors & blueberries, 463

# Index


Bacillus Calmette-Guerin, 338
Back pain & hydration, 514
Bael fruit, 479
Baicalein, (skullcap), 105
Baking soda & maple syrup cure, 593-594
*Bakuryokuso* barley, 426
Baobab pod fruit, 479
Barbados cherry, 479
Barbara Ann Karmanos Cancer Institute, 623
Barley & cancer, 484
Barley & tocotrienols, 484
*Barley Green*, 431
Barrett's esophagus, 301-302
  & cryospray, 598
Bartonella & vitamin C, 541
Basal body temperature, 499
Basal cell cancers, 383
Basal cell carcinoma & GDC-0449, 385-386
Basil, 562
Baycol, 39, 388
BBBD (intra-arterial platinum therapy), 352
B-cell biology, 35
B-cell lymphoma cure, 425
BCG, 332-333, 338
BCG & TB, 333
BCG test & urinary tract cancers, 332- 333
BCNU (in wafer form), 369, 370
Bee pollen & cancer, 553
Bee products, 552—556
Bee venom & cancer, 554
Behcet's Syndrome, 224
Bell's Palsy & Virastatin, 630
Bemer 3000, 36
Bentonite clay, 204
Benzaldehyde, 321,
  in figs, 483-484
Benzene & leukemia, 548
Benzodiazepine inhibitors, 36
Berberine, 151, 225, 385
Berberine & goldenseal, 332
Beres Drops Plus, 587
Berries & cancer, 75
Berry Young Juice, 461
Beta sitosterolemia, 162
Beta-carotene sources, 176, 478
Beta-cell regeneration, 457
Beta-glucan, 79
  & lymphoma, 406-407
Beta-Sitosterol, 105-106
Betulinic acid, 399
BHRT, 489-509
Bignay fruit, 479
Bile duct cancers, 267-268
Bilimbi, 480
Bindweed, 85, 397-398, 587-588
  dosing for, 587
Bindweed precautions, 587
Binzel Nutritional Program, 588
*Bio-Bran*, 612
BioCancell, 588
Bioenergy RIBOSE, 86
Bio-identical hormones, 489-509
Biological response modifier, 40
Biophosphonates, 93
BioPulse, 606
Biotherapy, 40
Bird flu & vitamin C, 541
Biriba, 479
Birth control pills, 505-506
  & liver cancer connection, 252
Birth defects & folic acid, 484
Biter orange, 260
Bitter melon, 36
Black cohosh, 72, 508-509
  precautions for, 508-509
Black cumin, 405-406
  & lymphoma, 405-406
Black sapote, 479
Black seed, 405-406
Black tea & anthrax, 567
Black walnut & parasites, 549
Bladder cancer, 331-348
  & alkalinity, 340
  & antineoplastons, 333
  & baicalein (skullcap), 342
  & berberine, 332
  & broccoli, 332
  & cat's claw, 333
  & chlorine danger, 334
  & cruciferous foods, 337
  & cumin, 566
  & CyberKnife, 334
  & EFAs, 335
  & Essiac tea, 335-336
  & fennel, 566
  & fruits in diet, 336
  & fungal (yeast) cure, 336
  & garlic taken orally, 336
  & grapes, 337
  & green tea, 337
  & inositol hexaphosphate, 338
  & intravesical immunotherapy, 338
  & IP-6, 338
  & LifeMel honey, 338
  & maitake, 339
  & pH, 559-560
  & Poly-MVA, 340, 375
  & polyporus umbellatus, 211
  & resveratrol, 337
  & *rhodiola rosea*, 341
  & selenium, 342
  & Ukrain, 342-343
  & vegetables in diet, 336
  & vitamin combo, 346-347
  & vitamin E, 345-346
  & water, 347-348
  advanced & Vitamin C, 343-344
  (recurring) & *Polyporus*, 340, 527
  & Rexin-G, 341
Bladder infections, 45
  & cranberries, 454
Bland embolization, 264-265
Blood clots:
  & ALA, 462-463
  & HRT, 495
  & quercetin, 471
  & reishi, 527-528
Blood electrification, 37
Blood pressure:
  & apple skins 483
  & cayenne, 364
  & genistein, 81-82
  & ginkgo biloba, 456
  & grapes, 77
  & hibiscus tea, 364
  & kombucha, 570
  & resveratrol, 364
  & rye bread, 364
  & seaweed, 433
  & sunshine, 523
  & vassourinha, 399
  & vitamin D, 345
Blood sugar:
  & anamu, 378
  & banaba leaf, 457
  & beta-sitosterol, 230
  & bilberry, 472
  & cinnamon, 563

& gymnema sylvestre, 457
& Hoelen, 526
& *rhodiola rosea*, 341
& vanadium, 457
& vassourinha, 378
Blood thinners – natural:
bilberry, 472
chlorophyll, 426
enoki mushroom, 528
Forskolin, 602
ginger, 414-415, 563
IP-6, 487
kiwi, 449
Lapacho, 376
mullaca, 232, 373
oyster mushroom, 528
papaya enzymes, 450, 481
quercetin, 159
red clover, 160, 257
reishi, 528
willow bark, 564
wood ear, 528
Blue Light Therapy, 588
Blueberries fight children's tumors, 463
BNCT, 36
Bob's Red Mill Products, 129
Boils & propolis, 556
Bolsa mullaca, 373
Bone cancer (also see under Ewing's & other types of bone cancer):
& antineoplastons, 230
& bupleurum, 452
& chlorella, 412
& flax, 413-414
& Radio Wave Therapy, 618
& selenium, 213
& vitamin A, 213
Bone loss & HRT, 498
Bone loss & ipriflavone, 498
Bone marrow transplants, 198-203
Borage oil, 296
& retina problems, 441
Boron Neutron Capture, 36
Boron, 106
Bottle gourd, 262
Botulism & vitamin C, 544
Bovine cartilage, 92
Bovine colostrum, 623
Bovine leukemia in milk, 535
Bowel cancer & Essiac, 58-59
Bowel growth & molasses, 543
Bowel tolerance level (of vitamin C), 423
Bowman-Birk inhibitor, 36
Brachytherapy, 99
Brain Cancer, 349-382 (also look under specific types of brain cancer)
& abajeru, 362
& anamu, 378
& antineoplastons, 349-356
& artemisinin, 362
& Budwig diet, 131-132
& cayenne, 364
& cell phone dangers, 382
& chaparral, 365
& citrus flavenols, 366
& CyberKnife, 379
& flax oil, 367, 443
& fungal <u>cure</u>, 592
& Gamma Knife, 379
& ginkgo biloba, 369
& graviola, 370
& lapacho, 376
& LifeMel Honey, 370-371
& Lodamin, 60
& macrobiotics 371
& mullaca, 373
& myrrh, 89, 374
& Noscapine, 614
& pau d'arco, 376
& Radio Wave Therapy, 618
& resveratrol, 365
& Ukrain, 377-378
& vassourinha, 378
& vitamin C, 70-71
& wormwood, 362
& GLA, 369
Brain cancer <u>cure</u> & Maitake D-Fraction, 374
Brain cell regeneration 88
Brain cells & green tea, 570
Brain damage & green tea, 280
Brain health & *Ecklonia Cava*, 630
Brain stem (inoperable) tumor <u>cure</u>, 352
Brain stem gliomas in Children, 373
symptoms of, 373
Brain stem tumors & antineoplastons, 352-353
Brain tumor:
(inoperable), 349
& Budwig diet, 368, 445-446
& berberine, 370
& folic acid, 359-360
& goldenseal, 370
& resveratrol, 370
& THC, 372
Brazilian ginseng, 153-154
Brazilian peppertree, 300
BRCA-1 mutation, 64, 65,74, 170-171, 192-193
BRCA-2, 65, 74, 170-171, 192-193
Breadfruit, 479
Breast Cancer, 51-101, 427-428
& abajeru, 71
& AHCC, 62
& algae, 71
& andrographis, 85
& artemisinin, 450-451
& aspilia, 85
& Avemar, 72
& beans, 482
& berries, 75
& Beta-Glucan, 79
& bindweed, 85
& black cohosh, 72
& broccoli, 65
& bromelain, 79, 752
& BSI-201, 60
& Calcium D-Glucarate, 92, 294
& Canelim, 594
& chaparral tea, 567-568
& clodronate, 92-93
& coffee, 86
& Coley's Toxins, 93
& concord grapes, 75
& CoQ10, 62-63, 248-249, 465
& coriander, 566
& cryoablation, 100
& Cytotron, 93-94
& dairy products, 57, 538
& dandelion, 86
& diet, 99
& DIM, 65
& dunaliella, 222-223
& Essiac, 58-59
& fenugreek, 87
& flax, 59-60, 84
& ginkgo biloba, 88, 369
& ginseng, 72
& GLA, 84, 488
& glutathione, 612-613
& grapes, 47
& green tea, 88

& Haelan, 81-83
& HRT, 489-509
& hydrazine sulfate, 94-95, 419-420
& IMRT, 95
& iodine, 63-64, 129
& IP6, 66
& Iscador, 458
& jamun berry, 66
& Laetrile, 586
& Lapatinib, 73
& LifeMel honey, 66-67
& limonene, 76
& Lodamin, 60
& Maitake D-fraction, 80
& mangosteen, 76
& marijuana extract, 96
& melatonin, 96
& milk thistle, 88-89
& milk, 532-533
& modified citrus, 68
& molasses, 543
& mushrooms, 81
& myrrh, 89
& Noscapine, 614
& O.J., 69
& olive oil, 74
& Onconase, 60-61
& oyster mushroom, 527
& papaya, 77, 481
& PARP inhibitors, 192-193
& Pau d'Arco, 89
& Peroxy Gel, 519
& pomegranate, 80-81
& PRIMA-1, 73
& quercetin, 69
& Ranpirnase, 60-61
& raw foods, 54-55
& resveratrol, 49
& Rexin-G, 97
& *rhodiola rosea*, 90, 341
& rosemary, 566
& selenium, 63-64
& shark cartilage, 92
& soy, 78
& St. John's Wort, 90
& statins, 155-156
& sunlight, 522
& TAP Technology, 99-100
& turmeric, 79-80, 91
& Tykerb, 74-75
& Ukrain, 98-99
& Visica2, 100
& vitamin C, 70-71
& vitamin D, 69-70, 77-78
& water, 100-101
& wormwood, 91
& zeolites, 100
Breast cancer awareness, 505
Breast cancer Stage IV, 54-55
Breast health & hormones, 61
Breast Specific Gamma Imaging, 51
Breuss Cancer Treatment, 588-589
Broccoli sprouts, 332
Bromelain, 79, 158-159, 616
& quercetin, 158-159
from pineapple), 452
precautions for use, 452
BSGI imaging, 51
BSI-201, 60
BTA STAT test (bladder), 331
Buckthorn bark, 234
Buckwheat:
& cancer, 484-485
& flavonoids, 484
& quercetin, 484-485
& rutin, 484-485
Budwig diet, 367-368, 413-414, 442-446
& cancer, Ch 36
& flax oil, 367-368
Budwig, Johanna, 439-440
Bulgar & nitrates, 485
Bulgar wheat & diabetics, 485
Bupleurum, 260, 452
*Bupleurum Chinense*, 452
precautions for, 452
Burkitt's lymphoma, 37
Burzynski website, 359
Burzynski's antineoplastons, 589-590
Butter vs. margarine, 439-440
Bypass surgery, 86

## C

CA-125, 169-170
Cabbage family, 78-79
Cabergolide, 381
Cachexia, 285,
& glutamine needs, 469
Cadscience MRI, 52
Caffeic acid, 45, 554, 572
in propolis, 556
Caffeine & skin protection, 392
Caffeine drinks, 510
Calabash, 479
Calcium:
& colon cancer, 154-155
& dairy, 530-531
loss of & acidity, 557-558
sources of, 530-531
Calcium bentonite clay, 548-549
Calcium D-Glucarate, 92, 294
Calmyra figs & parasites, 551
CAM, 132, 619-620
Camu-Camu, 480, 590
Cancel (Protocel), 590
Cancer (also look under cancer types in this index)
& 714X, 416
& ABM mushroom, 524-525
& ALA, 462-463
& beans, 482
& bee venom, 554
& berries, 221-222
& black tea, 567
& carotenoids, 477-478
& chlorella, 426-427
& chlorophyll, 596-597
& cigarettes, 182
& copper levels, 212
& cytotron therapy, 365
& dairy products, 531
& dehydration, 515
& eggplant, 468
& enoki mushroom, 525
& exercise, 518-523
& figs, 483-484
& fresh air, 520
& fungal cure, 591-594
& Gerson Treatment, 611-612
& ginger, 563, 569
& green drinks, 168
& green tea, 569-570
& hydration, 510-517
& iron, 608
& lentinan, 528
& maitake mushrooms, 526
& MSM, 612-613
& niacin, 425
& oregano, 565
& oxygen, 518-523
& papaya, 480-481
& parsley, 571
& peas, 482
& propolis, 556
& rest, 518-523
& Rooibos tea, 571

& shiitake, 528
& sunlight, 521-523
& Tarragon tea, 572
& tea (other types), 215-216
& the goji berry, 461
& the 1 461
& Virastatin, 630
& vitamin D, 69, 628
& willow bark, 564
& yeast, 171
Cancer anti-fungal cure, 561
Cancer caused by candida, 561
Cancer cure by killing yeast 561
Cancer diagnostics, 582-583
Cancer fungal cure, 55
Cancer in babies & blueberries, 463
Cancer prevention & paprika, 565-566
Cancer Tree, The (Xi Shu), 461
Canderel, warnings against, 455
Candida fungus & cancer, 304, 591-594
& acidity, 559
& green foods, 593
& oregano, 459
& Virastatin, 630
Canelim capsules, 594
Canistel, 480
Cannonball, 479
Cansema salve, 36
Cantron, 590
Cape gooseberry, 480
Caperberries, 480
Capsaicin & cancer, 389
Carambolas (starfruit), 479
Caraway & limonene, 281, 485, 566
Carboplatin, 619-620
Carcinoid cancers & Naltrexone, 610
Carcinoid tumors & phytoplankton, 611
Carcinoma:
& barley grass, 426
& Ukrain, 624
Carcinoma in-situ, 51
Carctol, 155, 594-595
Cardiac problems & tree bark, 605
Carica papaya, 481
Carnivore, 35
Carnosol, 89, 221
Carotenoids & healing foods, 477-488
Cartilage:
(precautions for usage), 92
Restoration of cartilage, 239,
& Cytotron, 403
Cascara sagrada, 452-453
Cashew apples, 479
Cat's Claw, 85-86, 289
& bladder cancer, 333
& precautions in usage, 640
& pycnogenols, 152-153, 463-464
Cataracts & ALA, 462-463
& bilberry, 472
Cationic Liposomes, 607
Cayenne & cholesterol, 364
CBD, 96
CCSA-2, 133
CD24, 133
CDA-II, 590
cDPCP, 36
CDX-110 vaccine, 360
Celebrex, 447
Celery, 485
& abdominal cancer, 485
& colon cancer, 485
Celiac disease, 132
Cell phone dangers, 382
Cell regeneration, 464-465
CellFeed Medical, 595
CellQuest, 595
Central nervous system cancers, 366
Cerebral palsy prevention, 67
Cernitin, 105
Cervical Cancer, 169-197
& AHCC, 175
& andiroba, 184
& antineoplastons, 189
& berries, 75, 175
& beta-carotene, 175-176
& broccoli, 176
& carrageenan, 176
& cartilage, 190-192
& cryotherapy, 390, 597-598
& cryptoxanthin, 483
& ellagic acid, 177
& emodin, 185-186
& flax, 178
& folate, 182
& fungus, 171
& glutathione, 183
& hydrazine sulfate, 190
& IMRT, 172
& Iscador, 188, 458
& seaweed, 176, 182-183
& snow fungus, 188
& the cancer bush, 185
& turmeric, 188-189
& Ukrain, 193
& vitamin C, 182-183
& vitamin E, 183
Cervical cells (abnormal) & andiroba oil, 415-416
Cervical dysplasia & vitamin C, 487
Cesium precautions, 595
Ceylon gooseberry, 479
CFS (Chronic Fatigue Syndrome), 86
& bindweed, 588
& ciwujia, 453
& HGH, 604-605
& IGF1, 605
& Lyprinol, 447
& suehirotake mushroom, 528
& the wolfberry (goji berry), 461
Chaga mushroom, 180, 181, 529
Chalta, 479
Chamomile (German), 187
Champedak, 479
*Champion* juicer, 429
Channeling, 12
Chaparral, 365
& Virastatin, 630
& neck cancer, 387-388
Chelation Therapy, 596
Chelators, cilantro, 453
Chelators, spirulina, 433-434
Chemluminescent hemoglobin, 331
Chemo combo, 203
Chemo, 34-35
Chemoembolization, 264-265
ChemoFX, 171
Chemokines, 36
Cherimoya, 479, 480
Cherries & cancer, 75
Cherries & gout, 75
CHF & CoQ10, 276-279, 466-467
CHI, 12
Chia seeds, 544
& EFAs, 488
Chicken-of-the-woods mushroom, 181, 529

Chicory root, 138
Children & CNS cancers, 366
Children & honey, precautions, 555
Chili peppers, 389
Chinese dates, 480
Chinese lantern, 480
Chinese red yeast rice, 486
& cancer, 486
Chinese wolfberry, 461
Chlordane, 362-363
Chlorella, 57, 427
& B12, 434, 478
& beta-carotene, 478
& candida, 593
*Chlorella vulgaris*, 426-427
Chlorella, highest in chlorophyll, 478
Chlorinated water, 510-511
Chlorophyll:
& candida, 593
& circulation, 426
& sprouts, 435
for cancer, 596-597
vs. hemoglobin, 435-436
Chlorophyllin, 146
for cancer, 596-597
Chocolate, 141
Cholangiocarcinoma, 592
Cholesterol (also see under "high Cholesterol")
& amla fruit, 260
& apple skins, 483
& barley, 155, 484
& beta-carotene, 478
& bilberry, 473
& Calcium-D-Glucarate, 155
& celery, 398, 485
& cernitin, 155
& Chinese red yeast rice, 364, 486
& citrus pectin, 177
& *Ecklonia cava*, 155, 630
& flax, 132, 438
& ginseng, 155, 456
& grapes 77
& guggul, 155, 226, 486
& hibiscus tea, 364
& kombucha, 570
& krill oil, 155, 446-447
& niacin, 155, 364, 424, 425, 486, 605
& olive oil, 614
& Policosanol, 364, 486
& pomegranate, 615-616
& red yeast rice, 155, 364
& reishi, 527-528
& resveratrol, 364, 605, 619
& rye bread, 364
& Seanol®, 630
& shiitake, 155, 528
& spirulina, 433-434
& low sodiumV8 Juice, 398
Cholesterol drug used for cancer, 597
Choline:
& bottle gourd, 262
& muscular dystrophy, 473-474
Choline sources, 473
Chondroitin sulfate, 507
Chondrosarcoma, 401
& Lovastatin, 389, 412
Chordomas, 373
Choroid plexus neoplasm, 359
Chronic dehydration, 511-512
Chronic diverticulitis & propolis, 556
Chronic Fatigue Syndrome
& Lyprinol, 447
& Wolfberry, 461
Chronic infections & bindweed, 588
Chronic sinus infections, 614
Chronic Subclinical Scurvy, 209-210
Chrysobalanus icaco, 71
Chymtrypsin, 616
Cilantro, 75
Cinnamon & e-coli, 562-563
Circulation:
& *Ecklonia cava*, 630
& ginkgo biloba, 456
& niacin, 486
Circulation miracles & chlorophyll, 426
Circulatory health & pycnogenols, 469
Cirrhosis & coffee, 238
Cisplatin, 267
Cisplatin-resistance, 624
Cisplatin-resistant cancers & Ukrain, 624
Citrus flavenols fight cancer, 366
Citrus pectin, 177
CLA, 83
*Classic Blend Tea*, 571
Cleansing tips, Ch 36
Clementine, 479
Clinical trials, 573-581, 619-620
Clodronate, 92-93
Cloud mushroom (yun zhi), 529
Cloves & parasites, 549
Cloves & worms, 563
CLT Therapy (Cytoluminescence), 599
C-MET/HGFR inhibitors, 36
CML & Dyer's woad root, 234
CML & Sprycel, 207
CML & vitamin A, 212
CNS cancers & Essiac tea, 366
CNS cancers, cure for, 366
CNS lymphoma, 373
CNS tumors in children, 351
Coco-plum (abajeru), 71, 86, 299
Cold sores & Virastatin, 630
Colds:
& ginger, 563
& horse radish, 564-565
Coley's Toxins, 93
Colitis, 427, 435,
& bee pollen, 552
& dehydration, 511-512
& Flor-Essence Essiac tea, 542
& pomegranate, 615-616
& probiotics, 542
Collagen loss & fluoride, 510-511
Colloid breast cancer 51
Colon cancer: 130-168, 594-595
& abajeru, 145
& AHCC, 136
& alkalinity, 542
& antineoplastons, 138, 162-163
& apple juice (cloudy) 136
& aronia berries, 136
& artemisinin, 145
& asparagus, 484
& Avanex 7-1037, 584-585
& bacteria, 162
& beans, 482
& beta-sitosterol, 162
& BioCancell, 588
& black raspberries, 137
& blackstrap molasses, 543
& blueberries, 137
& Budwig diet, 131-132

& calcium, 154-155
& cat's claw, 152-153
& celery, 398, 485
& chaparral tea, 567-568
& chicory root, 138
& chlorophyll, 146, 597
& citrus, 139
& coffee, 139
& cranberries, 139
& Echinacea, 455-456
& ellagic acid, 156
& Essiac, 147
& exercise, 165, 520
& fennel, 566
& fiber, 160
& flavenols, 141
& flax seed, 141
& ginger, 566
& goldenseal, 151
& grapes, 47
& graviola, 151-152
& *Hallelujah Acres* Diet, 130-131
& lutein, 160
& lycopene, 160
& milk thistle, 152
& modified citrus pectin, 68, 158
& Noscapine, 614
& olive oil, 143
& OncoVAX, 134
& oyster mushroom, 527
& PC-SPES, 153
& propolis, 554, 556
& proteolytic enzymes, 616
& PSK, 525
& quercetin, 158-159
& radio-immunotherapy, 135
& raisins, 143
& Rexin-G, 135
& snow rose, 153
& statin drugs, 138-139
& sulfur veggies, 160
& sunlight, 165, 522
& turmeric, 140, 143-144
& vegetables, 143-144
& vitamin D, 165, 167, 213
& water, 167-168
& wormwood, 145
& yeast, 133
Colon cancer screening, 133-134
Colon health & alkalinity, 542
Color & healing, Ch 36
Colorectal Cancer (also see under colon cancer), 130-168
& Avanex 7-1037, 137, 584-585
& B6, 154
& beta-carotene, 137
& folate (folic acid), 157
& ginger, 157-158
& hydrazine sulfate, 419-420
& 131-I, 135
& Labetuzumab, 135
& mushrooms that help, 161
& piceatannol, 396
& selenium, 159
& Sir-Spheres, 164
& SIRT, 164
& Ukrain, 165-166
& ZoonCan, 154
Colorectal cancer, advanced, 164
ColoSure, 133
Comedy & healing, Ch 36
Comfrey, 36
Complementary & alternative medicine, 619 (CAM)
Computed Ultrasound Risk Eval, 51-52
Concord grapes & cancer, 75
Confocal endomicroscopy, 133
Congestive heart failure, 62-63, 166-167
Congressional testimony: antineoplastons, 358-358
Conjugated linoleic acid, 83
Conk mushroom, 529
Constipation help:
& bee pollen, 552
& cascara, 452-453
& flax, 438
& ginger, 563
& pear juice, 563
Contortrostatin, 36
*Convolvulus arvensis* (bindweed), 587-588
CoQ10, 62-64
& Adriamycin, 215
& CHF, 62-63
& MS, 156
& selenium, 465
& sources of, 467
& statin drugs, 467
CoQ10 levels & melanoma risk, 389
Cord stem cells, 204
Cordycepin & HIV, 525
*Cordyceps sinensis* mushroom, 525
*Coriolus versicolor* mushroom, 81, 161, 525
Corn syrup, 488
Coronary artery disease & milk, 533
Cortisol, 502
*CORralen*, 86
Cranberries, 454
Craniopharyngioma, 359, 373
Creosote bush (chaparral tea), 387-388
Crohn's Disease, 41
& cat's claw, 463-464
& propolis, 556
& probiotics, 542
Cruciferous foods, 79, 486
Cryo Therapy, 108, 177, 390, 597-598
Cryoablation, 108, 177, 390 597-598
Cryospray Ablation, 301-302, 598
Cryptococal meningitis & garlic, 336
Cryptoxanthin, 483
CSS and vitamin C, 209-210
Curaderm BEC5 & skin cancer, 390
Curcumin (also look under turmeric)
Curcumin & MS, 475
CURE evaluation device, 51-52
Curing cancer by killing yeast, 561
Current testing, 30-31
Custard apple, 479
Customized vaccines, 600,613
Cutaneous T-cell lymphoma, 403, 602
CyberKnife therapy, 72, 109, 390, 598-599, 603
Cytoluminescent Therapy, 308, 599
Cytomegalovirus & Virastatin, 630
Cytotron Therapy, 93-94, 109, 171, 390-391, 599-600

## D

D.I.M., 65
Dairy:
& breast cancer, 57

& prostate cancer, 104
problems with, 530-539
D-alpha-tocopherol (vitamin E), 346
Dalton's ascitic lymphoma, 405-406
Dancing mushroom, 161
Dandelion, 86, 261
tea precautions, 568
DaVinci Surgical System, 600, 621
DCA (Dichloroacetate), 600
Death angel mushroom poisoning, 583-584
Deep breathing, 518
Degarelix, 36
De-glycrrhizinated licorice (DGL), 262, 458-459
Dehydration & cancer, 515
Dehydroepiandrosterone (DHEA), 231
Dementia:
& aluminum, 511
& ginkgo biloba, 456
Dendritic Cell Therapy, 600
Dengue fever cure, 361-362, 544, 551
Dental caries & green tea, 570
Depression & low-dose Dilantin, 658
Depression & HGH, 604-605
Dermatitis & propolis, 556
Dermatomyositis cure, 425
Desmoids tumors, 37
Detox & MSM, 612-613
Detox Program, Ch 35, 36
Detoxification, Ch 35, 36
Detoxing the body, Ch 35, 36
Detoxing with seaweed, 433
Devil's tongue, 270
Dexamethasone, 203
DGL & GERD, 262, 301-302
DGL licorice, 570-571
D-Glucarate, sources of, 92
DHEA, 109
Diabetes, 41, 69
& ALA, 462-463
& CoQ10, 464
& Gerson, 611-612
& jamun berry, 66
& milk, 504, 534-535
Diabetes (juvenile) & milk, 534-535
Diabetic PVD, 456
Diabetic sores & Manuka honey, 556
DiaGenic, 52
Diarrhea (help for):
& bee pollen, 552
& bilberry, 473
& honey, 555
& vitamin A, 479
Diabetic retinopathy & pine bark, 469
Dicer & Drosha genes, 36
Diclofenac, 527
Digestive diseases & Xi Shu, 461
Digestive disorders & bromelain, 452
Digestive tract cancers, 594-595 (also look under colon cancer & gastric)
DiGuglielmo's Syndrome, 37
Diindolymethane (DIM), 486
DIM, 78-79
sources of, 486
Dinoflagellates (phyto-plankton), 611
Diphtheria & Chinese asparagus, 453
Diphtheria & Echinacea, 455
Disc disease & HRT, 498
Disc herniations & hydration, 514
Diuretic, parsley tea, 459-460, 571
Diverticulosis & cascara, 452-453
D-Mannose & urinary tract health, 454
DNA protectant, wolfberry, 461
Double-blind trials, 574-577
Down's Syndrome, 473, 474
Dr. Burzynski's life-saving pump, 355-356
DR70 blood test, 36
D-ribose for energy, 86
Dries Cancer Diet, 36
Drug publicity, 579
Dry skin & natural progesterone, 498-499
Dry skin & vitamin A, 479
DS-6, 622-623
Ductal breast cancer, 100
Ductal cell carcinoma, 51, 54-55
Dunaliella bardawil, 222-223
Durian, 479
Dyer's woad root, 234

# E

Ear infections & dairy products, 537
Ear ache & wild oil of oregano, 456, 565
Ebola virus & vitamin C, 540
Ebola, 211
*Echinacea augustifolia*, 455-456
*Echinacea purpurea*, (best) 455-456
Echinacea, 147, 306, 455-456
*Ecklonia cava*, 630
E-coli, 294
& cinnamon, 562-563
ECT – Electro Chemical Therapy, 94
EDTA Liposomes, 596
EEA & pituitary tumors, 382
EFAs – best sources, 335
EFAs & ADD, 487-488
EGCG, 225-226, 337, 393
EGFR, 39
Eggplant & cancer, 390, 468
Eggplant extract (Curaderm BEC5), 390
Ehrlich's ascites carcinoma:
& ABM, 524
Electrical frequency generator, 549
Electrochemical Therapy (SEE ECT), 391
Elekta Body frame, 273-274
Elephant foot, 270
*Elephantopus scaber* & lymphoma, 406
Ellagic acid 45, 76, 110-111, 279, 302,468
sources of, 156, 177, 279, 302, 468
Ending the fast, 635-636
Endocrine cancers & macrobiotics, 541
Endocytoscopy, 133
Endometrial cancer (see ovarian too)
& beta-carotene, 175-176
& fiber, 194
& Haelan, 193
& lycopene, 179
& lymph nodes, 195
& milk thistle, 242, 395
& radiation, 195
Endonasal endoscopy, 382
Endoscopic trans-nasal brain

surgery, 382
Energy & the yun zhi mushroom, 529
Engraftment, 202
Enoki mushroom & cancer, 525
Enokitake mushroom, 181, 529
Ependymoma, , 358, 373
Epidermoid cancers, 393, 619
Epigenetic Therapy, 600-601
Epithelian ovarian carcinoma, 170-173
Epratuzumab, 37
Epstein-Barr Virus & the wolfberry, 461
Equal (see aspartame), 406
Equal, warnings against, 455
Erbitux, 37
ERCP, 267-268
Ergocalciferol, 522
Escoazul (blue scorpion venom), 621
Esinophilic granuloma, 423
Esophageal cancer, 299-314
& black raspberries, 300
& ellagic acid, 302
& garlic, 304
& green tea, 305
& molybdenum, 307
& niacinamide, 307
& riboflavin, 309
& Transfer Factor, 310-311
& Ukrain, 311-312
& zinc, 159
Espinheira santa, 391
Essential fatty acids, 487-488
Essiac tea, 57-58, 147-150, 568-569, 601
*Ester-C* (non-acidic Vitamin C), 344-345
Estradiol (synthetic estrogen), 489
Estriol (natural estrogen), 489, 492, 494
Estrogen, 489-509
& licorice, 458-459
blockers of estrogen, 486
in dairy products, 538
*Estrogen dominance*, 490-491, 497-498 504
Estrone (synthetic estrogen), 489
Ethanol injection, 314
Ethylene diamine tetra-acetic acid, 596
Etoposide, 424, 619-620
Eugenol in basil, 562
Evening primrose oil, 296, 487-488
EVOO, 143, 614
Ewing's sarcoma, 592
& niacinamide, 424
& Ukrain, 424
& vitamin C cure, 424-425
EWOT, 444
Exercise & cancer, 518-523
Extracorporeal photo-pheresis, 403, 600, 602
Eye tumors, 619-620


# F


Familial adenomatous polyposis, 143-144
Far Infrared Hyperthermia Treatment, 602
Fasting, 631-636
& alkalinity, 631-632
& Bible promises, 632-634
ending the fast safely, 635-636
precautions for, 635
Fatigue & schisandra, 90
Fatigue & vitamin A, 479
FDA, 59,122,406
& clinical trials, 574 578
Atrocities of, 31-35, 454, 484
attacks on Dr. Burzynski, 356-359
hypocrisy of FDA, 387-388
FDP test (bladder), 331
Feijoa, 479, 480
Fenugreek, 87
Fermented soy, 78, 509
Fermented wheat germ extract, 72
Ferrite Beads, 382
Ferulic acid, 485
Fever blisters & ginger, 563
Fibrinogen degradation products, 331
Fibrocystic breast cure, 499
Fibromyalgia, 86, 630
& *Ecklonia cava*, 630
Fibrosarcoma, 401
Fibrous histiocytoma, 358-359
Figs & cancer, 483-484
Fish (best type) for consumption, 335
Fish vs flax, 446
FIT Testing, 133-134
Flavenols, 173, 215-216
sources of, 215-216, 271
Flax:
& alkalinity, 438
& breast cancer, 59-60
& other miracle oils, 437-447
& varieties of, 439
Flax inhibits cancer, 437
Flax vs fish, 446
Flex-Het Drugs, 36
*Flor-Essence* Essiac Tea, 58-59, 366
Fluoride toxicity, 510-511
Folate & breast cancer, 65
Folate & ovarian cancer, 65
Folic acid & colorectal cancers, 157
Folic acid sources, 329
Food & parasites, 546
Formylmethionine, 295
Forskolin & cancer, 602
Forskolin source, 602
Fosamax, 93
Fostamatinib disodium, 204, 402-403
*Fosteronia refracta*, 36
Free radicals, 46, 427, 464-465
Freeze dried sprout extracts, 332
Fresh air & cancer cells, 520
Frontal anaplastic grade III astrocytoma, 378
Fucoidan (from kelp), 433
Fungal (yeast – Candida) cure, 369
Fungal cure for cancer, 403-404, 591-593
*Fungus japonicas* - (kombucha), 570


# G


Gac fruit, 479
Gac-Chi drink, 479
GADF, 77
Galectin inhibitors, 37
Gallstones:
& cascara, 452-453
& flax, 443
& parsley tea, 571
Gamma Knife, 603, 622
Gandaria fruit, 479
Ganglioneuroma, 373
*Ganoderma lucidum* (reishi), 527-528
Gardasil, 38-39, 41-42
*Garden of Life* Products,

211, 340, 604
Garlic, 87
& bladder cancer, 336
& esophageal cancer, 304
& yeast infections, 304
Gastric cancer (also see abdominal cancer)
& carctol, 155
& ECT, 140-141
& Essiac tea, 303
& magnesium, 129,141-142
& proteolytic enzymes, 143
& PSK, 525
& Tian Xian, 154
Gastric problems & ginger, 563
Gastroenteritis & honey, 555
Gc-MAF, 36
GDC-0449 & basal cell cancer, 385-386
GEMM, 36
Gene immunotherapy & melanoma, 383-384
Genipap, 479
Genomic testing, 52
Geraniol, 414-415
& pancreatic cancer, 321
in ginger, 564
sources of, 321
GERD, 301-302, 517, 598
& DGL, 301-302
& orange peel extract, 301-302
German New Medicine, 36
Gerson Therapy, 315-316, 611-612
Gerson, Max, 611-612
Giant granadilla, 479
Ginger, 563
Ginger & cancer, 563
Ginger tea, 569
Gingerol, 157-158
Ginkgo biloba, 88, 369
Ginseng, 72, 456
& cancer cell reversal, 456
GIST, 150
GKI (Polarizing Solution), 615
GLA, 487-488
Gland replenisher, royal jelly, 556
glandulars
Glaucoma:
& bilberry & pine bark, 470-471
& Forskolin, 602
Gleevec (or Glivec), 207
Glioblastoma:
& antineoplastons, 355
& garlic, 369
& the *Gliadel Wafer*, 369
& Lodamin, 60, 374
& Naltrexone, 610
& Neuradiab, 361
& vitamin C, 361-362
Glioblastoma multiforme:
& antineoplastons, 360
& CDX-110, 360
cure for, 360
Glioma, 349-382, 401
& chaparral tea, 567-568
& mullaca, 307, 373
& scorpion venom, 376, 621, 622
& the *Gliadel Wafer*, 369
& turmeric, 365
Glivec (or Gleevec), 150
Glucommanan, 279
Glucosamine, 507
Glutamine, 468
& cachexia prevention, 285, 469
sources of, 469
Glutathione, 262, 468
& milk thistle, 242
& MSM, 612-613
(reduced), 618
sources of, 242, 468
Gluten-sensitive enteropathy, 30, 132
Glyconutrition, 604
*Glycyrrhiza glabra* (licorice), 458-459
Glyoxylide, 609-610
GMO foods, 258, 287, 369-370, 504
horrors of, 503
GMO soy, 443
God's healing, 23-24
God's Word, 14
Goji berry (wolfberry), 461
Goji-Zen drink, 480
Gold, Dr. Joseph, 94-95, 417-420
Golden green tea, 570
Goldenseal, 225
Gossypol, 36
Goumi, 479
Gout, 75, 615
& autumn crocus, 224
& cherries for treating, 75
& gymnema sylvestre, 457
Graft vs. Host Disease, 202
Grape Antioxidant Dietary Fiber, 77
Grape seed extract, 65-66, 158, 280
Grapefruit juice & drugs, 40
Grapefruit seed extract, 204, 565
Grapes, 77
& abdominal cancer, 45
& cancer, 43-50
Graviola, 102, 322
Green drinks & cancer, 55
Green foods & calcium, 530-531
Green foods & wound healing, 426
Green grasses & drinks 426-436
*Green Magma*, 431
*Green Miracle*, 68-69, 431
Green powdered drinks, 431
*Green Power* juicer, 428
*Green Star* juicer, 428
Green tea, 88
& cancer, 569-570
Greenbriar, 36
Green-lipped mussel oil, 447
Grifola frondosa, 161
Ground ivy, 36
GRP receptors, 36
GTx, 114
Guacatonga, 415-416
Guanabana, 481
Guavas, 480-481
Guggul, 486
Guided Therapeutics, 114
Gullain-Barre Syndrome, 41-42
Gum disease, 278-279
& bindweed, 588
& CoQ10, 464
GVHD, 202
*Gynostemma pentaphyllum*, 458-459

# H

H19 gene, 588
Haelan, 78, 164-165, 476, 509
& skin problems, 398-399
Hair color restoration:
& kombucha, 570
& molasses, 543
Hair growth & kombucha, 570
Halitosis & green tea, 570

*Hallelujah Acres* diet, 54-55, 130-131
HAMA, 380-381
Hand-Schuller-Christian Disease, 423
Hanta virus & vitamin C, 541
Happy Tree, 461
Harmony healing, 9, 10
Harry Hoxsey, 393-394
Hay fever & bee pollen, 553
& horseradish, 564
HcG, 170-171
HCL & hoelen, 526
HDAC (Histone Deacetylase), 36
Head-&-Neck cancers, 299-314
& Advexin, 304
& chlorella, 301
& IMRT, 306
Healing through touch, Ch 36
Healthy tips, 638
Hearing loss & *rhodiola rosea*, 341
Heart attacks & HRT, 495
Heart disease:
& ALA, 462-463
& beta-carotene, 478
& CoQ10, 276-279, 464-465
& Gerson, 611-612
& HRT, 495
& quercetin, 171
Heart health & barley, 484
Heart health & olive oil, 614
Heartburn, 517
Heated liposomes (Thermo-Dox), 623
Heavy metal removal, 433-434
Heimlich Maneuver, 610-611
Hemangioblastomas, 374
Hemochromatosis, 88-89, 263
Hemoglobin dipstick, 331
Hen-of-the-woods, 161
Heparin, 507
Hepatic carcinoma 2, 592
Hepatitis:
& beet juice, 256
& bupleurum, 452
& licorice, 262
& milk thistle, 243
& picrorrhiza, 261
& schisandra, 261
(viral) & avocados, 469
Hepatitis C, 243, 246-247
& ALA, 463
Hepatitis-B, 256-257
HER-1, 39
HER-2, 73, 74-75
Herbal resources, 448-449
Herbalene, 571
Herceptin, 74
Herpes simplex & licorice, 458-459
Herpes virus & Virastatin, 630
HGH – human growth hormone, 604-605
& osteoporosis, 605
& stress, 521
HI-ART TOMO Therapy, 623
Hiatal hernia, 511-512
Hibiscus tea, 364
High blood pressure:
& bilberry, 473
& celery, 398, 485
& CoQ10, 464
& flax, 438
& hydration, 514, 515-516
& low sodium V8 Juice, 398
& rye, 485
High cholesterol (also look under "cholesterol")
& *Ecklonia cava*, 630
& flax, 438
High-grade gliomas, 359
Hiratake mushroom, 181, 529
Histamine, 501
regulation & asthma, 512-513
HIV:
& 714X, 416
& betulinic acid, 399
& bindweed, 588
& cordycepin, 525
& Hoxsey tea, 457-458
& kombucha tea, 570
& lentinan, 339
& macela, 261
& Maitake D-Fraction, 219-220
& oleander, 255
& olive leaf, 459
& PSK, 525
& red clover, 460
& selenium, 64
& skullcap, 185
& turmeric, 525
& vassourinha, 378
& Virastatin, 630
Hodgkin's vs. Non-Hodgkin's Lymphoma, 402
Hodgkin's cure & Resperin Essiac tea, 417
Hodgkin's disease (also, see lymphoma), 358-359, 402
& Budwig diet
& vitamin C, 207-208, 404
& flax, 413-414
& shark liver oil, 423
Hodgkin's lymphoma cure & 714X, 416-417
Hoelen mushroom, 526
Hogplum fruit, 479
Holt Microwave Therapy, 36
Homeopathy, 229-230
Homogenization, problems with, 533
Homogenized milk, 536-538
Honey, precautions for, 432
Hormonal cancers & HMR lignans, 605
Hormone Replacement, 489-509
Hormones:
testing for, 501-502
in cattle, 503-504
in meat & dairy, 490-491
in milk supply, 533, 538
Horseradish, 564
precautions for, 564
Horsetail herb, 460
*Host Defense*, 529
Hoxsey clinic, 458
Hoxsey, Harry, tea, 457-458
HPV & ellagic acid, 177
HPV virus, 39
H-pylori bacteria:
& cranberry, 91
& honey, 554
& wormwood, 91
HRT, 38
Hu zhang, 50
Huckleberries, 480
Human anti-mouse antibodies, 380-381
Hydrastine, 151
Hydration & cancer, 510-517
Hydration & salt, 513
Hydrazine Sulfate, 94-95, 417-420
Hydrogen peroxide gel, 519
Hydrogenated fats, 439-440
Hyperbaric oxygen therapy,

518, 520
Hyperforin, 90
Hyperthermia Therapy, 607-608
for treating cancer, 605-606
Hypofractionated Radiation, 95
Hysterectomies, 493-494
& HRT, 498

# I

I3C, 65, 106
IAT, 36
IBS (Irritable Bowel Syndrome):
& probiotics, 542
& propolis, 556
IC3, 78-79
Ice man mushroom, 181, 529
ICHT, 607
Ideal survival food, flax, 438
iFOBT, 134
IGF-I receptors, 35, 604-605
IHT, 606
Illuminated Ones, 12
Imiquimod (Aldara), 197
Immune-enhancer, glutamine, 469
Immunity:
& MGN-3, 612
& alkalinity, 559
& bee pollen, 553
& *Ecklonia cava*, 630
& LifeMel Honey, 520
& *MycoPhyto* Formula, 613
& Polyerga, 615
& rest, 520-521
& sunshine, 523
& Zun Zhi mushroom, 529
Immunokan, 37
Immunotherapy, 600, 613
& melanoma cure, 383-384
cure for AML, 606
cure for leukemia, 606
for brain tumors, 361
Transfer Factor, 623
Implanted magnetic sensing, 196
IMRT, 95, 114-115, 608-609, 623
Indian almond, 261
Indian ginseng, 451
Indian gooseberry, 260
Indian jujube fruit, 479
Indian sage, 571
Indigestion:
& bilberry, 473
& oregano, 456
Individualized vaccines, 361, 613
Indoles, 65, 79, 160, 337, 486
Infant botulism & honey, 432
Infertility cure, 499
Inflammation:
& *Ecklonia cava*, 630
& morels, 527
& Moxxor, 447
Inflammatory bowel & propolis, 556
Influenza & dairy products, 537
Inositol Hexaphosphate, 66, 608
Insomnia & vitamin A, 479
Insulin Potentiation Therapy (IPT), 607-608
Insulin-induced hypoglycemic Therapy (IHT), 606
Insulin-like growth factor:
in milk, 533
InSure FIT, 133-134
Insure Quik FIT, 133-134
Intensity Modulated Radiotherapy, 95, 608-609
Intercalating agents, 35
Interferon & kombucha, 526
Interstitial Radio Frequency, 605-606
Intestinal cancers & folate, 157
Intracellular Hyperthermia, 607
Intraoperative Electron Radiation, 96, 609
Intravesical Immunotherapy, 338
Inulin, 138, 258
Iodine, in milk, 533
IOERT (Mobetron), 96, 609
IP-6 & cancer, 115, 608, 486-487
Ipriflavone & osteoporosis, 155, 498
IPT, 607-608
IRE – NanoKnife, 630
Iressa, 36
Irinotecan, 461
Iron & cancer cells, 608
Irradiation of food, 332
Irreversible Electro-corporation (IRE), 630
Iscador (mistletoe), 458, 606
Isoprinosine, 291
Isosilybin-B, 115
Isothiocyanates, 65, 332
Israeli scorpion:
& gliomas, 376
Issel's Treatment Centers, 93, 156, 239, 403, 466, 584, 602, 613, 615
Ita palm, 479
ITC, 332
Itchy scalp, 435
IVDMIA, 36

# J

Jaboticaba, 479
Jackfruit, 479
Jambolana berry, 66
Jamun berry, 66
& diabetes, 66
Japanese plum balls, 561
Jaundice & dandelion, 261
Jellyfish & aloe vera, 450
Jesus' healing touch, Ch 36
Jiaogulun & liver health, 458
Johanna Budwig Diet, Ch. 36
Joint health:
& *Ecklonia cava*, 630
& MSM, 613
Joint pain & quercetin, 617
Joints & alkalinity, 559
Juicing:
juice-fasting, 560-561
& alkalinity, 560
& detoxing, 635
& juicer types, 428-430
what to choose, 530
*Just Barley*, 431
Juvenile pilocytic neuromas, 373

# K

Kakis fruit, 479
Kamunggay, 172-173
*Kamut*, 431
Kanamycin, 294
Kanga herbs, 37
Kansius Machine, 609
Kaposi's sarcoma & Virastatin, 630
Karawatake (coriolus) mushroom, 81, 525
Karmanos Cancer Center, 621

Karuki rhizome, 260
Karuna, 12
Kasha (roasted buckwheat), 485
Kelp, 433
& fucoidan, 433
Kepel, 479
Keshan's Disease, 64
Ketupa, 479
Ki, 12
Kidney ailments & Escoazul, 621
Kidney cancer, 331-348
& astragalus, 331
& cholesterol drugs, 334
& CyberKnife, 334
& Cytotron, 334-335
& Essiac tea, 335-336
& fungal (yeast) cure, 336
& LifeMel honey, 338
& Onconase, 60-61, 339
& Ranpirnase, 399
& saw palmetto, 341
& Ukrain, 343
& magnesium, 129, 339
& Rexin-G, 341
Kidney infections & Vitamin C, 344-345
Kidney problems & hoelen, 526
Kidney stones, 56
& dairy products, 537-538
Kidney stone tree, 256-257
Kiahiba (yellow reishi), 527
Kisshotake (reishi), 527-528
Koch Cancer Cure, 609-610
Kombu, 433
Kombucha tea, 526, 570
Konjac fiber, 270
Konjac-Mannan, 279
Konjaka, 270
Konnyaku, 270
Krebiozen, 36
Krill oil:
& arthritis, 446-447
& Omega-3, 446
& PMS, 446-447
Kudzu, 261
Kumquat, 479
Kundalini force, 12
Kuroshiba (black reishi), 527
*Kyolic* garlic, 256, 392

## L

Lack of tears & vitamin A, 479
Lactobacillus, 256
Lactoferrin, 36
Lactose intolerance, 536-537
Laetrile (Laevalin) (B17), 586, 610
dosing of, 585-586
resource for, 587
Laminaria, 227-228, 292
Lapacho, 89, 415-416
Lapatinib, 73
*Larrea diivericata* (chaparral tea), 387
*Larrea tridentate* (chaparral tea), 387, 630
Larynx cancer (also see neck, throat & esophageal cancer & head-and-neck cancers) 299-314
& abajeru, 299
Laser-Induced Thermo-therapy, 265-266
Laughter, 13-14
LCH, 37
Leiomyosarcoma, 401
Lemonade Diet, 558
Lentigo maligna melanoma, 37
Lentinan (from shiitake), 81, 161, 293, 386, 528
Lentinus edodes (shiitake) 280-281
Letterer-Siwe Disease, 423
Leukemia, 36, 198-236
& abajeru, 71, 222
& acai berry, 229
& Adriamycin, 215
& ALA, 462-463
& aloe, 223
& alpha lipoic acid, 229
& amargo, 232-233
& anamu, 232-233
& andrographis, 233-234
& anorexia, 210
& antineoplastons, 230
& arsenic, 229-230
& artemisinin, 223, 451
& autumn crocus, 224
& B12, 217-218
& B6, 217-218
& barley grass, 214
& beets, 214
& berberine, 225
& beta-sitosterol, 230
& Boswellia, 218
& buckthorn bark, 234
& butcher's broom, 224
& cascara sagrada, 452-453
& cat's claw, 224, 463-464
& chaparral, 224
& CoQ10, 214
& cranberries, 215, 454
& DHEA, 231
& dyer's woad root, 234
& feverfew, 220
& flax, 443
& folic acid, 208-209, 216, 217-218, 359-360
& Fostamatinib Disodium, 204, 402
& fungal cure, 205, 592
& garlic, 225
& GLA, 216-217
& goldenseal, 225
& grapes, 47
& green tea, 225-226, 570
& guggul, 226
& Kansius Machine, 609
& kiwi, 449
& Kudzu, 218
& lapacho, 226-227
& LifeMel honey, 218-219
& magnesium deficiency, 129, 210
& Maitake D-Fraction, 219-220
& mangosteen, 219
& milk, 534-535
& mullaca, 231-232
& Naltrexone, 610
& Noscapine, 614
& Onconase, 206
& parthenolide, 220
& pau d'arco, 89, 226-227
& Poly-MVA, 234
& *polyporus umbellatus* mushroom, 211, 340, 527
& processed meats, 236
& quercetin, 221
& resveratrol, 217
& RM-10, 211
& rosemary, 221
& royal jelly, 221
& saffron, 227, 566
& scutellaria, 227, 422
& shark liver oil, 234-235
& simarouba, 232-233
& spirulina, 434
& Sprycel, 207
& sulfated SKCF, 227-228
& taheebo, 226-227
& THC, 372
& Ukrain, 235

& vassourinha, 233, 378
& vitamin A, 212
& vitamin C, 209-210
& vitamin E, 212-213
& Viva Natural, 227-228
& wormwood, 223
& Xi Shu or Cancer Tree, 236, 461
& zinc, 212
& chlorella, 222-223
Leukemia cells in cow's
milk, 535
in dairy cattle, 236
Lewis lung carcinoma, 180,
& ABM, 524
Leydig cell tumor, 37
Libido & HGH, 604-605
Licorice, 262, 458-459, 570-571
precaution with, 458-459
LifeMel honey, 66-67, 281, 306, 394, 420, 555
Lifestyle & diet, 23-25
Light Infusion Therapy, 266
Light Therapy, 599
Lignans in barley, 484
Lignans in flax, 438
*Limaosinho maytenus*, 289
Limonene, 76, 485
& mint, 566
LINAC, 599
Linear accelerator, 599
Lip cancer, 303
Liposarcoma (adipose tissue), 401
Liposomal vitamin C, 544
*Liposome-encapsulated vitamin C*, 345, 347, 361-362, 519, 543, 544
LITT Therapy, 265-266
LITX, 266
Live cell therapy, 473
Liver cancer, 237-268
& ABM, 254-255
& actinidia root, 260, 449-450
& alkalinity, 253
& aloe emodin, 246
& apples, 247
& arginine, 258
& artichokes, 258
& BioCancell, 588
& bitter orange, 260
& bland embolization, 264-265
& blueberries, 248
& bupleurum, 260
& cartilage, 257
& cherries, 248
& chlorophyll, 146, 237, 238, 596-597
& chlorophyllin, 237-238
& choline, 256
& cinnamon, 248
& coffee, 238
& CoQ10, 238-239, 248-249
& coriander, 566
& cryotherapy, 390, 597-598
& CyberKnife, 239
& ECT therapy, 239-240
& Essiac Tea, 147, 249-250
& fungal cure, 240
& garlic, 256
& goldenseal, 250
& grapes, 47, 251
& holly mangrove, 240
& hormones, 252-253
& IP-6, 253
& lecithin, 256
& lentinan, 254
& light infusion therapy, 266
& limonene, 253
& LITT, 265-266
& LITX, 266
& Lodamin, 60, 245
& macela
& Maitake D-fraction, 254
& milk thistle, 240-245
& oleander, 255
& onions, 255-256
& phyllanthus, 256-257
& Poly-MVA, 266
& probiotics, 256
& radiofrequency ablation, 264
& reishi, 254
& resveratrol, 49, 251
& Rexin-G, 266-267
& scutellaria, 262
& selenium, 258
& shiitake, 528
& SIR-Spheres, 264-265
& SIRT, 164
& soy lecithin, 258
& TheraSphere, 259
& ThermoDox, 623
& Tian Xian, 259
& Ukrain, 267
& vitamin K, 259-260
Terminal liver cancer, 257
Liver flush, 641-642
Liver healing & ALA, 583-584
Liver health:
& AHCC, 237
& alpha lipoic acid, 246-247
& amla fruit, 260
& astragalus, 247
& beets, 247-248
& borage oil, 256
& bottle gourd, 262
& bupleurum, 452
& Chinese peony, 260-261
& dandelion tea, 261, 568
& glandulars, 604
& green foods, 251-252
& green tea, 252
& Indian almond, 261
& jiaogulan, 458
& kudzu, 261
& licorice, 262
& lycopene, 254
& picrorrhiza, 261
& red clover, 257
& schisandra, 90, 261
& snow fungus, 188
& tamarind juice, 262
Liver health products, 260-264
Liver inflammation, 90
Liver injury & bee pollen, 553
Liver problems & ALA, 462-463
Liver problems & cascara, 452-453
Liver protectors:
& artichokes, 484
& avocados, 469
& *rhodiola rosea*, 341
Liver stiffness test (LST), 237
Liver storage of vitamin A, 478-479
Liver tonic drink, 641-642
Liver tonic tea, 570-571
Liver transplants & ALA, 246-247, 268, 463
Lobular carcinoma, 51
Lodamin, 60
Loganberries, 480
Loquat, 479
Lorenzo's Oil, 472
Lovastatin, 389
& cancer therapy, 597
Low dose Naltrexone, 425, 610
LSM, liver stiffness measurement, 237

Lucky fungus (reishi), 527-528
Lucuma, 479
Lumpy breasts & HRT, 498
Lung cancer, 269-298
& abajeru, 288
& aloe vera juice, 288
& antineoplastons, 293-294
& apples, 274
& aspilia, 85, 288
& astragalus, 288
& bee pollen, 553
& beets, 274
& beta-carotene, 275-276
& Beta-Glucan, 293
& BioCancell, 588
& broccoli, 274
& Calcium D-Glucarate, 294
& Canelim, 594
& cat's claw, 289
& cayenne, 289
& cherries, 276
& Chinese asparagus, 453
& CoQ10, 276-279
& cranberries, 269-270, 279
& CyberKnife, 270
& dried wakame, 433
& ECT, 270
& espinheira santa, 289
& Essiac tea, 289-290
& flavenols, 271
& fungal cure, 271
& Gamma Knife, 622
& GLA, 488
& glucomannan, 279
& glutathione, 284-285
& grapes, 47, 283
& green tea, 280
& hydration, 296
& IMRT, 271-272
& IP-6, 280
& konjac-mannan, 279
& Laetrile, 586
& lentinan, 280-281
& LifeMel honey, 281
& limonene, 281
& Lodamin, 60
& lycopene, 281
& magnesium, 129, 272
& milk thistle, 290
& niacin, 282
& noni juice, 294
& Noscapine, 614
& oleander, 255, 290-291
& omega-3, 282-283
& Onconase, 60-61
& parsley, 291
& phytoplankton, 275
& Poly-MVA, 294-295
& pomegranate, 283
& proteolytic enzymes 273
& PSK, 525
& psoralea seed, 291, 421
& resveratrol, 283
& Rexin-G, 272
& *rhodiola rosea*, 90, 291, 341
& seaweed, 291-292
& selenium, 285-286
& shiitake, 280-281
& smoking, 296-297
& stereotactic therapy, 273-274
& sushi, 283
& tea, 290
& Tian Xian, 292
& Transfer Factor, 295
& turmeric, 292
& Ukrain, 295-296
& Uno de' Gato, 289
& vitamin C, 70-71, 282
& vitamin E, 287
(terminal) & vitamin C, 272
Lung tumors & Gamma Knife, 622
Lupus, 69, 358, 425, 436, 505-506
& beta-carotene, 478
& CoQ10, 436
& flax, 443
& hoelen for kidney disease, 526
& magnesium, 129, 436
& vitamin D connection, 436
Lupus Nephritis, 440
Lutein, 80
in avocados, 469
sources of, 160, 472
Lychee fruit, 479
Lycopene, 80
& prostate cancer, 115-116
in guavas, 482
sources of, 160, 179
Lymph node removal, 195
Lymphedema, help for, 101
Lymphocytic lymphoma, 358
Lymphoma, (& see Hodgkins), 401-425
& antineoplastons, 230-231
& black seed, 405-406
& Essiac Tea, 413
& Fostamatinib Disodium, 402
& Hoxsey formula, 420
& LifeMel honey, 420
& milk, 534-535
& monoclonal antibodies, 420-421
& nanotechnology, 420-421
& Nigella sativa 405-406
& scutellaria, 227, 422
& thymus extract, 423
& vitamin C, 404-405
fatal & selenium, 422-423
cure with antineoplastons, 230, 407, 412
staging of, 402
selenium & vitamin C, 422-423
& Fostamatinib Disodium, 204
& ginger, 414-415
& Naltrexone, 610
& Noscapine, 614
& willow bark, 414-415
Lymphosarcoma & Chinese asparagus, 453
*Lypo-Spheric C*, 551
*Lypo-Spherion* (vitamin C), 347
Lyprinol, 447

# M

Macela, 261
Macrobiotics, 541-542
Macular degeneration:
& Lodamin, 395
& lutein, 472
& zeaxanthin, 472
Magnascent Iodine, 129, 400
Magnesium, 67
& cancer, 129, 173
Magnesium, transdermal, 129, 400
Magnetic Resonance Elastography, 52
Magnetite Cationic Liposomes, 607
Magnetite Nanoparticles, 607
Magnolia, 220
Maitake, 161, 293
Maitake & cancer, 526

Maitake D-Fraction 80, 118, 161
& cancer, 526
Malaria:
& Echinacea, 455
& wormwood, 91, 450-451
As a cancer therapy, 610-611
Malay apple, 479
Malignant fibrous histiocytoma & Lovastatin, 389, 412
MALT tumors, 37
Mammaprint, 170-171
Mammogram, 53-54
Mammosite therapy, 99
Mammy apple, 479
Mammy sapote, 479
Mandarin, 479
Mangosteen, 76, 479
Mangosteen fruit, 479-480
Mango-Xan drink, 479-480
Mannatech (glyconutrition), 604
Mantle zone lymphoma, 358-359
mantle-cell-lymphoma, 37
Manuka honey, 555-556
Maple syrup cure, 593-594
MAO inhibitors, 90, 94-95, 418
Maple syrup, synthetic, 488
Margarine battle, 439-440
Marijuana & the brain, 372
Marine phytoplankton, 394
Maslinic acid, 143
MBI, 52
MCLs, 607
MDR cells & pawpaw, 482
MDX-1106, 36
Medlar, 479
Medullar metastatic compression, 592
Medullary breast cancer, 51
Medulloblastoma, 373
& antineoplastons, 350
& IMRT, 379-380
Megakaryoblastic leukemia, 37
Megamin (zeolites), 629
Melanoma (also see skin cancer) 383-400
& andiroba, 385
& antineoplastons, 386-387
& azelaic acid, 385
& berberine, 385
& chaparral tea, 387, 568
& cholesterol drugs, 389
& CoQ10 levels, 389
& *Ecklonia cava*, 630
& ginseng, 392-393
& Haelan, 398-399
& Lodamin, 60, 395
& *Neptune Krill Oil*, 394
& oregano, 459
& piceatannol, 396
& resveratrol, 396
& shark cartilage, 397-398
& Ukrain, 399
Melanoma (stage IV) cure, 383-384, 386-387
Melanoma of eye, 592
Melanoma, risk increase for transplants,384
Melatonin, 96, 285
& cachexia, 285
& cancer, 372-373
precautions for, 96-97, 285, 372-373
production of, 521
Myelodysplastic Syndrome, 601
Memory & HGH, 604-605
Meniere's Syndrome, 284
Meningeal carcinomatosis, 373
Meningiomas, 373
Meningitis, 41
& Echinacea, 455-456
& olive leaf, 459
& tree bark, 605
Menopause & weight, 507-508
MENS, 36
Mercury detox & bentonite clay, 548-549
Mercury fillings, dangers of, 546-547
Mercury vapors from fillings, 547-548
MERCK Cover up & hit list, 581
Merkel cell carcinoma, 37
Merlin, 36
Mesenchymous meso-dermal tumor, 400
Mesima mushroom, 180, 181, 529
Mesothelioma, 269, 297-298, 358-359
& antineoplastons, 297
& cholesterol drugs, 298
& Onconase, 60-61, 298
Metabolic Assessment Program, 363
Metabolism & Oolong tea, 571
Metal dentistry toxins, 546-547
Metastasis & Forskolin, 602
Metastatic cancers & Rexin-G, 375
Methanol (in Nutra-Sweet), 455
Mexican wild yam, 496
MGN-3, 528, 612
Microvascular Ultrasound, 170-171
Migraines, 315-316
& allergies, 500-501
& dehydration, 501
& feverfew, 501
& ginger, 563, 569
& hyssop, 501
& lecithin, 501
& natural progesterone, 400-501
& niacin, 501
& riboflavin, 500-501
Mijo (camu-camu), 590
Milk thistle, 88-89, 263-264, 459
Milk with added hormones, 538
Milk, bacteria content, 531-532
MINC, 382
Mind & healing, 9, 13-14
*Mineral Rich*, 63-64, 474, 643
Mini-transplant, 200
Minneolas, 479
Mint & limonene, 566
Miracle fruit berries, 480
*Miracle* juicers, 429
Mirtogenol, 470-471
MIS (minimally invasive surgery), 621
Miscarriages, 499
Miscellaneous Therapies, 582-630
Mistletoe extract, 606
Mixed gliomas, 373
Mixed mesodermal tumor, 401
Mixed olioma, 359
Mobetron (IOERT), 96, 609
Modified citrus pectin, 68
Moh's surgery (for skin cancer), 393-394
Molasses, 543
Molecular breast imaging, 36, 52
Molybdenum, 307

& sulfur allergies, 613
Monascus pigment, 486
MonaVie, 68, 479
Monkey bread, 479
Monoclonal antibodies, 622-623
Mono-laurin, 326
Mono-myristin, 326
Monoterpenes, 260
Morel mushrooms, 527
Morgellon's Disease, cure for, 657
Morinda, 479
Morning After Pill, 493
Mother's milk (tainted), 539
Motion sickness & ginger, 569
Mountain soursop, 479
Mouth cancer, 299-314 (also see head-and-neck and oral cancer), 299-314
& beta-carotene, 299-300, 478
& Blue Light Therapy, 588
& cell phone (dangers of), 382
& Essiac tea, 303
& fungal cure, 304
& lycopene, 306
& riboflavin, 309-310
& selenium, 309-310
& spirulina, 310, 434
& VELscope, 588
& zinc, 309-310
Moxxor & arthritis, 447
MPGC (bindweed), 184-185, 587-588
MPNSTs, 37
MR, 52
MRSA:
& agricur, 204
& bentonite clay, 204, 548-549
& cancer patients, 204
Multiple Sclerosis (MS), 69, 473, 488
& B12, 474
& CoQ10, 156
& dairy, 531
& IPT, 607-608
& milk supply, 504, 534-535
& nutrition concerns, 475
& spirulina, 434
& sunshine, 535
& vitamin D, 488
& the water cure, 475
& turmeric (curcumin), 475
& vegetarian diet, 515
& water hydration, 514-515
& the MS patch, Prokarin, 474-475
MSC, 72
MSM (Methyl Sulfanyl Methane), 612-613
Mucinous carcinoma, 51
Mucus production & dairy, 537
MUI, 170-171
Mullaca, 307
Multiple drug-resistant cells, 482
Multiple myeloma, 198-236
& CoQ10, 215
& proteolytic enzymes, 220
& Salinosporamide-A, 207
& Tian Xian, 235
& turmeric cure, 228, 467-468
Murasakishiba (purple reishi) 527
Musaceas plant & CellQuest, 595
Muscadine grapes, 480
Muscle spasms & basil, 562
Muscular dystrophy (MD), 473-474
& CoQ10, 473
& selenium, 473
& vitamin E, 473
Muscular weakness & dairy, 537-538
Mushroom poisoning, 583-584
& ALA, 462-463
& borage oil, 256
cure for, 243-245
Mushrooms, 524-529
& asthma, 517
& vitamin D, 522, 525
resources for, 525
Music & healing, Ch 36
MycoPhyto Formula, 613
Mycosis-fungoides-sezary syndrome, 38, 359
Myelofibrosis, 37
Myelogenous leukemia & vitamin C, 209-210
Myeloma (also see under multiple myeloma)
& antineoplastons, 230-231
& resveratrol, 217
& scutellaria, 227, 422
Myristicin, 291
Myrrh, 89
Mysosarcoma, 401
Myxopapillary Ependymoma & antineoplastons, 354
cure for, 354


# N


Naessens, Gaston, 629
& 714X, 416-417
Naltrexone, 610
Nance, 479
Nangka, 479
Nanobombs, 36
NanoKnife (IRE), 72, 630
Nanoparticles, 196, 609
Nanotechnology, 60
Narrow band imaging (NBI), 133
Nasal cancers, 299-314
& mullaca, 307
Nascent Iodine, 129, 400
Nashi (Asian pears), 479
Natural flavonoids, 188
Natural hormones, safety of, 504-505
Natural medicine opponents, 577-581
Natural progesterone:
creams, 497-498
dosing, 499-500
effects of, 495-496
for psoriasis, 398
precautions for use, 493
Natural vs. synthetic estrogen, 494
Nature's PCN, propolis, 556
*Nature's Way* brand, 468
Nausea (natural treatment for)
& basil, 562
& ginger, 569
NAVPSIPQ, 473
NDGA, 365, 387-388
& chaparral tea, 567
Neck cancers (also see throat, esophageal & head & neck cancers)
Neck cancer & antineoplastons, 301
& Sir Jason Winters Tea, 572
*Neptune Krill Oil*, 394, 446-447
Nettle root, 124
Neuradiab, 361
Neural tube defects, 209

Neuroblastoma, 349-382
& 3F8 monoclonal antibody, 380
& antineoplastons, 359
& astaxanthin, 363-364
& folic acid, 359-360
& IMRT, 379-380
& Lodamin, 60, 374
& turmeric, 365
& Ukrain, 377-378
& zeaxanthin, 379
cure with cartilage, 362-364
Neuro-endocrine tumors, 358-359
Neuropathy, 101
Neutropenia, 67
New Age, 12
*New Chapter* Products, 220, 254
Nexrutine, 119
Niacin:
& cancer, 425
for lowering cholesterol, 486
niacin flush, 425
Nieper therapy, 36
Nigella sativa seed oil extract, 323, 405-406
Night blindness & vitamin A, 479
Nitrates & bulgar, 485
Nitrosamines, 485
NMP22 (bladder test), 331
Node-positive breast cancer, 52
Non-Hodgkin's Lymphoma, 31, 200-201, 358-359, 402
& antineoplastons, 407-412
& fruits & vegetables, 414
cure for Non-Hodgkin's, 230-231, 407-412
& andrographis, 405
& Beta-Glucan, 406-407
& CDA-II, 402
& green tea, 415
Non-Hodgkin's lymphoma cure in R.N. 412
Noni juice, 294
Nordihydroguairetic acid (NDGA), 365, 387
Nori, 433
Noscapine, 614
NOVO-TTF device, 37
NRSTS, 37
*N-Tense*, 152
*N-Tense-2*, 233
Nutra-sweet (see aspartame), 406
dangers of, 455

# O

Obesity & resveratrol, 619
Obsessive-Compulsive disorders & low-dose Dilantin, 658
*OLA LOA*, 643
Olallieberries, 479
Oleic acid, 74
Oligodendrogliomas, 373
Olive oil, 614
Olive-skin pomace, 143
*Omega 8003* juicer, 428-429
Omega-3, 59-60
*Omega Essentials*, 444
Oncogenic proteins, 36
Onconase, 60-61, 339 (& See cancer-specific chapters)
Oncotype DX, 52, 170-171
Onions, 159
OnvoVAX, 134
Oolong tea, 571
OPCs (pycnogenols), 469-471
Optic nerve gliomas, 373
Optic pathway gliomas & antineoplastons, 359
Optical coherenc tomography, 133
ORAC – rated foods, 219, 475-476
Oral cancer 299, 314 (also see mouth cancer, throat cancer, esophageal & head & neck cancers)
& flavonoids, 304
& grapefruit, 305
& onions, 308
& photodynamic therapy, 308
& spirulina, 310
Oral leukoplakia reversed, 478
Orange peel extract & GERD, 301-302
Oregacyn & sinus problems, 614
Oregano oil, 565
Organic foods, 504
vs. non-organic, 618-619
Orphan drugs, 163, 589-590
Orthomolecular Medicine, 70, 132, 487, 540-541
Osiecki Therapy, 36
Osteoarthritis & Cytotron, 600
Osteogenic sarcoma, 401
Osteoporosis, 155, 494
& HGH, 604-605
& HRT, 498
& milk, 533
& natural hormone, 506-507
& red clover, 460
Osteosarcoma, 401 (also see other bone cancers in index)
& artemisinin, 450-451
& Lovastatin, 389, 412
& psoralea seed, 291, 421
& soda bicarb, 129
advanced & Budwig cure, 445
Otaheite gooseberry, 479
Ova & Parasite test, 546
Ovarian cancer, 169-197
advanced cases of, 173, 174, 186
& ABM mushroom, 179-180
& AHCC, 175
& antineoplastons, 189
& bindweed, 184-185, 587
& BioCancell, 588
& bromelain, 452
& BSI-201, 60, 189
& cartilage, 190-192
& cherries, 176
& coffee, 194
& dairy products, 194
& dietary fat, 194
& espinheira santa, 187
& Essiac tea, 186
& estrogen, 181-182
& fried foods, 171-172
& fungus, 171
& ginger, 178
& grapes, 178-179
& green tea, 187
& grilled foods, 171-172
& hydrazine sulfate, 419-420
& IMRT, 172
& Iscador, 188, 458
& kamunggay, 172-173
& Lodamin, 60, 194-195
& milk, 532-533
& moringa, 172-173

& nanoparticles, 196
& PET/CT, 173
& Rexin-G, 174
& RM-10, 173-174, 527
& rosemary, 172
& selenium, 182-183
& sunlight, 522
& talc danger, 195
& TAP Prodrug, 174-175
& tea, 179
& TGFBI, 195
& the cancer bush, 185
& vegetarians, 173
& vitamin C, 70-71, 181
cure with glyconutrition, 604
symptoms of, 169-171
& PARP inhibitors, 192-193
OvaSure, 169-170
OvPlex, 171
Oxalates & raw foods, 55-56
Oxalic acid, 614-615
Oxomate, 79
Oxygen & cancer, 518-523
Oxygen levels & pH, 558-559
Oxygen Radical Absorbance Capacity (ORAC), 219, 475
Oxygen therapies, 518-519
Oyster mushrooms, 527
Ozone treatment, 518-519

**P**

P4-D1, 426
p53 gene, 91, 292
Paclitaxel, 90, 196
PADMA-28, 36
Pain & willow bark, 564
Pain relief with ginger, 563
Palladium Lipoic Complex, 295, 308
Panax ginseng, 392-393
Pancreatic cancer, 315-330
& abajeru, 317
& ALA, 330
& antineoplastons, 318
& berries, 324
& beta-carotene, 323
& bindweed, 317-318, 587
& BioCancell, 588
& cherries, 318-319
& cholesterol drugs, 319
& CoQ10, 319-320
& CyberKnife, 320
& enzymes, 325-326
& Essiac tea, 320-321
& figs, 321
& folic acid, 329
& fungal cure, 321
& Gerson, 315
& GLA, 322
& grapes, 47
& green tea, 570
& hydrogen peroxide, 519
& IPT, 607-608
& LifeMel honey, 322-323
& limonene, 318-319
& lycopene, 323
& Naltrexone, 330, 610
& NanoKnife, 630
& nigella sativa oil, 323
& onions, 324
& PDT, 324-325
& resveratrol, 322
& Rexin-G, 326, 340-341
& saw palmetto, 326, 341
& Tian Xian, 327
& turmeric, 327
& Ukrain, 327-328
& vitamin B6, 329
& vitamin C, 70-71, 316-317, 329
& vitamin D, 330
& ZoonCan, 330
Pancreatitis & green foods, 426
Pangamic acid (B15), 36, 588
Papain, 273, 181, 616
& radiation protection, 481
Papaya, 77, 162, 480-481
chewables, 517
Papillary carcinoma, 51
Papillary thyroid cancer, 311
PAPIMI, 36
PAPION Magnetic Inductor, 36
Paralysis, 607-608
Parasites, 91, 416, 545-551
remedies for, 549-551
& alkalinity, 557
& black walnut, 549
& calmyra figs, 551
& cinnamon, 562-563
& cloves, 549, 563
& *Ecklonia cava*, 630
& fillings, 548
& honey, 554
& pets, 550
& wormwood, 549
Parkinson's Disease, 278
& Escoazul, 621
& Haelan, 82
PARP inhibitors, 74
Parsley, 291
& cancer, 571
precautions in using, 459-460, 571
Parsley tea, 571
Pasteurized milk, 536-538
Pau d' Arco tea, 89, 415-416
Pawpaw, 480-481
& MDR cells, 482
PBs (sodium phenyl-butrates), 163, 386-387, 589-590
PC-SPES, 153
PDT (Photo Dynamic Therapy), 267-268, 308
Peach palm, 479
Pear juice & constipation, 563
Pearl oyster (hiratake) mushroom, 181, 529
Peas & beans, 482
Pectin in apples, 483-484
Pelvic inflammation & Escoazul, 621
PEM, 52
Pepinos, 480
Peptide vaccines, 36
Perilla oil, 335, 447
Perillyl alcohol, 107, 161, 176
Periodontal disease, 278-279
Peritoneal cancer (also see under abdominal, uterine, cervical, etc)
Peritoneal cancer cure, 428
& cartilage, 190-192
Peritoneal carcinosis, 592
Pernicious anemia, 218, 465
Peroxy Gel, 519
Persimmons, 479
*Petroselinum crispum* (parsley), 459-460
Pets & parasites, 545, 550
Pfaffia (snow rose), 153-154
PFE (pomegranate fruit extract), 396
pH & fasting, 631-632
pH & MSM, 612-613
pH scale, 558
Pharynx cancer &

simarouba, 310
phenoxodiol, 36
Phenylalanines, warnings against, 455
Pheochromocytoma (adrenal tumor), 397
Philippine roseapple, 479
Phlebitis & ginkgo biloba, 456
Photocoagulation, 619-620
Photodynamic Therapy, 267-268, 308, 324-325, 599
Photon Beam Therapy, 616, 617
Phycocyanin (from spirulina) 433
Phyllanthus, 256-257
Physallis, 480
Phyto-estrogens, 508-509
Phytoplankton, 275, 394, 611
Piceatannol, 396
Picroliv, 261
Picrorrhiza, 261
Pine bark, 469-471
Pineal tumors, 373
Pineoblastomas:
  & antineoplastons, 356
  Pineoblastoma cure, 356
Pitachaya, 479
Pituitary adenoma, 373
Pituitary tumors, 373, 381-382
  & EEA, 382
  & Gamma Knife, 622
  symptoms of, 381
Plant estrogens, 489, 508-509
Plantains, 479
Plaque (arterial) & tea, 226
Plastic (dangers of), 508
Pleomorphic rhabdomyosarcoma, 38
Pleura-pulmonary blastoma, 37
PMG (bindweed), 587-588
Proteoglycan mixture, 184-185
PMS & krill oil, 446-447
PNET's, 37, 373
Polarizing Solutions, 615
Policosanol, 155-156, 364-486
Polio & vitamin C, 540
Polyerga Therapy, 615
Poly-MVA, 120, 375
Polypeptides, 615
Polypore mushroom, 181, 529
*Polyporus umbellatus* mushroom, 527
  & bladder, 340
Polyps, 143-144
  & vitamin C, 166-167
*Polysaccharide kureha*, 120, 180-181
*POM Wonderful* Juice, 471
Pom/dex, 203
Pomalidomide, 203
Pomegranates, 80-81, 107
  & cancer, 615-616
  Juice of, 471
Poppyseed & flax, 469
*Poria cocos* (hoelen) mushroom, 526
Poriatrin & kidney disease, 526
Positive Emission Mammogram, 52
Power Seed Mix recipe, 642-643
PPA, 388
Praise & prayer, Ch 36
Prayer & healing, 11-12, 14-15
Pregnant mare's urine, 492
Premarin, 492-493
PREMPRO, 495
Prescription HRT, 489-509
Preventing cancer in the womb, 359-360
PRIMA-1, 73
*Primal Defense* probiotics, 542
Primitive neuroectodermal tumors, 373
Proanthocyanidins (OPCs), 215, 393, 469-471
Probiotics, 542
Progesterone, 489-509
  (also see under natural progesterone)
  dosing for, 499-500
Progestin (synthetic progesterone), 495-496
  side effects, 495
Prolarix, 37
Promyelocytic leukemia & garlic, 225
Propionibacterium, 256
Propolis & cancer, 556
Propulsid, 37, 39
Prostate cancer, 102-129
  & Abiraterone, 103
  & Ablatherm, 103-104
  & AHCC, 104
  & antineoplastons, 106, 589
  & baicalein, 105, 342
  & beans, 105
  & bee pollen, 105, 553
  & beta-carotene, 105
  & beta-sitosterol, 105-106
  & boron, 106
  & BRCA-2, 65
  & cabbage, 106, 108
  & Calcium D-Glucarate, 107
  & cherries, 107
  & citrus pectin, 118
  & CoQ10, 108
  & cryotherapy, 108, 390, 597-598
  & cumin, 566
  & CyberKnife, 109
  & cytotron, 109
  & dairy products, 104, 538
  & DHEA, 109
  & diet, 109-110
  & dietary fat, 122
  & ellagic acid, 110-111
  & Essiac, 111
  & fennel, 566
  & fenugreek, 111
  & fish oils, 111-112
  & flax seed, 112
  & fungus, 112
  & garlic, 112-113
  & ginger, 113
  & ginseng, 113
  & GLA, 488
  & grapes, 47, 113
  & graviola, 102
  & GTx, 114
  & IMRT, 114-115
  & isosilybin-B, 115
  & Lodamin, 60, 118-119
  & lycopene, 115-116
  & magnesium, 116-117, 129
  & milk thistle, 117-118
  & mushrooms, 118
  & myrrh, 89, 118
  & Nexrutine, 119
  & Noscapine, 119, 614
  & Onconase, 60-61, 119-120
  & peas, 105
  & pomegranate, 80-81, 120-121, 471
  & PSK, 120
  & quercetin, 121
  & raspberries, 468
  & red clover, 121

& resveratrol, 122-123
& Rexin-G, 123-124
& Sagopilone, 124
& saw palmetto, 124
& selenium, 125
& soda bicarb cure, 129, 650-651
& skullcap, 342
& Sonablate, 103-104
& St. John's Wort, 125
& sunshine, 125
& tea, 114
& testosterone, 126
& turmeric, 127
& Ukrain, 127-128
& vitamin C, 102-103
& vitamin E, 345-346
& Zyflamend, 106
Prostate health:
& melatonin, 117
& pumpkin seeds, 121
& vitamin E, 128
& water, 128-129
Protease inhibitors, 544
in beans, 482
Proteases, 616
Proteolytic Enzymes, 143, 325-326, 480
Proteolytic enzyme therapy, 616
Proton Beam Therapy, 616-617
Pseudorabies, 261
Pseudo-tumor cerebri, 373
PSK (from karawatake) 161, 180-181, 525
& cancer, 525
& HIV, 525
*Psoralea corylifolia*, 421
Psoralea seed, 291, 421
Psoriasis, 255, 395, 398
& aloe vera, 398, 450
& beta-carotene, 398
& EFAs, 398
& fungal cause, 398
& green drinks, 398
& milk thistle, 395
& natural progesterone, 398, 506
& vitamin A, 398
Pterostilbene, 50, 248
PTPRD gene, 36
PTZ, 227-228
Pueraria Montana, 261
Pulmonary hypertension, 600
Pummelos, 480
Purines, 615
Purple coneflower (Echinacea), 455
PVD & ginkgo biloba, 456
PX-12, 37
Pycnogenols, 47, 280, 469-471
in cat's claw, 463-464

# Q

Qigong therapy, 36
QMR Therapy, 365,599-600
Quantum Magnetic Resonance, 365, 600
*Quackwatch*, 581
Quantum Touch, 12
Quercetin sources, 69, 221, 393, 471, 617

# R

R-A Therapy, 617-618
Radiation balloon implants, 37
Radiation exposure & Ukrain, 624
Radioactive iodine, 361
Radiofrequency ablation, 264, 314
Radio-immunotherapy, 135
Radiolabeled monoclonals, 37
Radiotherapy (Gamma Knife), 622
Radio Wave Therapy, 618
Rambai, 479
Rambutan, 479
Ranpirnase, 60 61, 339
Rashes, 416
Raspberries, 107
Raw food safety, 43-45
Raw foods & alkalinity, 557-558
Raw milk, 536-537
Reams Biological Ionization, 36
Recancostat, 618
Recipes, Ch 36
Rectal cancer (look under colon cancer, colorectal & intestinal cancer)
& Essiac, 149
& Ukrain, 166
Rectal polyps & vitamin C, 166-167
Recurring bladder neoplasm, 592
Red clover, 89, 508-509
& estrogen levels, 460
Red meat & cancer, 618-619
Red vs. white ginseng, 456
Red yeast rice, 155-156, 486
Reduced glutathione, 618
Reed Sternberg cells, 402
Reiki, 12
Reincarnation, 12
Reishi mushroom, 161, 527 528
& vitamin C, 528
Renal cancer (also, under kidney cancer & bladder cancer)
& Ukrain, 343
& vitamin D, 345
Reolysis, 36
Reossification therapy, 36
Resperin Canada Essiac Tea, 366
Respiratory illnesses & kiwi, 449
Respiratory problems & dairy, 537
Rest & cancer connection, 518-523
& healing, 9, 11-12
& immune system, 520-521
Restless legs & pine bark extract, 469
Resveratrol, 77, 43-50, 322, 619
& tree bark, 605
sources of, 50
studies using resveratrol, 46
Retinoblastoma, 177
& cryotherapy, 390, 597-598
treatment for, 390, 619-620
Retinoic acid (vitamin A), 300
Retroperitoneal sarcoma & Ukrain, 193-194
Revici Therapy, 286
Rexin-G, 97, 266-267, 375, 620
Rezulin, 39
Rhabdoid brain tumor in child, 351
Rhabdoid tumors of the CNS, 351
Rhabdomyolysis, 388
Rhabdomyosarcoma, 37, 401
& AHCC, 401-402
*Rhamnus purshiana*, 452
Rheumatic syndromes, 607-

608
Rheumatoid arthritis, 255
& beta-carotene, 478
& dairy, 531
& dehydration, 512
& Essiac tea, 512
& ginger, 563
& peroxide, 519
& Virastatin, 630
Rhodiola rosea, 90, 291, 341
Rhodiola, 90
Ricketts & vitamin D, 345, 521-522
Rife Machine, 620-621
Ringworm & oregano, 456
RM-10, 173-174
Robotic Technology, 621
Rodent tuber plant, 36
Rooibos tea & cancer, 571
Root canal problems, 544
Rosacea & natural progesterone, 506
Rose apple, 479
Roselle, 479
Rosemary, 89, 172, 414-415
Royal jelly, 556
Rumberry (camu-camu), 590
Ruthenium, 295
Rutin & cancer, 484-485
Rye & blood pressure, 485
Rye bread, 364

## S

S3I-201 & S3I-2001, 36
SAD diet, 591
Safer drugs, 27-29
Safer medicine, 629-630
Saffron & cancer, 566
Sagopilone, 124
Sakosides, 452
Sala, 479
Salba, 84, 447
Saliva alkalinity, 558
Saliva testing, 53, 501-502
Salivary gland tumors & cell phones, 382
SALLRSIPSA, 473
Salmonella, 294
Salvation, 17-19 & Appendix I
*Sampson* juicer, 428
Sansapote, 479
Santoli, 479
Sapodilla, 479
Sarcoma, 401-425
& andiroba, 415-416
& CyberKnife, 403
& Essiac tea, 413
& green tea, 421
& guacatonga, 415-416
& Lovastatin, 412
& reishi & green tea for, 421
& Rexin-G, 421-422
Sarcoma botryoides, 38
Sargassum kjellmaniaum, 227-228
SARS & vitamin C, 541
Satsuma, 479
Schisandra, 90, 261
Schizophrenia & niacinamide, 424-425
Schwannomas, 373, 622
Scorpion venom, 376, 621-622
Scurvy, 487
& leukemia connection, 207-210
& pine bark, 470
Scutellaria, 262
Sea grape, 479
Sea grasses, 432
Sea vegetables, 432
Seabuck-7 drink, 480
Seabuckthorn, 479
Seed foods, 544
Seichem, 12
Selective arteriography, 592
Selective internal radiation, 264-265
Selenium:
for BRCA-1, 64
for HIV, 64
for Keshan's Disease, 64
sources of, 63, 258, 286, 465
studies involving, 644-645
Seneca Valley Trials, 36
Senile dementia & yamabushiitake, 528
Serrapeptase, 616
Serratia peptidase, 616
Sertoli-cell tumor, 37
Sezary syndrome, 38
Shark cartilage, 92
precautions for using, 397-398
Sharons, 479
Shigella, 294
Shiitake, 79, 81, 161, 293
& cancer 528
Shingles:
& flax, 443
& olive leaf, 459
& Virastatin, 630
& vitamin C, 540
Shiroshiba (white reishi), 527
Siberian ginseng (ciwujia), 306, 453
Sickle cell anemia & B-17, 585
SIDS, 41
Silibinin & milk thistle, 393
Silymarin & skin cancer, 395
Simarouba, 232-233, 310
Sinus infections & grapefruit seed, 565
Sinusitis & dairy products, 537
*Sir Jason Winters' Tea*, 571
Sir-Spheres, 164, 264-265
SIRT (Sir-Spheres), 164, 264-265
Sjogren's, cure for, 425
Skenar, 36
Skin cancer (also see under melanoma), 383-400
& andiroba, 385, 415-416
& antioxidants, 384
& berberine, 385
& Beta-Glucan, 386
& betulinic acid, 399
& caffeine, 392
& chaparral tea, 387-388
& cryotherapy, 390, 597-598
& Curaderm BEC5, 390
& *Ecklonia cava*, 630
& ECT, 391
& EGCG, 393
& eggplant extract, 390
& espinheira santa, 391
& Essiac tea, 391-392
& fungus (candida), 392
& garlic, 392
& grape seed extract, 393
& grapes, 383, 393
& green tea, 393
& Hoxsey formula, 393-394
& kombucha-papaya, 481
& lentinan, 386
& LifeMel Honey, 394
& maitake, 386
& marine phytoplankton, 394
& milk thistle, 395
& Moh's surgery, 393-394
& *Neptune Krill Oil*, 394
& Noscapine, 614
& pomegranate extract,

396
& propolis, 554
& quercetin, 393
& Rexin-G, 396-397
& selenium, 397
& shiitake, 386
& silibinin, 393
& silymarin, 395, 484
& *Trinelle* Cream, 399
& vassourinha, 399
& vitamins, 384
& yucca root extract, 400
Skin cancer salve, 393-394
Skin carcinoma & barley, 426
Skin problems, 435
Skin rejuvenators, OPCs, 468
Sleep disorders & HGH, 604-605
Snake bites & vitamin C, 544
Snow fungus, 188
Soda bicarb cancer cure, 129, 591-594, 650-651
Sodium pyroglutamate, 255, 525
Solco SET-C21, 94, 391
Somatids, 416
Somocystinamide A (ScA), 36
Sonablate, 103 104
Soncoya, 479
Sore throats & dairy products, 537
Soursop tree, 481
South American holly, 187
Southern ginseng (jiaogulan), 458
Soy, 78
controversy over, 476
fermented soy, 81
Spectrum technology, 36
Spices for cancer, 562-566
Spinal cord tumors & CyberKnife, 403
Spinal tumors, 374
Spindle-cell carcinoma, 37
Spirit guides, 12
Spirulina, 310, 427
& B12, 433
Spirulina, chelator, 433
Split-gill mushroom, 180
Spreading cancers & Rexin-G, 375
Sprouts & sprouting, 434-435
Spruce Knot Heartwood, 605
Sprue, 132
Squalene, 234-235
Squamous cell cancers, 383
St. John's Wort, 90
Stage IV lymphoma & Beta-Glucan, 406-407
Stage IV Non-Hodgkins cure, 406-407
Stamina & HGH, 604-605
Staph germs & Manuka honey, 555-556
*Staphylococcus aureus*, 294
Star nut palm, 479
Starfruit (carambolas), 479
Statin drugs & CoQ10, 467
Steam-distilled water, 348
Stereotactic Body Radiotherapy, 273-274, 622
Stereotactic head frame, 602
Steroid sulfatase inhibitors, 36
Stevia, 454
Stilbene & tree bark, 605
Stinging nettle, 460
Stomach cancer (also see gastric cancer and abdominal cancer)
& cherries, 161
& Essiac, 147
& green tea, 305
Stroke (CVAs):
& cranberries, 279
& green tea, 280
& HRT risks, 496
& quercetin, 471
& recovery, 469, 607-608
Suehirotake & cancer, 528
Suehirotake in MGN-3, 528
Sulfated SKCF, 227-228
Sulfur allergies, 613
Sulfur veggies, 160, 487
Suma (pfaffia), 153-154
Sun exposure & the elderly, 523
Sun farm soups, 36
Sunburn:
& beta-carotene, 478
& aloe vera, 450
Sunlight exposure, 507
& cancer, 345, 518-523
& vitamin D, 507, 628
Supplement usage, 643
brand choices, 645-646
Surgery, 29
Surinam cherry, 479
Sutent, 150
Sutherlandia frutescens, 185
Sweet granadilla, 479
Sweetsop, 479
Symptoms of excess estrogen, 491
Synchrony (CyberKnife), 598-599
Syngeneic, 201
Synthetic estrogen, 489
side effects of, 493

# T

T.B. & Gerson, 611-612
T.B. & milk, 535
Tagamet, 289
Taheebo tea, 89, 376
Tainted breast milk, 539
Tamalaki, 260
Tamarind juice, 262
Tamoxifen, 72, 502-503
side effects of, 502-503
Tangelos, 479
Tangeretin, 468
Tangerines & tangeretin, 468
TAP Technology, 99-100, 622-623
Tarceva (Erlotinib), 39-40
Target GI, 35-36
Targeted Gene Therapy, 39
Targeted radiotherapy, 95
Targeted Therapy, 588
Tarragon tea & cancer, 572
Taxol, 196, 492
TB & BCG, 333
TBI (total body irradiation), 201
Tea & cancer, 215-216, 567-572
Teleomerase test, 582-583, 617-618
Teratoid tumor & antineoplastons, 351
Terminal cancer & bicarb, 593-594
Testicular cancers, 125-126
Tetraplex Binding Molecules, 36
TG-2, 36
The Cancer Tree (Xi Shu), 236
*The Maker's Diet*, 142
The Willett Study, 285-286
Thecomas, 37
TheraSphere, 259
ThermoDox, 623
Thermogram, 53-54
Third Eye Retroscope, 133
Thirst signals, 511-512
*THREELAC*, 593

Throat cancer, 299-314 (see Esophageal & neck cancer also)
& black raspberries, 300
& Brazilian peppertree, 300
& Canelim, 594
& cryospray ablation, 301-302, 598
& CyberKnife, 302
& Essiac tea, 303
& lycopene, 306
& mullaca, 307
& Rexin-G, 308-309
& selenium, 309-310
& simarouba, 310
& zinc, 309-310
Thrombocytopenia, 67
Thymoquinone, 323
Thymus extract & lymphomas, 423
Thymus health & glandulars, 604
Thyroid cancer 299-314 (also, see throat cancer)
& ablation, 314
& antineoplastons, 313
& hydrazine sulfate, 419-420
& IMRT, 314
& resveratrol, 308
& RFA, 314
& Transfer Factor, 311
Thyroid health & glandulars, 604
Tian Men Dong, 453
Tian Xian, 154, 259, 292 327
Tibetan Herbal Remedy, 36
Tinder polypore mushroom, 180
TM-601, 376, 622
Tomatoes, cooked vs raw, 468
TOMO Therapy (IMRT), 95, 271-272, 608-609, 623
Tong Ren, 36
Tongue cancer & molasses, 543 (also look under oral cancer & mouth cancers)
Tonsillitis & dairy products, 537
Toothaches & oregano, 456
Toothpaste toxicity, 511
Topotecan, 461
Touch & healing, 12, 13, Ch 36
Toxic enteritis, 536
Transfer Factor, 295, 310-311, 623
Transient elastography, 237
Transplant cases & melanoma risk, 384
Tree of Joy, 461
Tree tomato, 479
Tremella fuciformis, 188
Tribulus herb, 36
*Trinelle* Cream, 399
Trovax, 36
Trypsin, 616
TSACH, 36
Tuberous sclerosis, 373
Tubular carcinoma, 51
Tuckahoe bread (from hoelen), 526
Tumor-Activated Prodrug (TAP), 99-100, 622-623
Tumors in babies & blueberries, 463
Turkey tail, 81
Turmeric, 79-80, 91, 127, 467-468
& treating multiple myeloma, 228
in yellow mustard, 468
Turmeric vs curry powder, 454-455
TVZ-7, 36
Tykerb, 74-75
Typhoid & Echinacea, 455-456

# U

Ubiquinone, 155-156
Uethral cancer & Ukrain, 343
Ugli fruit, 479
Ukrain, 98-99, 377-378 (also, see under cancer specific chapters)
Ukrain & radiation exposure, 624
Ulcers, 427
& aloe vera, 450
& espinheira santa, 289
& flax, 438
& ginger, 564
& green foods, 426
& hydration, 511-512
& papaya, 481
& propolis, 556
Ulcers of the leg & Manuka honey, 556
Ultrasound hyperthermia, 605-606
Umbelliferae, 625
Ume plums, 561
Umeboshi, 561
*Uncaria tomentosa*, 306
Uno de Gato, 85-86
Urea, 36
Urethral cancer, 343
Urinary health:
& alkalinity, 558
& aronia berries, 136
& D-Mannose, 454
& RM-10, 211
Urinary infections & *polyporus*, 340, 527
Urinary Telomerase, 331
Urine alkalinity, 558
*UroSens*, 331
USP Progesterone, 506
Usui, 12
Uterine cancer, 169-197
& AHCC, 175
& antineoplastons, 189
& cartilage therapy, 190-192
& Essiac tea, 58-59,186-187
& flax, 178
& fungus, 171
& HRT, 491-493
& IMRT, 172
& Lodamin, 60, 194-195
& molasses, 543
& Tamoxifen, 502-503
Uterine fibroid cure, 499
UV Light Therapy, 403, 600, 602
UVA exposure & astaxanthin, 483

# V

V8 Juice, 398
Vaccine controversy, 41-42 196
Vaccines (custom made) 600
Vanadium, 457
Variscosities & grape seed/pine bark, 469
Vascular tumors, 373
VascuStatin/Angioblock (bindweed), 184-185, 587
Vassourinha, 233, 399
Velvet tamarind, 479
Vioxx, 31, 35, 37, 38, 39, 388, 574, 582
Virastatin & cancer, 630
Virtual colonoscopy, 134
Viruses:
Virus killer, Virastatin, 630
& horseradish, 564

& paprika, 565-566
Visica2, 100
Visual pathway gliomas, 359
*VitaCarte*, 362-364
Vitamin C:
& cancer, 625-628
& dosing amounts, 625-628
& grape seed extract, 643
& preventing bladder cancer, 344
& rectal polyps, 166-167
& reishi mushroom, 528
& skin cancer, 385
& sources – rose hips, 460
& studies, 643-644
Vitamin D, 69-71
& cancer, 345, 628
& lupus, 436
& MS link, 488
& sunlight, 628
in mushrooms, 81, 525
sources of, 507, 522
Vitamin D2 (ergocalciferol), 522
Vitamin D3 (calciferol), 522
Vitamin E:
best form, 183
different forms of, 474
sources of, 128, 183, 212-213, 287, 346, 474
studies involving, 643-644
Vitamin K, 426
sources of, 259-260
Voavanga, 479
Voodoo lily, 279
Vulva cancers, 169-197
& fungus, 171
& Aldara, 197
Vulvectomies, 554
Vytorin, 156

# W

Wakame, 291-292, 433
Wake-sleep cycle, 521
Waldenstrom's macroglobulinemia, 358
Wampee, 480
Wasabi, 36
Water:
& alkalinity, 560
& consumption, 510-511, 513-514
& hydration, 510-517
& intake and cancer, 196
& oxygenation, 516
& requirements for, 516
Water cure, 515
Water purity, 516-517
Weak tooth enamel & vitamin A, 479
West Nile virus, 211, 540
Wheat grass juice, 430
& alkalinity, 435
& benefits of, 427-430
Whitaker Wellness Center, 239, 466, 584, 602
White blood cell transfusions, 628-629
White jelly leaf, 188
White meat, 618-619
White tree ear, 188
White vs. red ginseng, 456
Wiedbrande Treatment, 36
Wigmore, Ann, 54, 427-428, 434-435
Wild coffee (guacatonga), 415-416
Wild sunflower, 85
Willow bark & aspirin, 564
Wilm's tumor, 37, 358-359
Winter cherry, 451
Wobenzyme, 101, 616
Wolfberry, 461
Wood apple, 479
Wood ear mushrooms, 528
Worms & cloves, 563
Wormwood, 91, 549-550
& parasites, 549
Worship, 19-23
Wound healing:
& green foods, 426
& honey, 554-555
Wrinkles & kombucha, 570

# X

Xanthine oxidase & milk, 533
Xeloda, 36, 74-75
Xenoestrogens, 489, 490
Xi Shu herb, 461

# Y

Yamabushiitake (lion's mane), 528
Yeast & alkalinity, 557-558
Yeast/cancer connection, 561
Yoshido's sarcoma, 89
Young children & blueberries, 463
Youngberries, 480
Yucca root, 400
Yuccalive, 36
Yun Zhi mushroom, 529

# Z

Zalypsis, 36
Zeaxanthin sources, 379, 472
Zeolites (Megamin), 100, 629
Zetia, 156
Zhi mushroom, 529
*Zhongiefeng Pian* (ZoonCan), 154
Zhu ling mushroom, 181, 529
ZoonCan, 154
*Zyflamend*, 106
Zymactive, 616

# Author Bio

Deanna Loftis is a licensed RN in several states. She spent many years working with med-surg and orthopedic patients in a clinical setting before returning to school for a B.B.A. (major in Managed Care), graduating Summa Cum Laude from Northwood University. She also worked many years in a managed care staff and supervisory position, which included following solid organ transplant patients and bone marrow (or stem cell) transplant patients for a major insurance company. Because of losing three family members to cancer, and the horrendous side effects that they (and many of her patients) suffered from chemo and radiation, she began an intensive study into alternative cancer therapies, which resulted in her first award-winning book, *PAINLESS CANCER CURES & Preventions Your Doctor May Not Be Aware Of.*

Deanna continues to research and study all forms of alternative cancer therapies, and now updates her readers with her newest book: ***GENTLE CURES FOR TOUGH CANCERS – Non-Toxic, God-Given Cures That Work,*** which covers the most current and effective alternative cancer therapies available today. Not only are some of the newest less toxic conventional treatments discussed, but the most promising and least toxic alternative cancer cures backed by many scientific research studies and testimonials of those who used them! There is also information on many other natural, effective treatments for disorders such as: Crohn's, viruses (e.g. West Nile and others), auto-immune disorders, high cholesterol, migraines, infertility, IBS, ADD, depression, high blood pressure, hepatitis, GERD, muscular dystrophy, multiple sclerosis, arthritis, Bell's Palsy, Meniere's Syndrome, Morgellon's Disease, HIV, lymphedema, osteoporosis, parasite infestation, menopausal problems, gum deterioration, COPD, CHF, CAD, chronic ear infections, circulation problems, chronic sinus infections, gout, ulcers, other liver disorders, acne, and many others too numerous to list here.

Lightning Source UK Ltd.
Milton Keynes UK
16 March 2011

169348UK00008B/199/P

9 781603 831154